$1

Quick

Reference Guide

for Using

Essential Oils

Connie and Alan Higley

This book has been designed to provide information to help educate the reader in regard to the subject matter covered. It is sold with the understanding that the publisher and the authors are not liable for the misconception or misuse of the information provided. It is not provided in order to diagnose, prescribe, or treat any disease, illness, or injured condition of the body. The authors and publisher shall have neither liability nor responsibility to any person or entity with respect to any loss, damage, or injury caused or alleged to be caused directly or indirectly by the information contained in this book. The information presented herein is in no way intended as a substitute for medical counseling. Anyone suffering from any disease, illness, or injury should consult a qualified health care professional.

Library of Congress Cataloging-in-Publication Data.

Higley, Connie.

> Reference guide for essential oils / Connie and Alan Higley
> > p. ill. cm.
> Includes bibliographical references.
> 1. Essences and essential oils–Therapeutic use–Handbooks, manuals, etc.
> 2. Aromatherapy–Handbooks, manuals, etc. 00-500404

Published and distributed by:

> **Abundant Health**
> 222 W. 3560 N.
> Spanish Fork, UT 84660
>
> **Phone:** 1-888-718-3068 (toll-free) / 801-798-0642 (local)
>
> **Internet:** www.AbundantHealth4u.com
> **E-Mail:** orders@abundanthealth4u.com

Printed and bound in the United States of America.

International Standard Book Number: 978-1-937702-45-8

DEDICATION

We, the authors (compilers) of this information, were introduced to Young Living Essential Oils in 1995. At that time, there was no compiled information on the use of these valuable oils, so together with Pat Leatham, we set out to find what we could. We gathered notes from lectures and seminars by D. Gary Young and product information from Young Living Essential Oils. Extensive research into the works of other aromatherapy experts have shown us that Gary Young, through his own research and clinical study, not only supports, but expands their solid foundation of knowledge and expertise. When this book was first made available in 1996, we made a conscious decision to keep the names of D. Gary Young and Young Living Essential Oils out of this book so as to remove all possibility of recrimination or harm to Gary Young or his company. However, all past, present, and future readers of this work need to understand that all of us, author and reader alike, are deeply indebted to Gary Young for his brilliant insight, extensive research, and incredible vision of the healing power of essential oils.

We, therefore, dedicate this book to D. Gary Young as a tribute to his vision of health for all who will embrace the oils and use them to their fullest potential. Gary Young is one of the foremost experts on the organic cultivation, distillation, and clinical use of essential oils in North America. His unwavering passion for maintaining the highest quality in his products have produced some astounding healing results. We applaud his heroic and often solitary effort to continue proving, by clinical study, the efficacy of essential oils as indispensable tools for combating disease.

ACKNOWLEDGMENTS

To our 6 children who demonstrate much patience and responsibility with the freedom they are given during the on-going compilation and updating of this book.

To the late Pat Leatham who provided the initial impetus for its creation.
Her many hours of research and meticulous note-taking will forever be appreciated.

And to all of you who are discovering, or re-discovering, for yourselves
the healing powers of essential oils. May this book provide quick access
to the information you need to help yourself, and those you love,
progress on the road to better health.

A special thanks goes to our families and to all of our "Essential Oil" friends! Without your love, friendship, suggestions, support, patience, and prodding, we would have crumbled under the strain of compiling a book such as this while trying to raise a family and have a life.

CONTENTS

The section tabs in the personal guide section correspond to the alphabetical listing of health topics. By holding the spine of the book in the left hand and bending the right side back with the right hand, section markings become visible along the right edge. This should allow you quick and easy reference to any particular topic.

BASIC INFORMATION

BASIC FACTS ABOUT ESSENTIAL OILS

How long have essential oils been around?

Essential oils were mankind's first medicine. From Egyptian hieroglyphics and Chinese manuscripts, we know that priests and physicians have been using essential oils for thousands of years. In Egypt, essential oils were used in the embalming process, and well-preserved oils were found in alabaster jars in King Tut's tomb. Egyptian temples were dedicated to the production and blending of the oils, and recipes were recorded on the walls in hieroglyphics. There is even a sacred room in the temple of Isis on the island of Philae where a ritual called "Cleansing the Flesh and Blood of Evil Deities" was practiced. This form of emotional clearing required 3 days of cleansing using particular essential oils and oil baths.

There are 188 references to essential oils in the Bible. Oils such as frankincense, myrrh, rosemary, hyssop, and spikenard were used for anointing and healing the sick. In Exodus, the Lord gave the following recipe to Moses for "an holy anointing oil":

> Myrrh ("five hundred shekels"— approximately 1 gallon)
> Sweet Cinnamon ("two hundred and fifty shekels"— approximately ½ gallon)
> Sweet Calamus ("two hundred and fifty shekels")
> Cassia ("five hundred shekels")
> Olive Oil ("an hin"— approximately 1 ⅓ gallons)

The 3 wise men presented the Christ child with essential oils of frankincense and myrrh. There are also accounts in the New Testament of the Bible where Jesus was anointed with spikenard oil: "And being in Bethany in the house of Simon the leper, as he sat at meat, there came a woman having an alabaster box of ointment of spikenard very precious; and she brake the box, and poured [it] on his head" (Mark 14:3). "Then took Mary a pound of ointment of spikenard, very costly, and anointed the feet of Jesus, and wiped his feet with her hair: and the house was filled with the odour of the ointment" (John 12:3). Some have even said that essential oils carry the consciousness of Christ.

What are *PURE, THERAPEUTIC-GRADE* essential oils?

Essential oils are the volatile liquids that are distilled from plants (including their respective parts such as seeds, bark, leaves, stems, roots, flowers, fruit, etc.). One of the factors that determines the purity and therapeutic value of an oil is its chemical constituents. These constituents can be affected by a vast number of variables including: the part(s) of the plant from which the oil was produced, soil condition, fertilizer (organic or chemical), geographical region, climate, altitude, harvest season and methods, and distillation process. For example, common thyme, or thyme vulgaris, produces several different chemotypes (biochemical specifics or simple species) depending on the conditions of its growth, climate, and altitude. High levels of thymol production depend on the time of year in which it is distilled. If distilled during mid-summer or late fall, there can be higher levels of carvacrol which can cause the oil to be more caustic or irritating to the skin. Low pressure and low temperature are also keys to maintaining the purity, the ultimate fragrance, and the therapeutic value of the oil.

As we begin to understand the power of essential oils in the realm of personal, holistic health care, we comprehend the absolute necessity for obtaining the purest therapeutic-grade essential oils possible. No matter how costly pure therapeutic-grade essential oils may be, there can be no substitutes. Chemists can replicate some of the known individual constituents, but they have yet to successfully recreate complete essential oils in the laboratory.

The information in this book is based upon the use of pure, therapeutic-grade essential oils. Those who are beginning their journey into the realm of aromatherapy and essential oils must actively seek for the purest quality and highest therapeutic-grade oils available. Anything less than pure, therapeutic-grade essential oil may not produce the desired results and can, in some cases, be extremely toxic.

Why is it so difficult to find *PURE, THERAPEUTIC-GRADE* essential oils?

Producing the purest of oils can be very costly because it may require several hundred pounds, or even several thousand pounds, of plant material to extract 1 pound of pure essential oil. For example, 1 pound of pure melissa oil sells for $9,000 - $15,000. Although this sounds quite expensive, one must realize that 3 tons of plant material are required to produce that single pound of oil. Because the vast majority of all the oils produced in the world today are used by the perfume industry, the oils are being purchased for their aromatic qualities only. High pressure, high temperatures, rapid processing, and the use of chemical solvents are often employed during the distillation process so that a greater *quantity* of oil can be produced at a faster rate. These oils may smell just as good and cost much less, but they will lack most, if not all, of the chemical constituents necessary to produce the expected therapeutic results.

What benefits do *PURE, THERAPEUTIC-GRADE* essential oils provide?

1. Essential oils are the regenerating, oxygenating, and immune defense properties of plants.
2. Essential oils are so small in molecular size that they can quickly penetrate the skin.
3. Essential oils are lipid-soluble and are capable of penetrating cell walls, even if they have hardened because of an oxygen deficiency. In fact, essential oils can affect every cell of the body within 20 minutes and then be metabolized like other nutrients.
4. Essential oils contain oxygen molecules which help to transport nutrients to the starving human cells. Because a nutritional deficiency is an oxygen deficiency, disease begins when the cells lack the oxygen for proper nutrient assimilation. By providing the needed oxygen, essential oils also work to stimulate the immune system.
5. Essential oils are very powerful antioxidants. Antioxidants create an unfriendly environment for free radicals. Antioxidants prevent all mutations, work as free radical scavengers, prevent fungus, and prevent oxidation in the cells.
6. Essential oils are antibacterial, anticancerous, antifungal, anti-infectious, antimicrobial, antitumor, antiparasitic, antiviral, and antiseptic. Essential oils have been shown to destroy all tested bacteria and viruses, while simultaneously restoring balance to the body.
7. Essential oils may detoxify the cells and blood in the body.
8. Essential oils containing sesquiterpenes have the ability to pass the blood-brain barrier, enabling them to be effective in the treatment of Alzheimer's disease, Lou Gehrig's disease, Parkinson's disease, and multiple sclerosis.
9. Essential oils are aromatic. When diffused, they provide **air purification** by:
    A. Removing metallic particles and toxins from the air;
    B. Increasing atmospheric oxygen;
    C. Increasing ozone and negative ions in the area, which inhibits bacterial growth;
    D. Destroying odors from mold, cigarettes, and animals; and
    E. Filling the air with a fresh, aromatic scent.
10. Essential oils help promote emotional, physical, and spiritual healing.
11. Essential oils have a bioelectrical frequency that is several times greater than the frequency of herbs, food, and even the human body. Clinical research has shown that essential oils can quickly raise the frequency of the human body, restoring it to its normal, healthy level.

What is frequency and how does it pertain to essential oils?

Frequency is a measurable rate of electrical energy that is constant between any 2 points. Everything has an electrical frequency. Bruce Tainio of Tainio Technology in Cheny, Washington, developed new equipment to measure the biofrequency of humans and foods. Bruce Tainio and D. Gary Young, a North American expert on essential oils, used this biofrequency monitor to determine the relationship between frequency and disease. Some of the results of their studies are show in the following table.

Human Brain	72-90 MHz	Processed/canned food	0 MHz
Human Body (day)	62-68 MHz	Fresh Produce	up to 15 MHz
Cold Symptoms	58 MHz	Dry Herbs	12-22 MHz
Flu Symptoms	57 MHz	Fresh Herbs	20-27 MHz
Candida	55 MHz	Essential Oils	52-320 MHz
Epstein-Barr	52 MHz	**Note:** Due to the sensitivity of the instruments, these results are not easily duplicable. What is important is the relativity of the numbers and the fact that the higher frequency of the essential oils can help raise the frequency of the human body to a more normal level.	
Cancer	42 MHz		
Death Begins	25 MHz		

Another part of this same study measured the frequency fluctuations within the human body as different substances were introduced. The chart shown below illustrates the frequency reaction of the human body to the introduction of coffee. The subsequent time necessary for the frequency to return to its original measurement was shown to be substantially reduced with the use of essential oils.

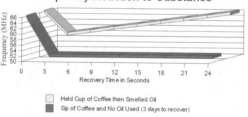

Frequency Reaction to Substance

☐ Held Cup of Coffee then Smelled Oil
■ Sip of Coffee and No Oil Used (3 days to recover)

Initially, the frequency of each of 2 different individuals—the first a 26-year-old male and the second a 24-year-old male—was measured at 66 MHz for both. The first individual held a cup of coffee (without drinking any), and his frequency dropped to 58 MHz in 3 seconds. He then removed the coffee and inhaled an aroma of essential oils. Within 21 seconds, his frequency had returned to 66 MHz. The second individual took a sip of coffee and his frequency dropped to 52 MHz in the same 3 seconds. However, no essential oils were used during the recovery time and it took 3 days for his frequency to return to the initial 66 MHz.

Another very interesting result of this study was the influence that thoughts have on our frequency as well. Negative thoughts lowered the measured frequency by 12 MHz and positive thoughts raised the measured frequency by 10 MHz. It was also found that prayer and meditation increased the measured frequency levels by 15 MHz.

How do *PURE, THERAPEUTIC-GRADE* essential oils affect the brain?

The blood-brain barrier is the barrier membrane between the circulating blood and the brain that prevents certain damaging substances from reaching brain tissue and cerebrospinal fluid. The American Medical Association (AMA) determined that if they could find an agent that would pass the blood-brain barrier, they would be able to cure Alzheimer's disease, Lou Gehrig's disease, multiple sclerosis, and Parkinson's disease. In June of 1994, it was documented by the Medical University of Berlin, Germany, and Vienna, Austria, that sesquiterpenes have the ability to go beyond the blood-brain barrier.

High levels of sesquiterpenes, found in the essential oils of frankincense and sandalwood, help increase the amount oxygen in the limbic system of the brain, particularly around the pineal and pituitary glands. This leads to an increase in secretions of antibodies, endorphins, and neurotransmitters.

Also present in the limbic system of the brain is a gland called the amygdala. In 1989, it was discovered that the amygdala plays a major role in the storing and releasing of emotional trauma. The only way to stimulate this gland is with fragrance or the sense of smell. Therefore, with aromatherapy and essential oils we are now able to release emotional trauma.

What enables *PURE, THERAPEUTIC-GRADE* essential oils to provide such incredible benefits?

Essential oils are chemically very heterogeneous—meaning they are very diverse in their effects and can perform several different functions. Synthetic chemicals are completely opposite in that they have basically one action. This heterogeneity gives essential oils a paradoxical nature which can be difficult to understand. However, essential oils can be compared to another paradoxical group—human beings. For example, a man can play many roles: father, husband, friend, coworker, accountant, school teacher, church volunteer, scout master, minister, etc. And so it is with essential oils: lavender can be used for burns, insect bites, headaches, PMS, insomnia, stress, and so forth.

The heterogeneous benefits of an oil depend greatly on its chemical constituents—and not only on the existence of specific constituents but also on the constituent amounts in proportion to the other constituents that are present in the same oil. Some individual oils may have anywhere from 200 to 800 different chemical constituents. However, of the possible 800 different constituents, only about 200 of those have so far been identified. Although not everything is known about all of the different constituents, most of them can be grouped into a few distinct families, each with some dominant characteristics. The following section provides greater insights into these constituent families.

ESSENTIAL OIL CONSTITUENTS

As was mentioned previously, the chemical constituents of an oil are affected by a vast number of variables. However, most of these variables are controlled by the oil producers. One thing that the student of aromatherapy can do is ask questions about the company from which they are purchasing the oils. Some of the most important questions should be, "Does the company utilize gas chromatography (GC) in their quality control process?" "Does their GC equipment utilize a column of at least 50 to 60 meters in length in order to properly identify the hundreds of natural constituents found in an essential oil?" A gas chromatogram shows a pattern of the separated constituents of an oil and helps a trained technician determine its purity and therapeutic quality. The following information can help us understand the functions of some of the main chemical constituents.

In general, *pure* essential oil constituents can be subdivided into 2 distinct groups: the **hydrocarbons,** which are made up almost exclusively of *terpenes* (monoterpenes, sesquiterpenes, and diterpenes), and the **oxygenated compounds,** which are mainly *esters, aldehydes, ketones, alcohols, phenols,* and *oxides.*

Terpenes

Terpenes are the largest family of natural products and are found throughout nature. High concentrations of terpenes are found directly after flowering[1]. The basic molecular structure of a terpene is an isoprene unit (which has a C_5H_8 molecular formula).

Classes of terpenes are named according to how many isoprene units are present.

- Monoterpenes (C10) = two isoprene units
- Sesquiterpenes (C15) = three isoprene units
- Triterpenes (C30) = six isoprene units
- Tetraterpenes (C40) = eight isoprene units

ISOPRENE UNIT (C_5H_8)

Figures such as the one shown at left represent the bonds between carbon (C) atoms in a molecule. Single lines represent a single bond, while double lines represent a double bond. Each intersecting point and the end of each line represents a carbon molecule along with any hydrogen molecules it is bonded to. Since each carbon molecule can have up to four bonds with other atoms, the number of hydrogen atoms can be determined by subtracting the number of bonds (lines) coming to each carbon atom from four. Thus, the shorthand figure at top represents the same molecule shown below it.

ISOPRENE UNIT (C_5H_8)

○ = CARBON

● = HYDROGEN

1   Paduch et al., 2007.

Terpenes may also have oxygen-containing functional groups. Terpenes with these oxygen-containing functional groups are referred to as terpenoids[2].

Monoterpenes—occur in practically all essential oils and have many different activities. Most tend to inhibit the accumulation of toxins and help discharge existing toxins from the liver and kidneys. Some are antiseptic, antibacterial, stimulating, analgesic (weak), and expectorant; while other specific terpenes have antifungal, antiviral, antihistaminic, antirheumatic, antitumor (antiblastic, anticarcinogenic), hypotensive, insecticidal, purgative, and pheromonal properties. Monoterpenes, in general, have a stimulating effect and can be very soothing to irritated tissues as well. Most citrus oils (not bergamot) and conifer oils contain a high proportion of terpenes.

Found as a Significant Constituent in ALL Essential Oils *Except*: Anise, basil, birch, calamus, cassia, cedarwood, German chamomile, cinnamon bark, clary sage, clove, blue cypress, davana, geranium, jasmine, melissa, lemon myrtle, onycha, palmarosa, patchouli, rosewood, sandalwood, vetiver, western red cedar, wintergreen, ylang ylang.

Pinenes (α- & β-) α- and β- pinene are isomers (meaning they have the same chemical formula but differing structures). They get their name because they are major constituents in pine resin or pine oil. They give off a resiny, piney smell. Pinenes have strong antiseptic, antibacterial, antifungal, and expectorant properties.

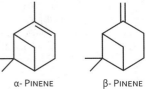

α- PINENE   β- PINENE

Bone Resorption Inhibition: α- and β-pinene (found in pine oil) were found in animal studies to inhibit bone resorption. Bone resorption is the process by which osteoclasts—macrophage cells that reside in the bones—break down bone and release the minerals, which can lead to the loss of bone, such as in osteoporosis. Further studies have indicated that while α- and β-pinene may not directly influence osteoclast activity and bone resorption rates, a metabolite (a product created by the body from the original molecule when taken internally) of the pinenes, cis-verbenol, did directly inhibit bone resorption and the formation of osteoclasts[3,4].

2   McGarvey et al., 1995.
3   Eriksson et al., 1996.
4   Muhlbauer et al., 2003.

Mosquito Larvicide: α-pinenes found in *Alpinia speciosa* and *Rosmarinus officinalis* (ginger and rosemary) demonstrated effective larvicidal activity against the mosquito *Aedes aegypti L.* The *A. aegypti* is a carrier of the dengue virus that causes dengue fever in tropical areas of the world[5].

Antibacterial: It has been observed that the larvae of the Douglas fir tussock moth have digestive systems that are relatively clear of bacterial flora. These larvae feed on terpenes found in the bark of Douglas fir trees, of which α-pinene is a major constituent. α-pinene inhibits the growth of *Bacillus* species (gram-positive bacteria). The concentration needed for maximum inhibition is well below the concentrations of α-pinene found in Douglas fir pine trees. Bacterial inhibition occurs because α-pinene disrupts the cytoplasmic membranes of the bacterial species. α-pinene seems to perform more effectively against gram-positive bacteria than gram-negative bacteria due to the extra outer membrane found in the cell walls of gram-negative bacteria[6,7].

Anti-inflammatory: NF_KB is an important transcription factor in the body that regulates proinflammatory responses (signals proteins, specifically cytokines, to cause inflammation). When NF_KB is activated, it goes to the nucleus of the cells, binds to DNA, and activates transcription needed to produce cytokines, chemokines, and cell adhesion molecules. These molecules all help in producing inflammation in the body.

α-pinene has been shown to inhibit/block NF_KB from going to the nucleus. LPS (lipopolysaccharide, an endotoxin produced by gram-negative bacteria that causes inflammation in the body) was introduced to the cell culture of THP-1 cells to induce the activation of NF_KB. However, when α-pinene was present, activation was markedly reduced.

α-pinene inhibits NF_KB by blocking the degradation of $I_KB\alpha$. $I_KB\alpha$ is a protein that binds to NF_KB to prevent it from constantly transcribing proinflammatory genes. If LPS, a virus, or some stimulant of the immune system is recognized, $I_KB\alpha$ will degrade and release/activate NF_KB. NF_KB will then transcribe genes to make proteins that cause inflammation at the site of "invasion," such as a

5   Freitas et al., 2010.
6   Andrews et al., 1980.
7   Uribe et al., 1985.

cut, scrape, or burn.

Even in the presence of an immune system stimulant (LPS), α-pinene blocks $I_\kappa B\alpha$. During experimentation, it was also noted that the THP-1 cells received no cytotoxicity from the addition of α-pinene[8,9].

Camphene Camphene is found in many oils, such as cypress, citronella, neroli, ginger, and others. It is an insect repellent. According to the *Phytochemical Dictionary*, it is "used to reduce cholesterol saturation index in the treatment of gallstones."

CAMPHENE

β-Myrcene β-Myrcene is found in oils such as lemongrass, verbena, and bay. It has cancer–preventative properties.

β-MYRCENE

> **Antioxidant:** Studies have elucidated that β-myrcene can reverse and prevent the damaging effects of TCDD (2,3,7,8-Tetrachloro-p-dibenzodioxin) to the liver of rats by increasing GSH (glutathione), SOD (superoxide dismutase), and catalase activation[10,11].

d-Limonene d-Limonene is found in 90% of the citrus peel oils and in caraway seeds and dill. It is anticancer, antibacterial, antifungal, antiseptic (5x phenol), and highly antiviral.

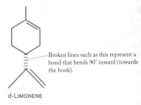

Broken lines such as this represent a bond that bends 90° inward (towards the book).

d-LIMONENE

> **Cancer Cell Inhibition:** d-Limonene has been found to be cancer-preventive in vitro and in human mammary cells. It acts as a selective isoprenylation inhibitor. d-Limonene specifically inhibits small g-proteins known as Ras p21 (or p21ras). p21ras is a critical protein for oncogenesis (formation of cancer cells) in the body. In order for oncogenesis to commence, the p21ras protein must be transferred within the cell to the plasma membrane. Once p21ras is able to interact with the plasma membrane of the cell, it causes abnormal cell growth, intracellular localization, and transformations.

8   Zhou et al., 2004.
9   Weaver, 2008.
10   Ciftci et al., 2011.
11   Gaetani et al., 1996.

d-Limonene inhibits the transferral of p21ras within the cell, blocking its access to the plasma membrane.

Researchers also found that d-Limonene is selectively inhibitive. It targets only the transferral of Ras proteins and leaves all other ordinary cell functions alone. This makes d-Limonene a potentially effective chemopreventive agent because it targets areas of high on-cogenic susceptibility and has no harmful side effects against critical cell components (low toxicity)[12,13,14].

Researchers have also observed that a continuous dose of limonene in the diets of rats with chemical-induced cancer helps inhibit the formation of secondary tumors and reduces the size of primary tumors. However, when limonene was removed from the rat's daily diet, tumors were more likely to return. This gives evidence that limonene works as a cytostatic agent (an agent that stops the tumor cells from creating new tumor cells) rather than a cytotoxic agent (an agent that kills the tumor cells). These researchers also observed that little toxicity occurred to the rats from the high doses of d-Limonene[15].

Cholesterol Suppression: Researchers have discovered that when d-Limonene is included in the daily diet of rats treated with a chemical (7,12-dimetylbenzantracene) that induced high cholesterol, there was a 45% decrease in hepatic HMG-CoA reductase activity. HMG-CoA reductase is an enzyme that converts HMG-CoA (93-hydroxy-3-methylglutaryl coenzyme A) to mevalonic acid, which acts as a precursor to the production of cholesterol. Inhibiting HMG-CoA reductase halts this process and, in effect, lowers cholesterol rates[16,17].

Sesquiterpenes Sesquiterpenes are found in great abundance in essential oils. They are antibacterial, strongly anti-inflammatory, slightly antiseptic and hypotensive, and sedative. Some have analgesic properties, while others are highly antispasmodic. They are soothing to irritated skin and tissue and are calming. They also work as liver and gland stimulants. Research from the universities of Berlin and Vienna shows that sesquiterpenes increase oxygenation around the pineal and pituitary glands. Further research has shown that ses-

12 Kato et al., 1992.
13 Crowell et al., 1991.
14 Morse et al., 1993.
15 Haag et al., 1992.
16 Sorentino et al., 2005.
17 Qureshi et al., 1988.

quiterpenes have the ability to surpass the blood-brain barrier and enter the brain tissue. They are larger molecules than monoterpenes and have a strong aroma.

Found as a Major Constituent In: Cedarwood, German chamomile, ginger, goldenrod, melissa, myrrh, patchouli, pepper, sandalwood, spikenard, vetiver, yarrow, ylang ylang.

Found as a Minor (but significant) Constituent In: Bergamot, carrot, cedar leaf, celery seed, Roman chamomile, cinnamon bark, clary sage, clove, cumin, cypress, blue cypress, elemi, *Eucalyptus citriadora* (lemon eucalyptus), *Eucalyptus globulus*, silver fir, white fir, frankincense, galbanum, geranium, helichrysum, hyssop, lavandin, lavender, ledum, lemongrass, *Melaleuca alternifolia* (tea tree), *Melaleuca ericifolia* (rosalina), *Melaleuca leucadendron* (cajeput), *Melaleuca quinquenervia* (niaouli), peppermint, pine, rosewood, sage, blue tansy, tsuga, valerian.

> **β-Caryophyllene** β-caryophyllene is found in clove and cinnamon essential oils and is found in high proportions in plants from the Labiatae family. It is antiedema, anti-inflammatory, antispasmodic, and an insect and termite repellent.
>
> β-CARYOPHYLLENE
>
> **Anesthetic:** β-caryophyllene has been shown to act as a local anesthetic in vitro and in vivo. In an in vitro experiment, β-caryophyllene reduced the number of contractions electrically invoked in rat phrenic nerve-hemidiaphragms. Phrenic nerves are found in the spine, specifically at the 3rd, 4th, and 5th cervical vertebrae. These nerves provide sole motor control to the diaphragm. In this experiment, electrical impulses through the phrenic nerves induced diaphragm contractions, but the addition of β-caryophyllene reduced the number of contractions[18].
>
> In an in vivo (real life) experiment, researchers performed a conjunctival reflex test on rabbits in which the conjunctival sac, found in the eye, was stimulated with a cat whisker to promote palpebral closure (or blinking). β-caryophyllene acted as a local anesthetic: when it was applied to the eye, more stimulation with the cat whisker was required in order to promote blinking in the rabbit[19].

18 Bulbring, 1946.
19 Ghelardini et al., 2001.

Chamazulene Chamazulene is found in chamomile oil and is very high in anti-inflammatory and antibacterial activity.

Farnesene Farnesene refers to several isomers with the chemical formula $C_{15}H_{24}$. Farnesene is found in ylang ylang, valerian, and German chamomile oil and is antiviral in action.

CHAMAZULENE

α-FARNESENE   β-FARNESENE

Alcohols

Alcohols are any organic molecule with a carbon atom bound to a hydroxyl group. A hydroxyl group is an oxygen and hydrogen molecule (-OH).

Alcohols are commonly recognized for their antibacterial, anti-infectious, and antiviral activities. They are somewhat stimulating and help to increase blood circulation. Because of their high resistance to oxidation and their low toxicity levels, they have been shown in animal studies to revert cells to normal function and activity. They create an uplifting quality and are regarded as safe and effective for young and old alike.

METHANOL (CH_3OH)
— OH

METHANOL (CH_3OH)

○ = CARBON
● = HYDROGEN
● = OXYGEN

Shorthand model of methanol, the simplest alcohol, and the molecular model it represents, below.

Monoterpene Alcohols (or Monoterpenols) Like monoterpenes, monoterpene alcohols are comprised of two isoprene units but have a hydroxyl group bound to one of the carbons instead of a hydrogen. Monoterpene alcohols are known for their ability to stimulate the immune system and to work as a diuretic and a general tonic. They are antibacterial and mildly antiseptic as well.

Linalool Linalool is found in rosewood, bergamot, coriander, rose, jasmine, and lavender essential oils. It has a flowery aroma and is used to scent soaps, shampoos, and perfumes. Linalool can help relieve discomfort. It has antibacterial, antifungal, antiseptic (5x phenol), antispasmodic, antiviral, and sedative properties.

LINALOOL

Anti-inflammatory: Linalool has been used to reduce paw swelling induced by carrageenan in mice. The effects of linalool work against swelling in a dose-dependent manner[1,2]. Linalool also mediates pain caused by inflammation. In a particular study, acetic acid was administered to mice via intraperitoneal (gut) injections. Mice that received a dose of linalool following administration of acetic acid exhibited less writhing (due to pain) than mice that acted as controls[3].

Antifungal: *Candida albicans* is the primary fungus responsible for yeast infections. Yeast infections are commonly exhibited as vulvovaginal candidiasis and thrush (oropharyngeal candidiasis, in the mouth). Thrush is commonly expressed in newborns and AIDS patients.

Candida albicans is also becoming a concern due to its emergence as a nosocomial infection (an infection contracted in a hospital) and its increasing resistance to fluconazole—an antifungal drug. *C. albicans* can form biofilms (aggregated colonies) on medical devices such as catheters and dentures[4,5].

Topical application of linalool to colonies of the polymorphic fungus *Candida albicans* results in growth inhibition and fungal death. Linalool affects growth by blocking passage beyond the G1 (cell growth) phase of the cell cycle[6].

Sedative: Linalool is a common sedative used in Brazilian folk medicine. According to studies using mice, inhaled linalool induces sleep or sedation[7,8].

Antiepileptic/Anticonvulsant: Epilepsy is characterized by seemingly spontaneous spasms of electrical activity in the brain. These spasms can cause seizures and convulsions. One hypothesis for the cause of epilepsy is excessive glutamate levels in neurons (nerve cells)[9,10,11,12]. Glutamates are a common form of neurotransmitter that are stored in special

1   Peana et al., 2002.
2   Skold et al., 2002.
3   Peana et al., 2003.
4   Mukherjee et al., 2003.
5   Microbiology. 9th ed, 2007.
6   Zore et al., 2011.
7   Linck et al., 2009.
8   de Almeida et al., 2009.
9   Chapman et al., 2000.
10 Meldrum et al., 1999.
11 Meldrum, 1994.
12 Chapman, 1998.

vesicles (storage containers) near nerve synapses (locations where nerve cells come close to each other in order to pass along electrical impulses and signals). Impulses along the nerve cause one nerve cell to release glutamate across the synapse where it is received by receptors on the second nerve cell, opening channels in that cell to allow it to pass ions through the cell membrane, changing the electrical potential of that cell[13].

Studies have shown that the release of large concentrations of glutamate will lead to too many open channels, which will cause high, intense depolarization sequences of the action potential. Disproportionate depolarizations are the basis for seizures and convulsions in epilepsy[14,15,16].

Using mouse models, researchers have found that applications of linalool on cortical synaptosomes (isolated nerve terminals, or synapses) significantly inhibited glutamate uptake. Inhibition of glutamate is a method to reduce occurrences of epileptic seizures. These observations provide significant evidence for linalool acting as a possible antiepileptic agent[17,18].

Citronellol Citronellol is found in citronella, rose, melissa, and eucalyptus essential oils. It has antibacterial, antifungal, antiseptic (3.8x phenol), and sedative properties.

Anticonvulsant Activity: Administered doses of citronellol given via the intraperitoneal cavity (gut) to rodents have been observed to reduce the convulsive effects in induced epileptic attacks. Epilepsy is studied in animal models by inducing convulsions with compounds such as pentylenetetrazol (PTZ) and picrotoxin. Citronel-

---

13 Medical Physiology. 10th ed, 2000.
14 Chapman et al., 2000.
15 Meldrum et al., 1994.
16 Paolette et al., 2007.
17 Silva Brum et al., 2001a.
18 Silva Brum et al., 2001b.

lol, over time, reduces the amplitude of the compound action potential (CAP) in neurons. This decreases the effect and intensity of convulsions[19].

Blood Pressure: Injections of citronellol into the blood were found by researchers to reduce blood pressure in animal models. Citronellol is theorized to decrease the flux of Ca^{2+} ions into smooth vascular muscle cells by deactivating VOCCs (voltage-operated calcium channels). Calcium is the principle regulator of tension in vascular smooth muscle (blood vessels). When the transport of Ca^{2+} into the cell is blocked, smooth muscle relaxation occurs. This leads to increased vasodilation (an increase in the diameter of the blood vessels, allowing a higher volume of blood flow) and, thus, lowered blood pressure[20,21,22].

Geraniol Geraniol is found in rose, citronella, and lemon essential oils. It has antifungal, antiseptic (7x phenol), cancer preventative, and sedative properties.

GERANIOL

Other Monoterpene Alcohols Other monoterpene alcohols include borneol, menthol, nerol, terpineol (which Dr. Gattefosse considered to be a decongestant), vetiverol, and cedrol.

Sesquiterpene Alcohols (Sesquiterpenols) are antiallergenic, antibacterial, anti-inflammatory, ulcer-protective (preventative), and a liver and glandular stimulant.

Farnesol Farnesol is found in rose, neroli, ylang ylang, and Roman chamomile essential oils. It is known to be good for the mucous membranes and to help prevent bacterial growth from perspiration.

FARNESOL

Bisabolol Bisabolol is found in German chamomile essential oil. It is one of the strongest sesquiterpene alcohols.

Other Sesquiterpene Alcohols Others include nerolidol and zingiberol.

BISABOLOL

---

19 de Sousa et al., 2006.
20 Bastos et al., 2009.
21 Gurney, 1994.
22 Munzel et al., 2003.

Found as a Significant Constituent in ALL Essential Oils *Except*: Anise, birch, calamus, cassia, celery seed, clove, cumin, davana, dill, *Eucalyptus polybractea*, balsam fir, silver fir, white fir, galbanum, goldenrod, grapefruit, hyssop, juniper, melissa, mugwort, lemon myrtle, myrrh, onycha, oregano, pepper, pine, rosemary (CT verbenon), spruce, blue tansy, Idaho tansy, tarragon, tsuga, western red cedar, wintergreen, yarrow.

Esters

Esters are the compounds resulting from the reaction of an alcohol with an acid (known as esterification). Esters consist of a carboxyl group (a carbon atom double bonded to an oxygen atom) bound to a hydrocarbon group on one side and bound to an oxygen and a hydrocarbon group on the opposite side.

METHYL ACETATE (CH$_3$OOCH$_3$)

Methyl acetate (shown here) is a simple organic ester molecule.

METHYL ACETATE (CH$_3$OOCH$_3$)

○ = CARBON
● = HYDROGEN
● = OXYGEN

Esters are very common and are found in the mildest essential oils. Mostly free of toxicity and irritants, they tend to be the most calming, relaxing, and balancing of all the essential oil constituents. They are also antifungal and antispasmodic. They have a balancing or regulatory effect, especially on the nervous system. Some examples are linalyl acetate, geranyl acetate (with strong antifungal properties), and bornyl acetate (effective on bronchial candida). Other esters include eugenyl acetate, lavendulyl acetate, and methyl salicylate.

Found as a Major Constituent In: Birch, bergamot, cardamom, Roman chamomile (85%), clary sage, geranium, helichrysum, jasmine, lavandin, lavender, onycha, petit-grain, spruce, tsuga, valerian, wintergreen, ylang ylang.

Found as a Minor (but significant) Constituent In: Angelica, carrot, cassia, cedar leaf, celery seed, cistus, clove, coriander, cypress, dill, *Eucalyptus citriadora* (lemon eucalyptus), balsam fir, Douglas fir, silver fir, white fir, fleabane, juniper, *Laurus nobilis*, lemon, lemongrass, mandarin, marjoram, melissa, myrtle, neroli, orange, palmarosa, rosemary (CT verbenon), sage lavender.

Aldehydes

Aldehydes are often responsible for the fragrance of an oil. They exert powerful aromas and are often calming to the emotions. They are highly reactive and are characterized by a carboxyl group (a carbon atom double bonded to an oxygen atom) with a hydrogen atom on one side and a hydrocarbon group on the opposite side. In general, aldehydes are anti-infectious, anti-inflammatory, calming to the central nervous system, fever-reducing, hypotensive, and tonic. Some are antiseptic, antimicrobial, and antifungal, while others act as vasodilators. They can be quite irritating when applied topically (citrals being an example). However, it has been shown that adding an essential oil with an equal amount of d-Limonene can negate the irritant properties of a high citral oil.

ACETALDEHYDE (CH₃CHO)

Acetaldehyde (shown here) is a simple organic aldehyde molecule.

ACETALDEHYDE (CH₃CHO)

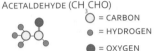

○ = CARBON
● = HYDROGEN
● = OXYGEN

Found as a Major Constituent In: Cassia, cinnamon bark, cumin, *Eucalyptus citriadora* (lemon eucalyptus), lemongrass, lemon myrtle, lemon verbena.

Found as a Minor (but significant) Constituent In: Calamus, cistus, citronella, *Eucalyptus radiata*, grapefruit, lemon, lime, mandarin, myrrh, orange, tangerine.

Citrals Citrals (like neral, geranial, and citronellal) are very common and have a distinct antiseptic action. They also show antiviral properties (as is the case with melissa oil) when applied topically on herpes simplex.

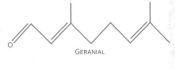

GERANIAL

Other Aldehydes include benzaldehyde, cinnamic aldehyde, cuminic aldehyde, and perillaldehyde.

Ketones

Ketones are organic compounds characterized by a carboxyl group (a carbon atom double bonded to an oxygen atom) with a hydrocarbon on both sides. Ketones are sometimes mucolytic and neurotoxic when isolated from other constituents. However, all recorded toxic effects come from laboratory testing on guinea pigs and rats. No documented cases exist where oils with

ACETONE (CH₃COCH₃)

Acetone (shown here) is a simple ketone molecule.

ACETONE (CH₃COCH₃)

○ = CARBON
● = HYDROGEN
● = OXYGEN

a high concentration of ketones (such as mugwort, tansy, sage, and wormwood) have ever caused a toxic effect on a human being. Also, large amounts of these oils would have to be consumed for them to result in a toxic neurological effect. Ketones stimulate cell regeneration, promote the formation of tissue, and liquefy mucous. They are helpful with conditions such as dry asthma, colds, flu, and dry cough and are largely found in oils used for the upper respiratory system, such as hyssop, rosemary, and sage.

Found as a Major Constituent In: Calamus, cedar leaf, davana, dill, *Eucalyptus dives*, hyssop, rosemary (CT cineol), rosemary (CT verbenon), sage, sage lavender, spearmint, Idaho tansy, Western red cedar.

Found as a Minor (but significant) Constituent In: Cedarwood, Roman chamomile, cistus, coriander, *Eucalyptus polybractea*, fennel, geranium, helichrysum, juniper, lavandin, lemongrass, melissa, mugwort, myrrh, peppermint, spikenard, blue tansy, vetiver, yarrow.

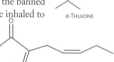

α-THUJONE

Thujone Thujone is one of the most toxic members of the ketone family. It can be an irritant and upsetting to the central nervous system and may be neurotoxic when taken internally, such as in the banned drink absinthe. Although oils containing thujone may be inhaled to relieve respiratory distress and may stimulate the immune system, they should usually be used in dilution (1–2%) and/or for only short periods of time.

Jasmone is found in jasmine essential oil and is nontoxic.

Fenchone Fenchone is found in fennel essential oil and is nontoxic.

JASMONE

Other Ketones include camphor, carvone, menthone, methyl nonyl ketone, and pinocamphone.

FENCHONE

Phenols

Phenols are a diverse group of compounds derived from a phenol group, which is comprised of a benzene ring (six carbon atoms bound in a circle) and a hydroxyl group (oxygen and hydrogen).

Phenols comprise some of the most powerful antibacterial, anti-infectious, and antiseptic constituents in the plant world. They are also very stimulating to both the nervous and immune systems. They contain high levels of oxygenating molecules and have antioxidant properties. However, they can be quite caustic to the skin, and they present some concerns regarding liver toxicity. Essential oils that contain a high proportion of phenols should be diluted and/or used only for short periods of time.

PHENOL (C_6H_6OH)
OH

Phenol (shown here) is a simple phenol molecule.

PHENOL (C_6H_6OH)

○ = CARBON
● = HYDROGEN
● = OXYGEN

Found as a Major Constituent In: Anise, basil, birch, cinnamon bark, clove, fennel, *Melaleuca alternifolia* (tea tree), mountain savory, oregano, peppermint, tarragon, thyme, wintergreen.

Found as a Minor (but significant) Constituent In: Cassia, citronella, cumin, *Eucalyptus citriadora* (lemon eucalyptus), *Laurus nobilis*, marjoram, nutmeg, ylang ylang.

Eugenol Eugenol is found in clove, nutmeg, cinnamon, bay, and basil essential oils. It has analgesic, anesthetic (in dentistry), anticonvulsant, antifungal, anti-inflammatory, antioxidant, antiseptic, cancer-preventative, and sedative properties.

EUGENOL

> **Vasodilator:** Eugenol was found to increase vasodilation (increase the diameter of the opening through the blood vessels) in animal models. When blood vessels expand, the result is larger amounts of blood flow and, thus, a decrease in heart rate. In these particular studies, it was observed that heart rate decreased in conjunction with increased vasodilation, as compared to controls[23,24].
>
> Eugenol is thought to increase vasodilation by inhibiting the action of calcium (Ca^{2+}) in voltage-operated calcium channels (VOCCs). Ca^{2+} is the main regulator of vascular smooth muscle (blood vessel) tension. When Ca^{2+} is blocked, blood vessels relax and widen, allowing for an increase in blood flow[25,26].

Thymol Thymol is found in thyme and oregano essential oils. It may not be as caustic as other phenols. It has antibacterial, antifungal, anti-inflammatory, antioxidant, antiplaque, antirheumatic, antiseptic (20x phenol), antispasmodic, deodorizing, and expectorant properties.

THYMOL

> **Antibacterial:** Thymol has been shown to inhibit the growth of microorganisms such as *Escherichia coli*, *Campylobacter jejuni*, *Porphyromonas gingivalis*, *Staphylococcus aureus*, and *Pseudomonas aeruginosa*. Thymol is thought to disrupt (or impair) the cytoplasmic membranes of mi-

---

23 Lahlou et al., 2004.
24 Damiani et al., 2003.
25 Gurney, 1994.
26 Munzel et al., 2003.

crobes, causing cell leakage. Without the protective barrier of the cytoplasmic membrane, viability of these microorganisms significantly decreases[27,28,29,30].

Carvacrol Carvacrol is a product of auto-oxidation of d-Limonene. It is antibacterial, antifungal, anti-inflammatory, antiseptic (1.5x phenol), antispasmodic, and expectorant. Researchers believe it may possibly have some anticancer properties as well.

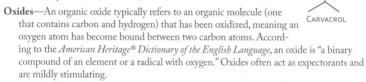

CARVACROL

Other Phenols Others in the phenol family include methyl eugenol, methyl chavicol, anethole, and safrole.

Oxides—An organic oxide typically refers to an organic molecule (one that contains carbon and hydrogen) that has been oxidized, meaning an oxygen atom has become bound between two carbon atoms. According to the *American Heritage® Dictionary of the English Language*, an oxide is "a binary compound of an element or a radical with oxygen." Oxides often act as expectorants and are mildly stimulating.

Found as a Major Constituent In: Cardamom, German chamomile, *Eucalyptus globulus*, *Eucalyptus polybractea*, *Eucalyptus radiata*, *Laurus nobilis*, *Melaleuca leucadendron* (Cajeput), *Melaleuca quinquenervia* (Niaouli), myrtle, ravensara, rosemary (CT cineol).

Found as a Minor (but significant) Constituent In: Basil, carrot, *Eucalyptus citriadora* (lemon eucalyptus), lavandin, lemongrass, lime, *Melaleuca alternifolia* (tea tree), *Melaleuca ericifolia* (rosalina), melissa, mugwort, pepper, rosemary (CT verbenon), rosewood, sage, sage lavender, thyme, ylang ylang.

1,8-Cineol (Eucalyptol) 1,8-cineol is, by far, the most prevalent member of the oxide family and virtually exists in a class of its own. It is anesthetic, antiseptic, and works as a strong mucolytic as it thins mucus in respiratory tract infections.

1,8-CINEOL
(EUCALYPTOL)

Anti-Inflammatory: Researchers found in an animal experiment that rats that were given oral doses of 1,8-cineole before injection with lambda carrageenan (a sweetener that causes inflammation) had markedly decreased swelling when compared to rats that were given the injection without a dosage of 1,8-cineole.

27 Shapiro et al., 1995.
28 Xu et al., 2008.
29 Lambert et al., 2001.
30 Evans et al., 2000.

It has been suggested by scientists that 1,8-cineole inhibits cytokine production. Inhibiting cytokine production would decrease inflammation despite having a stimulant present (such a carrageenan)[31,32].

Asthma: Asthma is a chronic inflammatory disease that restricts air flow to the lungs (specifically in the bronchial tubes). A double-blind, placebo-controlled study was performed to test the ability of 1,8-cineole to alleviate asthmatic symptoms. All subjects in the study suffered from bronchial asthma and required daily administration of oral glucocorticosteroids in order to maintain stable conditions.

At the conclusion of the study, which lasted over a course of 12 weeks, patients who received daily doses of 1,8-cineole were able to maintain stable conditions despite significantly reduced oral doses of glucocorticosteroids, as compared to the placebo group. Proper lung function was also maintained four times longer in the test group than in the placebo group[33,34].

Pain: In one study, mice were injected in the hind paw with a dose of 1% formalin (a common substance used to model pain in experimental studies)/99% saline solution. A portion of mice were given 1,8-cineole. It was observed that these mice who received 1,8-cineole licked their paw substantially less (meaning they did not feel as much pain) than mice that did not receive the 1,8-cineole treatment. In this study, researchers found that 1,8-cineole treatment produced antinociceptive (pain-blocking) effects comparable to those observed for morphine[35,36].

Other Oxides Linalool oxide, ascaridol, bisabolol oxide, 1,4-cineol, and bisabolone oxide.

All pure essential oils have some antibacterial properties. They increase the production of white blood cells, which help fight infectious illnesses. It is because of these properties that aromatic herbs have been esteemed so highly throughout the ages and so widely used during the onsets of malaria, typhoid, and, of course, the epidemic plagues during the 16th century. Research has found that people who consistently use pure essential oils have a higher level of resistance to illnesses, colds, flues, and diseases than does the average person. Further indications show that such individuals after contracting a cold, flu, or other illness will recover 60–75 percent faster than those who do not use essential oils.

---

31 Santos et al., 2000.
32 Juergens et al., 2003.
33 Juergens et al., 2003.
34 Goodwin et al., 1986.
35 Santos et al., 2000.
36 Shibata et al., 1989.

THE ART OF BLENDING

Blending essential oils is an art and usually requires a little bit of training and experimentation. If you choose to create your own blends, it is important to understand that the order in which the oils are blended is key to maintaining the desired therapeutic properties in a synergistic blend. An alteration in the sequence of adding selected oils to a blend may change the chemical properties, the fragrance, and the desired results. The "Blend Classification", and "Blends With" listings under each oil in the Single Oils section of this book should assist one in the blending process. In general, oils that are from the same botanical family usually blend well together. In addition, oils with similar constituents also mix well.

Depending upon the topical application of your blend, you will want to add some carrier/base oil. When creating a **therapeutic essential oil blend**, you may want to use about **28 drops of essential oil to ½ oz. of V-6 Oil**. When creating a **body massage blend**, you will want to use a total of about **50 drops of essential oils to 4 oz. of V-6 Oil**. Remember to store your fragrant creation in dark-colored glass bottles.

As essential oils can vary in thickness, the following are approximate measurements:

25-30 drops	= 1/4 teaspoon	= 1-2 milliliters	= 5/8 dram
45-50 drops	= 1/2 teaspoon	= 2-3 milliliters	= 1 dram
75-80 drops	= 3/4 teaspoon	= 3-4 milliliters	= 1/8 oz.
100-120 drops	= 1 teaspoon	= 5 milliliters	= 1/6 oz.
160 drops	= 1½ teaspoons	= 6-8 milliliters	= 1/4 oz.
320-400 drops	= 3 teaspoons	= 13-15 milliliters	= 1/2 oz.
600-650 drops	= 6 teaspoons	= 25-30 milliliters	= 1 oz.

Learn to trust your nose as it can help you decide which classification an oil should be in. More detailed information about these methods of blending is beyond the scope of this revision of the book. For additional information on using these classifications in your blending, we highly recommend Marcel Lavabre's *Aromatherapy Workbook*. Another very simple book about blending, with recipes and easy-to-follow guidelines, is Mindy Green's *Natural Perfumes*, which uses perfume notes (top, middle, base), odor, and odor intensity to help guide you in making your own fragrant blend creations (1-lightest to 5-strongest—refer to the chart on the following page).

ESSENTIAL OILS ODOR CHART

Essential Oil	Scent	Intensity
Top Notes	(5-20% of the blend)	
orange	Fresh, citrusy, fruity, sweet, light	1
bergamot	Sweet, lively, citrus, fruity	2
grapefruit	Clean, fresh, bitter, citrusy	2
citronella	Citrusy, slightly fruity, fresh, sweet	3
lemon	Sweet, sharp, clear, citrusy	3
lime	Sweet, tart, intense, lively	3
mandarin	Very sweet, citrusy, fruity	3
petitgrain	Fresh, floral, citrusy, slightly woody	3
ravensara	Slightly medicinal, eucalyptus-like	3
spearmint	Minty, slightly fruity	3
tangerine	Fresh, sweet, citrusy	3
euc. polybrac.	Fresh, woody, earthy	4
lemongrass	Grassy, lemony, pungent, earthy	4
euc. globulus	Fresh, medicinal, woody, earthy	5
galbanum	Warm, earthy, green, woody, spicy	5
lemon myrtle	Extremely lemony and crisp	5
Top to Middle Notes	(20-80% of the blend)	
anise	Licorice-like, rich, sweet	3
laurel	Sweet, fresh, spicy, medicinal	3
lavandin	Fresh, sweet, floral, herbaceous	3
myrtle	Sweet, slightly camphorous, floral hint	3
palmarosa	Lemony, fresh, green, hints of rose	3
angelica	Earthy, peppery, green, spicy	4
basil	Spicy, anise-like, camphorous, lively	4
fennel	Sweet, somewhat spicy, licorice-like	4
Middle Notes	(50-80% of the blend)	
carrot seed	Sweet, fruity, warm, earthy	2
dill	Fresh, sweet, herbaceous, slight earthy	2
fir, balsam	Fresh, clean, green, balsamic, sweet	2
lavender	Floral, sweet, balsamic, slightly woody	2
melissa	Delicate, lemony	2
cajeput	Fresh, camphorous, with fruity note	3
coriander	Woody, spicy, sweet	3
cypress	Fresh, herbaceous, slightly woody	3
elemi	Balsamic, fresh, citrusy, peppery, spicy	3
euc. citriodora	Sweet, lemony, fresh, slightly woody	3
euc. radiata	Slightly camphorous, sweet, fruity	3
fir	Fresh, woody, earthy, sweet	3
geranium	Sweet, green, citrus-rosy, fresh	3

Essential Oil	Scent	Intensity
Middle Notes (continued)	(50-80% of the blend)	
helichrysum	Rich, sweet, fruity, slightly honey-like	3
hyssop	Fresh, earthy, woody, fruity	3
juniper	Sweet, musky, tenacious	3
marjoram	Herbaceous, green, spicy	3
melaleuca	Medicinal, fresh, woody, earthy	3
neroli	Floral, citrusy, semi-sweet, delicate	3
niaouli	Earthy, musty, harsh	3
black pepper	Spicy, peppery, musky, warm	3
rosemary cin.	Strong, camphorous, slightly woody	3
rosewood	Sweet, woody, fruity, floral	3
spruce	Fresh, woody, earthy, sweet	3
cardamom	Sweet, spicy, balsamic, slightly floral	4
G. chamomile	Deep, rich, tenacious, cocoa-like	4
R. chamomile	Fresh, sweet, fruity, apple-like	4
ginger	Sweet, spicy-woody, warm, fresh, sharp	4
nutmeg	Sweet, musky, spicy	4
pine, scotch	Fresh, woody, earthy, balsamic	4
thyme	Fresh, medicinal, herbaceous	4
yarrow	Sharp, woody, herbaceous, slight floral	4
oregano	Herbaceous, sharp	5
peppermint	Minty, sharp, intense	5
Middle to Base Notes	(20-80% of the blend)	
clary sage	Spicy, hay-like, sharp, fixative	3
rose	Floral, spicy, rich, deep, sensual, green	3
clove bud	Spicy, warming, slightly bitter, woody	5
ylang ylang	Sweet, heavy, narcotic, tropical floral	5
Base Notes	(5-20% of the blend)	
onycha	Rich, warm, slightly woody, creamy	1
cedarwood	Warm, soft, woody	3
cypress, blue	Long-lasting, warm, woody, earthy	3
frankincense	Rich, deep, warm, balsamic, sweet	3
sandalwood	Soft, woody, sweet, earthy, balsamic	3
jasmine	Powerful, sweet, tenacious, floral	4
myrrh	Warm, earthy, woody, balsamic	4
patchouli	Earthy, sweet-balsamic, rich, wood-like	4
vanilla	Sweet, balsamic, heavy, warm	4
spikenard	Heavy, earthy, animal-like	5
vetiver	Heavy, earthy, balsamic, smoky	5

APPLICATION OF ESSENTIAL OILS

1. **Direct Application.** Apply the oils directly on the area of concern using 1 to 6 drops of oil. More oil is not necessarily better, since a large amount of oil can trigger a detoxification of the surrounding tissue and blood. Such a quick detoxification can be somewhat uncomfortable. To achieve the desired results, 1 to 3 drops of oil is usually adequate. A few guidelines for direct application of the oils are as follows:

   ✓ The feet are the second fastest area of the body to absorb oils because of the large pores. Other quick-absorbing areas include behind the ears and on the wrists.

   ✓ To experience a feeling of peace, relaxation, or energy, 3 to 6 drops per foot are adequate.

   ✓ When massaging a large area of the body, always dilute the oils by 15% to 30% with the V-6 Oil.

   ✓ When applying oils to infants and small children, dilute with V-6 Oil. Use 1 to 3 drops of an essential oil to 1 tablespoon (Tbs.) of V-6 Oil for infants and 1 to 3 drops of an essential oil to 1 teaspoon (tsp.) V-6 Oil for children from 2- to 5-years-old.

   ✓ <u>Do not mix</u> oil blends. Commercially available blends have been specially formulated by someone who understands the chemical constituents of each oil and which oils blend well. The chemical properties of the oils can be altered when mixed improperly, resulting in some undesirable reactions.

   ✓ Layering individual oils is preferred over mixing your own blends. Layering refers to the process of applying one oil, rubbing it in, and then applying another oil. There is no need to wait more than a couple of seconds between each oil as absorption occurs quite rapidly. If dilution is necessary, the V-6 Oil may be applied on top. The layering technique is not only useful in physical healing, but also when doing emotional clearing.

   ✓ Hot Moist compresses can be applied over top of the application area. The moist heat will force the oils deeper into the tissues.

   ✓ The FDA has approved some essential oils for internal use and given them the designation of GRAS (Generally Regarded As Safe for internal consumption). *This designation is listed in the Single Oil Summary Information chart in the Appendix of this book under Safety Data.* **Oils without this designation should never be used internally.**

2. **Baths.** Add 3-6 drops of your favorite essential oil to the bath water as the tub is filling. Adding the oils to a bath and shower gel base first allows one to obtain the greatest benefit from the oils as they are more evenly dispersed throughout the water and not allowed to immediately separate.

3. **Diffuse.** A diffuser will disperse the essential oils into a micro-mist that will stay suspended for several hours to reduce bacteria, fungus, mold, and freshen the air with natural fragrances. Diffusing releases oxygenating molecules, antiviral, antibacterial, and antiseptic properties, as well as negative ions, which kill bacteria.When diffused, essential oils have been found to reduce airborne chemicals, bacteria, and metalics in the air as well as help to create great spiritual, physical, and emotional harmony. It is usually best to diffuse an oil 15-30 minutes at a time as you can become accustomed to them. You may mix the single oils, but do not mix the blends together.

4. **Feet Massage.** Your feet are the second fastest area of the body to absorb oils because of the large pores. Three to six drops per foot are adequate to experience a feeling of peace, relaxation or energy.

5. **Body Massage.** If massaging a large area of the body, always dilute the oils by 15 to 30 percent with V-6 Oil.

6. **Vita Flex Therapy.** One to three drops of the oil may be applied to the Vita Flex points (contact points) on the foot. Refer to the pages on Vita Flex therapy for more details.

7. **Auricular Therapy.** This is a method of applying the oils to the rim of the ears. This technique works extremely well for emotional clearing. Some physical benefits can also be obtained from this technique. See the pages on Auricular Therapy in this section of the *Quick Reference Guide for Using Essential Oils* for more details.

8. **Raindrop Technique.** This is a simple application of dropping certain oils like little drops of rain from about 6 inches above the body along the entire length of the spine. This particular application technique helps bring the body into balance, align the energy centers of the body, and release them if blocked. The oils used in this technique will continue to work in the body for about 5 to 7 days after treatment with continued realignment taking place during this time. The following oils are used: Thyme, oregano, cypress, birch/wintergreen, basil, peppermint, marjoram, Aroma Siez, Valor, Ortho Ease Massage Oil, and V-6 Oil. For more information about this technique, see the Raindrop Technique section of this book. The video entitled *Raindrop Technique* by D. Gary Young (available from Abundant Health) provides step-by-step instructions for this technique.

9. **Perfume or Cologne.** Wearing the oils as a perfume or cologne can provide wonderful emotional and physical support—not just a beautiful fragrance. (For some simple, yet exquisite, perfume/cologne blends, refer to the book *Natural Perfumes*, by Mindy Green).

10. Cooking. Essential oils can easily be incorporated into your cooking, as long as you remember that they are very concentrated. Usually only 1 drop is necessary, and sometimes even less. Use a toothpick to help control the addition of smaller amounts of oil by dipping the toothpick into the oil (more oil on the toothpick = stronger flavor, etc.) and then stirring it into the food. Here are a couple examples of recipes where people have used the essential oils for flavoring.

Lemon Tarragon Dressing

1 tablespoon fresh tarragon diced, or 1 teaspoon dried tarragon
1 tablespoon fresh or 1 teaspoon dried basil leaves
1 cup organic extra virgin cold pressed olive oil
dash of pepper
dash of red pepper
6 drops lemon essential oil

Mix well, and drizzle on salad or fish or anything! Keep unused portion in the fridge.

**-Submitted by Jill Burk,
Saginaw, Michigan (July 2004)**

Cream Cheese Icing

8 oz. package of cream cheese
1½ cups of powdered sugar
1 stick of butter
3 drops of tangerine essential oil

Thoroughly cream together the cream cheese, powdered sugar, and butter with an electric beater. Stir in the tangerine oil. Enjoy!

-Submitted by Ellie Ayers (July 2004)

> *I love to add a drop or two of lemon oil to the Joy blend! It's a wonderful perfume. If you want the blend to last longer and cool you off for the summer, fill a small spray bottle with distilled water, ten drop of Joy, and two drops of lemon. I like to spray it on after I shower.*
> *-Submitted by Nancy Dutton (July 2004)*

KEY PRINCIPLES OF VITA FLEX THERAPY

1. **To reduce any discomfort, fingernails should be cut and filed as short as possible**.

2. Remove all jewelry and watches to prevent an interference of energy.

3. Always **DROP** the oils into the palm of your non-dominant hand, and use the dominant hand to stir the oils clockwise 3 times before application. This method will increase the electrical frequency of the oils and significantly improve the results. **To prevent contamination of the oils, do not touch the top of the bottle with any part of your body.**

4. Put a drop of <u>White Angelica</u> on each of your shoulders to protect yourself against any negative energies from the person you are working on.

5. Always start on the bottoms of the feet. Put 3 to 6 drops of <u>Valor</u> on the bottom of each foot. Some may be applied to the area above the brain stem if desired. Hold the bottoms of the feet with your hands: right hand to right foot and left hand to left foot. Continue holding the feet until you feel the body's energy balance. This usually feels like an energy pulse beating in both feet. Another way to balance, which may be preferable to some, is to put 1 drop of <u>Valor</u> on the wrists and hold the wrists crossed together for a few minutes until you feel a pulse in the tips of the thumb and index finger.

6. Use the Vita Flex charts (*shown on the next couple of pages*) to determine where the oils should be placed during the therapy. One to three drops of oil may be applied to the specific Vita Flex points of the foot. Vita Flex points on the hand can be used as an alternative to extremely sensitive or sore feet. Apply the oil(s).

7. Apply the Vita Flex technique as follows: Starting with the fingers on their pads, curl the fingers up and over onto the nails (see photo examples on the next page). Increasing pressure is applied until the fingers are curled almost completely over on the nails. Pressure is then immediately released to create the spark of energy and send it on its way. The curling should be one continuous motion, not jerky, with medium to heavy pressure being placed on the contact point. Never press and hold while performing this technique. This may be done several times on the same spot to obtain the desired results. Some leverage can be achieved by placing the thumb of the same hand around to the other side of the foot or hand on which the Vita Flex is being performed. This allows the hand to operate in a fashion similar to a pipe wrench, which increases pressure on the pipe as it is twisted.

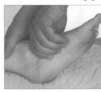 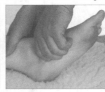 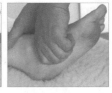

Comments: For a detailed explanation of the entire Vita Flex system, refer to Stanley Burrough's book, *Healing for the Age of Enlightenment*.

For step-by-step instructions of the full Vita Flex treatment, refer to the video, *Vita Flex Instruction* with Tom Woloshyn. This video teaches the proper Vita Flex technique as developed by Stanley Burroughs, including the Atlas Adjustment (a non-chiropractic technique used to quickly and efficiently re-align the spine or any other misalignment in the body). Another excellent tool for use with this technique is the Vita flex Roller or "Relax-a-Roller." This unique massage roller was specifically designed by Stanley Burroughs to provide the same stimulating effect as the fingers of teh hand. It is excellent for personal use (Both of these products are available from Abundant Health)

VITA FLEX HAND CHART

Vita Flex points in this hand chart correspond to those in the feet. Occasionally the feet n be too sensitive for typical Vita Flex therapy. Working with the hands will not only affect the ecific body points, but may also help to provide some pain relief to the corresponding points the feet. (Refer to Stanley Burroughs' book, *Healing for the Age of Enlightenment*, p. 78 for a ore detailed explanation.)

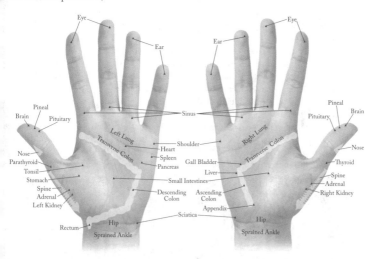

VITA FLEX FEET CHART

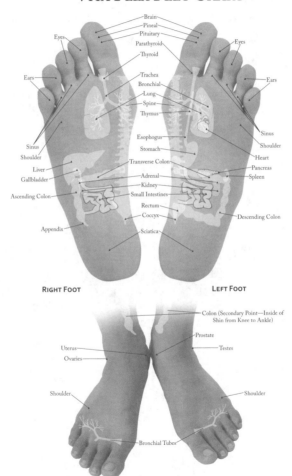

RIGHT FOOT   **LEFT FOOT**

AURICULAR EMOTIONAL THERAPY POINTS

f more than one oil/blend is indicated, layer them on one at a time.

When working on the ear, apply Harmony and Forgiveness to the entire ear, and apply Valor on the Feet.

YMPATHY & GUILT
Use Joy and Inspiration.

ELF PITY
Use Acceptance.

EJECTION
Use Forgiveness and Acceptance. Work the rejection points on both ears. For rejection from Mother, use Geranium. For rejection from Father, use Lavender. While applying the oils say, "I choose to accept my Mother/Father for what they have done or not done. It is their life and not mine."

YES & VISION
To Improve Eyesight, use 10 drops Lemongrass, 5 Cypress, and 3 Eucalyptus in ½ oz. (1 Tbsp) of V-6 Mixing Oil.

IEART
Use Joy to stimulate the pituitary. Use Valor and Release to release the anger.

PEN THE MIND
Use Valor and Motivation. Take deep breaths to express oneself.

MOTHER: Geranium
Sexual Abuse: Geranium, Ylang Ylang.
Abandonment: Geranium, Forgiveness, Acceptance.

FATHER: Lavender
Sexual Abuse: Lavender, Ylang Ylang.
Male Abuse: Helichrysum, Lavender.

DEPRESSION
Any of the following: Valor, Joy, Hope, White Angelica, Peace & Calming, Citrus Fresh, Christmas Spirit, Gentle Baby.
Use whichever blend(s) work for you.

OVERWHELMED
Use Hope and Acceptance.

BEARING BURDENS OF THE WORLD
Use Release and Valor.

ANGER & HATE
Use Joy to stimulate the pituitary.
Use Valor and Release to release the anger.

SELF EXPRESSION
Use Valor and Motivation. Take deep breaths to express oneself.

FEAR
Apply Valor, Release, Joy.

RAINDROP TECHNIQUE

This application technique was developed by D. Gary Young, aromatologist and one of North America's leading experts on the art and science of aromatherapy. This technique involves dropping the oils directly onto the spine from about six inches above the body. The oils are then worked into the spine using light strokes with the fingers, which stimulate energy impulses and disperse the oils along the nervous system throughout the entire body. In this way, the body can be brought into balance and the energy centers can be cleared and realigned. This method also helps to reduce spinal inflammations and to kill viruses that hibernate along the spinal column, as well as to help straighten any spinal curvatures. Although a session only lasts from about 45 minutes to an hour, the oils will continue to work in the body for a week or more following the treatment. The Raindrop Technique that is explained below is an abbreviated form. The video entitled *Raindrop Technique* by D. Gary Young (*available from Abundant Health*) provides step-by-step instructions for this technique.

Oils used in the Raindrop Technique

Valor—is the first and most important oil used in this technique because it helps balance the electrical energies within the body. It also helps create an environment where structural alignment can occur.

Thyme—is used for its ability to support the immune system by attacking any bacteria, fungus, infection, or virus that may be present. It may also help one overcome fatigue and physical weakness after an illness.

Oregano—works in conjunction with thyme to strengthen the immune system and to attack bacteria and viruses. It may also act as an antiseptic for the respiratory system, help balance metabolism, and help strengthen the vital centers of the body.

Cypress—is used for its antibacterial, anti-infectious, antimicrobial, and diuretic properties. In addition, it may function as a decongestant for the circulatory and lymphatic systems.

Birch/Wintergreen—is great for removing discomfort associated with the inflammation of bones, muscles, and joints. It may also help cleanse the lymphatic system.

Basil—is relaxing to spastic muscles and is stimulating to the nerves and to the adrenal cortex.

Peppermint—is used to calm and strengthen the nerves, reduce inflammation, and is highly effective when dealing with conditions related to the respiratory system. It also has a synergistic and enhancing effect on all other oils.

Marjoram—is used to relax spastic muscles, soothe the nerves, relieve cramps, aches, and pains, and to help calm the respiratory system.

Aroma Siez—may help to relax, calm, and relieve the tension of spastic muscles resulting from sports injury, fatigue, or stress.

Ortho Ease—is the crowning oil to this application. It is used to help relax all the muscles of the back and legs and to help reduce any stress, arthritic pain, or tension that may exist.

V-6 Oil—is used to help dilute any of the oils that may be somewhat caustic to the skin. It should always be used with oregano and thyme and can be used with any of the other oils based upon the person's skin sensitivity.

Note: The oils listed above have many more benefits. *For more specific information, please refer to the sections in this book on Singles and Blends.*

Raindrop Technique

1. Remove all jewelry or metal to allow the energy to flow freely. Put a drop of **White Angelica** on each of your shoulders to protect yourself against any negative energies coming from the person receiving the treatment.

2. Have the person lie face up on a table with their body as straight as possible on the table. The person receiving the treatment should be as comfortable as possible, so the arms can be resting along side the body or resting on the top of their hips, whichever they prefer (don't let their hands touch each other as this will tend to short circuit the flow of energy through their body). Cover the person with a sheet to protect their privacy and to keep them warm as you roll them over and alternate between working on their back and working on their legs and feet.

3. Apply **3** drops of **Valor** on each shoulder as well as 6 drops on each foot. Hold right foot/shoulder with right hand and left foot/shoulder with left hand (crossing hands if necessary – see the photo illustration entitled, "Valor Balance on Feet") for 5 to 10 minutes or until you can feel an energy pulse in the person's feet. For this part of the application, it works best if there is another person assisting in the treatment. If you are working by yourself, do the feet only. **Valor** is used to balance, and it works well on the energy alignment of the body. **This is the most important oil that is used in this application.**

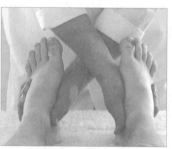

Valor Balance on Feet

4. First apply 2 drops of **thyme** to the Vita Flex spine points along the inside edge of each foot, working it in 3 times with the Vita Flex technique (*refer to Vita Flex Technique in this same section, Key Principle #7 and photo illustrations for an explanation of this technique*). Repeat this procedure with each of the following oils, one at a time: **oregano, cypress, birch/wintergreen, basil,** and **peppermint**. Then, have the person roll over onto their stomach, and perform steps 5 through 14 on their spine.

5. Hold the bottle of **thyme** about 6 inches from the spine, and evenly space **4 to 5** drops from the sacrum (tailbone) to the neck. Work it in evenly along the curvature of the spine with gentle upward strokes. Apply **5** drops of **oregano,** and work it in the same way. Then, apply **10 to 15** drops of **V-6 Oil** to prevent any discomfort, since both these oils can be quite caustic.

6. Using the very tips of the fingers, alternate between left hand and right hand as you very lightly work up the spine from the sacrum to the base of the neck with short, brush-like strokes. Follow the curvature of the spine, and repeat 2 more times.

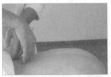 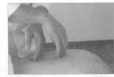 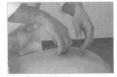

7. Using your finger tips again, softly brush up a few inches from the sacrum and then out to either side of the body; right hand to the right and left hand to the left.

Repeat this step from the sacrum, but go a few more inches up the spine and then out to the sides. Then again from the sacrum, go up a few more inches and then out. Then do it again, each time going further up the spine until you reach the base of the neck and flare out along the shoulders. This entire step should then be repeated 2 more times.

8. Using your finger tips again, start at the sacrum and, in full-length strokes, lightly brush all the way up the spine to the base of the neck and then out over the shoulders. Repeat 2 more times.

9. Evenly space **4 to 5** drops of **cypress** from the sacrum to the neck. Work it in evenly along the curvature of the spine with gentle upward strokes. Then apply the oils of **birch/wintergreen, basil, and peppermint** in the same manner.

10. Place both hands side by side (parallel to the spine) and, using the tips of the fingers, massage in a circular, clock-wise motion, just off to one side of the spine, from the sacrum up to the neck. **Remember to never work directly on the spine**. Apply moderate pressure, and move a finger's width at a time. This will help to loosen the muscles and allow the spine to straighten itself. After doing one side of the spine, move around the person, and work the other side of the spine from the sacrum to the neck in the same manner. Repeat 2 more times on either side.

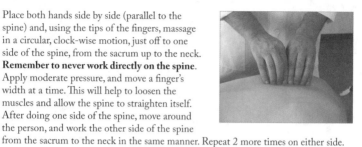

11. Using whichever hand is most comfortable to you, place the index and middle finger on either side of the spine at the sacrum. Place the other hand on top of the first, part way down the 2 fingers. Apply moderate pressure and, with a quick, forward and back continued sawing motion of the hand on top, slide the fingers a little at a time up the spine to the skull. Move the fingers upward slowly during the sawing motion. Once the skull is reached, apply gentle but firm pressure to push the skull forward, stretching the spine. Return to the sacrum, and repeat 2 more times.

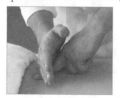 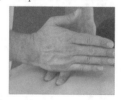 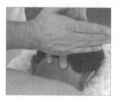

12. Place the thumbs of each hand on either side of the spine at the sacrum, and point them towards each other. Next, using the Vita Flex technique, roll the thumbs up and over onto the thumbnails, applying some pressure straight down during the roll. Then release and slide the thumbs up an inch or so, and repeat the roll with pressure. Continue up to the base of the neck, then return to the sacrum and repeat 2 more times. This will become easier with practice.

13. Apply 5 to 6 drops of **marjoram** up the spine, and work it in. Then apply 5 to 6 drops of **Aroma Siez** to each side and away from the spine. Gently massage these oils into the muscle tissue all over the back to soothe and relax the patient. After the oils have been massaged in well, you may cover the person with the sheet and rest for approximately 5 minutes. Apply **Ortho Ease** over the entire area of the back, and gently massage it in. Then cover the person to keep them warm, and massage **Ortho Ease** into the legs. This will help to relax the muscles that may be pulling on the spine.

14. Fold a hand towel, soak it in hot water, wring it out, and lay it along the entire length of the spine. Take a dry bath towel, fold it in half lengthwise, and place it over the hot wet towel. Be extremely sensitive to the feelings of the person as the heat may build along the spine. The heat will gradually build for 5 to 8 minutes and then cool right down to normal. If the heat becomes too uncomfortable, remove the towels and apply V-6 Oil. Then replace the towels and continue until the wet towel becomes cold. If the person's back is still hot, cover with a dry towel and allow the back to cool down slowly.

15. After the person's back begins to cool down, gently stretch the spine by crossing hands and straddling the spine with your hands—one pointing towards the top of the spine and the other towards the bottom as shown in the adjacent photo. Starting in the middle, gently press the hands downwards and apart towards opposite ends of the spine. Then move the hands apart more, and repeat the stretch. Continue until the ends of the spine are reached.

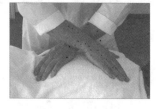

16. Remove the wet towels and have the person roll over onto their back. Apply 2 to 3 drops of **birch/wintergreen** along the inside of each leg from the knee to the heel and up the inside of the foot to the big toe. Layer it in, and apply the oils of **cypress, basil, and peppermint** in the same fashion. Then work the same area using the Vita Flex technique. The inside of the shin corresponds to the colon. By working this area, you are opening the colon and allowing it to expel any toxins released during the Raindrop Technique.

17. The final step is to perform another gentle stretching of the spine. If you are working alone, put your right hand behind the base of the head and your left hand under the chin. Very gently pull to create a slight tension and release. Do this 3 times, and then move to the feet. Hold above the ankles, and gently pull and release 3 times. If you have an assistant, one person can hold the head and the other hold the feet. Then together, apply a gentle tension and hold for a few minutes. This is then completed by the person at the head doing a very slight pull and release 3 times.

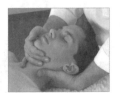 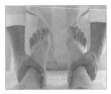

18. If certain systems of the body need work, have the person roll back over onto their stomach, and use the applicable blends and/or singles with the Vita Flex technique on the spine. Refer to the chart of the autonomic nervous system to help with placement of the oils along the spine.

By stimulating the Central Nervous System, you have just given someone a total treatment, affecting every system in the body, including emotional release and support. Even though the oils continue to work in the body for a week or more, one application may last months, or it may be necessary to repeat the application every week until the body begins to respond. The object is to develop a new memory in the tissues of the body and to train them to hold themselves in place. **(For a list of videos that effectively demonstrate this valuable application technique, refer to the *Video Listing* in the Bibliography section of this book.)**

Another aspect to the Raindrop Technique is the ability to **customize it** to the needs of the receiver. Each Raindrop Technique session should begin with the **<u>Valor</u>** essential oil blend, and the single oils of **oregano** (*Origanum compactum* CT carvacrol), and **thyme** (*Thymus vulgaris* CT thymol). However, after that, the remaining oils can be replace with others more specific to the condition or body system needing to be affected. To assist with this customization, the following chart is a partial list of single oils and oil blends under the particular body system which they affect. This chart is a condensed excerpt from the Body System Chart shown in the Appendix of this book *(Refer to the full chart in the Appendix for other products that can assist in strengthening a particular body system)*.

> *Mom had worn a narcotic pain patch for the past two years for her "chronic back pain" due to osteoarthritis, spurring of the spine, and numerous back surgeries. By using PanAway, we were able to discontinue the pain patch. We continued to alternate PanAway with Wintergreen, Peppermint, Clove, and V-6 Oil to her back and feet with warm compresses once or twice a day as needed for complete relief. Six weeks after she started receiving weekly Raindrop massages, she no longer complained of back pain. She continues to receive weekly or bi-weekly Raindrop massages, and its been 6 months since she has complained of back pain! Praise God!*
>
> *-Submitted by E. Pinar (July 2004)*

PERSONAL GUIDE

APPLICATION NOTES AND EXPLANATIONS

1. Next to each oil or blend listed in this section is a symbol (or symbols) that indicates the recommended application method(s) of that oil for the specific condition.

   A: **Aromatic** means that the oils are inhaled through the mouth and nose. This could include inhaling the aroma of the oil directly from the bottle or inhaling the aroma of the oil after it has been applied to the hands or to another material, such as a tissue or a cotton wick. It could also mean breathing in the vapor or mist of an oil that has been diffused or sprayed into the surrounding air.

   T: **Topical** means that the oils are applied directly to the skin, hair, or other surface of the body. This can be through massage, bath, direct application of the oils, or application of the oils within a cream, lotion, bath gel, or soap. While many oils can be applied neat (without dilution), others may need to be diluted with V-6 Oil or with another vegetable or carrier oil before topical application, especially in cases of young or sensitive skin. Refer to the Single Oil section of this book for recommended dilutions.

   I: **Internal** means that the oils are taken orally as a dietary supplement. This is done either by adding the oil to a food or beverage that is then consumed or by swallowing a capsule with the oil inside.

   Specific application instructions are usually listed for each condition, and further detailed information on application techniques can be found in the Science & Application section of this book.

2. Oils and application recommendations are color-coded as **Primary Recommendations** (listed in order of highest recommendation to lowest recommendation when research and consensus between essential oil experts warrants such an ordering) and Other Recommendations (listed alphabetically). It is not necessary to use all of the oils listed. Try one oil at a time. If you do not see a change soon, try a different one. What one person needs may be different from what another person needs. (Hint: Use kinesiology testing to determine which oils are right for you.)

3. A subscripted "F" (i.e. $_F$clary sage) means the oil has been used medicinally in France.

A=Aromatic **T**=Topical **I**=Internal | 43

4. *Neat* means to apply the oil without diluting it with a vegetable oil.

5. If essential oils get into your eyes by accident or if they burn the skin a little, do not try to remove the oils with water. Water will only drive the oils deeper into the tissue. It is best to dilute the essential oils with a pure vegetable oil.

6. The FDA has approved some essential oils for internal use and given them the following designations: GRAS (Generally Regarded As Safe for human consumption), FA (Food Additive), or FL (FLavoring agent). *These designations are listed in the Single Oil Summary Information chart in the Appendix of this book under Safety Data.*

7. Using some oils such as lemon, orange, grapefruit, mandarin, bergamot, angelica, etc. before or during exposure to direct sunlight or UV rays (tanning beds, etc.) may cause a rash, pigmentation, or even severe burns. These oils are designated as photosensitive (PH) or extremely photosensitive (PH*) in the Single Oil or Blend Summary Information in the Appendix of this book. It is best to check the safety data for the oils to be used and then either dilute the oils and test on a small area or avoid their use altogether.

8. Caution should be used with oils such as clary sage, sage, and fennel during pregnancy. These oils contain active constituents with hormone-like activity and could possibly stimulate adverse reactions in the mother, although there are no recorded cases in humans.

9. Particular care should be taken when using cinnamon bark, lemongrass, oregano, and thyme—as they are some of the strongest and most caustic oils. It is best to dilute them with a pure vegetable oil.

10. In this document, several homemade blends are suggested. However, this is done with great hesitancy. Some of the blends listed come from individuals who may not be experts in the field of essential oils and aromatherapy. Rather than mix the oils together, it may be better to layer the oils; that is, apply a drop or two of one oil, rub it in, and then apply another oil. If dilution is necessary, a pure vegetable oil can be applied on top.

11. When someone is out of electrical balance, try the following:

    A. Place a drop or two of Harmony in one hand, and then rub the palms of both hands together in a clockwise motion.

    B. Place one hand over the thymus (heart chakra) and the other hand over the navel.

    C. Take 3 deep breaths and switch hands; then take 3 more deep breaths. (Refer to Allergies in this section for more information).

12. Less is often better; use 1–3 drops of oil and no more than 6 drops at a time. Stir and rub on in a clockwise direction.

13. When applying oils to **infants** and to **small children**, dilute 1–2 drops of pure essential oil with ½–1 teaspoon (tsp.) of a pure vegetable oil (V-6 Oil). If the oils are used in

the bath, always use a bath gel base as a dispersing agent for the oils. See **Babies/Children** for more information about the recommended list of oils for babies and children.

14. The body absorbs oils the fastest through inhalation (breathing) and second fastest through application to the feet or to the ears. Testing on the thyroid, heart, and pancreas showed that the oils reached these organs in three seconds. Layering oils can increase the rate of **absorption**.

15. When an oil causes **discomfort,** it is because it is pulling toxins, heavy metals, chemicals, poisons, parasites, and mucus from the system. Either stop applying the oils for a short time, to make sure your body isn't eliminating (detoxifying) too fast, or dilute the oils until the body catches up with the releasing. Toxins go back into the system if they cannot be released.

16. When the cell wall thickens, oxygen cannot get in. The life expectancy of a cell is 120 days (4 months). Cells also divide, making duplicate cells. If the cell is diseased, new diseased cells will be made. When we stop the mutation of the diseased cells (create healthy cells), we stop the disease. Essential oils have the ability to penetrate and carry nutrients through the cell wall to the nucleus and improve the health of the cell.

17. Each oil has a **frequency**, and each of our organs and body parts has a frequency. The frequency of an oil is attracted by a like frequency within the body. Lower oil frequencies become a sponge for negative energy. The frequency is what stays in the body to maintain the longer-lasting effects of the oil.

    Low frequencies can make physical changes in the body.

    Middle frequencies can make emotional changes in the body.

    High frequencies can make spiritual changes in the body.

    A. Average frequency of the human body during the day time is between 62 and 68 Megahertz (MHz). Bone frequency is 38 to 43 MHz. Frequencies from the neck down vary between 62 and 68 MHz.

    B. Spiritual frequencies range from 92 to 360 MHz.

18. *Use extreme caution when diffusing cinnamon bark* because it may burn the nostrils if you put your nose directly next to the nebulizer of the diffuser.

19. When traveling by air, you should always have your oils hand-checked. X-ray machines may interfere with the frequency of the oils. *See Comments under Asthma for a discussion on plastic nasal inhalers for using oils on the airplane instead of taking the bottles of oil.*

20. Keep oils away from the light and heat, although they seem to do fine in temperatures up to 90 degrees. If stored properly, they can maintain their maximum potency for many years.

A=Aromatic **T**=Topical **I**=Internal

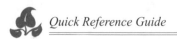

Abandoned: *See also Emotions.*

Oils—^{AT}<u>Acceptance</u>, ^{AT}<u>Forgiveness</u>, ^{AT}<u>Valor</u>.

A—Diffuse into the air. Inhale directly or applied to a tissue or a cotton wick.

T—Dilute, and use as massage oil. Apply to auricular emotional points.

Abscess: *See also Antifungal,*
Antibacterial, Infection, or Oral
Conditions: ABSCESS.

Oils—^{TA}<u>Thieves</u>, ^{TA}tea tree, ^Tthyme,
^{TA}<u>Purification</u>, ^Tbergamot, ^Telemi,
^Tfrankincense, ^Tgalbanum, ^{TA}lav-
ender, ^{TA}<u>Melrose</u>, ^Tmyrrh, ^TRoman
chamomile, ^Twintergreen.

> *I had an abscess tooth. The dentist and the specialist he referred me*
> *to insisted I have a root canal. I used 3 to 4 drops of Thieves in a*
> *glass of water to gargle with. Then I used a mixture of half Thieves*
> *and half olive oil and rubbed this on both sides of my gums on the*
> *infected area. I then used the Dentarome Plus toothpaste. It has*
> *been 2 months and my mouth is fine.*
>
> *–Submitted by K. Ernst (July 2004)*

Blend #1—**Dilute equal parts** Roman chamomile, lavender, and tea tree (tea tree) in V-6
Oil, and apply on location.

Supplements—Life 5 (probiotic), Super B.

***Comments—Some sources recommend a nontoxic diet and an increase in liquid intake.

—MOUTH

Oils—^T_FLavender.

T—To reduce swelling, pain, inflammation, and to draw out toxins, it may help to apply
the oil(s) with a hot compress. Put <u>Thieves</u> on a rolled up gauze, and place over abscess
to pull out the infection.

A—Diffuse into the air.

Absent Minded: *See also Memory.*

Oils—^ARosemary[1], ^Apeppermint[2], ^Asage lavender[3], ^A<u>Brain Power</u>, ^A<u>Clarity</u>, ^Abasil, ^Acarda-
mom, ^Afrankincense, ^Alemongrass, ^A<u>M-Grain</u>, ^Asandalwood.

Supplements—Mineral Essence, MultiGreens, Omega Blue, OmegaGize[3], Power Meal,
Sulfurzyme, Master Formula (whole food multi-nutrient), Ultra Young+.

A—Diffuse into the air. Inhale directly or applied to a tissue or a cotton wick.

Abundance:

Oils—^{AT}<u>Abundance</u>, ^{AT}<u>Oola Finance</u>, ^{AT}cinnamon bark, ^{AT}<u>Acceptance</u>, ^{AT}bergamot,
^{AT}cypress, ^{AT}<u>Harmony</u>, ^{AT}<u>Gathering</u>.

—ATTRACTS

    Oils—^{AT}<u>Abundance</u>, ^{AT}<u>Oola Finance</u>, ^{AT}cinnamon bark.

—MONEY

    Oils—^{AT}Ginger, ^{AT}<u>Oola Finance</u>, ^{AT}patchouli.

*****Comments**—One waitress demonstrated her luck when she wore <u>Abundance</u> and <u>Harmony</u> together; she received a whopping $120.00 tip! Who knows, it may work for you too!

A—Diffuse into the air.

T—Wear oil as perfume or cologne.

Abuse:

≫ *Abuse is the harmful treatment or use of something or someone. Abuse has many different forms: physical, sexual, verbal, spiritual, psychological, etc. Abuse in all of its forms often has long-lasting negative effects on the person or thing abused.*

    Oils—^{TA}<u>SARA</u> (releases memory and trauma of sexual or ritual abuse), ^{TA}<u>Trauma Life</u>, ^{TA}<u>Release</u>, ^{TA}melissa, ^{TA}<u>Acceptance</u>, ^{TA}<u>Brain Power</u>, ^{TA}<u>Citrus Fresh</u>, ^{TA}<u>Christmas Spirit</u>, ^{TA}geranium, ^{TA}<u>Forgiveness</u>, ^{TA}<u>Grounding</u>, ^{TA}<u>Harmony</u>, ^{TA}<u>Hope</u>, ^{TA}<u>Humility</u>, ^{TA}<u>Inner Child</u>, ^{TA}<u>Joy</u>, ^{TA}lavender, ^{TA}<u>Peace & Calming</u>, ^{TA}<u>3 Wise Men</u>, ^{TA}sandalwood, ^{TA}<u>Surrender</u>, ^T<u>Tranquil</u> (roll-on), ^{TA}<u>Valor</u>, ^{TA}ylang ylang.

    Supplements—Power Meal, Super B, Super C / Super C Chewable.

—BY FATHER

    Oils—^{AT}<u>Sacred Mountain</u> (empowers self), ^{AT}<u>Forgiveness</u>, ^{AT}lavender.

—BY MOTHER

    Oils—<u>Forgiveness</u>, geranium, lavender.

    *****Comments**—*Refer to the page on Auricular Emotional Therapy in the Science & Application section of this book for the points where oils can be applied.*

—FEELINGS OF REVENGE

    Oils—^T<u>Forgiveness</u> (around navel), ^T<u>Present Time</u> (on thymus), ^T<u>Surrender</u> (on sternum over heart), ^T<u>Tranquil</u> (roll-on).

—PROTECTION OR BALANCE

    Oils—^T<u>Harmony</u> (over thymus; on energy centers/chakras), ^T<u>White Angelica</u> (on shoulders).

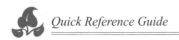

—SEXUAL/RITUAL

  Oils—ᵀForgiveness (around navel), ᵀRelease (liver Vita Flex point on feet; under
  nose), ᵀSARA (over area of abuse), ᵀᴬHarmony, ᵀᴬJoy, ᵀᴬPresent Time, ᵀᴬsage, ᵀᴬ3
  Wise Men, ᵀᴬTrauma Life, ᵀᴬValor, and ᵀᴬWhite Angelica.

—ESPOUSAL

  Oils—ᵀᴬRelease, ᵀᴬForgiveness, ᵀᴬValor, ᵀᴬAcceptance, ᵀᴬEnvision, ᵀᴬJoy, ᵀᴬTrauma
  Life.

—SUICIDAL

  Oils—ᵀHope (on rim of ears),ᵀᴬBrain Power, ᵀᴬmelissa, ᵀᴬPresent Time.

T—Apply 1 drop in area indicated, or apply 1 drop of the desired oils on each chakra to
allow blocked emotions to come out. Apply to auricular emotional points. Dilute, and
use as massage oil.

A—Diffuse into the air. Inhale directly.

Accidents: *See Emotions.*

  Oils—ᴬᵀTrauma Life.

A—Diffuse into the air. Inhale directly.

T—Apply 1 drop of the desired oils on each chakra to allow blocked emotions to come
out. Apply to auricular emotional points. Dilute, and use as massage oil.

Aches/Pains: *See Pain*

Acidosis: *See also Alkaline and pH
  Balance.*

  Oils—ᴵLemon, ᵀᴵThieves (dissolves
  and digests acid in the interstitial
  tissues), ᵀmyrrh, ᵀᴵpeppermint.

  I—Add 1 drop to 8 oz. rice milk or
  other beverage and drink. Add 3–5
  drops oil to 3–5 drops V-6 Oil in
  capsule, and swallow.

  T—Dilute, and apply 1 drop of the
  desired oils on location. Add 3–5
  drops to 1 Tbs. V-6 Oil, and massage on location. Apply to Vita-Flex
  points.

> *Acidosis is a condition of over-acidity in the blood and body
> tissues. When the body loses its alkaline reserve, pleomorphic virus,
> bacteria, yeast, and fungus take over and cause degenerative
> diseases such as, diabetes, cancer, AIDS, arteriosclerosis, arthritis,
> osteoporosis, chronic fatigue, etc.*
>
> ***Symptoms of acidosis*** *may include frequent sighing, insomnia,
> water retention, recessed eyes, rheumatoid arthritis, migraine
> headaches, abnormally low blood pressure, and alternating
> constipation and diarrhea.*
>
> ***Causes of acidosis*** *may include improper diet, kidney, liver, and
> adrenal disorders, emotional disturbances, fever, and an excess of
> niacin, vitamin C, and aspirin.*
>
> ***Oxygen*** *reduces the acidity of the blood. All essential oils contain
> oxygen. We like to flavor our water with 1-2 drops of lemon or
> peppermint oil. Lemon has the ability to counteract acidity in
> the body. The citric acid found in lemons is neutralized during
> digestion, giving off carbonates and bicarbonates of potassium and
> calcium, which helps maintain the alkalinity of the system.*

Supplements—**AlkaLime** (acid-neutralizing mineral), Balance Complete, JuvaPower (loaded with acid-binding foods), Life 5 (probiotic) Mineral Essence, MultiGreens (for alkaline/acid balance), Power Meal.

*****Comments**—Cancer and candida need an acid condition in order to thrive and spread. In acidic conditions, the oils will neutralize the acid but are consumed in the process and are not able to perform their physiological functions. Increase your use of the oils and take other measures to reduce acid levels in the body. The body can only heal in an alkaline state.

ACID-FORMING FOODS—Avoid meat, dairy products, whole wheat or rye bread, coffee, tea, wine, beer, root beer, cider, yeast products, soy sauce, cold cereals, potato chips, etc.

NEUTRALIZING FOODS—Raw apple cider vinegar is an acid neutralizer. Add a few drops of <u>Thieves</u> to 2 oz. of raw apple cider vinegar and drink in the morning and evening to help reduce acid levels in the body.

Acne: *See also Hormonal Imbalance, Scarring, Skin, and Stress.*

» *Acne is a deep blockage of a skin pore by dead skin cells, tiny hairs, and oil secreted by the sebaceous glands located near the hair follicles in the face, neck, and back. This blockage causes red, irritating blemishes (pimples) on the skin (most commonly found on the oil-producing parts of the body such as the face, chest, back, upper arms, and back of neck).*

> *Acne is often a result of seborrhea (an overproduction of fat from the sebaceous glands), which can oftentimes be traced back to a hormonal imbalance. Stress is another reason for increased sebum production. Consequently, it may be of help to use oils that balance the hormones and reduce stress.*
>
> *Essential oil treatments combined with a good diet (lots of vegetables and lots of water), exercise, and increased lymphatic and circulatory flow, will allow the toxic wastes to leave the body as the oxygen and nutrients reach the skin in greater proportions.*
>
> *One of the best ways to release toxins through the skin is to sweat. Chamomile, hyssop, juniper, lavender, rosemary, and thyme contain sudorific properties and may facilitate the sweating process. The antibacterial and anti-inflammatory oils may assist in the healing process.*

Oils—^TTea tree (tea tree)[4], ^T_FGerman chamomile, ^T_Fjuniper, ^T_Flavender, ^T_Frosewood, ^T<u>Melrose</u>, ^Tbergamot, ^Tcedarwood, ^T<u>Clarity</u> (on temples), ^Tclary sage, ^Tclove, ^Teucalyptus, ^TEucalyptus radiata, ^Tfrankincense, ^T<u>Gentle Baby</u>, ^Tgeranium, ^T<u>ImmuPower</u> (pimples in ears), ^Tlemon, ^Tlemongrass, ^Tmarjoram, ^Tmyrtle, ^Tpatchouli, ^Tpetitgrain, ^T<u>Purification</u>, ^T<u>Raven</u>, ^Travintsara, ^T<u>RC</u>, ^Trosemary, ^Tsage, ^Tsage lavender, ^Tsandalwood, ^T<u>Sensation</u>, ^Tspearmint, ^Tthyme, ^Tvetiver, ^Tyarrow.

Personal Care—**Essential Beauty Serum - Acne-Prone Skin Blend**, A·R·T Skin Care System, Prenolone/Prenolone+, Progessence/Progessence Plus, Rose Ointment, Sensation Massage Oil.

Supplements—ComforTone, Digest + Cleanse, ICP, Essentialzyme, Essentialzymes-4, JuvaTone, and Sulfurzyme. Cleansing the colon may help (*See Cleansing*).

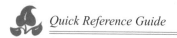
—Adult Onset

>> *Adult-onset acne affects many men and women at some point in their adult lives. Possible causes are thought to be hormones, cosmetic products, stress, and increased bacteria. Women often experience increased breakouts with the onset of menstruation each month.*

Personal Care—Prenolone/Prenolone+, Progessence/Progessence Plus if the acne stems from a hormonal imbalance.

—Cellular Regenerative

>> *When an injury occurs to the skin, such as the irritation caused by acne, scar tissue will form if the cells are unable to regenerate (replace) themselves.*

Oils—[T]Palmarosa, [T]rosewood.

—Healing

Oils—Use antibacterial and anti-inflammatory oils like [T]tea tree (tea tree)[4], [T]Melrose, [T]geranium, and [T]rosewood.

—Infectious

Oils—[T]Clove.

—Menstrual

Premenstrual or mid-menstrual cycle acne may be helped by balancing the hormones.

Personal Care—Prenolone/Prenolone+, Progessence/Progessence Plus.

Supplements—CortiStop (Women's), FemiGen, Super B.

—Rosacea (Acne Rosacea)

Oils—[T]Lavender. Dilute with V-6 Oil and apply daily after washing face with Orange Blossom Facial Wash and before applying Sandalwood Moisture Cream. Can also add extra lavender oil to Sandalwood Moisture Cream.

> *Rosacea is a chronic, acne-like condition of the facial skin that typically first appears as a flushing or subtle redness on the cheeks, nose, chin or forehead that comes and goes. Left untreated, the condition progresses and the redness becomes more persistent, bumps and pimples appear, and small dilated blood vessels may become visible. In some cases the eyes may be affected, causing them to be irritated and bloodshot and, according to some doctors, even blindness can occur. In the more advanced cases, the nose becomes red and swollen from excess tissue. Currently, this condition can only be controlled.*

Personal Care—Essential Beauty Serum - Acne-Prone Skin Blend, Orange Blossom Facial Wash, Sandalwood Moisture Cream.

—Toxin Release

Oils—Use sudorific oils like [T]chamomile, [T]hyssop, [T]juniper, [T]lavender, [T]rosemary, and [T]thyme to help promote sweating.

T—Apply one of the above oils on location; or try putting about 10 drops of an oil into a small spray bottle with distilled water, and mist your face several times a day.

ADD/ADHD (Attention Deficit Disorder/Attention Deficit Hyperactive Disorder): *See also Hyperactivity.*

>> *Attention Deficit Disorder or Attention Deficit/Hyperactive Disorder is a psychological condition characterized by inattentiveness, restlessness, and difficulty concentrating. Although most individuals exhibit all of these symptoms at some point, ADD is characterized by a frequency and duration of these symptoms that are inappropriate to an individual's age.*

Oils—^{AT}Reconnect, ^{AT}InTouch, ^{TA}Lavender[6], ^{TA}Citrus Fresh, ^TRutaVaLa, ^TTranquil (roll-on), ^{TA}ledum.

Blend Ideas—Lavender with basil (on crown), Harmony, or Peace & Calming; Basil with Clarity; Frankincense with Valor. Apply 1–3 drops of any of these blends on the bottoms of the feet and on the spine; Diffuse.

Supplements—NingXia Red (provides a full range of vitamins, trace minerals, amino acids, and essential fatty acids), **Omega Blue** (absolutely necessary), OmegaGize³, Allerzyme (aids the digestion of sugars, starches, fats, and proteins), Digest + Cleanse, Mineral Essence.

***Comments—Avoid sweeteners such as sugar and corn syrup. Eliminate caffeine and food additives from diet. Individuals who have ADD often have high aluminum toxicity.

—CHELATING AGENT

   Oils—^THelichrysum.

—SLEEPING

   Oils—^{AT}Reconnect, ^{AT}InTouch, ^APeace & Calming or ^AGentle Baby.

T—Dilute 3–5 drops of oil in 1 Tbs. V-6 Oil and use as a massage oil. Add 1–2 drops to warm bathwater (or combine with 1/4 cup bath salts and add to warm bathwater) and bathe.

A—Diffuse into the air.

Addictions:

>> *An addiction is an obsession, compulsion, or extreme psychological dependence that interferes with an individual's ability or desire to function normally. Common addictions include drugs, alcohol, coffee, tobacco, sugar, video games, work, gambling, money, explicit images, compulsive overeating, etc.*

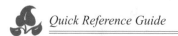

Oils—^{TA}<u>Acceptance</u>, ^{TA}<u>JuvaFlex</u>, ^{TA}bergamot (helps with over indulgences), ^{TA}<u>Peace & Calming</u>, ^{TA}<u>Purification</u>, ^{TA}calamus (tobacco), ^{TA}<u>GLF</u>.

Supplements—**JuvaTone,** Digest + Cleanse, Mineral Essence, Super C / Super C Chewable.

Recipe #1—This recipe has worked for individuals who are trying to break addictions. Use JuvaPower, JuvaTone, ComforTone, <u>JuvaFlex</u> and <u>Acceptance</u> together.

—**ALCOHOL** (to stop drinking):

Oils—^{TA}<u>Purification</u>, ^{TA}<u>Peace & Calming</u>. Do not use clary sage and alcohol together; it may result in nightmares. For professional assistance, contact the local chapter of Alcoholics Anonymous.

—**ALCOHOLISM**

▸▸ *Alcoholism is an extreme dependence on alcohol that interferes with an individual's social, physical, and mental health.*

Oils—^{AT}Rosemary, ^{AT}fennel, ^{AT}juniper (<u>Alternative Medicine—A Definitive Guide</u>, p. 492). Can also use ^{AT}<u>Acceptance</u>, ^{AT}elemi, ^{AT}<u>Forgiveness</u>, ^{AT}<u>GLF</u>, ^{AT}helichrysum, ^{AT}<u>Joy</u>, ^{AT}<u>JuvaFlex</u>, ^{AT}lavender, ^{AT}<u>Motivation</u>, ^{AT}orange, ^{AT}Roman chamomile, ^{AT}rosemary verbenon, ^{AT}<u>Transformation</u>, ^{AT}<u>Surrender</u>.

Supplements—Work on cleaning out the colon and liver with **JuvaPower/JuvaSpice,** Balance Complete or the Cleansing Trio, Digest + Cleanse, and JuvaTone or the Master Cleanser (*See Cleansing*). Mineral Essence, Power Meal, Thyromin.

—**COFFEE**

Oils—^{AT}Bergamot, ^{AT}calamus.

—**DRUGS**

Oils—^{TA}Cumin[6], ^{TA}<u>Peace & Calming</u>, ^{TA}<u>Purification</u>, ^{TA}grapefruit (withdrawal)[7], ^{TA}basil, ^{TA}bergamot, ^{TA}eucalyptus, ^{TA}fennel, ^{TA}lavender, ^{TA}marjoram, ^{TA}nutmeg, ^{TA}orange, ^{TA}Roman chamomile, ^{TA}sandalwood, ^{TA}wintergreen.

Supplements—Super C / Super C Chewable (at least 250 mg per day).

—**SMOKING/TOBACCO**

Oils—^ABlack pepper[8]. Use **Recipe #1** above. Applying either **clove** or <u>Thieves</u> to the tongue before lighting up helps remove the desire to smoke. Calamus may also help.

***COMMENTS—*One individual used JuvaTone to break a habit of smoking 2 ½ packs of cigarettes a day for 20 years. It only took him 3–5 days!*

—SUGAR

    Oils—^T**Dill** (on wrists to help remove addiction to sweets), ^{TA}**Purification,** ^{TA}Peace & Calming.

    Supplements—Allerzyme (aids the digestion of sugars, starches, fats, and proteins), Cleansing Trio (ComforTone, Essentialzyme, Essentialzymes-4, and ICP).

—WITHDRAWAL

    Oils—^{AT}**Grapefruit,** ^{TA}**cumin,** ^T**dill** (to the wrists helps reduce the sweating that often accompanies withdrawal), ^{TA}lavender, ^{TA}marjoram, ^{TA}nutmeg, ^{TA}orange, ^{TA}sandalwood.

T—Apply to temples and to Vita Flex points on the feet. Apply to stomach, abdomen, liver area, and feet.

A—Diffuse into the air. Inhale directly or applied to tissue or a cotton wick.

Addison's Disease: *See Adrenal Glands: ADDISON'S DISEASE.*

Adenitis: *See also Lymphatic System.*

    » *Adenitis is an acute or chronic inflammation of the lymph glands or nodes. Drink a lot of water to help remove the toxins from the body.*

    Oils—^T**Rosemary,** ^Tpine, ^Tsage. Could also try ^Tgarlic or ^Tonion.

    T—Dilute as recommended, and apply on location.

Adrenal Glands: *See also Endocrine System, Lupus, Thyroid.*

    » *The adrenal glands are two small glands located on top of the kidneys. The inner part of the adrenal gland, called the medulla, is responsible for producing adrenalin, a hormone that helps control blood pressure, heart rate, and sweating. The outer part of the adrenal gland, called the cortex, is responsible for producing corticosteroids, hormones that help control metabolism and help regulate inflammation, water levels, and levels of electrolytes such as sodium and potassium. Nutmeg displays properties similar to these hormones. When the adrenal glands are working properly, it is easier to correct low thyroid function.*

    Oils—^T**Nutmeg** (increases energy; supports adrenal glands), ^TEndoFlex, ^TEn-R-Gee, ^TForgiveness, ^TJoy.

    Blend #1—Add 3 drops clove, 4 drops nutmeg, and 6 drops rosemary to 1 tsp. V-6 Oil. Apply 4–5 drops of this mixture to kidney areas, and cover with a hot compress. Also apply 1–2 drops of mixture to Vita Flex kidney points on the feet, and work in with fingers using the Vita Flex technique.

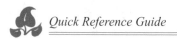

—**Addison's Disease:**

>> *Addison's disease is an autoimmune disease where the body's own immune cells attack the adrenal glands and either severely limit or completely shut down the production of the adrenal cortex hormones. Extreme fluid and mineral loss are the life-threatening results.*

Oils—ᵀ**Nutmeg** (increases energy; supports adrenal glands), ᵀEn-R-Gee, ᵀEndo-Flex, ᵀJoy, ᵀsage (combine with nutmeg).

Supplements—**Sulfurzyme** (shown to slow or reverse autoimmune diseases), **Endo-Gize,** ImmuPro, Master Formula, Mineral Essence (help supplement mineral loss), MultiGreens, Super B.

—**Cushing's Disease**

>> *Cushing's disease is characterized by an overabundance of corticosteroids (such as cortisol) in the body—typically caused by over-production of these steroids by the adrenal glands. This overproduction can be caused by a growth in the adrenal glands or by a tumor in the thyroid, causing production of too much corticotropin (the hormone that stimulates production of corticosteroids in the adrenal gland). This syndrome can also be caused by taking artificial cortisone or cortisone-like substances. Symptoms of excessive corticosteroids include weight gain, muscle loss and weakness, bruising, and osteoporosis.*

Oils—ᵀ**Lemon,** ᵀbasil, ᵀForgiveness, ᵀImmuPower, ᵀJoy, ᵀThieves.

Supplements—ImmuPro, Inner Defense.

—**Schmidt's Syndrome** *See also Addison's Disease above.*

>> *This syndrome refers specifically to an auto-immune disorder that causes Addison's disease in combination with decreased thyroid function.*

Oils—ᵀ**Nutmeg** (increases energy; supports adrenal glands), ᵀEn-R-Gee, ᵀEndo-Flex, ᵀJoy, ᵀsage (combine with nutmeg).

Supplements—**Sulfurzyme** (shown to slow or reverse autoimmune diseases), EndoGize, ImmuPro, Inner Defense, Master Formula, (3 times a day), Mineral Essence (help supplement mineral loss), MultiGreens, Super B (after each meal), Thyromin (first thing in morning).

—**Stimulant**

Oils—ᵀ_F_Basil, ᵀ_F_sage, ᵀrosemary, ᵀclove, ᵀgeranium, ᵀpine.

—**Strengthen**

Oils—ᵀSpruce (black), ᵀpeppermint.

—**Underactive Adrenals** *See Addison's Disease.*

Supplements—Thyromin (1–4 tablets daily. *See Suggested Use under Thyromin in the Supplements section of the <u>Reference Guide for Essential Oils</u>*), Master Formula, Mineral Essence, MultiGreens, Super B.

T—Apply as a warm compress over kidney area. Dilute as recommended, and apply on location or on Vita-Flex points on the feet.

Aftershave: *See also Skin.*

Oils—[T]<u>Awaken</u> (can be used instead of aftershave lotion), [T]<u>Valor</u>.

Comments—Try adding <u>Awaken</u> to Sandalwood Moisture Cream, Lavender Hand & Body Lotion, Sensation Hand & Body Lotion, or Genesis Hand & Body Lotion as an aftershave.

T—Dilute with V-6 Oil and apply on skin. *See Comments above for additional applications.*

Personal Care—Genesis Hand & Body Lotion, Sensation Hand & Body Lotion, Sandalwood Moisture Cream, Lavender Hand & Body Lotion, KidScents Lotion (soothes and rehydrates the skin—and smells great too), Prenolone/Prenolone+, Rose Ointment.

Agent Orange Poisoning:

»» *Agent Orange is a toxic herbicide that was used to defoliate areas of the forest during the Vietnam War.*

Oils—[T]<u>GLF</u> or [T]<u>JuvaFlex</u> (over liver), [T]<u>EndoFlex</u> (over adrenal glands/kidneys).

T—Apply 1–2 drops to areas indicated above with a hot compress.

Bath—Add 1 cup Epsom salts and 4 oz. of food grade hydrogen peroxide to warm bathwater.

Supplements—Balance Complete, ComforTone, Digest + Cleanse, EndoGize, Essentialzyme, Essentialzymes-4, ICP, ImmuPro, Thyromin.

Recipe #1—3 drops <u>EndoFlex</u> on throat, feet (under big toes and on kidney Vita Flex point). Also across the back over the kidneys. After 90 days, start the Cleansing Trio (ComforTone, Essentialzyme, and ICP), and continue using it for one year.

Recipe #2—1 ImmuPro three times a day, 2 Thyromin at bedtime. After 90 days, start the Cleansing Trio (ComforTone, Essentialzyme, and ICP), and continue for one year.

Aging: *See also Wrinkles.*

Oils—[I]Thyme[9], [I]<u>Longevity</u>, [I]lemon[10], [T]carrot, [T]frankincense, [T]rosehip, [T]rosewood, [T]sandalwood.

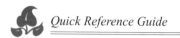

Supplements—**NingXia Red, Longevity Capsules, Ningxia Wolfberries** (dried), Master Formula.

I—Add 1–3 drops to an empty capsule with 1–3 drops V-6 Oil, and swallow.

T—Dilute as recommended, and apply on skin.

—**Moisturizers**

Personal Care—**A·R·T Skin Care System** (builds collagen, repairs DNA damage, and smooths wrinkles), Boswellia Wrinkle Cream, Essential Beauty Serums (Dry & Acne-Prone Skin Blends), Satin Facial Scrub—Mint, Prenolone/Prenolone+, Progessence/Progessence Plus, Rose Ointment, Sandalwood Moisture Cream, Sensation Hand & Body Lotion, Wolfberry Eye Cream.

Supplements—**Wolfberry Crisp Bars** *(Refer to the Wolfberry Crisp Bar in the Supplements section of the <u>Reference Guide for Essential Oils</u> for more information on the benefits of the Ningxia Wolfberry)*, Essentialzyme, Essentialzymes-4, Mineral Essence (antioxidant).

Agitation: *See Calming: AGITATION.*

AIDS: *See also Antiviral.*

⠠⠠ *Acquired immune deficiency syndrome (AIDS) is a disease of the human immune system. AIDS progressively inhibits the effectiveness of the immune system, leaving the human body susceptible to both infections and tumors. AIDS is caused by the human immunodeficiency virus (HIV), which is acquired by direct contact of the bloodstream or mucous membrane with a bodily fluid (such as blood, breast milk, vaginal fluid, semen, and preseminal fluid) containing HIV.*

Oils—[TA]Helichrysum[11], [TA]cumin **(supports immune system; inhibits HIV virus)**, [TA]<u>Thieves</u>, [TA]<u>Brain Power</u>, [TA]cistus, [TA]<u>Exodus II</u>, [TA]<u>ImmuPower</u>, [TA]lemon, [TA]bergamot[12], [TA]nutmeg, [TA]<u>Valor</u>.

T—Apply to thymus and to bottoms of feet.

A—Diffuse into the air.

Supplements—Balance Complete, Cleansing Trio (ComforTone, Essentialzyme, and ICP), Digest + Cleanse, ImmuPro, Inner Defense, Mineral Essence, MultiGreens, NingXia Red, Power Meal (contains wolfberry which is an immune stimulator), Super B, Super C / Super C Chewable, Thyromin, Master Formula, Ultra Young+.

***Comments—Refer to the chapter entitled "How to Use—The Personal Usage Reference" in the Essential Oils Desk Reference under "AIDS" for specific oil blend and supplement recommendations.

Airborne Bacteria: *See also Antibacterial.*

Oils—[A]Cinnamon bark, [A]mountain savory, [A]oregano, [A]<u>Thieves</u>, [A]lemongrass[13], [A]geranium[13], [A]fir, [A]balsam fir, [A]<u>Purification</u>.

A—Diffuse into the air.

Air Pollution:

Oils—[A]<u>Purification</u>, [A]<u>Thieves</u>, [A]lemon (sterilize air), [A]<u>Abundance</u>, [A]<u>Christmas Spirit</u>, [A]cypress, [A]eucalyptus, [A]fir, [A]grapefruit, [A]<u>Immu-Power</u>, [A]lavender, [A]lime, [A]rosemary.

—**DISINFECTANTS**

Oils—[A]<u>Purification</u>, [A][F]lemon, [A]eucalyptus, [A]clove, [A]citronella, [A]grapefruit, [A]peppermint, [A]sage, [A]spruce, [A]wintergreen.

A—Diffuse into the air.

> *Diffusing essential oils in the home or workplace is one of the best ways to purify our environment. The antiviral, antibacterial, and antiseptic properties of the oils, along with the negative ions and oxygenating molecules that are released when essential oils are diffused, all help to reduce chemicals, bacteria, and metallics in the air.*
>
> *Cinnamon bark, mountain savory, oregano, and <u>Thieves</u> were all tested by Weber State University and were shown to kill 100% of the airborne bacteria present. This was all done by diffusing the oils into the atmosphere.*
>
> *(KID-Radio with Lance Richardson and D. Gary Young, March 5, 1996)*

Alcoholism: *See Addictions: ALCOHOL.*

Alertness:

Oils—[AT]Peppermint[14], [ITA]sage lavender[15], [TA]basil, [TA]<u>Citrus Fresh</u>, [TA]<u>Clarity</u>, [TA]lemon, [TA]rosemary. Apply to temples and to bottoms of feet.

A—Diffuse into the air. Inhale directly or applied to a tissue or a cotton wick.

T—Apply 1–2 drops to temples and to bottoms of feet.

I—Add 1–2 drops to an empty capsule, and swallow.

Alkaline: *See Acidosis, pH Balance.*

ALKALI-FORMING FOODS—Dark green and yellow vegetables, sprouted grains, legumes, seeds, nuts, essential fats (omega-3 and 6), and low sugar fruits like avocados and lemons.

Personal Care—Genesis Hand & Body Lotion balances pH on the skin.

> *Alkaline refers to a substance or solution that has a pH of 7.0 or above. The optimum pH for our blood and body tissues is about 7.2 (The use of saliva and urine test strips will show a much lower pH level due to the protein present in the solution. Saliva and urine tests from a healthy body should be about 6.6 to 6.8).*
>
> *The body heals best when it is slightly alkaline. To keep the blood and body tissue at an optimum pH, avoid acid-forming food. See Acidosis. Make sure your food intake is 80 percent alkaline, and drink plenty of water.*

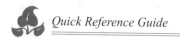
Supplements—AlkaLime, JuvaPower (contains many acid-binding foods), Life 5 (probiotic), Mineral Essence, MultiGreens (helps normalize blood pH levels), Omega Blue and OmegaGize[3] (loaded with omega-3 fatty acids of EPA and DHA), Power Meal (predigested protein).

Alkalosis: *See pH Balance.*

>> *Alkalosis refers to a condition where the blood and intestinal tract becomes excessively alkaline. Slight alkalinity is important for a healthy body, but excessive alkalinity can cause depression, fatigue, and sickness.*

Oils—[TI]Anise, [TI]Di-Gize, [TI]ginger, [TI]tarragon.

Supplements—Digest + Cleanse, Essentialzyme, Essentialzymes-4, Life 5 (probiotic), Mineral Essence, MultiGreens (helps normalize blood pH levels), Power Meal (predigested protein), Sulfurzyme.

T—Apply 1–2 drops to Vita Flex points on feet.

I—Add 1–2 drops to an empty capsule, and swallow.

Allergies:

>> *An allergy is a damaging immune system response to a substance that does not bother most other people. Allergy symptoms vary greatly, but common allergic responses include itching, swelling, runny nose, asthma, and sneezing.*

Oils—[T]Tea tree[16], [TF]lavender[17], [A]peppermint[18], [TF]patchouli, [T]elemi (rashes), [T]eucalyptus, [T]Harmony, [T]ledum, [T]Tea tree ericifolia, [T]Tea tree quinquenervia, [TA]melissa (skin and respiratory), [T]ImmuPower, [T]Raven, [T]RC, [T]Roman chamomile, [T]spikenard.

***Comments—According to the <u>Essential Oils Desk Reference</u>, "Rub three drops [Harmony] on sternum, breathing deeply" (<u>EDR</u>–June 2002).

Supplements—AlkaLime, ComforTone, ICP fiber beverage (beneficial when there is an allergy to psyllium), ImmuPro, Mineral Essence, Super C / Super C Chewable, Super Cal.

Recipe #1—Apply 1 drop of peppermint on the base of the neck two times a day. Tap the thymus (located just below the notch in the neck) with pointer and index fingers (energy fingers). Diffuse peppermint. For some individuals, the use of peppermint oil has eliminated the need for allergy shots!

Recipe #2—Apply 1 drop of <u>RC</u> and 1 drop of <u>Raven</u> on the base of the neck two times a day. Tap on thymus; massage chest and back with 5 drops <u>Raven</u>, 5 drops <u>RC</u>, and 2 tsp. V-6 Oil. Diffuse <u>RC</u> and <u>Raven</u>.

Recipe #3—For allergy rashes and skin sensitivity, D. Gary Young applies 3 lavender, 6 Roman chamomile, 2 myrrh, and 1 peppermint on location.

—**ANTIHISTAMINE**

    »» *An antihistamine is a substance that inhibits the effects of histamine. Histamine is a chemical released as a result of an allergic reaction, causing sneezing, itching, increased mucus, swelling, wheezing, cramps, and burning.*

    Oils—[TA]Tea tree[16], [TA]lavender[17], [TA]Roman chamomile.

—**COUGHING**

    Oils—[A]Purification.

—**HAY FEVER**

    »» *Hay fever, also known as allergic rhinitis, is an allergic reaction to airborne allergens: pollen, pet dander, dust mites, etc.*

    Oils—[AT]Lavender[17], [AT]Roman chamomile, [AT]Cajeput, [AT]eucalyptus, [AT]Juva Cleanse, [AT]rose.

—**PSYCHOLOGICAL ALLERGIES (IN THE MIND)**

    Recipe #4—Put <u>Harmony</u> on feet, neck, navel, or in your shoes for one to five days.

—**TO OILS**

Put one drop of the oil to which there is an allergy reaction on a cotton ball, and place it in the allergic person's shoe. Add a drop each day until

> *If you have a reaction to the oils, it is only a reaction to all of the chemicals you have been dumping into your body throughout the years. The oils are merely reacting with the toxins in the sub-dermal tissues and beginning their removal.* **Cleanse the body!**

the allergy to that particular oil is gone. Since allergies often indicate an electrical imbalance, try the following:

    A. Place a drop or two of <u>Harmony</u> in one hand; then rub the palms of both hands together in a clockwise motion.

    B. Place one hand over the thymus (heart chakra) and the other hand over the navel.

    C. Take three deep breaths and switch hands; then take three more deep breaths.

    Oils—[T]<u>Harmony</u> (helps open the energy meridians and balance the bioelectric field of the body).

T—Apply 1–2 drops to sinuses or to Vita Flex points.

A—Diffuse into the air. Inhale directly or applied to a tissue or a cotton wick.

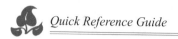
Alone (feeling): *See also Emotions.*

Oils—[AT]Acceptance, [AT]Valor.

A—Diffuse into the air. Inhale directly or applied to a tissue or a cotton wick.

T—Dilute, and use as massage oil. Apply to auricular emotional points.

Alopecia Areata: *(Inflammatory hair loss disease) See Hair: Loss.*

Aluminum Toxicity: *See also Alzheimer's Disease, Attention Deficit Disorder.*

Oils—[IT]Juva Cleanse.

I—Add 1–2 drops to an empty capsule, and swallow.

T—Dilute with V-6 Oil, and massage over spine.

> *Aluminum is one of the most abundant elements on Earth; therefore, we are constantly exposed to it. Some estimate that an average person consumes between three and ten milligrams of aluminum every day. Aluminum toxicity may contribute to the cause of colic, rickets, kidney and liver dysfunction, speech and memory problems, osteoporosis, and Alzheimer's disease.*

Alzheimer's Disease: *See also Brain, Memory, Pineal Gland, Pituitary Gland.*

>> *Alzheimer's is a progressive and fatal disease that attacks and kills brain cells, causing a loss of memory and a loss of other intellectual capacities. Alzheimer's is most commonly diagnosed in individuals over the age of 65. As the disease progresses, sufferers often experience mood swings, long-term memory loss, confusion, irritability, aggression, and a decreased ability to communicate.*

> *Autopsies have revealed that victims of **Alzheimer's disease** have four times the normal amount of aluminum in the nerve cells of their brain.*
>
> ***Prevention:*** *Use glass, iron, or stainless steel cookware. Avoid products containing aluminum, bentonite, or dihydroxyaluminum. Some of these products are aluminum cookware, foil, antacids, baking powders, buffered aspirin, most city water, antiperspirants, deodorants, beer, bleached flour, table salt, tobacco smoke, cream of tartar, Parmesan and grated cheeses, aluminum salts, douches, and canned goods.*

Oils—[I]coriander[19], [IT]lemon[20].

Supplements—**Omega Blue, OmegaGize[3],** Cleansing Trio (ComforTone, Essentialzyme, and ICP), Digest + Cleanse, JuvaTone, PD 80/20, Power Meal, Sulfurzyme, Master Formula.

***Comments**—The gingko biloba that is found in Power Meal has been shown to help improve memory loss, brain function, depression, cerebral and peripheral circulation, oxygenation, and blood flow.*

—**Blood-Brain Barrier**

>> *The blood-brain barrier is the body's filtering mechanism that allows necessary substances, such as blood, to freely enter the brain and spine, while preventing other substances, such as*

certain drugs, from entering. Studies have shown that sesquiterpenes can pass the blood-brain barrier.

Oils—Oils that are high in sesquiterpenes include cedarwood, vetiver, sandalwood[21], black pepper, patchouli, myrrh, ginger, German chamomile, spikenard, galbanum, and frankincense. Some essential oil blends containing some of these oils include: <u>3 Wise Men</u>, <u>Acceptance</u>, <u>Brain Power</u>, <u>Forgiveness</u>, <u>Gathering</u>, <u>Harmony</u>, <u>Inspiration</u>, <u>Into the Future</u>, <u>Transformation</u>, and <u>Trauma Life</u>. Apply to temples and to bottoms of feet; diffuse.

*****Comments**—*Oils that pass through the blood-brain barrier cannot carry unwanted substances with them.*

—**BRAIN FUNCTION**

Oils—^ASage[22], ^A<u>Clarity</u>.

Supplements—Omega Blue, OmegaGize[3].

—**EMOTIONS**

Oils—^A <u>Peace & Calming</u>, ^{AT}<u>3 Wise Men</u> (crown), ^{AT}<u>Acceptance</u>, ^Acypress.

A—Diffuse into the air. Inhale directly.

T—Dilute as recommended, and apply over brain stem on back of neck. Dilute with V-6 Oil, and use for massage.

Amino Acids:

Oils—^ALavender.

> *Amino acids have the ability to neutralize and to help eliminate free radicals in the body's system.*

A—Diffuse into the air. Inhale directly or applied to a tissue or a cotton wick.

Supplements—Pure Protein Complete (has a complete array of ultra-bioactive amino acids), NingXia Red (18 amino acids in whole food form), Cleansing Trio (Comfor-Tone, Essentialzyme, and ICP), FemiGen, JuvaTone, KidScents MightyVites, Master Formula, Mineral Essence, Power Meal, Thyromin.

Amnesia: *See Memory.*

Analgesic: *See Pain.*

Anemia:

>> *Anemia is a condition marked by a decreased number of red blood cells or by a deficiency of hemoglobin in the blood. The most common signs of anemia are fatigue, pallor, physical weakness,*

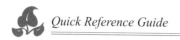

poor concentration, and shortness of breath on exertion. Anemia is most common in infants and in small children and is often caused by a deficiency of iron in the diet.

Oils—^T_FLemon, ^Tcarrot, ^T<u>ImmuPower</u>, ^T<u>Juva Cleanse</u>, ^Tlavender.

T—Apply to bottoms of feet and to stomach.

—Food

> Oils—Flavor water with a drop of **lemon**.
>
> Supplements—**Rehemogen tincture** (10 drops twice a day) and **JuvaTone** together help raise blood cell count.

Anesthesia: *See Pain:ANESTHESIA, Pain:ANALGESIC.*

Aneurysm: *See also Blood, Cardiovascular System.*

>> *An Aneurysm is a swelling or dilation of a blood vessel in the area of a weakened blood vessel wall.*

Oils—^{TA}Cypress (strengthens the capillary walls and increases circulation), ^{TA}<u>Aroma Life</u> (chelates plaque), ^{TA}helichrysum, ^{TA}frankincense, ^{TA}Idaho tansy.

T—Apply to temples, heart, and Vita Flex heart points.

A—Diffuse into the air. Inhale directly.

Blend #1—5 frankincense, 1 helichrysum, and 1 cypress. **Diffuse**.

Herbs—Cayenne pepper, garlic, hawthorn berry.

Personal Care—Cel-Lite Magic dilates blood vessels for better circulation.

Supplements—Cleansing Trio (ComforTone, Essentialzyme, and ICP), Sulfurzyme, Super C / Super C Chewable, Master Formula.

Anger: *See also Calming, Liver.*

Oils—^{AT}Lavender[23], ^{AT}ylang ylang[24], ^{TA}rose[25], ^{TA}melissa[26], ^T<u>Tranquil</u> (roll-on), orange, ^{AT}<u>Peace & Calming</u>, ^{AT}<u>Australian Blue</u>, ^{AT}bergamot, ^{AT}cedarwood, ^{AT}cypress, ^{AT}<u>Forgiveness</u>, ^{AT}frankincense, ^{AT}geranium, ^{AT}German chamomile, ^{AT}<u>Grounding</u>, ^{AT}<u>Joy</u>, ^{AT}<u>Harmony</u>, ^{AT}helichrysum, ^{AT}<u>Hope</u>, ^{AT}<u>Humility</u>, ^{AT}<u>Inspiration</u>, ^{AT}lemon, ^{AT}mandarin, ^{AT}marjoram, ^{AT}myrrh (soothes), ^{AT}myrtle, ^{AT}petitgrain, ^{AT}<u>Present Time</u>, ^{AT}<u>Release</u>, ^{AT}Roman chamomile, ^{AT}<u>Sacred Mountain</u>, ^{AT}sandalwood, ^{AT}<u>Surrender</u>, ^{AT}<u>Trauma Life</u>, ^{AT}<u>Valor</u>.

*****Comments**—Refer to the Emotional Release part of the Science and Application section of the <u>Reference Guide for Essential Oils</u>.

—CALMS ANGER

    Oils—^{AT}<u>Peace & Calming</u>, ^T<u>Tranquil</u> (roll-on), ^{AT}<u>Australian Blue</u>, ^{AT}<u>Inspiration</u>, spruce, ^{AT}<u>Trauma Life</u>.

—CLEANSING AFTER ARGUMENT AND PHYSICAL FIGHTING

    Oils—^{AT}Eucalyptus.

—CLEANSE THE LIVER

    Oils—(Anger is stored in the liver) ^{AT}<u>JuvaFlex</u>, ^{AT}_Igeranium (cleanses and detoxifies the liver), ^{AT}<u>GLF</u>, ^{AT}grapefruit (liver disorders).

—DISPELS ANGER

    Oils—^{AT}Ylang ylang[24], ^T<u>Tranquil</u> (roll-on).

—FOR COMMUNICATION WITHOUT ANGER

    Oils—^{AT}Roman chamomile.

—LESSENS ANGER

    Oils—^{AT}Myrrh.

—OVERCOME

    Oils—^{AT}_ICedarwood, ^{AT}bergamot, ^{AT}<u>Release</u>, ^{AT}Roman chamomile.

—RELEASES LOCKED UP ANGER AND FRUSTRATION

    Oils—^{AT}<u>Release</u> (together with <u>JuvaFlex</u>), ^{AT}<u>Surrender</u>, ^{AT}<u>Transformation</u>, ^{AT}<u>Valor</u>, ^{AT}Roman or German chamomile, ^{AT}<u>Sacred Mountain</u>, ^{AT}sandalwood.

    Supplements—JuvaTone, Thyromin, Super B.

    Blend #1—4 drops lavender, 3 geranium, 3 rosewood, 3 rosemary, 2 tangerine, 1 spearmint, 2 Idaho tansy, 1 German chamomile, and 1 oz. V-6 Oil. Apply to back of neck, wrist, and heart.

A—Diffuse into the air. Inhale directly or applied to a tissue or a cotton wick.

T—Dilute, and massage onto the skin. Apply to temples or auricular emotion points.

Angina: *See Cardiovascular System.*

Animals:

    Only 1–2 drops of oil is all that is necessary on animals as they respond much more quickly to the oils than do humans. V-6 Oil can be added to extend oil over larger areas and to heavily dilute the essential oil for use on smaller animals, especially cats.

    Oils—^{TA}<u>PuriClean</u>, ^{TA}<u>Infect Away</u>, ^{TA}<u>MendWell</u>, ^{IT}<u>ParaGize</u>, ^{AT}<u>RepelAroma</u>, ^{AT}<u>T-Away</u>

Personal Care—Animal Scents Pet Shampoo, Animal Scents Pet Ointment. Other alkaline shampoos without chemicals are good for animals.

Supplements—Ningxia Red to help support the liver and enhance energy and healing. BLM (added to their food; can help speed the healing of bones), Power Meal, and Sulfurzyme.

> *I have a large brown tabby cat that was limping bad, so I took him to the vet. The vet said he had a knee injury (he compared it to a football player's injured knee–"cruciate ligament rupture") and said it would need surgery. He wanted me to bring my cat back in a week to see his son (who is also a vet) to make arrangements for the surgery. Later, using V-6 as my carrier oil and combining it with a couple drops of lavender oil, I rubbed my cat from the bottom of the paw up to his hip area. The next day I could see an improvement, and by the time I took him back to the vet he was walking on his leg with only a slight limp. The vet said he would heal nicely on his own and there would be no need for surgery. Today he walks, runs, and is even now jumping with no problems.*
>
> *–Submitted by M. Rynicki*

—BLEEDING

> **Oils**— ᵀᴬPuriClean, ᵀᴬInfect Away, ᵀᴬMendWell, ᵀHelichrysum, ᵀgeranium.
>
> **T**—Dilute, and apply on location.

—BONES (PAIN)

> **Oils**—ᵀPanAway , ᵀwintergreen, ᵀlemongrass, ᵀspruce.
>
> **T**—Dilute, and apply on location.
>
> **Personal Care**—Ortho Ease or Ortho Sport Massage Oils.
>
> **Supplements**—BLM (added to their food; can help speed the healing of bones), Power Meal and Sulfurzyme.

—CALM

> **Oils**— ᴬᵀT-Away, ᴬᵀLavender, ᴬᵀPeace & Calming, ᵀTranquil (roll-on), ᴬᵀCitrus Fresh, ᴬᵀRoman chamomile (for horses, add to feed), ᴬᵀTrauma Life. Dilute well for cats.
>
> **A**—Diffuse into the air.
>
> **T**—Dilute, and apply on back.

—CANCER

> **–SKIN**
>
> > **Oils**—ᵀFrankincense, ᵀcumin.
> >
> > **T**—Dilute, and apply on location.

—CATS

> Valerie Worwood says that you can treat a cat like you would a child (see Babies). Dilute oils heavily with V-6 Oil. Avoid tea tree.

***Comments—*Cat physiology is so different from other animals and from humans that oils should be used with extreme caution on cats. In fact, tea tree (or tea tree oil) should never be used on a cat as death can result. Some cases exist where a blend of oils containing tea tree has killed cats.*

—COLDS AND COUGHS

Oils—ᵀEucalyptus, ᵀtea tree (not for cats).

T—Apply on fur or on stomach.

—COWS

Recipe #1—For scours, use 5 drops <u>Di-Gize</u> on stomach (can mix with V-6 Oil to cover a larger area); repeat 2 hours later.

—CUTS AND SORES

Oils— ᵀᴬ<u>PuriClean</u>, ᵀᴬ<u>Infect Away</u>, ᵀᴬ<u>MendWell</u>, ᵀ<u>Melrose</u> (not on cats).

T—Apply 1 drop on location. Work in with finger.

—DOGS

***Comments—There was a dog that walked with its head down and its tail between its legs. <u>Valor</u> was put on its feet and <u>3 Wise Men</u> and <u>Joy</u> on its crown. The next day its head was up, and it was happy.

–ANXIETY/NERVOUSNESS

Oils— ᴬᵀ<u>T-Away</u>, ᵀLavender, ᵀ<u>Peace & Calming</u>, ᵀ<u>Tranquil</u> (roll-on), ᵀvalerian, ᵀ<u>Valor</u>.

T—Rub 1–2 drops between hands, and apply to muzzle, between toes, on top of feet to smell when nose is down, and on edges of ears.

–ARTHRITIS

Oils—ᵀCopaiba.

Blend #1—A blend of rosemary, lavender, and ginger diluted with V-6 Oil.

Personal Care—Ortho Ease Massage Oil applied to arthritic areas.

> One Saturday in February, my husband woke me up by yelling from the living room for me to bring my oils and any oil books I had at hand to him immediately. Our dog, Buddy, (a mutt from the pound, age approx. 7+ years) was lying on the floor, and all of his muscles were completely seized up and tensed to the point where we couldn't move any part of his body. I had most of my oils in my large case and the Higley *Reference Guide* at my side. I put 4 or 5 drops of lavender oil in my husband's hand and he put that on Buddy's paws, ears, and all over his back and legs—anywhere he was tense that we could reach. We followed the lavender with Peace & Calming, Valor, and frankincense, applied the same way. Those four were the oils I was drawn to by instinct. We massaged him and continued to stroke and pet him during and after the application of oils, and after about 10 minutes he was able to get up and go to the door to go outside and run around. In between applying oils I looked up the info on animals as well as the info on seizures and strokes (we weren't sure what kind of episode he was having), just to make sure my instincts were near to on target (which they were). We had plans to travel about an hour out of town to visit with family, and we kept Buddy with us the whole day just to be sure he was ok. When I tell this story to other people they tell me about how their dog(s) had seizures and had to be put on steroids and eventually put down because of the seizures. I am very thankful for Young Living and the oils that allowed me to go the natural route for the care of our dog.
>
> *-Submitted by A. Cornn*
> *Machesney Park, Illinois*

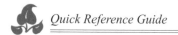

Supplements—Add **Sulfurzyme** (powder) or vitamin C to their food.

–BONE INJURY

Oils—ᵀWintergreen.

T—Apply 1 drop on location. Work in with finger.

Personal Care—Ortho Ease Massage Oil on injury.

Supplements—Add **Sulfurzyme** (powder) and BLM in food.

–CHEWING ON FURNITURE

Supplements—**Mineral Essence** (helps satisfy mineral deficiency).

–DIGESTION

Oils—ᴵᵀ**ParaGize**

Supplements— Essentialzymes-4, **Essentialzyme**.

–HEART PROBLEMS

Oils—ᵀPeppermint

T—Apply on paws.

Recipe #1—Myrtle, ravintsara, and Thieves on back using Raindrop Technique with warm wet pack.

> I went to visit my son in Ft. Lauderdale, FL . . . and was also happy to see his dog, Luna, who I've known for 7 years, since she was a puppy. I could tell she was in pain, as she was not as active as usual and was limping. My son, Jason, told me that she is part German Shepherd—a breed that is prone to hip dysplasia. It broke my heart to see her in such pain. Jason had been giving her various vitamins and other supplements for several months, without much success. I myself have had success with Sulfurzyme for an arthritic knee, and I asked if he would like to try that for Luna. We began to give her 1/4 tsp. twice a day with her meals. Within two days, we began to see a change. My son was amazed! As the two weeks passed while I was visiting, we saw a huge change. She was running like her old self, and you could sense that the pain was almost (if not totally) gone. Within a month, Jason told me that she was now even jumping up on furniture, which she was unable to do when we started with the Sulfurzyme. That was 18 months ago, and Luna is still taking Sulfurzyme . . . and still doing great!
> **–Submitted by Linda Griffith**
> **Dixon, New Mexico**

–LIMPING

Supplements—**Sulfurzyme** (powder with food).

–PAIN AND STRESS

***Comments**—Do Raindrop Technique. (*The video "Essential Tips for Happy, Healthy Pets" demonstrates this technique on a dog and a horse.*) This technique helps relieve stress on the back, shoulders, and legs and also raises immune function and protects against illness.

–SLEEP

Oils— ᴬᵀT-Away, ᵀLavender (on paws), ᵀPeace & Calming (on stomach).

T—Apply on indicated areas.

–STROKE

   Oils—^TBrain Power (on head), ^Tfrankincense (on brain stem area/back of neck), ^TValor (on each paw).

   T—Apply on indicated areas.

–TICKS AND BUG BITES

   Oils—^{AT}RepelAroma, ^{TA}PuriClean, ^{TA}Infect Away, ^{TA}MendWell

   Recipe #2—Apply 1 drop Purification directly on live tick. Can also be applied to untreated tick wound and worked in with finger.

–TRAVEL SICKNESS

   Oils—^TPeppermint.

   T—Dilute with V-6 Oil, and rub on stomach. Also helps calm stomachaches.

–TRAUMATIZED

   Oils— ^{AT}T-Away, ^ATrauma Life.

   A—Rub 1–2 drops between hands, and cup over nose and mouth for dog to inhale.

—EARACHE

   Blend #2—1 drop Melrose or a blend of 1 drop tea tree (tea tree), 1 drop lavender, and 1 drop Roman chamomile diluted in V-6 Oil. Put in ear, and rub around the ear.

—EAR INFECTIONS

   Oils—^TImmuPower, ^TPurification (helps ward off insects too).

   T—Dip cotton swab in oil, and apply to inside and front of ear.

—FLEAS

   Oils—^{AT}RepelAroma, ^TCitronella, ^TMelrose, ^TIdaho tansy, ^Teucalyptus, ^Tlemongrass, ^Tpine.

   T—Add 1–2 drops of oil to shampoo.

   Blend #3—Combine eucalyptus, orange, citronella, and cedarwood. Add blend to distilled water in a spray bottle, shake well, and mist over entire animal.

—HEMORRHAGING

   Oils— ^{TA}PuriClean, ^{TA}Infect Away, ^{TA}MendWell, ^TCistus (stops internal bleeding)

   I—Take 1-2 drops orally.

—**HORSES**

　–**ANXIETY/NERVOUSNESS**

　　　Oils— ^{AT}T-Away, ^TPeace &Calming.

　　　T—Rub 1–2 drops between hands, and apply to nose and on front of chest, knees, and tongue.

　–**FLIES**

　　　Oils—^{AT}RepelAroma, ^TIdaho tansy.

　　　T—Add 1–5 drops to 1 oz. water in a small spray bottle, and mist over animal to keep flies away.

> *I have a 21 year old gelding who was diagnosed with "kidney colic" back in January. He would be down one day, up the next, down the next, up for several days, down again, etc. He would show all the general signs of colic but was also wanting to urinate frequently, passing little or nothing. This went on for about four weeks, and the vet thought he probably was trying to pass kidney stones. Since it was happening so often, I was wanting something to give him for the pain instead of using Banamine so much. I had used marjoram, clary sage, and lavender successfully on an intestinal colic, so I tried them; but they just didn't work as well on the kidneys. So I tried JuvaFlex, and the results were dramatic! Four drops over each kidney, with or without a warm compress, would get him up and back to eating and drinking in 10–20 minutes. The pain-killing effects would last from 2–4 hours and seemed to be cumulative. After I had done this for two separate "episodes," the symptoms went away completely. I don't know if the stones dissolved or if he passed them, but he's been pain free for six months.*
>
> *–Submitted by Jan Early*
> *Tallahassee, Florida*

　–**HOOF ROT**

　　　▸▸ *Hoof Rot is a hoof infection commonly found in cattle, sheep, horses, and goats. Hoof Rot attacks the area between the two toes and begins to literally rot away the animal's hoof. This infection is identified by a swelling of the skin between the claws of the hoof and by a foul odor. If not treated, Hoof Rot can easily be spread to other animals.*

　　　Blend #4—Blend Roman chamomile, thyme, and melissa in V-6 Oil, and apply on location.

　–**INFECTION**

　　　Oils— ^{TA}PuriClean, ^{TA}Infect Away, ^{TA}MendWell, ^TMelrose, ^TThieves.

　　　T—Dilute, and apply on location.

　–**INJURIES**

　　　*****Comments**—Do Raindrop Technique. (*The video "Essential Tips for Happy, Healthy Pets" demonstrates this technique on a dog and a horse.*) When a frisky race horse took a fall and was unable to walk, application of the oils using the Raindrop Technique brought the horse out of it in a matter of days.

　–**LEG FRACTURES**

　　　Recipe #2—Apply ginger and V-6 Oil. Wrap the leg with a hot compress. Massage leg after the fracture is healed with a blend of rosemary and thyme with V-6 Oil. This may strengthen the ligaments and prevent calcification.

–MUSCLE TISSUE/LIGAMENTS

> **Blend #5**—Equal parts lemongrass and lavender on location; wrap to help regenerate torn muscle tissue.

–SADDLE SORES

> **Oils**—ᵀMelrose
>
> **T**—Apply on location.
>
> **Personal Care**—Rose Ointment.

–WOUNDS

> **Oils**— ᵀᴬPuriClean, ᵀᴬInfect Away, ᵀᴬMendWell, ᵀHelichrysum, ᵀMelrose
>
> **T**—Dilute as recommended, and apply on location.
>
> **Personal Care**—Rose Ointment.

> *One couple had a horse that got kicked in the flank, creating a large wound. The Vet treated the wound and gave her some medication. Unfortunately, the wound became reinfected and worsened to the point that the horse almost died. The Vet came over and reopened the wound and flushed out nearly two gallons of blood clots. However, the Vet had no medication with him and would not be able to deliver any more for a couple of days. So, the wife put 15 drops of Thieves in about ¼ cup of olive oil, and while the husband held open the horse's mouth, she poured the oil down its throat. This was repeated 3 or 4 times, and within just a few days the horse was fully recovered.*

—INFECTION

> **Oils**— ᵀᴬPuriClean, ᵀᴬInfect Away, ᵀᴬMendWell, ᵀDi-Gize, ᵀImmuPower.
>
> **T**—Apply on the paws.

—PARASITES

> **Oils**— ᴵᵀParaGize, ᴬᵀRepelAroma, ᵀLavender, ᵀDi-Gize, ᵀCedarwood.
>
> **T**—Rub on paws to release parasites.
>
> **Supplements**—ParaFree.

—SNAKE BITES (VENOMOUS WOUNDS)

> ***Comments**—Do Raindrop Technique. (The video "Essential Tips for Happy, Healthy Pets" demonstrates this technique on a dog and a horse.)

Anorexia: *See Eating Disorders: ANOREXIA.*

Anthrax: *See also Antibacterial.*

≫ *Anthrax is a serious, sometimes deadly, infectious disease caused by the bacteria Bacillus anthracis. The disease has three main forms: cutaneous anthrax (the bacteria enter through a cut or sore on the body), gastrointestinal anthrax (the bacteria enter by eating improperly cooked meat from an*

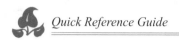

infected animal), and inhalation anthrax (caused by inhaling anthrax bacteria spores). Symptoms vary with each form.

Oils—[IAT]$_F$ Thyme.

I—Add 2–3 drops to an empty capsule with 2–3 drops V-6 Oil; swallow.

A—Diffuse into the air.

T—Dilute, and apply on location.

Antibacterial:

>> *The term antibacterial refers to anything that kills bacteria or that limits its ability to grow or to reproduce.*

Oils—Oils high in thymol (a phenol), such as [TA]$_F$thyme[27] and [T]mountain savory, tend to be highly antibacterial. Other effective antibacterial oils include [TA]Thieves (annihilates bacteria), [T]tea tree[28], [TA]$_F$cinnamon bark[29], [TA]lemongrass[30], [T]peppermint[31], [T]$_F$oregano[32], [T]lemon myrtle[33], [T]$_F$basil[34], [TA]$_F$clove[35], [T]$_F$spearmint[36], [TA]plectranthus oregano, [TA]Purification, [T]$_F$rosemary[37], [T]$_F$cypress[38], [TA]$_F$rosewood, [TA]rose[39], [T]pink pepper[40], [A]RC, [TA]micromeria, [A]geranium[41], [T]bergamot, [T]caraway[42], [T]cassia[43], [T]cedarwood, [TA]citronella[44], [TA]Christmas Spirit, [TA]Citrus Fresh, [T]clary sage, [T]copaiba, [T]cumin[45], [T]Egyptian Gold, [TA]eucalyptus, [T]Evergreen Essence, [TA]fir, [T]goldenrod[46], [T]grapefruit, [T]Idaho tansy, [TA]juniper, [T]lavender[47], [TA]lemon, [T]marjoram, [T]Tea tree ericifolia, [T]neroli, [T]ocotea, [T]palmarosa, [T]petitgrain, [TA]pine, [AT]ravintsara, [T]Roman chamomile, [T]Sacred Mountain, [T]tarragon, [T]valerian, [T]western red cedar.

*****Comments—**See the "Single Oil Property Chart" in the Appendix of this book for additional antibacterial oils and their strengths.

—AIRBORNE

    Oils—[A]Cinnamon bark, [A]mountain savory, [A]oregano, [A]Thieves, [A]lemongrass[30], [A]fir, [A]Purification.

—CLEANSING

    Oils—[TA]Purification.

—INFECTION

    Oils—[T]Nutmeg (fights).

—MRSA (*METHICILLIN RESISTANT STAPHYLOCOCCUS AUREUS*)

> *Dr. Terry Friedmann, MD, would often recommend the following* **Essential Oil Antibiotic Regimen:**
>
> *In a "00" capsule put 12 drops of Thieves, 6 drops of oregano, and 2 drops of frankincense. Ingest one capsule every 4 hours for 3 days, then every 8 hours for 4 days.*

> *Research at Weber State University has shown that out of 67 oils tested, 66 of them were powerful antibacterial agents. Oregano, cinnamon bark, mountain savory, ravintsara, and peppermint were all more powerful as antibacterial agents than penicillin or ampicillin. Thieves was shown to be 60 percent higher in activity against bacteria, germs, and antimicrobial action than either ampicillin or penicillin!*
>
> *(KID-Radio with Lance Richardson and D. Gary Young, March 5, 1996)*

Oils—[T]Tea tree[28], [T]oregano[32], [T]geranium[41], [T]lemon myrtle[33], [T]cinnamon bark, [T]peppermint[36], [T]spearmint[36], [T]lemongrass, [T]clove, [T]Eucalyptus radiata, [T]grapefruit, [T]lavender, [T]mountain savory, [T]orange, [T]patchouli, [T]thyme.

—PREVENTS GROWTH OF

Oils—[T]Melrose.

—STAPH INFECTION *See also MRSA above.*

>> *Staph infection is any of a number of infections caused by Staphylococcus bacteria. These condition can vary from mild skin infections to severe and life-threatening blood and respiratory illnesses.*

Recipe #1—Use oregano and hyssop; alternate with oregano and thyme to relieve the pain.

Oils—[T]Helichrysum, [T]lavender, [T]Purification.

***Comments—Black pepper or peppermint may make it more painful.

T—Apply on location, liver area, or bottoms of feet

A—Diffuse into the air.

I—Add oils to 00 capsule; swallow.

Antibiotic: *See Antibacterial.*

Anticancerous: *See Cancer: ANTICANCEROUS.*

Anticatarrhal: *See also Congestion.*

>> *Catarrh is an excessive buildup of mucus in the nose or throat.*

Oils—[TA]Eucalyptus[48], [TA]cypress, [TA]fir, [TA]helichrysum (discharges mucus), [TA]Thieves (dissolves excess mucus), [TA]RC, [TA]Raven, [TA]black pepper, [TA]cajeput, [TA]cistus, [TA]dill, [TA]elemi, [TA]frankincense, [TA]ginger, [TA]hyssop (opens respiratory system and discharges toxins and mucous), [TA]jasmine, [TA]myrrh, [TA]onycha (benzoin), [TA]ravintsara, [TA]rosemary.

T—Apply on lung area, feet, around nose, and Vita Flex lung points

A—Diffuse into the air.

***Comments—See the "Single Oil Property Chart" in the Appendix of this book for additional anticatarrhal oils and their strengths.

Anticoagulant: *See Blood: ANTICOAGULANT.*

Antidepressant: *See Depression: ANTIDEPRESSANT.*

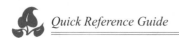

Antifungal:

>> *Antifungal refers to any substance that kills or inhibits the growth, metabolism, function, or reproductive ability of fungi. Fungi are a broad range of organisms such as yeast, mold, and mushrooms. While many fungi are safe and beneficial, some create mycotoxins, which are chemicals that can be toxic to plants and animals, including humans. Examples of fungi that can be detrimental to humans include black mold, candida, and ringworm.*

> *I had developed a **fungus** on my big toenails. The fungus was bad enough that the white, thick toenail was making shoes painful. I went to a podiatric doctor. The doctor removed the inside edge of the left big toenail down to the nail bed. He then prescribed some medicine that was $80 a tube to get rid of the rest. It continued to get worse and was spreading all over the nails and was headed for the rest of the nail beds. I decided to use Animal Scents Ointment on my toes 3 times a day. Now my nails are normal and the thickness is gone.*
>
> *–Submitted by K. Ernst*

Oils—**TA**_FTea tree[49], **TAr**Thieves, **TA**_Fcinnamon bark[50], **TA**_Fclove[51], **IAT**_Foregano[52], **T**_Fthyme[53], **T**pink pepper[54], **T**lemon myrtle[55], **T**_Fspearmint, **T**_Frosewood, **TA**lemon[56], **T**mountain savory[57], **T**carrot[58], **T**Melrose, **TA**micromeria, **T**Abundance, **T**cajeput, **T**cumin[59], **T**dorado azul[60], **T**Egyptian Gold, **T**fennel, **T**fleabane[61], **T**geranium, **T**German chamomile[62], **TA**ImmuPower, **TA**juniper, **T**lavender, **TA**lemongrass, **T**mandarin, **TA**Tea tree ericifolia, **T**palmarosa, **T**RC, **T**Raven, **T**Roman chamomile, **T**rosemary verbenon, **TA**sage.

***Comments—See the "Single Oil Property Chart" in the Appendix of this book for additional antifungal oils and their strengths.

Blend #1—2 myrrh and 2 lavender. Rub on location.

Supplements—**AlkaLime** (designed to combat yeast and fungus overgrowth and to preserve the body's proper pH balance), **Essentialzyme, Essentialzymes-4, Life 5** (probiotic), **Digest + Cleanse** (contains coconut oil with capric acid, which has been shown to inhibit the growth of three different strains of *Candida*), Balance Complete, MultiGreens, Super C / Super C Chewable, Thyromin.

***Comments—Refer to the chapter entitled "How to Use—The Personal Usage Reference" in the <u>Essential Oils Desk Reference</u> under "Fungal Infections" for some excellent blends and tips for combating systemic fungal infections.

—ATHLETE'S FOOT

>> *Athlete's foot (tinea pedis) is a fungal infection that develops on the skin of the feet. This infection causes itching, redness, and scaling of the skin, and in severe cases it can cause painful blistering or cracking of the skin.*

Oils—**T**_FTea tree[46], **T**cajeput, **T**cypress, **T**Eucalyptus citriodora, **T**geranium, **T**lavender, **T**myrrh, **T**thyme.

Blend #2—Combine 2 oz. of Genesis Hand & Body Lotion with 10 drops thyme, 10 drops lavender, and 10 drops tea tree. Rub on feet.

—CANDIDA *See also: Acidosis, Alkaline, Blood, Diet, Food, Thyroid, pH Balance*

>> *Candida refers to a genus of yeast that are normally found in the digestive tract and on the skin of humans. These yeast are typically symbiotically beneficial to humans. However, several species of Candida, most commonly Candida albicans, can cause infections such as vaginal candidiasis or thrush (oral candidiasis) that cause local-ized itching, soreness, and redness (see Vaginal:Candida for further application methods). In immune system–compromised individuals, these infection-causing species of Candida can spread further, leading to serious, life-threatening complications..*

> *Candida is caused by the fermentation of yeast and sugar, antibiot-ics, thyroid shut down, stress, chlorinated water, etc. When there is Candida there is usually hypoglycemia and hypothyroidism. It is usually a digestive problem; putrefaction in the system causes Candida overgrowth. Candida is a natural fungus in the stomach; we need some, but it becomes a problem when there is an overgrowth. Yeast is not the problem; the problem is the fermentation of the yeast. The fermentation exists because of a mineral imbalance and an enzyme imbalance in the digestive system. The enzymes needed for digestion are secreted by the thyroid, so it is necessary to support both the thyroid and the digestive system. Also, maintaining a slightly alkaline state in the blood and body can help to slow the overgrowth of Candida.*

Oils—[T]F Tea tree[49] (dilute with V-6 Oil for body massage), [T]Flavender[64], [IT]oregano[52], [TAI]Thieves, [T]clove[51], [T]dill[65], [T]lemon myrtle[55], [T]mountain savory[57] (dilute with V-6 Oil; can be hot), [AT]peppermint[66], [T]cinnamon bark, [T]Feucalyptus, [T]Frosewood, [T]Fspearmint, [T]Fspruce, [TA]micromeria, [T]bergamot, [T]Di-Gize, [T]EndoFlex, [T]Im-muPower, [T]laurel, [T]marjoram, [T]Tea tree quinquenervia, [T]Melrose (+ rosemary), [T]ocotea, [T]palmarosa (skin), [T]rose, [T]rosemary, [T]tarragon (prevents fermentation), [T]thyme.

Supplements—Life 5 (probiotic, prevents overgrowth), Allerzyme (aids the digestion of sugars, starches, fats, proteins), AlkaLime (combats yeast and fungus overgrowth and preserves the body's proper pH balance), Balance Complete, ComforTone, Detoxzyme (helps maintain and support a healthy intestinal environment), Digest + Cleanse, EndoGize, Essentialzyme (increases digestion), Essentialzymes-4, ICP, Mineral Essence, MultiGreens (balances the alkaline/acid condition in the body and provides chlorophyll and oxygen), ParaFree, Power Meal (vegetable protein), Super C / Super C Chewable, Thyromin (to help the thyroid).

–DIGESTIVE CANDIDA

Oils—[T]Di-Gize (hot compresses over abdomen; in a retention enema at night), [T]ImmuPower, [T]Thieves.

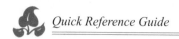

–Vaginal Candida

Oils—^T_FTea tree[49], ^{IT}oregano[52], ^T_Fthyme[53], ^T_Fmyrrh, ^T_Fbergamot, ^{T}geranium, ^{T}patchouli, ^{T}rosemary, ^{T}spikenard.

Blend #3—2 Tbs. garlic oil, 8 drops lavender, 8 drops tea tree, 1 ml (1 softgel) vitamin E oil. Apply to irritated area.

Supplements—AlkaLime, Life 5 (probiotic). Yogurt, mixed with a little bit of water and some probiotic powder, may be applied directly to relieve the pain associated with candida.

***Comments**—*Focus on the underlying problem of system-wide yeast infection. Also, refer to the chapter entitled "How to Use—The Personal Usage Reference" in the* Essential Oils Desk Reference *under "Fungal Infections" for some excellent blend recipes for dealing with vaginal yeast infections.*

—Fungal Infections

Oils—^{T}Tea tree, ^{T}Eucalyptus citriodora, ^{T}geranium, ^{T}patchouli.

—Mold

➤➤ *Mold are a type of microscopic multi-cellular fungi that grow together to form filaments. Mold is found throughout the world and can survive in extreme conditions. While most mold does not adversely affect humans, an over-abundance of mold spores can cause allergies or other problems within the respiratory system. Additionally, some types of mold produce toxins that can be harmful to humans or to animals.*

Oils—^{AT}Purification, ^{AT}Thieves.

–Toxic Black

Oils—^{TA}Thieves (on feet, as rectal implant, with Raindrop Technique on back).

***Comments**—One young boy had toxic black mold infection. His parents gave him a rectal implant of 8 ml myrrh, 2 ml oregano, 5 ml *Melaleuca alternifolia*, and 5 ml *Eucalyptus globulus*. They followed up with Thieves, as described above, to help clear him of the infection.

—Prevents Growth Of

Oils—^{T}Melrose (two times a day for seven days), ^{TA}Purification.

—Ringworm

➤➤ *Ringworm (or tinea) is a fungal infection of the skin that can cause itching, redness, and scaling of the skin. The name comes from the ring-shaped patches that often form on the skin.*

Oils—^{T}Tea tree, ^{T}Melrose, ^{T}peppermint, ^{T}thyme, ^{T}bergamot[67], ^{T}Purification, ^{T}geranium, ^{T}lavender, ^{T}myrrh, ^{T}RC, ^{T}Raven, ^{T}rosemary verbenon.

Blend #1—2 drops lavender, 2 drops tea tree, and 2 drops thyme, or ,

Blend #2—3 drops tea tree, 2 drops peppermint, and 3 drops spearmint. Apply 1–2 drops of blend (#s 1 or 2 above) or <u>Melrose</u> on ringworm 3 times a day for 10 days. Then mix 30 drops of tea tree (tea tree) or <u>Melrose</u> with 2 Tbs. V-6 Oil, and use daily until ringworm is gone.

> *My friend's eight-month-old little boy had a* **ringworm** *the size of a quarter on his head. After putting lavender neat on it several times, it started to go away; and after a few more times, it was gone altogether. Shortly after that he got a* **tick** *in his head, and by putting peppermint right on the back of the tick that nasty thing backed right out. I guess [the tick] could not breath. Whatever it was, it got the tick out without us trying to pull it out and perhaps getting only part of the critter out.*
>
> *–Submitted by V. Frierdich*

Personal Care—**Rose Ointment,** Ortho Ease, Ortho Sport Massage Oils.

—**Thrush** See *Candida*, above.

T—Dilute as recommended, and apply on location or on bottoms of feet. Apply on location with a hot compress.

A—Diffuse into the air.

I—Place oils in empty 00 capsule; swallow.

Antihemorrhaging: *See Blood: Hemorrhaging.*

Antihistamine: *See Allergies: Antihistamine.*

Anti-infectious: *See Infection: Anti-infectious. See also Antibacterial, Antifungal, Antiviral.*

Anti-inflammatory: *See also Antioxidant.*

Oils—Oils high in carvacrol (a phenol), like **Toregano, Tmountain savory,** and **Tthyme,** are very effective as anti-inflammatory agents. Other effective oils include **Tfrankincense**[68], **TAtea tree**[69], **TAeucalyptus**[70], **T<u>PanAway</u>, T<u>Deep Relief</u> (roll-on), T_Flavender**[71], **T_Fmyrrh**[72], **T_FGerman chamomile**[73], **Tcopaiba, T<u>Relieve It</u>, TIwintergreen**[74], **ATdorado azul, T_Fspruce, TAeucalyptus blue, ATeucalyptus citriodora**[75], **T_Ftarragon, T_Fpatchouli, T_FRoman chamomile, Tocotea**[76], **TIApeppermint**[77], **Tbalsam fir,** Tblack pepper, Tblue cypress, Tblue tansy, TIcalamus (gastrointestinal), Tcaraway, Tcitronella, Tclove, Tcoriander, Tcypress, Telemi (breast and uterus), Thelichrysum[78], Thinoki[79], TAhyssop (of the pulmonary), Tjuniper, Tlemongrass, Ttea tree, Tonycha (benzoin), Tpalo santo, T<u>Peace & Calming</u>, Tpetitgrain, Travintsara, Tspearmint, Tspikenard, Ttangerine.

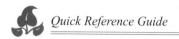
T—Apply on location and on brain stem area (*this helps stop pain and reduces the production of noradrenaline and cortisol).*

I—Place oils in empty 00 capsule, and swallow.

A—Diffuse into the air.

*****Comments**—One study showed that oils that inhibit the production of nitric oxide (NO) could greatly reduce the resulting inflammation and tissue damage. The six oils which showed the greatest percentage of NO inhibition were oregano, nutmeg, lemongrass, *Tea tree ericifolia*, dill, and peppermint.

*****Comments**—See the "Single Oil Property Chart" in the Appendix of this book for additional anti-inflammatory oils and their strengths.

Personal Care—Ortho Sport Massage Oil.

Supplements—According to Dr. David Hill, "Inflammation and oxidation go hand-in-hand." **NingXia Red** and **Longevity Capsules** on a daily basis are a powerful combination to help fight oxidation and inflammation system-wide. Also, **Omega Blue and OmegaGize³** contain clove oil and fish oil, which have been shown to work together to reduce inflammation by up to 30%! **Majestic Essence Chocolates** contain high levels of boswellic acids that have demonstrated an ability to alleviate inflammation[68]. **Slique Tea** contains flavinoids and polyphenols which have been studied for their abilities to fight inflammation.

*****Comments**—Refer to the chapter entitled "How to Use—The Personal Usage Reference" in the <u>Essential Oils Desk Reference</u> under "Inflammation" for some excellent blend recipes.

Antimicrobial: *See also Antibacterial, Antifungal, Antiviral.*

Oils—ᵀTea tree ericifolia (powerful), ᵀmelissa (shown in lab tests to be effective against Streptococcus haemolyticus), ᵀcinnamon bark, ᵀlemongrass, ᵀcypress, ᵀrosemary, ᵀthyme, ᵀ<u>Abundance</u>, ᵀhelichrysum, ᵀjasmine, ᵀlavender, ᵀmyrrh, ᵀpalmarosa, ᵀpine, ᵀrosewood, ᵀsage.

T—Apply on location

*****Comments**—See the "Single Oil Property Chart" in the Appendix of this book for additional antimicrobial oils and their strengths.

Antioxidant:

Oils—ᵀᴬClove[80], ᴵᵀᴬthyme[81], ᵀᴬrosemary[82], ᵀᴬpeppermint[83], ᵀᴬtea tree[84], ᵀᴬhelichrysum[85], ᵀᴬfir[86], ᵀᴬlemon[87],

> *Antioxidants create an unfriendly environment for free radicals. They can help prevent mutations, work as free radical scavengers, prevent fungus, prevent oxidation in the cells, and help to oxygenate the cells.*

Acinnamon bark, [T]Di-Gize, [TA]Exodus II, [TA]frankincense, [TA]goldenrod[88], [TA]hyssop, [TA]ImmuPower, [TA]JuvaFlex, [I]Longevity (take as a dietary supplement to promote longevity), [TA]Melrose, onycha (benzoin), [TA]oregano[89], [TA]PanAway, [TA]Purification, [TA]ravintsara, [TA]RC, [TA]Relieve It, [TA]Roman chamomile, [TA]Thieves.

T—Dilute as recommended, and apply on location or on Vita Flex points on feet.

A—Diffuse into the air. Inhale directly.

I—Place oils in empty 00 capsule; swallow.

Supplements—NingXia Red (tested at Brunswick Laboratories with S-ORAC score of 363 per oz. The next closest "functional drink" competitor was tested at 8.6), **Longevity Capsules** (contains clove oil, which has the highest known ORAC score, and thyme oil, which increases antioxidant levels in heart, liver, & kidneys and doubles antioxidant activity in the entire body), **Ningxia Wolfberries** (dried), Essentialzyme, Essentialzymes-4, JuvaTone, Majestic Essence Chocolates, Master Formula, Mineral Essence, MultiGreens, Super C / Super C Chewable, Super B, Master Formula, Wolfberry Crisp Bars (*Refer to the Wolfberry Crisp Bar in the Supplements section of the* Reference Guide for Essential Oils *for more information on the benefits of the Ningxia Wolfberry*).

Antiparasitic: *See Parasite: ANTIPARASITIC.*

Antirheumatic: *See also Arthritis: RHEUMATOID.*

▸▸ *Rheumatism is an older term used to describe many different painful conditions of the muscles, tendons, bones, and joints. Common rheumatic disorders include rheumatoid arthritis, osteoarthritis, lupus, tendinitis, and fibromyalgia.*

Oils—[T]Wintergreen, [T]eucalyptus, [T]juniper, [T]onycha (benzoin), [T]oregano, [T]rosemary, [T]thyme.

T—Dilute as necessary, and apply on location.

***Comments—See the "Single Oil Property Chart" in the Appendix of this book for additional antirheumatic oils and their strengths.

Antiseptic: *See also Antibacterial, Antifungal, Antiviral.*

▸▸ *An antiseptic is a substance applied on a surface that kills or inhibits the growth of disease-causing microorganisms.*

Oils—[T]Di-Gize (all oils in this blend are antiseptic), [T,F]pine (pulmonary, urinary, hepatic), [T,F]thyme, [T,F]oregano, [T,F]peppermint, [T,F]cedarwood, [T]Purification, [T]cinnamon bark, [T]tea tree, [T,F]fir, [T,F]sage, [T,F]sandalwood, [T,F]spearmint, [T,F]myrtle (skin), [T,F]nutmeg (intestinal), [T,F]patchouli, [T]bergamot, [T]citronella, [T]clove, [T]copaiba, [T]cumin, [T]elemi, [T]eucalyptus,

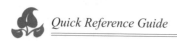

ᵀUnderline:Evergreen Essence, ᵀfennel, ᵀbalsam fir, ᵀfrankincense, ᵀlavender, ᵀlemon, ᵀmandarin, ᵀmarjoram, ᵀMelrose, ᵀmountain savory, ᵀmugwort, ᵀorange, ᵀonycha (benzoin), ᵀravintsara, ᵀRoman chamomile, ᵀrosemary cineol, ᵀrosemary verbenon, ᵀthyme linalol, ᵀwestern red cedar, ᵀylang ylang.

T—Apply on location.

***Comments**—Most oils can be used as antiseptics. See the "Single Oil Property Chart" in the Appendix of this book for additional antiseptic oils and their strengths.

Personal Care—Rose Ointment (apply over oils to increase antiseptic properties and to extend effectiveness).

Supplements—Super C / Super C Chewable.

Antisexual:

Oils—ᴬᵀ_FMarjoram (helps balance sexual desires).

A—Diffuse into the air. Inhale directly or applied to hands, tissue, or a cotton wick.

T—Dilute with V-6 Oil and massage into skin.

Antispasmodic:

>> *An antispasmodic is an agent that is used to reduce or prevent muscle spasms, cramps, and convulsions.*

Oils—ᵀᴵ_FBasil, ᵀᴵ_Fpeppermint[90], ᵀ_Flavender[91], ᵀ_FGerman chamomile, ᴵᵀ_FRoman chamomile (relaxes spastic muscles of the colon wall), ᵀᴵ_Frosemary, ᵀ_Fsage, ᵀ_Fmarjoram, ᵀmugwort[92], ᵀ_Fspruce, ᵀanise, ᵀcalamus, ᵀcitronella, ᵀcumin, ᵀᴵfennel, ᵀhelichrysum, ᵀmandarin, ᵀpetitgrain, ᵀRutaVaLa, ᵀspearmint, ᵀspikenard, ᵀᴵtarragon, ᵀvalerian, ᵀylang ylang.

***Comments**—See the "Single Oil Property Chart" in the Appendix of this book for additional antispasmodic oils.

T—Apply on location. Dilute, and massage on location.

I—Add 2–5 drops to an empty capsule with 2–5 drops V-6 Oil; swallow.

Antitumoral: *See Tumors: ANTITUMORAL. See also Cancer.*

Antiviral:

>> *Antiviral refers to a substance that is able to inhibit or stop the development, function, or replication of an infection-causing virus. A virus is a tiny microorganism that can only grow and replicate by living on a host cell. Viruses are responsible for causing numerous human infections and diseases.*

Oils—[TA]Melissa[93] oil has shown some of the strongest antiviral activity. Oils high in limonene (a monoterpene), like [TA]grapefruit, [TA]orange, [TA]tangerine, [TA]palo santo, [AT]eucalyptus blue, [TA]mandarin, and [TA]lemon, may be effective antiviral agents. Other effective antiviral oils include [TA]helichrysum[94], [TA_F]tea tree[95], [TA_F]clove[96], [AT]Thieves (diffuse with extra cinnamon bark to help fight viral conditions), [TA_F]cinnamon bark, [T]lemon myrtle[97], [TA]manuka[98], [TA]peppermint[99], [TA_F]ravintsara (viral infection), [TA_F]oregano, [TA_F]thyme, [TA_F]rosewood, [A]RC, [TA]myrrh (both internally and externally—reported 75% effective), [TA]Abundance, [TA]blue cypress (especially for HPV), [TA]bergamot[100], [TA]clary sage, [TA]cypress, [TA]Egyptian Gold, [TA]Eucalyptus radiata, [TA]galbanum, [TA]geranium, [TA]hinoki, [TA]hyssop, [TA]Idaho tansy, [TA]ImmuPower, [TA]juniper, [TA]lavender, [TA]Tea tree quinquenervia (viral and fungal infection), [TA]mountain savory, [TA]palmarosa, [TA]pine, [TA]sandalwood, [TA]tarragon.

***Comments—(Viruses often hibernate along the spine) **Do the Raindrop Technique!** Dr. J. C. Lapraz found that viruses cannot live in the presence of cinnamon oil. However, because of its high phenol content, it must be diluted before being applied to the skin. See the "Single Oil Property Chart" in the Appendix of this book for additional antiviral oils and their strengths.

> *When my friend contracted the West Nile virus from a mosquito bite last summer, her neck became stiff, and she had swelling in her ears and behind her ears at the base of her brain. She was in great pain and her ears felt "full" all of the time. We applied an oil blend from Young Living Oils called Thieves. We placed the oil at the base of her head and down both sides of her neck and jaw area. This gave her relief from the intense pain in her neck and reduced the swelling in her ears and head. She also drank a couple of drops of the Thieves oil blend in fluids several times a day. She continued doing this for at least a month while she fought this disease. We both agree this probably kept her from more serious complications due to the severity of the illness. We also believe it kept her out of the hospital.*
>
> *-Submitted by C. Ness*

Recipe #1—Massage ImmuPower and oregano along the spine.

Supplements—ImmuPro, Inner Defense, Thieves Lozenges, Life 5 (probiotic), ParaFree.

—**Airborne Viruses**

Recipe #2—ImmuPower on throat and chest, Thieves on feet. Diffuse.

—**Asthma** *See Asthma.*

—**Ebola Virus**

Oils—This virus cannot live in the presence of [TA]cinnamon bark or [TA]oregano.

—**Epstein–Barr Virus** *See Epstein–Barr.*

***Comments—Strengthen immune system, ensure proper thyroid function, and work on hypoglycemia. Use ImmuPower, Thieves.

Supplements—Inner Defense, ImmuPro, NingXia Red, Wolfberry Crisp Bars.

—**Respiratory**

Oils—[A]Eucalyptus radiata (diffuse with Thieves; add spruce to push lower in lungs).

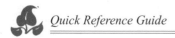

—SPINE

Blend #1—5 drops oregano and 5 drops thyme. Put on bottoms of the feet and up the spine using the Raindrop Technique.

—VIRAL DISEASE *SEE ALSO CHILDHOOD DISEASES*

>> *A viral disease is any of a large number of diseases caused by a virus. The list of viral diseases includes AIDS/HIV, chicken pox, adenovirus, Epstein-Barr virus, hepatitis, herpes, measles, meningitis, Ebola virus, and many others.*

Oils—[AT]Cinnamon bark.

Supplements—Inner Defense, ImmuPro, ParaFree, Super C/Super C Chewable, Master Formula,.

–INFECTION

Oils—[TA]Tea tree, [TA]oregano, [AT]ravintsara, [TA]thyme, [TA]cajeput.

Blend #2—Mix one drop each of lavender, orange, and spruce, and apply to chest. Then put 10 drops of frankincense in a cap full of Evening Peace Bath Gel; add to bath as a bubble bath, and soak.

T—Dilute as recommended, and apply on location or to the Vita Flex points on the bottoms of the feet. Apply along the spine.

A—Diffuse into the air. Inhale oil directly or applied to hands, tissue, or a cotton wick.

Anxiety: *See also Calming.*

>> *Anxiety is the body's way of preparing itself to deal with a threat or to deal with future stressful events. While this response is normal, and happens as part of the body's natural response to stress, this response can also happen at inappropriate times or too frequently, as in the case of anxiety disorders. Anxiety can include both physical and mental symptoms such as fear, nervousness, nausea, sweating, increased blood pressure and heart rate, feelings of apprehension or dread, difficulty concentrating, irritability, restlessness, panic attacks, and many others.*

Oils—[AT]Lavender[101], [AT]orange[102], [AT]lemon[103], [TA]Roman chamomile[104], [AT]valerian[105], [AT]melissa[106], [AT]copaiba[107], [AT]ylang ylang, [AT]angelica[108], [AT]basil, [AT]bergamot[109], [AT]cedarwood, [AT]clary sage[110], [AT]cypress[111], [AT]Evergreen Essence, [AT]frankincense[112], [AT]geranium, [AT]hinoki[113], [AT]hyssop, [AT]jasmine, [AT]juniper, [AT]lime, [AT]marjoram, [TA]onycha (combine with rose for massage), [AT]patchouli, [AT]pine, [AT]Release, [AT]rose, [AT]sandalwood, [AT]Surrender, [AT]tangerine, [AT]tsuga (grounding).

—PANIC

>> *Panic is a sudden overwhelming feeling of fear and anxiety that tends to dominate a person's thoughts, leading to wild, irrational, and unthinking behavior.*

Oils—^{AT}Lavender[101], ^{AT}Roman chamomile[104], ^{AT}ylang ylang, ^{AT}<u>Awaken</u>, ^{AT}bergamot, ^{AT}fir, ^{AT}balsam fir, ^{AT}frankincense, ^{AT}<u>Gathering</u>, ^{AT}<u>Harmony</u>, ^{AT}marjoram, ^{AT}myrrh, ^{AT}rosemary, ^{AT}sandalwood, ^{AT}spruce, ^{AT}thyme[114], ^{AT}<u>Valor</u>, ^{AT}<u>White Angelica</u>, ^{AT}wintergreen.

A—Diffuse into the air. Inhale directly or applied to hands, tissue, or a cotton wick.

T—Dilute in V-6 Oil, and massage[115] into the skin. Dilute as recommended, and apply to back of neck, temples, or Vita Flex points on the feet. Apply to auricular emotional points. Add 1–2 drops to 1/4 cup bath salts or to 1 Tbs. bath and shower gel, and dissolve in warm bathwater.

Apathy: *See also Depression.*

Oils—^A<u>Joy</u>, ^A<u>Transformation</u>, ^A<u>Valor</u>, ^Aorange, ^Apeppermint, ^Afrankincense, ^Ageranium, ^A<u>Harmony</u>, ^A<u>Highest Potential</u>, ^A<u>Hope</u>, ^Ajasmine, ^Amarjoram, ^Arose, ^Arosemary, ^Arosewood, ^Asandalwood, ^A<u>3 Wise Men</u>, ^Athyme, ^A<u>White Angelica</u>, ^Aylang ylang.

A—Diffuse into the air. Inhale directly or applied to hands, tissue, or a cotton wick.

Aphrodisiac:

Oils—^{AT}_FSandalwood, ^{AT}rose, ^AIdaho blue spruce, ^{AT}<u>Sensation</u>, ^{AT}<u>Lady Sclareol</u>, ^Acinnamon bark, ^{AT}clary sage, ^{AT}ginger, ^{AT}jasmine, ^{AT}patchouli, ^{AT}neroli, ^{AT}ylang ylang.

Personal Care—Sensation Bath & Shower Gel, Sensation Massage Oil, Sensation Hand & Body Lotion.

> *An Aphrodisiac is a substance used to stimulate feelings of love or sexual desire. Many books of aromatherapy tout the **aphrodisiac** qualities of a number of oils. Perhaps an aphrodisiac to one individual may not be to another. The most important factor is to find an oil that brings balance to the mind and body. A balanced individual is more likely to extend love.*

A—Diffuse into the air. Wear as perfume or cologne.

T—Dilute in 1 Tbs. V-6 Oil, and use as massage oil. Add 1–2 drops to 1/4 cup bath salts or to 1 Tbs. bath and shower gel, and dissolve in warm bathwater.

Apnea:

Oils—^T<u>Valor</u> (on feet), ^A<u>Clarity</u> (diffuse), ^{AT}<u>Brain Power</u>, ^A<u>Raven</u>, ^A<u>RC</u>.

A—Inhale directly or applied to hands, tissue, or a cotton wick. Diffuse into the air.

> *Apnea is the cessation of breathing. During sleep, periods of apnea can occur for a few seconds before breathing resumes. May be due to irregular heartbeats, high blood pressure, obesity, or damage to the area of the brain responsible for controlling respiration.*

T—Dilute as recommended, and apply to Vita Flex points on the feet.

A=Aromatic   **T**=Topical   **I**=Internal

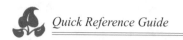
Supplements—MultiGreens, Super B, Thyromin.

Recipe #1—Try 3 MultiGreens twice per day, 1 Super B three times per day with meals, and 1 Thyromin before bed.

Appetite:

—Loss Of

Oils—^{TA}_FBergamot, ^{TA}_Fnutmeg, ^{TA}ginger, ^{TA}spearmint, ^{TA}calamus, ^{TA}cardamom, ^{TA}hyssop, ^{TA}lemon, ^{TA}myrrh, ^{TA}orange.

T—Apply to stomach, bottoms of feet.

A—Diffuse into the air.

Supplements—ComforTone, Essentialzyme, Essentialzymes-4.

—Suppressant

Oils—^{TA}Slique Essence·

Supplements—Slique Bar, Slique Tea, **Slique Gum, Slique Slim Caps.**

Argumentative: *See also Calming.*

Oils—^{AT}Peace & Calming, ^{AT}ylang ylang, ^{AT}orange, ^TTranquil (roll-on), ^{AT}Roman chamomile, ^{AT}Harmony, ^{AT}Acceptance, ^{AT}cedarwood, ^{AT}eucalyptus, ^{AT}frankincense, ^{AT}Hope, ^{AT}Humility, ^{AT}jasmine, ^{AT}Joy, ^{AT}thyme, ^{AT}Transformation, ^{AT}Trauma Life, ^{AT}Valor.

A—Inhale directly. Diffuse into the air.

T—Apply to auricular emotional points. Dilute in V-6 Oil, and apply as massage oil.

Arms-flabby:

Oils—^TCypress, ^Tfennel, ^Tjuniper, ^Tlavender.

T—Dilute in V-6 Oil, and massage into skin on location.

Arterial Vasodilator: *See Arteries: Vasodilator. See also Cardiovascular System.*

Arteries:

Oils—^{TA}Aroma Life, ^{TA}lavender, ^{TA}Melrose.

T—Dilute as recommended, and apply to carotid arteries in neck, over heart, and to reflex points on the feet.

A—Diffuse into the air. Inhale directly or applied to hands.

Personal Care—Cel-Lite Magic and drink Chamomile Tea.

Supplements—Cleansing Trio (ComforTone, Essentialzyme, and ICP).

—Arteriosclerosis *See Also Cardiovascular System: Atherosclerosis.*

>> *Arteriosclerosis is a hardening, stiffening, or loss of elasticity of the arteries that occurs over time as the artery walls experience excessive pressure.*

Oils—[T]Aroma Life, [T][F]cedarwood, [T]lemon[116] (increase white and red blood cells), [T]ginger, [T]juniper, [T]rosemary, [T]thyme, [T]wintergreen.

T—Apply to heart and Vita Flex points on feet.

–**Blood Clots** *See also Blood: Clots*

Oils—[I]Ocotea[117], [I]fennel[118], [I][T]clove[119], [T]balsam fir, [T]grapefruit, [T]helichrysum.

Supplements—In addition to vitamins E and C, all supplements containing essential oils should help increase the supply of oxygen in the blood stream. Rehemogen (tincture) together with JuvaTone may help build blood and hemoglobin platelets (raise cell count); also Master Formula.

I—Place 2–3 drops in an empty capsule with V-6 Oil; swallow.

T—Dilute as recommended, and apply to carotid arteries, over heart, and to Vita Flex points on the feet.

—Strengthens

Oils—[T][A]Aroma Life

T—Dilute as recommended, and apply to carotid arteries in neck, over heart, and to reflex points on the feet.

A—Diffuse into the air. Inhale directly or applied to hands.

—Vasodilator

>> *A vasodilator is a substance that causes a blood vessel to dilate (increase in diameter) through the relaxation of the endometrial cells lining the vessel walls. This gives the blood more room to flow and lowers the blood pressure.*

Oils—[T]Eucalyptus[120], [T]rosemary[120], [T][F]marjoram, [T]Aroma Life.

T—Apply to carotid arteries in neck, over heart, and to Vita Flex points on feet.

Arteriosclerosis: *See Arteries: Arteriosclerosis.*

Arthritis: *See also Acidosis.*

>> *Arthritis is the painful swelling, inflammation, and stiffness of the joints*

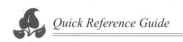

Oils—[TA]Frankincense[121], [TA]rosemary[122], [TA]marjoram[122], [TA]Aroma Siez, [TA]PanAway, [TA]spruce, [TA]cypress, [TA]wintergreen (drains toxins that cause pain), [TA]fir (has cortisone-like action), [TA]Aroma Life, [TA]basil, [TA]cedarwood, [TA]clove[123], [TA]eucalyptus[122], [TA]balsam fir, [TA]ginger, [TA]Harmony (with Valor), [TA]helichrysum, [TA]hyssop, [TA]Idaho tansy, [TA]Immu-Power, [TA]lavender, [TA]Melrose, [TA]nutmeg, [TA]onycha (benzoin), [TA]palo santo, [TA]Peace & Calming, [TA]peppermint, [TA]pine, [TA]Purification, [TA]Roman chamomile, [TA]sage lavender, [TA]Valor, [TA]white fir (has cortisone-like action).

T—Apply oils on location.

A—Diffuse into the air.

Blend #1—Combine 1 oz. Ortho Ease with 25 drops wintergreen, 12 drops cypress, 9 drops Roman chamomile, and 3 drops juniper. Massage on location.

Blend #2—Combine Ortho Ease with wintergreen alone, and apply on location.

Blend #3—Wintergreen with PanAway.

Personal Care—**Ortho Ease Massage Oil,** Prenolone/Prenolone+, Progessence/Progessence Plus, Regenolone.

Supplements—AlkaLime, BLM, Mineral Essence, MultiGreens, NingXia Red, Power Meal (contains wolfberry), Slique Tea, Sulfurzyme (contains wolfberry), Super C / Super C Chewable, Super Cal, Thyromin (improves thyroid function and energy levels).

—Arthritic Pain

   Oils—[T]Wintergreen, [T]PanAway, [T]palo santo, [T]spruce, [T]ginger.

   T—Dilute as recommended, and apply on location.

—Osteoarthritis

   ›› *Osteoarthritis is a degenerative arthritis where the cartilage that provides lubrication between the bones in a joint begins to break down, becoming rough and uneven. This causes the bones in the joint to wear and create rough deposits that can become extremely painful.*

   > *Detoxify with cypress, fennel, and lemon. Massage affected joints with rosemary, chamomile, juniper and lavender (Alternative Medicine—A Definitive Guide, p. 537).*

   Oils—[T]Wintergreen, [T]eucalyptus, [T]basil, [T]lavender, [T]lemon, [T]marjoram, [T]thyme.

   T—Dilute as recommended, and apply on location.

—Rheumatoid Arthritis

   ›› *Rheumatoid arthritis: Rheumatoid arthritis is arthritis caused by inflammation within the joint, causing pain and possibly causing the joint to degenerate.*

Oils—[TA]F Spruce, [TA]F marjoram, [TA]F cypress, [TA]PanAway, [TA]F pine, [TA]F nutmeg, [TA]F lemon, [TA]F bergamot, [TA]F ginger, [TA]angelica, [TA]black pepper, [TA]cajeput, [TA]cinnamon bark[124], [TA]coriander[125], [TA]eucalyptus, [TA]fennel, [TA]fir, [TA]balsam fir, [TA]galbanum, [TA]geranium, [TA]hyssop, [TA]juniper, [TA]lavender, [TA]oregano (chronic), [TA]palo santo, [TA]Peace & Calming, [TA]peppermint, [TA]Roman chamomile, [TA]rosemary, [TA]tarragon, [TA]thyme, [TA]wintergreen.

T—Dilute as recommended, and apply on location.

A—Diffuse into the air.

Personal Care—Prenolone/Prenolone+, Progessence/Progessence Plus, Regenolone.

Blend #4—Combine 2 oz. of Ortho Ease with 7 drops wintergreen, 6 drops ginger, 19 drops eucalyptus, 6 drops juniper, 8 drops marjoram, and 3 drops peppermint. Rub on location.

Ashamed: *See Emotions.*

Oils—[AT]Acceptance, [AT]Forgiveness, [AT]Valor.

A—Diffuse into the air. Inhale directly or applied to hands, tissue, or a cotton wick.

T—Apply to auricular emotional points.

Assault: *See Emotions.*

Oils—[AT]Trauma Life.

A—Diffuse into the air. Inhale directly or applied to hands, tissue, or a cotton wick.

T—Apply to auricular emotional points.

Assimilating Food:

Supplements—Enzyme products: **Allerzyme** (aids the digestion of sugars, starches, fats, and proteins), **Detoxzyme** (helps maintain and support a healthy intestinal environment), **Essentialzyme**, **Essentialzymes-4**. Also Balance Complete, Digest + Cleanse, Power Meal (predigested protein), and Super B.

Asthma: *See Respiratory System.*

 ›› *Asthma is a disease that causes the lung's airways to narrow, making it difficult to breathe. Episodes (or attacks) of asthma can be triggered by any number of things, including smoke, pollution, dust mites, and other allergens. Asthma causes reoccurring periods of tightness in the chest, coughing, shortness of breath, and wheezing.*

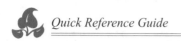

Oils—$^{AT}_F$Eucalyptus[126], $^{AT}_F$peppermint[127], $^{AT}_F$frankincense (on crown), ^{AT}<u>Raven</u> (diffuse), ^{AT}<u>RC</u> (some people use <u>RC</u> or <u>Raven</u> instead of inhaler), ^{AT}dorado azul, ^{AT}rose[128], $^{AT}_F$thyme[126], $^{AT}_F$lemon, $^{AT}_F$marjoram, $^{AT}_F$oregano, $^{AT}_F$pine, $^{AT}_F$sage, ^{AT}cajeput, ^{AT}calamus, ^{AT}clary sage, ^{AT}cypress, ^{AT}<u>Evergreen Essence</u>, ^{AT}fir, ^{AT}hyssop, ^{AT}laurel[129], ^{AT}lavender[130], ^{AT}mugwort[131], ^{AT}myrrh, ^{AT}myrtle, ^{AT}onycha (benzoin), ^{AT}ravintsara, ^{AT}rose, ^{AT}rosemary, ^{AT}sage, ^{AT}tsuga (opens respiratory tract).

A—Avoid steam inhalation. Drop on pillow or diffuse into the air.

T—Dilute as necessary, and apply over lungs and throat.

Recipe #1—May insert <u>RC</u> and <u>Raven</u> with 1 tsp. V-6 Oil in rectum. **Or** <u>Raven</u> rectally with <u>RC</u> on chest and back. Reverse each night. **Or** *Eucalyptus radiata* and frankincense in rectum.

***Comments—Plastic nasal inhalers work very well for breathing in the essential oils. Nasal inhaler blanks (empty inhalers) are available from Abundant Health to fill with your choice of oil. Just saturate an absorbent wick with the essential oil or blend, insert wick into the inhaler blank, and plug the end. Then just unscrew the cap, place inhaler next to or inside each nostril, and breathe deeply. Replace the cap to prevent evaporation. These are great to take on airplanes instead of the messy, bulky oil bottles.

Blend #1—Combine 10 drops cedarwood, 10 drops eucalyptus, 2 drops Roman chamomile, and 2 oz. water. Put on hanky and inhale. Can also be used to gargle.

Blend #2—Combine 10 drops <u>Raven</u>, 5 drops hyssop, and 2 tsp. V-6 Oil. Massage on spine and chest.

Personal Care—Prenolone/Prenolone+.

Supplements—Super C / Super C Chewable, Thyromin.

***Comments—Do a colon and liver cleanse with either the Master Cleanser (see Cleansing) or with the Cleansing Trio supplements (ComforTone, ICP, Essentialzyme) and JuvaTone.

—Attack

    Oils—^{A}<u>RC</u> or ^{A}<u>Raven</u>.

    A—Just smelling from the bottle has stopped attacks.

    Recipe #1—<u>3 Wise Men</u> on crown, <u>Raven</u> on throat, <u>RC</u> on lungs, <u>Thieves</u> on feet, <u>ImmuPower</u> on spine. May insert <u>RC</u> and <u>Raven</u> with V-6 Oil in rectum, **or** <u>Raven</u> rectally with <u>RC</u> on chest and back; reverse each night.

    Recipe #2—Inhale or diffuse bergamot, eucalyptus, hyssop, lavender, or marjoram. Try frankincense for calming. (*Alternative Medicine—The Definitive Guide*, p. 824).

Recipe #3—Apply frankincense to the crown, <u>RC</u> on the throat and chest, and <u>Raven</u>
on the back. Then inhale the aroma of the oils from your hands.

Astringent:

>> *An astringent is a substance that controls bleeding by causing the body's tissues and vessels to*
contract.

Oils—^TLemon, ^Tonycha (benzoin).

T—Dilute as necessary, and apply on location.

Athletes Foot: *See Antifungal: ATHLETE'S FOOT.*

Attention Deficit Disorder: *See ADD. See also Hyperactivity.*

Aura:

Oils—^{AT}<u>White Angelica</u>, ^{AT}<u>Awaken</u>, ^{AT}<u>Joy</u>, ^{AT}<u>Sacred Mountain</u>.

—INCREASE AURA AROUND BODY

Oils—^{AT}<u>White Angelica</u> (use with <u>Awaken</u> and <u>Sacred Mountain</u>).

—PROTECTION OF

Oils—^{AT}<u>White Angelica</u>.

—STRENGTHEN

Oils—^{AT}<u>White Angelica</u>.

A—Wear as perfume or cologne. Diffuse into the air.

T—Dilute as necessary, and apply on chakras.

Autism:

>> *Autism is a developmental disorder that impairs the normal development of communication,*
sociality, and human interaction.

Oils—^{AT}<u>Reconnect</u>, ^{AT}<u>InTouch</u>

—REDUCE ANXIETY/FEAR

Blend #1—Bergamot, geranium, and clary sage. Layer or dilute in V-6 Oil for a
massage.

—STIMULATE THE SENSES

Blend #2—Basil, lemon, peppermint, and rosemary. Layer or dilute in V-6 Oil for a
massage.

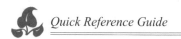

*****Comments**—Make sure that no negativity exists when the oils are used because the autistic child will make those associations when the oil is used again.

Autoimmune System: *For Autoimmune diseases, see AIDS, Grave's Disease, Hashimoto's Disease, and Lupus.*

Oils—^{AT}<u>ImmuPower</u>, ^{AT}cistus.

A—Diffuse into the air.

T—Dilute as necessary, and apply to Vita Flex points on the feet. Dilute with V-6 Oil, and massage into skin.

Supplements—ImmuPro, MultiGreens, NingXia Red, Sulfurzyme (helps mitigate effects of autoimmune diseases), Thyromin, Master Formula,.

Avoidance: *See Emotions.*

Oils—^{AT}<u>Magnify Your Purpose</u>, ^{AT}<u>Motivation</u>.

A—Diffuse into the air. Inhale directly or applied to hands, tissue, or a cotton wick.

T—Apply to auricular emotional points.

Awake: *See also Alertness.*

—Jet Lag *See Jet Lag*

—Staying Awake While Driving

Blend #1—<u>Clarity</u> and <u>En-R-Gee</u> together. Diffuse.

Awaken the Mind, Spirit:

Oils—^{AT}<u>Awaken</u>, ^{AT}myrrh.

A—Diffuse into the air. Inhale directly or applied to hands, tissue, or a cotton wick.

T—Apply to auricular emotional points.

Awaken the Past:

Oils—^{AT}Cypress.

A—Diffuse into the air. Inhale directly or applied to hands, tissue, or a cotton wick.

T—Apply to auricular emotional points.

Awareness:

—Greater Awareness of Ones Potential

Oils—^{AT}<u>Believe</u>, ^{AT}<u>Into the Future</u>, ^{AT}<u>Oola Friends</u>, ^{AT}<u>White Angelica</u>.

A
B

—INCREASES SENSORY SYSTEM

Oils—^{AT}Awaken, ^{AT}wintergreen.

—OPENS SENSORY SYSTEM

Oils—^{AT}Peppermint, ^{AT}wintergreen.

—REVITALIZES

Oils—^{AT}Lemongrass.

—SELF

Oils—^{AT}Acceptance, ^{AT}Believe, ^{AT}Oola Friends.

—SPIRITUAL

Oils—^{AT}Believe, ^{AT}frankincense, ^{AT}Inspiration (enhances spiritual mood), ^{AT}myrrh, ^{AT}3 Wise Men.

A—Diffuse into the air. Inhale directly or applied to hands, tissue, or a cotton wick.

T—Apply to auricular emotional points. Dilute with V-6 Oil, and massage into skin.

Babies: *See Children/Infants.*

Back:

Oils—^TPanAway, ^TEndoFlex, ^TRelieve It, ^TValor (aligns; a chiropractor in a bottle), ^Tthyme (for virus in spine), ^Twintergreen, ^Tbasil, ^Tblack pepper, ^Tcypress, ^Teucalyptus, ^Tgeranium, ^Tginger, ^Tjuniper, ^Tlavender, ^Toregano, ^Tpeppermint, ^TRoman chamomile, ^Trosemary, ^Tsage, ^Ttangerine.

Supplements—BLM, EndoGize.

—CALCIFIED (SPINE)

    ›› *Calcification occurs when calcium builds up in tissue and causes the tissue to harden. As people age, calcification can cause the ligaments of the spine to thicken and harden, making the spinal canal narrow, creating pressure on the spinal nerve.*

    Oils—^TPanAway, ^Trosemary, ^Tgeranium.

> *I was about 8½ hours into a 10 hour round trip drive and my back started to seize up. I have an old muscle injury, and I knew I was in trouble. I had my oils on the seat next to me and grabbed my PanAway at a stoplight and poured it in my hand. I was in a hurry. I had planned on putting on about 5 drops, but the oil was warm, and I think I ended up with about 20 in my hand. Rather than waste it, I put it all on my lower back and sat back in my seat. Within a few minutes my spine did a complete correction starting at the base and going up to the back of my head. I felt each click as it ran up my spine. Needless to say, my back no longer hurt, and I had no stiffness when I finally got out of the car!*
>   **-Submitted by Andrea Safford**
>   **Warrenton, Virginia (July 2004)**

Personal Care—Ortho Ease Massage Oil (combine with <u>PanAway</u> on spine).

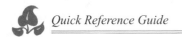

Supplements—Super C / Super C Chewable.

—Deteriorating Discs

>> *Deteriorating disc disease occurs as people age and their spinal discs begin to deteriorate. As deterioration progresses, movement becomes restricted and pain in the neck and back increases. Although most commonly associated with aging, disc deterioration can be caused by back injuries as well.*

Recipe #1—Do raindrop therapy with just the application of the oils, none of the working along the spine.

Personal Care—Ortho Ease Massage Oil.

Supplements—BLM, Super C / Super C Chewable.

—Herniated Discs

>> *A herniated disc is caused when one of the discs of the spine is damaged and either bulges or breaks open. When the herniated disc presses on a nerve, it causes pain in the buttock, thigh, and calf. Herniated discs can be caused by spinal injuries or by the wear and tear that come with age as the discs begin to dry out.*

Oils—ᵀ<u>Valor</u> (3 drops on location may help relieve pressure) ᵀ<u>PanAway</u>, ᵀ<u>Relieve It</u>, (massage up disc area three times to help with pain), ᵀcypress (strengthens blood capillary walls, improves circulation, powerful anti-inflammatory), ᵀblack pepper, ᵀpeppermint.

Recipe #2—Do raindrop therapy with just the application of the oils, none of the working along the spine.

Blend #1—Lemongrass with Idaho tansy; then marjoram with balsam fir or frankincense to help repair the damage.

Personal Care—Ortho Ease Massage Oil.

Supplements—BLM, Super C / Super C Chewable.

—Low Back Pains

Oils—ᵀ<u>Deep Relief</u> (roll-on), ᵀsandalwood.

Recipe #3—Rub <u>Valor</u> on top and bottoms of feet, <u>Di-Gize</u> on colon, and Ortho Ease up the back. Massage cypress up the disc area three times. Cypress strengthens blood capillary walls, improves circulation, and is a powerful anti-inflammatory. Use helichrysum to increase circulation, decongest, and reduce inflammation and pain. Use peppermint to stimulate the nerves (may need to dilute with Ortho Ease). Layer basil, <u>Aroma Siez</u>, <u>Relieve It</u>, and spruce.

Supplements—BLM

—MUSCULAR FATIGUE

Oils—^TMarjoram, ^Trosemary, ^Tclary sage, ^Tlavender.

—PAIN

Oils—^T<u>Deep Relief</u> (roll-on), ^T<u>Valor</u>, ^T<u>PanAway</u>.

Personal Care—^TOrtho Sport Massage Oil.

Blend #2—5 to 10 drops each of rosemary, marjoram, and sage **or**

Blend #3—5 to 10 drops each of lavender, eucalyptus, and ginger **or**

Blend #4—5 to 10 drops each of peppermint, rosemary, and basil.

Recipe #4—Apply <u>PanAway</u> and <u>Valor</u> on the shoulders. If the individual being worked on is lying on their stomach, the person applying the oils to the shoulders should cross their arms so the electrical frequency is not broken (right to right etc.). Apply the following oils **up** the spine, one at a time, using a probe on each vertebra if possible; stroke with fingers, feathering gently in 4" strokes three times for each oil: Peppermint (excites the back), cypress (anti-inflammatory), <u>Aroma Siez</u>, <u>Relieve It</u>, and spruce. Follow the procedure with a hot compress. The blends above have also been used with success. Follow the same stroking procedure, and dilute the blends with a little V-6 Oil for a massage.

Supplements—BLM.

—SCOLIOSIS

  ▸▸ *Scoliosis is an abnormal sideways curvature of the spine. Scoliosis can cause back pain and uneven shoulders or hips. Severe cases of scoliosis can be disabling.*

Recipe #5—May be caused by a virus. **Do the Raindrop Technique!**

***COMMENT—The videos listed in the Bibliography are highly recommended for a professional visual presentation of the Raindrop Technique.

Blend #5—8 drops basil, 12 drops wintergreen, 5 drops cypress, 10 drops marjoram, and 2 drops peppermint.

–CORRECT

Oils—Do the following (a variation of the Raindrop Technique) every 7 to 10 days for a minimum of 8 times to help get rid of **scoliosis**:

1. Rub <u>Valor</u> on feet.

2. Apply oregano and thyme using the Raindrop Technique up the spine.

3. Apply **blend #5** (shown above) along the spine. Push or pull in the direction that the spine needs to be strengthened. Knead fingers

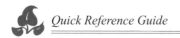

clockwise three times. Then work two fingers up the spine with the other hand on top of the hand that is doing the kneading (do this three times).

4. Apply <u>Aroma Siez</u> and marjoram on the muscles on each side of the spine. Apply warm wet towel to back, and have individual lay on their back.

5. Work the Vita Flex areas down the leg to the feet with basil, wintergreen, cypress, and peppermint in V-6 Oil.

6. Work the spine Vita Flex areas on the feet; then give feet a mild pull.

7. Put one hand under the chin and the other hand at the back of the neck. Have the person receiving the massage breathe in and out as you gently rock and pull the neck in time with their breathing.

8. Take towel off. If the back gets too hot during massage, apply V-6 Oil.

9. Measure the spine to see how much it has changed.

—STIFFNESS

    Oils—^TMarjoram, ^T<u>Valor</u>.

    ***Comments—Do the Raindrop Technique.

    Personal Care—Ortho Sport Massage Oil.

—VIRUSES ALONG SPINE *See Also Antiviral*

    Recipe #6—Layer *Eucalyptus radiata*, <u>ImmuPower</u>, oregano, and Ortho Ease on spine. Viruses tend to hibernate along the spine.

T—Dilute as necessary, and apply along the spine, on affected muscles, or on reflex points on the feet. Do the Raindrop Technique. Dilute in V-6 Oil, and massage into muscles on the back or along the spine. Apply as a hot compress over the affected area.

Bacteria: *See Antibacterial.*

Balance:

    Oils—^{TA}<u>Valor</u>, ^{TA}frankincense (balances electrical field), ^{TA}vetiver (is shown to have a balancing effect on the whole body when applied to the brain stem), ^{TA}Oola Balance, ^{TA}<u>Acceptance</u>, ^{AT}AromaEase, ^{TA}<u>Aroma Siez</u>, ^{TA}<u>Awaken</u>, ^{AT}AromaEase, ^{TA}cedarwood, ^{TA}<u>Harmony</u>, ^{TA}<u>Mister</u>, ^{TA}palo santo, ^{TA}Roman chamomile, ^{TA}ylang ylang.

—BALANCE MALE/FEMALE ENERGIES

    Oils—^{TA}<u>Acceptance</u>, ^{TA}ylang ylang.

—CHAKRAS

Oils—[TA]Harmony, [TA]Valor.

—EMOTIONAL

Oils—[TA]Envision.

—ELECTRICAL ENERGIES

Oils—[TA]Valor, [TA]frankincense, [TA]Harmony.

—FEELING OF

Oils—[TA]Envision, [TA]spruce.

—HARMONIC BALANCE TO ENERGY CENTER

Oils—[TA]Acceptance, [TA]Harmony.

Supplements— Master Formula.

T—Dilute as necessary, and apply on location. To balance energies, start by applying 3–6 drops Valor on the bottom of each foot. Some may be applied to the neck and shoulders if desired. When working on someone else, place the palms of the hands on the bottom of each foot (left hand to left foot and right hand to right foot), and hold for 5 to 15 minutes. If working on yourself, perform the Cook's Hookup by lifting the right foot and placing the right ankle on top of the left knee in cross-legged fashion. Next place the left hand on the right ankle, and cup the front of the ankle with the fingers. Then cross the right hand over the left; and with the right hand, grasp the heel of the right foot (with thumb around the back and fingers cupping the bottom of the heel). Hold this for 5 to 15 minutes. The balancing of the electrical energies can be felt by either a pulse in the hands and feet or by a warming sensation.

A—Inhale directly or applied to the hands. Diffuse into the air.

Baldness: *See Hair: BALDNESS, LOSS.*

Bath:

Oils—While tub is filling, add oils to the water (oils will be drawn to your skin quickly from the top of the water, so use gentle oils like lavender, Roman chamomile, rosewood, sage, ylang ylang, etc). For the most benefit, add 5–10 drops of your favorite essential oil to 1/2 ounce Bath and Shower Gel Base. You can also add 3–5 drops to 1/4–1/2 cup bath or Epsom salts or Dead Sea Bath Salts before dissolving in warm bathwater.

Personal Care—Evening Peace, Relaxation, and Sensation Bath and Shower Gels, Dead Sea Bath Salts, as well as Lavender Rosewood, Sacred Mountain, and Peppermint Cedarwood Moisturizing, and Dead Sea Mud Soaps are all wonderfully soothing in

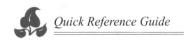

the evening. Morning Start Bath and Shower Gel as well as Lemon Sandalwood and Thieves Cleansing Soaps are all terrific ways to jump-start your day.

Bed Wetting: *See Bladder: Bed Wetting and Incontinence.*

Belching:

Oils—**ᵀ**<u>Di-Gize</u>.

T—Apply to stomach and on Vita Flex points.

Bereavement (Mourning):

Oils—**ᴬᵀ**Basil, **ᴬᵀ**cypress.

A—Diffuse into the air. Inhale directly or applied to hands, tissue, or a cotton wick.

T—Apply to auricular emotional points.

Betrayed (Feeling): *See also Emotions.*

Oils—**ᴬᵀ**<u>Acceptance</u>, **ᴬᵀ** <u>Forgiveness</u>, **ᴬᵀ**<u>Transformation</u>, **ᴬᵀ**<u>Valor</u>.

A—Diffuse into the air. Inhale directly or applied to hands, tissue, or a cotton wick.

T—Apply to auricular emotional points.

Birthing: *See Pregnancy.*

Bites: *See also Insect.*

Oils—**ᵀ**Basil, **ᵀ**cinnamon bark, **ᵀ**lavender, **ᵀ**lemon, **ᵀ**sage, **ᵀ**thyme (all have antitoxic and antivenomous properties). Can also try fresh **ᵀ**garlic oil.

—Allergic

Oils—**ᵀ**<u>Purification</u>.

—Bees and Hornets

Recipe #1—Remove the stinger; apply a cold compress of Roman chamomile to area for several hours or for as long as possible. Then apply 1 drop of Roman chamomile three times a day for two days. Idaho tansy may also work.

—Gnats and Midges

Recipe #2—Lavender; or 3 drops thyme in 1 tsp. cider vinegar or lemon juice. Apply to bites to stop irritation.

—Insect

Oils—**ᵀ**Cajeput, **ᵀ**patchouli.

— Mosquito

> Oils—^THelichrysum, ^Tlavender.

— Snake

> Oils—^TBasil, ^Tpatchouli.

— Spiders, Brown Recluse, Bee Stings, Ants, Fire Ants

> Oils—^TBasil (neutralizes), ^T<u>Purification</u>, ^Tthyme, ^Tcinnamon bark, ^Tlavender, ^Tlemon, ^Tlemongrass, ^Tpeppermint.

> **Recipe #3**—(For Spiders) 3 drops lavender and 2 drops Roman chamomile in 1 tsp. alcohol. Mix well in clockwise motion, and apply to area three times a day.

— Ticks

> **Recipe #4**—After getting the tick out, apply 1 drop lavender every 5 minutes for 30 minutes.

> **How to remove:**
>
> * Do not apply mineral oil, Vaseline, or anything else to remove the tick, as this may cause it to inject the spirochetes into the wound.
> * Be sure to remove the entire tick. Get as close to the mouth as possible, and firmly tug on the tick until it releases its grip. Don't twist. If available, use a magnifying glass to make sure that you have removed the entire tick.
> * Save the tick in a jar, and label it with the date, where you were bitten on your body, and the location or address where you were bitten for proper identification by your doctor, especially if you develop any symptoms.
> * Do not handle the tick.
> * Wash hands immediately.
> * Check the site of the bite occasionally to see if any rash develops. If it does, seek medical advice promptly.

— Wasps (are alkaline)

> **Recipe #5**—1 drop basil, 2 drops Roman chamomile, 2 drops lavender, and 1 tsp. cider vinegar. Mix in clockwise motion; put on area three times a day.

Bitterness: *See also Emotions.*

Oils—^{AT}<u>Acceptance</u>, ^{AT}<u>Forgiveness</u>, ^{AT}Roman chamomile, ^{AT}<u>Valor</u>.

A—Diffuse into the air. Inhale directly or applied to hands, tissue, or a cotton wick.

T—Apply to auricular emotional points.

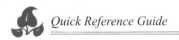

Bladder:

▸▸ *The urinary bladder is a hollow organ that collects urine before it is disposed of by urination. The bladder sits on the pelvic floor.*

Oils—ᵀEndoFlex

T—Apply over kidneys as a hot compress.

—**BED WETTING AND INCONTINENCE**

> **Recipe #1**—Before bed, rub cypress mixed with V-6 Oil on abdomen.

—**INFECTION/CYSTITIS**

▸▸ *Cystitis is a bladder infection characterized by urinary burning, urgency, and increased frequency. Other possible symptoms include blood in the urine, pelvic discomfort, and a low-grade fever.*

Oils—ᴵᵀ_FLemongrass, ᴵᵀThieves, ᵀ_FGerman chamomile, ᵀ_Fspearmint, ᵀ_Fthyme, ᵀbasil, ᵀbergamot, ᵀcajeput, ᵀcedarwood, ᵀcinnamon bark, ᵀclove, ᵀeucalyptus, ᵀfennel, ᵀfrankincense, ᵀhyssop, ᵀInspiration, ᵀjuniper, ᵀlavender, ᵀmarjoram, ᵀonycha (benzoin), ᵀoregano, ᵀpine, ᵀsage, ᵀsandalwood (for 1st stages of bladder infection), ᵀrosewood.

T—Massage or bathe with one of these oils.

I—Add 1 drop lemongrass or 1 drop Thieves to 8 oz. juice or water; drink three times a day.

Supplements—NingXia Red (½ cup followed by a full cup of water has brought relief within 10 minutes when taken at the first sign of discomfort).

***Comments**—One individual who had a bladder infection took 1 oz. NingXia Red (followed by 6–8 oz. water) every four hours. They were over the infection in two days.

—**HANGING DOWN**

> **Recipe #3**—Valor on feet; 3 drops ravintsara and 1 drop lavender on calves (bladder should pull up).

Blame: *See Emotions.*

Oils—ᴬᵀAcceptance, ᴬᵀForgiveness, ᴬᵀValor.

A—Diffuse into the air. Inhale directly or applied to hands, tissue, or a cotton wick.

T—Apply to auricular emotional points.

B

Blister: *(on lips from sun)*

> Oils—ᵀLavender

> **T**—Apply as often as needed. (It should take fever out and return lip to normal.)

Bloating: *See Digestive System: BLOATING.*

Blocked (Emotionally): *See Emotions.*

Blood:

⯈ *Blood is the fluid inside the body that transports oxygen and nutrients to the cells and carries waste away from the cells. It also transports cells involved in the immune and inflammatory response, hormones and other chemical messengers that regulate the body's functions, and platelets that help facilitate the blood clotting necessary to repair damaged blood vessels. Blood is primarily composed of plasma (water with dissolved nutrients, minerals, and carbon dioxide) that carries red blood cells (the most numerous type of cells in blood, responsible for transporting oxygen), white blood cells (cells involved in the immune system and immune response), and platelet cells. Blood is circulated in the body by the pumping action of the heart propelling blood through various blood vessels. Proper and healthy circulation and function of blood throughout the body is critical for health, and even for the sustaining of life.*

BLOOD TYPES—Different blood types have different dominating glands.

> **Type A:** more prone to be alkaline pH balanced. Natural vegetarians. A type A child living in the home of a type O parent is affected by parents' programing or conditioning or visa versa. They have problems with their thyroids, may have a tendency to gain weight, and need exercise.

> **Type AB:** may want to be a vegetarian on some days but not on others. Can go either way, like A or O types. They may be affected by either the A or O parent. AB types haven't decided whether to be an A or B type. They may even need more protein than O types.

> **Type B:** down the middle, more balanced. Takes them about 3 years to convert to being a vegetarian.

> **Type O:** more prone to acidic condition in blood. AlkaLime is an acid-neutralizing mineral formulation and may help preserve the body's proper pH balance. Big eaters may need to take more supplements because they are not assimilating the nutrients. If they are not assimilating their food, they eat and get full quick and one hour later they are hungry again. They get more gas because they lack enzyme secretion. They may need **Essentialzyme** for the enzymes, and **Digest + Cleanse** to improve digestion and assimilation of nutrients. They eat more, digest less, but

don't gain weight. May take 8 years to totally convert to vegetarian diet. Need more protein; **Pure Protein Complete, Vitagreen** and **Power Meal** are mainstays for O types as they are high protein and high energy formulas; nuts and seeds are good too. Nutrients in purest form reduces the need to eat. They have a harder time structuring their diet and they get cold because of poor circulation. If an O type is slender, has high energy, is compulsive in behavior, and/or is a hard worker, they may need as many as 16 MultiGreens and 10 Master Formulas per day.

—ANTICOAGULANT

>> *An Anticoagulant is a substance that keeps blood from clotting.*

Oils—^{TI}Clove[132], ^{IT}fennel[133], ^{TA}_Fhelichrysum, ^{TA}angelica, ^{TA}cassia, ^{TA}lavender, ^{TA}tangerine, ^{TA}tarragon.

T—Apply on location or on bottoms of feet.

I—Place 1–3 drops of oil in an empty capsule, and ingest up to 3 times per day.

A—Diffuse into the air. Apply oils to hands, and inhale oils from hands cupped over the nose. Inhale oil applied to a tissue or a cotton wick.

—BLOOD PRESSURE

–HIGH (HYPERTENSION)

Oils—^{AT}_FYlang ylang[134] (arterial; put in hand, rub palms together, cup over nose, and breathe deeply for 5 minutes and/or put on feet), <u>Aroma Life</u>, ^{TA}_Fmarjoram[135] (regulates), ^{TA}eucalyptus[135], ^{TA}_Flavender, ^{TA}_Fspearmint, ^{TA}clary sage, ^{TA}clove, ^{TA}balsam fir (lowers), ^{TA}goldenrod, ^{TA}lemon, ^{TA}nutmeg, ^{TA}wintergreen.

> ### *OILS TO AVOID IF HYPERTENSIVE*
>
> **Single oils:** *Hyssop, rosemary, sage, thyme, and possibly peppermint.*
>
> **This list is a compilation of the safety data contained in aromatherapy books written by the following authors:*
> *Ann Berwick, Julia Lawless, Shirley & Len Price, Jeanne Rose, Robert Tisserand, and Tony Balacs.*

T—Place oils on heart points on left arm, hand, foot, and over heart.

A—Can also smell from palms of hands, diffuse, or place a few drops on a cotton ball and put in a vent. *See Comments under Asthma for a discussion on using plastic nasal inhalers.*

*****Comments**—Refer to the chapter entitled "How to Use—The Personal Usage Reference" in the <u>Essential Oils Desk Reference</u> under "Blood Pressure, High" for specific product recommendations.

Recipe #1—3 ylang ylang and 3 marjoram in bathwater. Bathe in the evening twice a week.

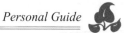

B

Blend #1—5 geranium, 8 lemongrass, 3 lavender, and 1 oz. V-6 Oil. Rub over heart and heart Vita Flex points on left foot and hand.

Blend #2—10 ylang ylang, 5 marjoram, 5 cypress, and 1 oz. V-6 Oil. Rub over heart and on heart Vita Flex points on left foot and hand.

–LOW

Oils—**AT**_FRosemary[136], **AT**<u>Aroma Life</u>, **AT**hyssop (raises), **AT**pine, **AT**ylang ylang.

T—Place oils on heart points on left arm, hand, foot, and over heart.

A—Can also smell from palms of hands, diffuse, or place a few drops on a cotton ball and put in a vent. *See Comments under Asthma for a discussion on using plastic nasal inhalers*.

—BLOOD PROTEIN

Supplements—MultiGreens.

—BLEEDING (STOPS)

Oils—**T**Helichrysum, **T**<u>Aroma Life</u>, **T**geranium (will increase bleeding first to eliminate toxins and then stop it), **T**cistus, **T**onycha (benzoin), **T**rose. Can also use **T**cayenne pepper tincture.

T—Dilute as necessary, and apply on location.

*****Comments**—Some have found that taking 14 capsules of helichrysum internally over a 24 hour period, right before surgery, can help prep the blood so that bleeding is reduced. Can also topically apply helichrysum to the surgical location before surgery.

—BROKEN BLOOD VESSELS

Oils—**T**Helichrysum, **T**grapefruit.

T—Dilute as necessary, and apply on location.

*****Comments**—One woman had some blood vessels break in her brain, which effected her short-term memory, concentration, focus, and emotions. She used the oils of <u>Clarity</u>, basil, rosemary, peppermint, and cardamom. Not only did her blood vessels heal, but her concentration, awareness, focus, and self-esteem increased.

—BUILD

Recipe #1—Rehemogen (tincture) together with JuvaTone and <u>Juva Cleanse</u> may help build blood and hemoglobin platelets (raise cell count).

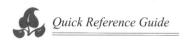
—CHOLESTEROL

>> *Cholesterol is a soft, waxy substance found in the bloodstream and in all of the body's cells. The body requires some cholesterol to function properly, but high levels of cholesterol narrow and block the arteries and increase the risk of heart disease.*

Oils—[TI]Helichrysum (regulates), [IT]dill[137].

T—Dilute as necessary, and apply on heart Vita Flex points on the feet.

I—Add 3–5 drops essential oil to 3–5 drops V-6 Oil in an empty capsule; swallow.

—CLEANSING

Oils—[T][F]Helichrysum, [T]Juva Cleanse, [T]Roman chamomile.

T—Dilute as necessary, and apply to bottoms of feet.

Supplements—MultiGreens, Rehemogen Tincture (purifier).

—CLOTS

>> *Blood Clots occur as a natural bodily defense to repair damaged blood vessels and to keep the body from losing excessive amounts of blood. However, clotting can become dangerous if an internal blood clot breaks lose in the circulatory system and blocks the flow of blood to vital organs.*

Oils—[TI]Clove[138], [IT]fennel[133], [TA][F]helichrysum, [TA]balsam fir (reduces pressure), [TA]grapefruit.

T—Apply on location or on bottoms of feet.

I—Place 1–3 drops of oil in an empty capsule; ingest up to 3 times per day.

A—Diffuse into the air. Apply oils to hands, and inhale oils from hands cupped over the nose. Inhale oil applied to a tissue or a cotton wick.

Recipe #2—Balsam fir, helichrysum, and cistus together (both topically and internally 3–4 times per day) help to dissolve blood clots.

—HEMORRHAGING *See also Female Specific Conditions: HEMORRHAGING.*

Oils—[T]Helichrysum, [T]cistus, [T]rose. Can also use [T]cayenne pepper.

T—Dilute as necessary, and apply on location or on bottoms of feet.

—LOW BLOOD SUGAR *See also Hypoglycemia*

>> *When the level of glucose in the blood drops below its normal level, this is called "low blood sugar" or "hypoglycemia." Since glucose is such an important source of energy for the body, low blood sugar can result in light-headedness, hunger, shakiness, anxiety, weakness, confusion, nervousness, difficulty speaking, and anxiety.*

Oils—[T][T]<u>Thieves</u> (balances blood sugar), [T]cinnamon bark, [T]clove, [T]thyme.

T—Dilute as necessary, and apply on location or on bottoms of feet.

I—Place 1–3 drops of oil in an empty capsule; ingest.

Supplements—AlkaLime, Mineral Essence, MultiGreens (balances blood sugar).

B

—STICKY

Oils—[IT]Clove[138], [IT]thyme (inhibits blood platelet aggregation)

I—Place 1–3 drops of oil in an empty capsule; ingest.

T—Dilute as necessary, and apply on location or on bottoms of feet.

Supplements—Longevity Capsules (contains both clove and thyme oils)

—STIMULATES

Oils—[IT]Peppermint[139], [IT][F]lemon (helps with the formation of red and white blood cells).

I—Place 1–3 drops of oil in an empty capsule; ingest.

T—Dilute as necessary, and apply on location or on bottoms of feet.

—VASODILATOR

›› *A vasodilator is a substance that causes a blood vessel to dilate (increase in diameter) through the relaxation of the endometrial cells lining the vessel walls. This gives the blood more room to flow and lowers the blood pressure.*

Oils—[T]Eucalyptus[120], [T]rosemary[120], [T][F]marjoram, [T]<u>Aroma Life</u>, [T]lemongrass.

T—Apply to carotid arteries in neck, over heart, and to Vita Flex points on feet.

—VESSELS *SEE ALSO ARTERIES, CARDIOVASCULAR SYSTEM, CAPILLARIES, VEINS*

Oils—[T]<u>Aroma Life</u>, [T]cypress (strengthens the capillary walls and increases circulation), [T]lemongrass (vasodilator).

T—Dilute as necessary, and apply on location or on bottoms of feet.

Supplements—Cel-Lite Magic dilates blood vessels for better circulation.

Body Systems: *See Bones, Cardiovascular System, Digestive System, Emotions, Hormonal System, Immune System, Muscles, Nervous System, Respiratory System, Skin.*

—BALANCE

Oils—[AT]<u>Valor</u>, [AT]<u>Harmony</u>, [AT]<u>Joy</u>, [AT]lavender, [AT]spruce.

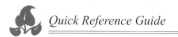

—CONTROL

    Oils—^{AT}Cedarwood.

—ODORS

    Oils—^{AT}<u>Purification</u> (obnoxious odors), ^{AT}sage.

—STRENGTHEN VITAL CENTERS

    Oils—^{AT}Oregano.

—SUPPORT

    Oils—^{AT}Fir, ^{AT}ledum, ^{AT}<u>Valor</u>.

    A—Inhale directly or applied to cupped hands.

    T—Dilute as necessary, and apply to Vita-Flex points on feet or to auricular points. Dilute with V-6 Oil, and use as massage oil.

Boils:

>> *A boil is a skin infection that forms in a hair follicle or oil gland. The boil starts as a red, tender lump that after a few days forms a white or yellow point in the center as it fills with pus. Boils commonly occur on the face, neck, armpits, buttock, and shoulders and can be very painful.*

    Oils—^TTea tree[140], ^T<u>Melrose</u>, ^T<u>Purification</u>, ^Tbergamot, ^Tclary sage, ^Tfrankincense,^Tgalbanum, ^T<u>Gentle Baby</u>, ^Tlavender, ^Tlemon, ^Tlemongrass, ^T<u>Raven</u>, ^Travintsara, ^T<u>RC</u>, ^TRoman chamomile.

    Personal Care—Rose Ointment.

    *****Comments**—One individual put lemon oil on a sore that looked like a boil. The next day it turned black, puss came out, and it got smaller and finally disappeared.

> *I have suffered from large boils on the tops of my legs for about 30 years, and nobody could help me get rid of them. Last fall I counted 12 boils. I started using Lavender and did the Master Cleanser, lemonade cleanse. On the third day, my boils opened and ran freely. This was in January of this year. Now I only occasionally get them, and they are many times smaller than before. I know if I continue the regimen, they will eventually leave altogether.*
>
> *-Submitted by K. Ernst (July 2004)*

Bonding: *See Emotions.*

    Oils—^{AT}<u>Gentle Baby</u>.

    A—Diffuse into the air. Inhale directly or applied to hands, tissue, or a cotton wick.

    T—Apply to auricular emotional points.

    *****Comments**—Use <u>Release</u> or other oils listed under Emotional Release in the Science and Application section of the <u>Reference Guide for Essential Oils</u> to help release emotional connections to one who has passed on. Also, to help children create good bonds with others, tell them about the person when working with the oils.

Bones:

Oils—ᵀWintergreen, ᵀ<u>PanAway</u> (bone pain), ᵀspruce, ᵀcedarwood, ᵀcypress, ᵀfir, ᵀjuniper, ᵀlavender, ᵀlemongrass, ᵀmarjoram, ᵀpeppermint, ᵀ<u>Relieve It</u>, ᵀsandalwood.

Supplements—BLM, **Super Cal**, Mineral Essence, Power Meal, Sulfurzyme, Master Formula,.

—BONE SPURS

>> *A bone spur (osteophyte) is a bony projection formed on a normal bone. Bone spurs form as the body tries to repair itself by building extra bone in response to continued pressure, stress, or rubbing. Bone spurs can cause pain if they rub against soft tissues or other bones.*

> *One lady had a heel spur flare up one evening, so she took a bath with birch and cypress before retiring. The next morning, the pain was a little better. She then put 6 drops birch, 6 drops cypress, and, on top of that, 5 drops RC on a cotton pad and applied it to her heel. In 10 minutes all pain was gone, and even after four days the pain had not returned.*

Oils—ᵀWintergreen,ᵀcypress, ᵀmarjoram, ᵀRC (dissolves).

—BROKEN (HEAL)

Recipe #1—Wintergreen and cypress (before bed); helichrysum, oregano, and <u>Valor</u> (in morning). Frankincense and balsam fir can also be used internally and externally.

Blend #1—9 drops wintergreen, 8 drops each of spruce, white fir, and helichrysum, and 7 drops clove (good when inflammation is causing the pain).

Blend #2—Equal parts lemongrass, clove, *Eucalyptus radiata*, and *Melaleuca alternifolia* (tea tree). Has been used to heal an infected bone fracture in as little as 3 months.

Personal Care—Ortho Ease mixed with lavender, lemongrass, and <u>PanAway</u>. Ortho Sport with juniper, lemongrass, and marjoram (apply over broken bones).

Supplements—BLM and **Super Cal**.

—BRUISED

Oils—ᵀHelichrysum, ᵀ<u>Relieve It</u>, ᵀ<u>PanAway</u>.

—CARTILAGE

>> *Cartilage is a type of connective tissue in the body that provides structure and support for other tissues without being hard and rigid like bone. Unlike other connective tissues, cartilage does not have blood vessels. Cartilage is found in many areas of the body, including the joints, ears, nose, bronchial tubes, and intervertebral disks.*

Oils—ᵀSandalwood (regenerates), ᵀwhite fir (pain from inflammation).

A=Aromatic **T**=Topical **I**=Internal

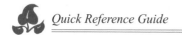

—**D**EGENERATION

  Recipe #1—Apply Ortho Ease and then peppermint.

  Supplements—Super C / Super C Chewable.

—**D**EVELOPMENT

  Supplements—**Ultra Young+** (may help boost bone formation), Super C / Super C Chewable, Master Formula.

—**O**STEOMYELITIS *SEE ALSO ANTIBACTERIAL*

  ▸▸ *Osteomyelitis is a bone infection usually caused by bacteria. The infection often starts in another area of the body and then spreads to the bone. Symptoms include fever, pain, swelling, nausea, drainage of pus, and uneasiness. Diabetes, hemodialysis, recent trauma, and IV drug abuse are risk factors for osteomyelitis.*

  Recipe #2—Equal parts lemongrass, clove, *Eucalyptus radiata*, and *Melaleuca alternifolia* (tea tree), either blended together or applied individually, on the direct topical location.

  *****Comments**—Osteomyelitis is infection in the bones. Often, the original site of infection is elsewhere in the body and spreads to the bone by the blood. Bacteria or fungus may sometimes be responsible for osteomyelitis.

—**O**STEOPOROSIS *SEE ALSO HORMONAL IMBALANCE*

  ▸▸ *Osteoporosis is a disease characterized by a loss of bone density, making the bones extremely fragile and susceptible to fractures and breaking. Osteoporosis develops when bone resorption exceeds bone formation. Osteoporosis is significantly more common in women then in men, especially after menopause; but the disease does occur in both genders.*

  Oils—ᵀPanAway, ᵀwintergreen, ᵀclove, ᵀspruce, ᵀthyme, ᵀgeranium, ᵀpeppermint, ᵀrosemary[141], ᵀAroma Siez, ᵀchamomile (Roman and German), ᵀcypress, ᵀfennel, fir (cortisone-like action), ᵀginger, ᵀhyssop, ᵀlemon, ᵀnutmeg, ᵀoregano, ᵀPeace & Calming, ᵀpine, ᵀRelieve It, ᵀrosemary.

> *Studies and clinical experience by Dr. John R. Lee indicate that bone mass can be reversed (regained) by as much as 41% with the use of Natural Progesterone. For information on Dr. Lee's book,* see Hormonal Imbalance.

  Supplements—**Super Cal, BLM,** FemiGen, PD 80/20, Prenolone/Prenolone+, Progessence/
  Progessence Plus.

—**P**AIN

  Oils—ᵀPanAway, ᵀwhite fir, ᵀwintergreen.

B

—ROTATOR CUFF (SORE) *SEE ALSO SHOULDER*

>> *The rotator cuff is the group of muscles and tendons that encircles and supports the arm at the shoulder joint.*

Oils—ᵀWintergreen (bone), ᵀlemongrass (torn or pulled ligaments), ᵀPanAway, ᵀpeppermint (nerves), ᵀwhite fir (inflammation), ᵀRelieve It, ᵀspruce.

T—Dilute as necessary, and apply on location or on Vita Flex points on the feet.

Boredom:

Oils—ᴬAwaken, ᴬMotivation, ᴬValor, ᴬBelieve, ᴬcedarwood, ᴬcypress, ᴬDream Catcher, ᴬfir, ᴬfrankincense, ᴬGathering, ᴬjuniper, ᴬlavender, ᴬpepper, ᴬRoman chamomile, ᴬrosemary, ᴬsandalwood, ᴬspruce, ᴬthyme, ᴬylang ylang.

A—Diffuse into the air. Inhale directly.

Bowel: See Digestive System.

Boxed in (Feeling):

Oils—ᴬᵀPeace & Calming, ᴬᵀValor, ᵀTranquil (roll-on).

A—Diffuse into the air. Inhale directly or applied to hands, tissue, or a cotton wick.

T—Apply to auricular emotional points.

Brain:

>> *The Brain is the central part of the nervous system. It is responsible for processing sensory stimuli and directing appropriate behavioral responses to each stimulus, or set of stimuli. The brain also stores memories and is the center of thought.*

Oils—ᴬᵀLavender[142], ᴬᵀlemon[143], ᴬᵀlemongrass, ᴬᵀAroma Life, ᴬᵀblue cypress (improves circulation), ᴬᵀclary sage (opens brain, euphoria), ᴬᵀsacred frankincense, ᴬmyrrh[144], ᴬrose[145], ᴬᵀcypress, ᴬᵀdorado azul (stimulates hypothalamus), ᴬᵀgeranium, ᴬᵀspearmint, ᴬᵀTransformation

Supplements—MindWise, Longevity Capsules (contains thyme oil, which helps preserve omega-3s in

> *The **blood-brain barrier** is the barrier membrane between the circulating blood and the brain that prevents certain damaging substances from reaching brain tissue and cerebrospinal fluid. The American Medical Association (AMA) determined that if they could find an agent that would pass the blood-brain barrier, they would be able to heal **Alzheimer's, Lou Gehrig's, Multiple Sclerosis, and Parkinson's disease.** In June of 1994, it was documented by the Medical University of Berlin, Germany and Vienna, Austria that **sesquiterpenes have the ability to go beyond the blood-brain barrier. High levels of sesquiterpenes** are found in the essential oils of cedarwood, vetiver, sandalwood, black pepper, patchouli, myrrh, ginger, vitex, German chamomile, spikenard, galbanum, and frankincense. Some blends containing these oils include: 3 Wise Men, Acceptance, Brain Power, Forgiveness, Gathering, Harmony, Inspiration, Into the Future, and Trauma Life (refer to Single Oil Chart in the Appendix for other blends that contain these oils).*

A=Aromatic **T**=Topical **I**=Internal

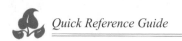

the brain; and contains clove oil, which helps to protect the neurons), **Omega Blue or OmegaGize**³ (contain pure fish oil with naturally occurring ratios of EPA and DHA), Master Formula.

—**ACTIVATES RIGHT BRAIN.**

> Oils—^{AT}Bergamot, ^{AT}geranium, ^{AT}grapefruit, ^{AT}helichrysum, ^{AT}Roman chamomile, ^{AT}wintergreen.

—**BROKEN BLOOD VESSELS** *See Blood: BROKEN BLOOD VESSELS.*

—**CEREBRAL (BRAIN)**

> Oils—^{AT}ₚNutmeg.

—**CONCUSSION** *See Concussion*

—**FOOD**

> **Recipe #1**—Omega-3 fatty acids found in Flax Seed Oil and Sesame Oil (taken internally).

—**INJURY**

> Oils—^{AT}Sacred frankincense/frankincense[146], ^{AT}bergamot[147], ^{AT}Valor, ^{AT}peppermint[148], ^{AT}lemon[149].

—**INTEGRATION**

> Oils—^{AT}Valor, ^{AT}helichrysum (increases neurotransmitter activity), ^{AT}clary sage, ^{AT}cypress, ^{AT}geranium, ^{AT}lemongrass, ^{AT}spearmint.

—**NEUROLOGICAL INJURY (BREAKDOWN OF MYELIN SHEATH)**

> ›› *The myelin sheath is an insulating layer of protein and fatty substances that forms around nerves (including those in the brain), increasing the speed of nerve impulses. Damage to the myelin sheath interrupts these nerve impulses and can cause diseases such as multiple sclerosis, peripheral neuropathy, central pontine myelinolysis, and other neurological diseases.*

> Oils—^{AT}Peppermint[148], ^{AT}frankincense, ^{AT}lemongrass[150], ^{AT}Valor.

—**OXYGENATE**

> Oils—^AEucalyptus[151], ^Arosemary[151], ^Ablack pepper[152], ^{TA}helichrysum, ^{TA}sandalwood, ^{TA}blue cypress.

> **Recipe #2**—3 drops each of helichrysum and sandalwood once or twice a day on the back of neck, temples, and behind ears down to jaw. Also blue cypress.

—**TUMOR** *See Cancer: BRAIN*

> Oils—^{TA}Frankincense[153], ^{TA}Valor.

A—Diffuse into the air. Inhale directly or applied to a tissue or a cotton wick.

T—Dilute as recommended, and rub onto the brain stem area, back of neck, temples, behind ears down to jaw, or on reflex points on the feet. Apply as a cold compress.

Breast: *See also Cancer: BREAST, Pregnancy/Motherhood: LACTATION.*

Oils—^TClary sage, ^Tgeranium, ^Tcypress, ^Telemi (inflammation), ^Tfennel, ^Tlemongrass, ^Tsage, ^Tspearmint, ^Tvetiver.

Personal Care—ClaraDerm, Prenolone/Prenolone+/Progessence/Progessence Plus (for tenderness and swelling).

—ENLARGE AND FIRM

Oils—^TClary sage, ^Tfennel, ^Tsage, ^TSclarEssence.

Blend #1—Equal parts vetiver, geranium, and ylang ylang.

Personal Care—A·R·T Purifying Toner (to tone and tighten skin)

—LACTATION *See Pregnancy/Motherhood.*

—MASTITIS (BREAST INFECTION) *See also Antibacterial*

Oils—^TCitrus Fresh (with lavender), ^TExodus II, ^Tlavender, ^Ttangerine.

Blend #2—Equal amounts of lavender and tangerine. Dilute with some V-6 Oil, and apply to breasts and under arms twice a day.

—MILK PRODUCTION *See Pregnancy/Motherhood.*

—SORE NIPPLES

Oils—^TRoman chamomile.

Personal Care—Animal Scents Pet Ointment

—STRETCH MARKS

Oils—^TGentle Baby.

T—Dilute as necessary, and apply on location or on Vita Flex points on the feet.

Breath(ing): *See Respiratory System.*

Bronchitis: *See also Respiratory System.*

» *Bronchitis is a disease of the respiratory system, marked by inflamed and narrowed bronchial tubes. Symptoms include coughing, breathlessness, and thick phlegm. Bronchitis occurs in two forms: Acute (lasting six weeks or less) and Chronic (reoccurring frequently over two or more years).*

Oils—^{AT}Eucalyptus[154], ^{AT}Eucalyptus radiata[154], ^{AT}_Fthyme[155], ^TBreathe Again, ^{AIT}Thieves, ^{AT}_Ffir (obstructions of bronchi), ^{AT}_Ftea tree, ^{AT}RC, ^{AT}Raven, ^{AT}ravintsara, ^{AT}_Fpeppermint, ^{AT}_Fpine, ^{AT}_Fcedarwood, ^{AT}_Frosemary, ^{AT}_Fclary sage, ^{AT}_Fcypress, ^{AT}_Fmarjoram,

^{AT}_Fspearmint, ^{AT}_Fmyrtle, ^{AT}<u>Abundance</u>, ^{AT}basil, ^{AT}bergamot, ^{AT}cajeput, ^{AT}clove, ^{AT}elemi, ^{AT}frankincense, ^{AT}ginger, ^{AT}hinoki, ^{AT}<u>ImmuPower</u>, ^{AT}lavender, ^{AT}ledum, ^{AT}lemon, ^{AT}Tea tree ericifolia, ^{AT}myrrh, ^{AT}nutmeg, ^{AT}onycha (benzoin), ^{AT}Roman chamomile, ^{AT}rose, ^{AT}sage lavender, ^{AT}sandalwood, ^{AT}tsuga (opens respiratory tract), ^{AT}wintergreen.

Blend #1—10 drops cedarwood, 10 drops eucalyptus, 2 drops Roman chamomile, and 2 oz. water. Put on hanky and inhale. Blend can also be added to water for gargling.

Blend #2—Clove, cinnamon bark, melissa, and lavender (<u>Alternative Medicine—The Definitive Guide</u>, p. 55).

***Comments—Refer to the chapter entitled "How to Use—The Personal Usage Reference" in the <u>Essential Oils Desk Reference</u> under "Bronchitis" for specific oil blend and supplement recommendations.

Recipe #1—According to Dr. Daniel Pénoël, bronchitis can be broken down into three separate areas, each of which should be considered separately. Following are the three areas and the specific blends recommended by Dr. Pénoël:

> ***Inflammation***—Mix equal portions of *Eucalyptus citriodora* and lemongrass. Apply 36 drops per foot to the sinus and lung Vita Flex points. Add to V-6 Oil, and apply over the chest.

> ***Infection***—Mix 1 tsp. tea tree, 25 drops palmarosa or geranium, 3 drops peppermint, 1 drop thyme. Apply 3–6 drops per foot to the sinus and lung Vita Flex points. Add to V-6 Oil, and apply over the chest.

> ***Accumulation of Fluids (mucus)***—Mix 25 drops each of *Eucalyptus dives*, peppermint, and dill. Apply 3–6 drops per foot to the sinus and lung Vita Flex points.

—CHRONIC

> **Oils**—^{AT}Eucalyptus[154], ^{AT}_Fravintsara, ^{AT}_Fsage, ^{AT}_Fsandalwood, ^{AT}_Foregano, ^{AT}elemi, ^{AT}laurel.

—CHILDREN

> **Oils**—^{AT}Eucalyptus[154], ^{AT}tea tree, ^{AT}lavender, ^{AT}Tea tree ericifolia, ^{AT}Roman chamomile, ^{AT}rosemary, ^{AT}thyme (CT linalol).

—CLEAR MUCUS

> **Oils**—^{AT}Eucalyptus[154], ^{AT}onycha (benzoin), ^{AT}<u>Thieves</u>, ^{AT}bergamot, ^{AT}sandalwood, and ^{AT}thyme (*Alternative Medicine—The Definitive Guide*, p. 824).

> *****Comments**—*Diffusing the oils is a great way to handle a respiratory problem.*

A—Diffuse the oils into the air. Inhale directly or from a tissue or a cotton wick. *See Comments under Asthma for a discussion on using* **plastic nasal inhalers**.

T—Dilute as necessary, and rub on chest. Add 2–3 drops to water; gargle.

I—Add 1–2 drops to 8 oz.; drink. Add 3–5 drops to an empty capsule with 3–5 drops V-6 Oil; swallow.

B

Bruises:

›› *A bruise is a tissue injury that results in blood capillaries breaking and spilling blood into the tissue. This can cause swelling, soreness, and a visible discoloration when the bruise is near the skin.*

Oils—^THelichrysum, ^Tgeranium, ^TPanAway, ^Tfennel, ^Tangelica, ^Thyssop, ^Tlavender, ^TMelrose, ^TThieves.

T—Dilute as necessary, and apply on location.

*****Comments**—Refer to the chapter entitled "How to Use—The Personal Usage Reference" in the Essential Oils Desk Reference under "Bruising" for some excellent blend recipes and supplement recommendations.

Bugged (Feeling): *See Emotions.*

Oils—^{AT}Acceptance, ^{AT}Forgiveness, ^{AT}Peace & Calming, ^{AT}Valor.

A—Diffuse into the air. Inhale directly or applied to hands, tissue, or a cotton wick.

T—Apply to auricular emotional points.

Bugs (Repel): *See Bites and Insect: REPELLENT.*

Bulimia: *See Eating Disorders: BULIMIA.*

Bumps:

Oils—^TFrankincense, ^TMelrose, ^TPanAway, ^TPeace & Calming.

T—Dilute as necessary, and apply on location.

Bunions: *See Bursitis: Bunions.*

Burdens: *See Emotions.*

Oils—^{AT}Acceptance, ^{AT}Hope, ^{AT}Release, ^{AT}Transformation, ^{AT}Valor.

A—Diffuse into the air. Inhale directly or applied to hands, tissue, or a cotton wick.

T—Apply to auricular emotional points.

A=Aromatic **T**=Topical **I**=Internal

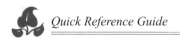

Burns:

>> *A burn is an injury to tissue (often the skin) caused by heat, chemicals, or radiation. Minor burns are painful and red, while more serious burns can blister, cause swelling, and char or destroy the skin and underlying tissues. Minor burns can be treated by immersing them in cool water, while more serious burns require medical treatment.*

*Dr. Alex Schauss, a prominent mineral researcher, has discovered that **burns** are painful because certain trace minerals are depleted from the skin and surrounding tissue. If the trace minerals are replenished to the affected area, then the pain will subside almost immediately. Many people have received instant pain relief when Mineral Essence was either taken internally or topically applied on the sunburn or burn.*

Oils—ᵀ_F Lavender (cell renewal), ᵀravintsara (healing), ᵀtamanu (mix with helichrysum), ᵀeucalyptus, ᵀgeranium, ᵀhelichrysum, ᵀIdaho tansy, ᵀtea tree, ᵀpeppermint, ᵀRoman chamomile, ᵀrosehip.

Personal Care—LavaDerm Cooling Mist (soothing and cooling for all burns), Lavender Hand & Body Lotion (moisturizes and promotes healing).

Supplements—**Mineral Essence** (can be taken internally and applied topically).

Blend #1—Put 3 drops of lavender in some Lavender Hand & Body Lotion, and apply. This is effective for pain, healing, peeling, and sunburns.

Blend #2—10 drops German chamomile, 5 drops Roman chamomile, and 10 drops lavender. Mix together, and add 1 drop to each square inch of burn after it has been soaked in ice water. If you don't have the chamomile, lavender will do great. Can top with LavaDerm Cooling Mist to keep skin cool and moist.

—Cleansing

　　Oils—ᵀMelrose.

—Infected

　　Oils—ᵀPurification.

—Pain

　　Blend #1 (above)

　　Supplements—**Mineral Essence** (apply topically).

—Healing *See Scarring.*

　　Oils—ᵀRosehip.

　　Blend #1 (above)

　　Blend #3—Ravintsara or geranium mixed with helichrysum.

René Maurice Gattefossé, PhD, a French cosmetic chemist who coined the phrase "Aromatherapy," severely burned his hand in a laboratory accident. The continual application of lavender oil soothed the pain, nullified the effects of gas gangrene, and healed his hand without a scar.

B

C

—Peeling

Blend #1, Blend #2 (both shown above).

—Sunburn *See Sunburn.*

—Sun Screen

Oils—^T_FHelichrysum, ^{T}tamanu.

T—Dilute as necessary, and apply on location. Place 2–3 drops with 1 oz. distilled water in a misting spray bottle, shake well, and mist on location.

Bursitis:

➤➤ *Bursitis is the inflammation of the fluid-filled sack located close to joints that provides lubrication for tendons, skin, and ligaments rubbing against the bone. Bursitis is caused by infection, injury, or diseases such as arthritis and gout. Bursitis causes tenderness and pain, which can limit movement.*

Oils—^{T}PanAway, ^{T}Aroma Siez, ^{T}cypress, ^{T}cajeput, ^{T}ginger, ^{T}hyssop, ^{T}juniper, ^{T}onycha (benzoin), ^{T}Roman chamomile.

Blend #1—Apply 6 drops of marjoram on shoulders and arms; wait 6 minutes. Then apply 3 drops of wintergreen; wait 6 minutes. Then apply 3 drops of cypress.

Personal Care—Ortho Ease, Ortho Sport.

Supplements—BLM

—Bunions

➤➤ *Bunions are bursitis located at the base of a toe, often caused by constrictive footwear.*

Oils—^{T}Aroma Siez, ^{T}M-Grain, ^{T}cypress, ^{T}carrot, ^{T}German chamomile, ^{T}juniper.

Blend #2—6 drops eucalyptus, 3 drops lemon, 4 drops ravintsara, and 1 drop wintergreen in 1 oz. V-6 Oil. Apply a couple drops of this blend directly on area of concern as often as desired.

T—Dilute as necessary, and apply on location.

Calcium: *See Hormonal Imbalance.*

Supplements—Allerzyme (aids the digestion of sugars, starches, fats, and proteins), Digest + Cleanse, Super Cal, Mineral Essence.

Calluses: *See Skin: Calluses.*

According to Dr. John R. Lee, processed food, carbonated soft drink, caffeine, high protein, sugar, and salt consumption all contribute to increased calcium deficiency in the human body (Burton Goldberg Group, Alt. Med., The Definitive Guide, pp 773-4). Sulfur cannot be metabolized if there is a calcium deficiency. This can cause poor nail and hair growth, falling hair, eczema, dermatitis, poor muscle tone, acne, pimples, gout, rheumatism, arthritis, and a weakening of the nervous system.

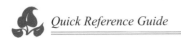

Calming:

> Oils—^AT^<u>Peace & Calming</u>, ^AT^lavender^156^, ^AT^ylang ylang^157^, ^T^<u>Stress Away</u>, ^AT^rose^158^, ^AT^<u>Citrus Fresh</u>,
> ^AT^melissa^159^, ^AT^orange^160^, ^AT^~F~cedarwood, ^AT^hinoki, ^AT^yuzu, ^AT^hong kuai, ^AT^bergamot^161^,
> ^AT^sacred frankincense, ^A^clary sage, ^AT^<u>Gentle Baby</u>, ^AT^jasmine, ^AT^Tea tree ericifolia,
> ^AT^myrrh, ^AT^onycha (benzoin), ^AT^<u>Release</u>, ^AT^<u>Surrender</u>, ^AT^tangerine, ^AT^<u>Trauma Life</u>,
> ^AT^western red cedar.

> Supplements—SleepEssence (short-term only).

—AGITATION

> Oils—^AT^Lavender^156^, ^AT^rose^158^, ^AT^ylang ylang^157^, ^AT^~F~bergamot^161^, ^AT^<u>Peace & Calming</u>,
> ^AT^<u>Trauma Life</u> (calms), ^AT^cedarwood, ^AT^clary sage, ^AT^<u>Forgiveness</u>, ^AT^frankincense,
> ^AT^geranium, ^AT^<u>Harmony</u>, ^AT^<u>Joy</u>, ^AT^juniper, ^AT^marjoram, ^AT^myrrh, ^AT^rosewood,
> ^AT^sandalwood, ^AT^<u>Transformation</u>, ^AT^<u>Valor</u>.

—HYPERACTIVITY

> Oils—^AT^Lavender^162^, ^AT^<u>Peace & Calming</u> (gets them off Ritalin), ^AT^<u>Citrus Fresh</u>, ^AT^<u>RutaVaLa</u>, ^AT^<u>Valor</u> (sometimes works better than <u>Peace & Calming</u>) ^AT^Roman chamomile, ^AT^<u>Trauma Life</u> (calming).

> *Hyperactivity* may indicate a trace mineral deficiency. Get off Prozac and Ritalin and use Mineral Essence. It is interesting to note that 48 out of 49 death row inmates were tested and found to be deficient in the same trace minerals.

> Supplements—ComforTone, Essentialzyme, Essentialzymes-4, ICP, Mineral Essence, **healthy diet**.

—SEDATIVE

> ≫ *A sedative is a calming or sleep-inducing agent*

> Oils—^AT^Lavender^163^, ^AT^<u>Peace & Calming</u>, ^AT^<u>RutaVaLa</u>, ^T^<u>Tranquil</u> (roll-on), ^AT^bergamot, ^AT^<u>Citrus Fresh</u>^164^, ^AT^valerian^165^, ^AT^neroli, ^AT^mastrante, ^AT^angelica, ^AT^cedarwood, ^AT^clary sage, ^AT^coriander, ^AT^cypress, ^AT^elemi, ^AT^frankincense, ^AT^geranium, ^AT^hyssop, ^AT^jasmine, ^AT^juniper, ^AT^lemongrass, ^AT^melissa, ^AT^marjoram, ^AT^onycha (benzoin), ^AT^orange, ^AT^patchouli, ^AT^Roman chamomile, ^AT^rose, ^AT^sandalwood, ^AT^tangerine, ^AT^<u>Trauma Life</u>, ^AT^vetiver (nervous system), ^AT^ylang ylang. Use intuition as to which one may be best for the given situation. In addition, check the safety data for each of the oils in the Appendix of this book.

> ***Comments—*Refer to BLEND #3 under Insomnia for a blend of oils that can either be taken internally in water or applied to the back of the neck to help relax the body.*

A—Diffuse into the air. Inhale directly, or apply to hands, tissue, or a cotton wick, and inhale.

T—Dilute as recommended, and apply 1–2 drops to back of neck, temples, chest, shoulders, wrist, back, or reflex points on the feet. Dilute in V-6 Oil, and massage into the back, shoulders, neck, or arms.

Cancer: *See Chemicals, Tumors, Radiation.*

C

>> *Cancer can be any of many different conditions where the body's cells duplicate and grow uncontrollably, invade healthy tissues, and possibly spread throughout the body. It is estimated that 95% of cancers result from damage to DNA during a person's lifetime rather than from a preexisting genetic condition (American Cancer Society, 2008). The most important factor leading to this DNA damage is DNA mutation. DNA mutation can be caused by radiation, environmental chemicals we take into our bodies, free radical damage, or DNA copying or division errors. If the body is working properly, it can correct these mutations either by repairing the DNA or by causing the mutated cell to die. When the DNA mutation is severe enough that it allows the cell to bypass these controls, however, the mutated DNA can be copied to new cells that continue to replicate and create more and more new cells uncontrollably, leading to a cancerous growth within an individual.,*

Oils—^{AIT}Frankincense[166] (combine with ledum and take internally), ^{ATI}sandalwood[167], ^{AT}lavender[168], ^{TAI}rosemary[169], ^{AT}caraway[170], ^{ATI}lemongrass[171], ^{AIT}clove[172], ^{AT}basil[173], ^{TIA}geranium[174], ^{ATI}clary sage[175], ^Torange[176], ^{TA}myrrh[177], ^{TA}ₑtarragon,

> *When the cell wall thickens, oxygen cannot get in. The life expectancy of a cell is 120 days (4 months). Cells also divide, making duplicate cells. If the cell is diseased, new diseased cells will be made. When we stop the mutation of the diseased cells (create healthy cells), we stop the disease. Essential oils have the ability to penetrate and carry nutrients through the cell wall to the nucleus and improve the health of the cell.*

^T<u>Di-Gize</u> (rub on feet and stomach), ^{TA}<u>ImmuPower</u> (put on throat and all over feet, three times a day), ^{TA}<u>Melrose</u> (cancer sores, fights infection), ^{TA}<u>Juva Cleanse</u>, ^{TA}rose, ^{TA}sage.

*****Comments**—Since it is very important to maintain a positive attitude while healing, it may be helpful to address the emotions using <u>Acceptance</u>, <u>Believe</u>, <u>Envision</u>, <u>Forgiveness</u>, <u>Gathering</u>, <u>Gratitude</u>, <u>Hope</u>, <u>Joy</u>, <u>Live with Passion</u>, and/or ravintsara (*refer to the emotional therapies in the Science and Application section of the <u>Reference Guide for Essential Oils</u>*). One of the most common emotions cancer patients have to deal with is anger or a pattern of resentment. Others are fear, judgement, and doubt. Doubt limits God and restricts His ability to work miracles in our lives. Praying for all those with cancer can help release these emotions. Also, work on recognizing why cancer was chosen.

*****Comments**—All conifer oils have great value in fighting cancers, while balsam fir and white fir have more specific actions.

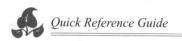

***Comments—Oils high in limonene (like grapefruit, tangerine, orange, palo santo, mandarin, fleabane, and lemon) have been shown to be effective in fighting cancer.

***Comments—Refer to the chapter entitled "How to Use—The Personal Usage Reference" in the <u>Essential Oils Desk Reference</u> under "Cancer" for some excellent blend recipes, supplement recommendations, and cleansing and maintenance programs for many different kinds of cancer.

***Important Notice: Health care professionals are emphatic about avoiding heavy massage when working with cancer patients. Light massage may be used, but never over the trauma area. Also, the information in this section should not be perceived as a cure for cancer. Always consult with your health care professional.

Supplements—Cleansing Trio (ComforTone, Essentialzyme, and ICP), AlkaLime (acid-neutralizing mineral formulation), Balance Complete, Digest + Cleanse, ImmuPro, Inner Defense, MultiGreens, NingXia Red (nutrient powerhouse), NingXia Wolfberries (dried), Power Meal, Sulfurzyme, Super C / Super C Chewable, Master Formula, Wolfberry Crisp Bars (*Refer to the Wolfberry Crisp Bar in the Supplements section of the Reference Guide for Essential Oils for more information on the benefits of the Ningxia Wolfberry*).

***Comments—One lady who was receiving chemotherapy treatments for cancer of the spleen used <u>Di-Gize</u> to promote elimination through the colon. Her doctors wondered why her chemotherapy treatments had not made her sick.

> *There must be an acid condition in the body for cancer to thrive and spread. See pH Balance. Power Meal contains predigested proteins and helps the body move towards an alkaline balance. AlkaLime combats yeast and fungus overgrowth and helps preserve the body's proper pH balance.*
>
> *Cancer cells also have a very low frequency.*

When she felt any discomfort (light nausea or cramps in the descending colon), she rubbed 4–6 drops of Di-Gize on her abdomen, and within 10 minutes all discomfort stopped.

The following are recipes that some individuals have used successfully:

Recipe #1—For the first month, supplement with the following: 6 MultiGreens three times a day,
6 Super C / Super C Chewable three times a day, and 1 ImmuPro three times a day. After remission, apply <u>ImmuPower</u> on the spine three times a day. Do a *light* full body massage with 6 clove and
15 frankincense in 1 oz. V-6 Oil.

Recipe #2—Supplement with the following: Cleansing Trio (ComforTone, Essentialzyme, and ICP),
12 Super C / Super C Chewable, and 9 MultiGreens. Drink ½ gallon of carrot juice

each day. Eliminate white flour, white sugar, and red meat from the diet. Rub <u>Thieves</u> on the feet, and do a *light* full body massage with frankincense.

Recipe #3—Supplement with the following: 1 Master Formula, 2 MultiGreens, 6 Super C / Super C Chewable. Do a *light* full body massage with frankincense, clove, and V-6 Oil. Apply <u>ImmuPower</u> to the spine and feet twice a day.

—BONE

Oils—[T]Frankincense

Recipe #1—Cleansing Trio (ComforTone, Essentialzyme, and ICP) for a week, then JuvaTone was added for six days, then Super B was added morning and evening. Other vitamin supplements included Super C / Super C Chewable, MegaCal, and Super Cal. All processed foods were eliminated, and a strict vegetarian diet was followed, including 8 glasses of water each day. Birch was applied on location for pain. Frankincense and lavender were applied on the feet.

—BRAIN

Oils—[AT]Frankincense[178], [AT]myrrh[179], [AT]clove

> *Frankincense contains sesquiterpenes which allow it to go beyond the blood-brain barrier. Sesquiterpenes are also found in many of the emotional blends. ImmuPower builds the immune system. Clove is antiparasitic and antitumoral.*

The following are recipes that some individuals have used successfully:

Recipe #4—*Light* massage daily on spine with 1 oz. V-6 Oil, 15 drops frankincense, and 6 drops clove. Rub brain stem area with <u>ImmuPower</u>. Diffuse 15 drops frankincense and 6 drops clove for ½ hour three times a day.

Recipe #5—Diffuse frankincense 24 hours a day, and massage the brain stem area with frankincense.

—BREAST

Oils—[TA]Rosemary[180], [TA]lavender[181], [TA]frankincense, [TA]clove, [TA]clary sage[182], [TA]basil[183].

Supplements—FemiGen.

Personal Care—Progessence/Progessence Plus.

***Comments—Often there is an emotional issue of self-worth that must be dealt with as well.

—CERVICAL

Oils—[TA]Frankincense, [TA]geranium, [TA]clove, [TA]cypress, [TA]lavender, [TA]lemon.

—COLON

Oils—[ITA]Lavender[184], [TA]geranium[185], [TA]frankincense[186], [TA]lemongrass[187].

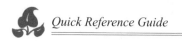

Supplements—ICP (fiber beverage that helps prevent), Super Cal (studies have shown that taking calcium supplements at night helps protect the colon from polyps and cancer).

—DIET

Fast 21 days (*See Fasting or Cleansing*); then have soup. *See Diet.*

—HEART

Supplements—HRT

—LIVER

> *One woman had **cancer of the heart**, which literally ate a hole in the heart. She took the tincture HRT, and the tissue of her heart regenerated and the cancer disappeared!*
>
> ***JuvaTone** and **Rehemogen** build blood and hemoglobin platelets One individual had total **liver regeneration** by using JuvaTone, Rehemogen, and JuvaFlex.*

Oils—^{TA}Frankincense[186] (hot compress over liver), ^{TA}lemongrass[187], ^{TA}lavender[188], ^{TA}GLF, ^{TA}JuvaFlex, ^{TA}Juva Cleanse, ^{TA}myrrh.

Supplements—JuvaTone was formulated to fight cancer in the liver.

—LUNG

Oils—^{TA}Frankincense (rub on chest, or add 15 drops to 1 tsp. V-6 Oil for nightly retention enema), ^{TA}lavender[189].

Blend #1—15 drops frankincense, 5 drops clove, 6 drops ravintsara, 4 drops myrrh, and 2 drops sage. This blend can be mixed with 1 tsp. V-6 Oil if it is too strong. It is best when inserted into rectum.

—LYMPHOMA

>> *Lymphoma is a cancer of the lymphatic system (part of the immune system). Hodgkin's disease is a form of lymphoma, and lymphomas are generally classified in two categories: Hodgkin lymphoma and non-Hodgkin lymphomas.*

Nodes or small tumors in neck and groin. Cleanse liver.

Blend #2—10 drops frankincense, 5 drops myrrh, and 3 drops sage. Mix with small amount of V-6 Oil, and apply daily over nodes or tumor areas and rectally. Every other day, apply frankincense neat.

–HODGKIN'S DISEASE

>> *Hodgkin's disease (or Hodgkin's lymphoma) is a type of cancer that affects lymphocytes (white blood cells). It can cause enlarged lymph nodes and cause fever, sweating, fatigue, and weight loss.*

Oils—^TClove (Apply to liver, kidney, and Vita Flex points on feet).

—Lymphoma Stage 4 (bone marrow)

Extreme fatigue: eat vegetables and fruits; no meat.

Oils—ᵀImmuPower (on the spine).

Recipe #6—Life 5 (probiotic), Cleansing Trio (ComforTone, Essentialzyme, and ICP), 6 Super C / Super C Chewable three times a day, 6 MultiGreens three times a day. After remission, continue one more month; then reduce amounts for maintenance.

—Melanoma *See also Corns, Warts.*

>> *Melanoma is the most serious type of skin cancer. It is a malignant tumor that affects the melanocytes (the cells that produce the pigment melanin that colors our skin, hair, and eyes) in our skin. Melanoma often manifests itself in the forms of moles—new moles or ones that already exist. It can be spotted by*

Aloha! I have been using essential oil for many years, resulting in many amazingly wonderful results. One of the best took place when a dear friend was being consumed by cancer. She was in stage 4 for 4 years—amazing in itself. RC and frankincense were used the most. When she was put into the hospice, with only days left, the oils were still used, and she remained in the hospice for another year and a half. Others at the hospice got sick with colds and flu, including the workers, but my friend never got any of the passing bugs... Amazing to say the least, but this was a true testimonial to the antiviral and antibiotic effects of the oils.
-Submitted by Yvonne Vnuk-Nielsen
Kailua, Hawaii (July 2004)

noticing changes in the moles such as symmetry, edges, color, and size. Melanoma can be cured if treated early; but if it spreads, it can cause death.

Oils—ᵀᴵSandalwood[190], ᵀfrankincense[191], ᵀlavender.

—Ovarian

Oils—ᵀImmuPower (on spine three times a day).

Blend #3—15 drops frankincense, 6 drops geranium, and 5 drops myrrh in ½ tsp. V-6 Oil; alternate: one night in vagina (tampon to retain), next in rectum.

Recipe #7—6 FemiGen a day, 8 Super C / Super C Chewable a day. Those with "A" type blood should take 8 MultiGreens a day while those with "O" type blood should take 12 or more a day; MultiGreens is a mainstay, it is a predigested protein and helps maintain an alkaline balance.

—Prostate

Oils—ᵀAnise (blend with frankincense, fennel, ImmuPower, Mister, sage, and/or yarrow). ᴵJuva Cleanse.

T—Apply to posterior scrotum, ankles, lower back, and bottoms of feet.

I—Add 3–5 drops to empty capsule; swallow.

Personal Care—Protec was designed to accompany the night-long retention enema. It helps buffer the prostate from inflammation, enlargement, and tumor activity.

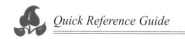
Recipe #1—Diffuse <u>ImmuPower</u>. Do a spinal massage and Vita Flex on the feet with <u>ImmuPower</u>. Blend 5 drops frankincense, 15 drops <u>Mister</u>, and 2 tsp. V-6 Oil together **or** 15 drops <u>ImmuPower</u> with 2 tsp. V-6 Oil. Insert and retain in the rectum throughout the night.

Case History #1—A 71-year-old man had prostate cancer and bone metastasis. After three weeks of using frankincense, sage, myrrh, and cumin in rectal implants, he was free of cancer.

—THROAT

Oils—^{TA}Frankincense, ^{TA}lavender.

—UTERINE

Oils—^{TA}Geranium, ^{TA}ImmuPower.

Blend #4—2–5 drops cedarwood **or** 2–5 drops lemon **or** 2–5 drops myrrh in 1 tsp. V-6 Oil.

Personal Care—Progessence/Progessence Plus.

T—Dilute as necessary, and apply 1–5 drops on location and on Vita Flex points on the feet and hands. Apply as a warm compress over affected area.

A—Diffuse into the air. Inhale oil directly or applied to hands, tissue, or a cotton wick.

I—Add 3–5 drops of oil in an empty capsule; swallow

Candida: *See Antifungal: Candida*

Cankers: *See Acidosis.*

»» *Canker sores are small, round sores that develop in the mouth, typically inside the lips and cheeks or on the tongue.*

Oils—^T<u>Thieves</u>, ^Ttea tree, ^T<u>Australian Blue</u>, ^Tchamomile (both German and Roman), ^T<u>Envision</u>, ^Thyssop, ^Tlaurel, ^T<u>Melrose</u>, ^Tmyrrh, ^Toregano, ^Tsage lavender.

> *Canker sores are occasionally associated with Crohn's disease, which affects the bowels. Deficiencies of iron, vitamin B12, and folic acid have been linked to this disease in some people. Stress and allergies are usually the cause of open sores in the mouth. To avoid getting canker sores, it is important to have a body chemistry that is balanced in minerals, acidity, and alkalinity (Prescription for Nutritional Healing, p. 126).*

T—Dilute as necessary, and apply on location.

Blend #1—Sage with clove and lavender.

Blend #2—Sage with <u>Thieves</u>.

Supplements—**Inner Defense,** AlkaLime (combats yeast and fungus overgrowth and preserves the body's proper pH balance), ImmuPro, Mineral Essence, MultiGreens.

Capillaries: *See also Cardiovascular System.*

>> *Capillaries are the small, thin blood vessels that allow the exchange of oxygen and other nutrients from the blood to cells throughout the body and allow the exchange of carbon dioxide and other waste materials from these tissues back to the blood. The capillaries connect the arteries (that carry blood away from the heart) and veins (that carry blood back to the heart).*

—BROKEN *SEE ALSO BRUISES*

Oils—[T]**Geranium,** [T]**cypress,** [T]hyssop, [T]lime (soothes), [T]Roman chamomile.

T—Dilute as necessary, and apply on location.

Blend #1—Apply 1 drop lavender and 1 drop Roman chamomile.

Carbuncles: *See also Boils.*

>> *A carbuncle is a swollen, puss-filled lump or mass under the skin, varying from the size of a pea to the size of a golf ball. Carbuncles form in infected hair follicles*

Oils—[T]**Tea tree.**

T—Dilute as necessary, and apply on location.

Cardiotonic: *See Cardiovascular System: HEART.*

Cardiovascular System: *See also Arteries, Blood, Capillaries, Veins.*

Oils—[TA]F**Orange** (cardiac spasms), [TA]**cypress** (strengthens the capillary walls and increases circulation), [TA]**valerian**[192], [TA]**thyme**[193], [TA]**anise,** [TA]Aroma Life (cardiac spasms), [TA]cinnamon bark (strengthens), [TA]clary sage, [TA]clove, [TA]En-R-Gee, [TA]fleabane (dilates), [TA]goldenrod, [TA]helichrysum, [TA]marjoram, [TA]onycha (benzoin), [TA]palmarosa (supports), [TA]PanAway, [TA]rosemary, [TA]sandalwood (strengthns), [TA]tsuga (opens and dilates for better oxygen exchange), [TA]ylang ylang.

Supplements— **Omega Blue, OmegaGize**[3]**, MindWise,**FemiGen, ICP, Majestic Essence Chocolates, Mineral Essence, Slique Tea, Super B, Super Cal, Master Formula.

Personal Care—Progessence/Progessence Plus.

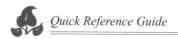
—ANGINA

Oils—**TA**F Ginger, **ITA**valerian[192], **TA**F orange (for false angina), **TA**Aroma Life, **TA**laurel.

> *Angina pectoris is a severe spasmodic pain in the chest that is due to an insufficient supply of blood to the heart.*

Supplements— Master Formula.

—CIRCULATION

Oils—**TA**F Cypress, **TA**eucalyptus[194], **TA**valerian[192], **TA**Aroma Life, **TA**basil, **TA**cinnamon bark, **TA**Citrus Fresh, **TA**clary sage, **TA**copaiba (stimulates), **TA**cumin, **TA**geranium, **TA**helichrysum, **TA**hyssop, **TA**Juva Cleanse, **TA**nutmeg, **TA**onycha (benzoin), **TA**oregano, **TA**peppermint, **TA**Peace & Calming, **TA**RC, **TA**rosemary, **TA**sage lavender, **TA**thyme, **TA**wintergreen.

–CAPILLARIES

Oils—**TA**Cypress (strengthens the capillary walls, and increases circulation), **TA**oregano, **TA**thyme.

–PROMOTES HEALTHY

Oils—**TA**Onycha (benzoin), **TA**PanAway, **IA**melissa[195], **IA**dill[196].

Personal Care—**Cel-Lite Magic** dilates the blood vessels for better circulation; may add grapefruit or cypress to enhance. Also Ortho Ease and Ortho Sport.

Supplements—Cleansing Trio (ComforTone, ICP, Essentialzyme), JuvaTone, NingXia Red, Thyromin.

***Comments—*Constipation affects circulation. Improving the circulation in the colon and liver improves the circulation in the blood.*

—HEART .

Oils—**TA**Aroma Life (on heart and all Vita Flex heart points), **TA**ylang ylang (balances heart function), **TA**marjoram, **TA**geranium, **TA**Joy, **TA**Valor (on feet), **TA**Citrus Fresh, **TA**Clarity, **TA**cypress, **TA**Dragon Time, **TA**fleabane, **TA**Forgiveness, **TA**Gentle Baby, **TA**ginger, **TA**Harmony, **TA**Hope, **TA**hyssop, **TA**lavender, **TA**Mister, **TA**M-Grain, **TA**PanAway, **TA**Relieve It, **TA**rosemary, **TA**White Angelica

> **HEART PUMP FOR HEART STRESS**
>
> *Using your thumbs, apply pressure in an alternating "pumping" fashion between the following two heart points: (1) on the left hand at the lifeline under the ring finger; and (2) just inside the elbow. Also apply Aroma Life to the chest and to the hand and heart points. And of course, GET HELP FAST!*

Supplements—**Longevity Capsules** (contains thyme oil to help preserve omega-3 fatty acids in the heart), **Omega Blue, OmegaGize³,** Mineral Essence, NingXia Red, Power Meal, Rehemogen Tincture, Slique Tea, Sulfurzyme, Super B, Ultra Young+ (may help reverse heart disease), Master Formula, Wolfberry Crisp Bars.

–ANGINA *See ANGINA above*

–ARRHYTHMIA

C

>> *Arrhythmia is an irregular heart beat rhythm: the heart either beats too slow, too fast, or in an irregular pattern. Arrhythmia can be a symptom of a larger problem.*

Recipe #1—<u>PanAway</u> on heart and <u>Relieve It</u> on left foot Vita Flex heart point (rotate each application). Goldenrod and lavender are also good. Research done by Dr. Pénoël indicates that ylang ylang may be beneficial in preventing or correcting an irregularity in the force or rhythm of the heart.

–BRINGS JOY TO HEART

Oils—^A<u>Christmas Spirit</u>, ^A<u>Citrus Fresh</u>, ^A<u>Joy</u>.

–CARDIOTONIC

Oils—^{TA}Lavender, ^{TA}thyme.

Supplements— Master Formula.

–CORONARY ARTERY

Personal Care—Prenolone/Prenolone+, Progessence/Progessence Plus.

***Comments—*Research has shown that natural progesterone protects the coronary artery from going into spasms. Provera, a synthetic progestin, offers no protection from coronary artery spasms. In fact, it promotes the spasm to the point of completely shutting off the flow of blood. This may explain the increase in heart attacks in women 5 to 10 years after menopause, many of whom are on synthetic progestin.*

Supplements—FemiGen, Super B.

–HEART TISSUE

Oils—^{TA}Marjoram (has been found to help rejuvenate the smooth muscle tissue of the heart).

–HYPERTENSION (HIGH BLOOD PRESSURE) *See Blood.*

–LARGE VALVE

Oils—^{TA}<u>Aroma Life</u> (shortness of breath).

–Palpitations

   >> *Palpitations are irregular, pounding, sporadic, or fluttering heart beats. The heart beats are irregular enough that the person becomes aware of them.*

    Oils—^{TA}<u>Aroma Life</u>, ^{TA}_Forange, ^{TA}_Fylang ylang, ^{TA}lavender, ^{TA}melissa, ^{TA}peppermint.

–Prolapsed Mitral Valve

   >> *Mitral valve prolapse (MVP) is a condition where the valve between the upper and lower chambers of the heart does not close correctly, sometimes allowing leakage of blood through the valve opening.*

    Oils—^{TA}Marjoram.

–Stimulant

    Oils—^{TA}Coriander, ^{TA}cumin.

–Strengthens Heart Muscle

    Oils—^{TA}Lavender, ^{TA}marjoram, ^{TA}peppermint, ^{TA}rose, ^{TA}rosemary (<u>Alternative Medicine—A Definitive Guide</u>, p. 722).

–Strengthening

    Oils—^{TA}Cinnamon bark.

    Supplements— MindWise, Wolfberry Crisp Bars.

–Tachycardia *See also Anxiety, Shock, Stress*

   >> *Tachycardia is an abnormally rapid resting heart rate, indicating a possible overworking of the heart.*

    Oils—^{TA}_FLavender, ^{TA}_Fylang ylang (smell on tissue or straight from bottle in emergency), ^{TA}<u>Aroma Life</u> (combine with ylang ylang), ^{TA}<u>Australian Blue</u>, ^{TA}goldenrod, ^{TA}Idaho tansy, ^{TA}lavender, ^{TA}neroli, ^{TA}orange, ^{TA}PanAway, ^{TA}<u>Relieve It</u>, ^{TA}spikenard.

    Supplements—Power Meal, Sulfurzyme, Master Formula, Wolfberry Crisp Bars.

—Phlebitis

   >> *Phlebitis is the inflammation of a superficial vein, typically in the legs or groin area. Wearing support hose or a compression bandage over the affected area can help aid in healing.*

    Oils—^{TA}_FHelichrysum (prevents), ^{TA}_Flavender, ^{TA}cypress, ^{TA}geranium, ^{TA}grapefruit, ^{TA}Roman chamomile, ^{TA}<u>Valor</u>.

Recipe #1—Massage toward heart, and wear support hose until healed, possibly two to three months. Use <u>Aroma Life</u> every morning and night. Do the Raindrop Technique on leg.

—Stimulant

Oils—^{TA}$_F$Nutmeg, ^{TA}onycha (benzoin), ^{TA}pine.

—Support

Oils—^{TA}Goldenrod.

T—Dilute oils as necessary, and apply oils to area: to carotid arteries, heart, feet, under left ring finger, above elbow, behind ring toe on left foot, and to Vita Flex points on the feet. Add 1–2 drops to bathwater for a bath. Dilute with V-6 Oil, and massage on location or on chest, neck, or feet.

A—Diffuse into the air. Inhale directly or applied to hands, tissue, or a cotton wick.

Carpal Tunnel Syndrome: *See also Inflammation.*

▸▸ *Carpal Tunnel Syndrome is a condition where inflamed carpal ligaments at the wrist press upon the median nerve. Indications include tingling or numbness in the palm or thumb and first three fingers of the hand, weak grip, or impaired finger movement.*

Oils—^T<u>Deep Relief</u> (roll-on), ^Tbasil, ^Tcypress, ^Teucalyptus, ^Tlavender, ^Tlemongrass, ^Tmarjoram, ^Toregano, ^Tpeppermint.

T—Apply oils on location, and either use massage or Vita Flex to work them in.

Recipe #1—First start with basil and marjoram on the shoulder to help release any energy blockages. Then use lemongrass on the wrist and oregano on the rotator cup in the shoulder. Next apply marjoram and cypress on the wrist and then cypress on the neck and down to the shoulder. Lastly, apply peppermint from the shoulder down the arm to the wrist then out to the tips of each finger.

***Comments—Make sure it really is carpal tunnel syndrome, because many people who think they have carpal tunnel syndrome (one report says up to 90%) really have problems with muscles in the neck and shoulder that create similar symptoms.

Blend #1—Layer geranium, balsam fir, juniper, peppermint, and sandalwood on the wrist. Apply several times per day for an extended period to give the nerves time to heal.

Personal Care—**Ortho Ease** or **Ortho Sport Massage Oils**. Massage into neck, shoulder, and wrist. Prenolone/Prenolone+ / Progessence/Progessence Plus (on shoulder and wrist).

Supplements—BLM, Mineral Essence, Sulfurzyme, Super Cal.

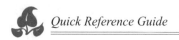

Cataracts: *See Eyes.*

Catarrh (Mucus): *See Anticatarrhal, Congestion.*

Cavities: *See Oral Conditions.*

Celibacy (vow not to marry):

Oils—**A**Marjoram.

A—Diffuse into the air. Inhale directly or applied to tissue or to a cotton wick.

Cells:

Oils—All essential oils restore cells to original state. Need to change the RNA and DNA to change the habit.

Supplements—NingXia Red (nutrients promote cellular health).

—**DNA (CELL CHEMISTRY)**

»» *DNA is the genetic material of the cell. DNA contains all of the codes that enable the cell to build the materials needed for proper cell structure and function. Mutation of DNA can lead to cell death or to cancer.*

Supplements— Master Formula, MultiGreens, Super B, Thyromin.

—**FREQUENCY**

Oils—**AT**Rose (enhances frequency of every cell, which brings balance and harmony to body).

—**LIVER**

Oils—**TA**Helichrysum (stimulates cell function).

—**OXYGENATION**

Oils—**AT**Black pepper.

—**REGULATING**

Oils—**AT**Clary sage (removes negative programming).

—**RNA (CELL MEMORY)**

»» *Ribonucleic acid (RNA) is a molecule similar to DNA. RNA is transcribed from DNA and is used in the production of proteins, as well as in regulating gene expression of the DNA*

–**STIMULATES**

Oils—**AT**<u>Abundance</u>.

T—Dilute as necessary, and apply to area of concern. Dilute with V-6 Oil, and massage on location.

A—Diffuse into the air. Inhale directly or applied to cupped hands, tissue, or a cotton wick.

Cellulite: *See also Weight.*

>> *Cellulite refers to deposits of fat under the skin of the thighs, abdomen, and buttocks that cause the skin to appear dimpled.*

Try flavoring 1 gallon of water with 5 drops grapefruit and 5 drops lemon. Adjust to taste, and drink. This may also improve energy levels.

Oils—ᵀ_F Grapefruit, ᵀ_F cedarwood, ᵀ_F rosemary, ᵀbasil, ᵀcumin, ᵀcypress, ᵀfennel, ᵀgeranium, ᵀjuniper, ᵀlavender, ᵀlemon, ᵀlime, ᵀorange, ᵀoregano, ᵀpatchouli, ᵀrosewood, ᵀsage, ᵀspikenard (increases metabolism to burn fat), ᵀtangerine (dissolves), ᵀthyme. *Refer to the chapter entitled "How to Use—The Personal Usage Reference" in the* Essential Oils Desk Reference *under "Cellulite" for some excellent blend recipes and recommendations.*

Supplements—Allerzyme (aids the digestion of sugars, starches, fats, and proteins), Digest + Cleanse, Power Meal (eat for breakfast).

—**ATTACKS FAT AND CELLULITE**

Oils—ᵀGrapefruit, ᵀbasil, ᵀlavender, ᵀlemongrass, ᵀrosemary, ᵀsage, ᵀthyme.

Personal Care—Cel-Lite Magic (add grapefruit to increase activity and to dissolve cellulite even faster).

Chakras (Energy Centers): *(Refer to the chart at the end of the Science and Application section of the* Reference Guide for Essential Oils.*)*

Oils—ᵀᴬHarmony (apply 1 drop on each chakra to open the energy centers and to balance the electrical field of the chakras, starting at the base chakra located on the coccyx at the end of the spinal column and working up), ᵀᴬlavender (brings harmony to chakras), ᵀᴬrosemary (opens chakras), ᵀᴬsandalwood (affects each chakra differently).

—**UNITES HEAD AND HEART**

Oils—ᵀᴬHelichrysum.

—**ANGELIC CHAKRA (#8—LOCATED ABOVE THE CROWN OF THE HEAD)**

Oils—ᵀᴬAngelica, ᵀᴬneroli.

—**CROWN CHAKRA (#7)**

Oils—ᵀᴬ3 Wise Men (to replace void with good/positives), ᵀᴬangelica (links 7-8, 7-1), ᵀᴬbasil, ᵀᴬcistus, ᵀᴬfrankincense (links 1-7), ᵀᴬlavender, ᵀᴬmyrrh, ᵀᴬonycha, ᵀᴬravintsara, ᵀᴬrose, ᵀᴬrosemary, ᵀᴬrosewood (links 7-1), ᵀᴬsandalwood (links 7-1), ᵀᴬspikenard, ᵀᴬspruce.

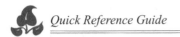

–BALANCE

    Oils—^{TA}<u>Highest Potential</u>.

–OPEN

    Oils—^{TA}<u>Forgiveness</u>, ^{TA}<u>Harmony</u>.

—BROW CHAKRA (3RD EYE -#6)

    Oils—^{TA}<u>Acceptance</u>, ^{TA}<u>Awaken</u>, and ^{TA}<u>Dream Catcher</u> (rub on lobe of ear to increase vision and spiritual vision); ^{TA}cedar leaf (western red cedar), ^{TA}cedarwood, ^{TA}clary sage, ^{TA}frankincense, ^{TA}<u>Harmony</u>, ^{TA}helichrysum, ^{TA}juniper, ^{TA}mugwort, ^{TA}palo santo, ^{TA}peppermint, ^{TA}pine, ^{TA}rose, ^{TA}rosemary, ^{TA}spruce, ^{TA}thymes, ^{TA}<u>Transformation</u>, ^{TA}tsuga.

  –OPEN

    Oils—^{TA}Frankincense, ^{TA}<u>Harmony</u>.

—THROAT CHAKRA (#5)

    Oils—^{TA}Carrot seed, ^{TA}chamomile (Roman and German), ^{TA}cypress, ^{TA}frankincense, ^{TA}geranium, ^{TA}lavender, ^{TA}rose geranium, ^{TA}sandalwood, ^{TA}spearmint, ^{TA}spruce.

  –OPEN

    Oils—^{TA}<u>Harmony</u>.

—HEART CHAKRA (#4)

    Oils—^{TA}Bergamot, ^{TA}carrot seed, ^{TA}cinnamon bark, ^{TA}frankincense, ^{TA}helichrysum, ^{TA}hyssop, ^{TA}inula, ^{TA}laurel, ^{TA}lavandin, ^{TA}lavender, ^{TA}marjoram, ^{TA}melissa, ^{TA}neroli, ^{TA}onycha, ^{TA}oregano, ^{TA}pepper (black), ^{TA}rose, sage, ^{TA}sandalwood, ^{TA}spikenard, ^{TA}tansy.

  –OPENS A CLOSED HEART

    Oils—^{TA}Bergamot, ^{TA}<u>Harmony</u>.

—SOLAR PLEXUS CHAKRA (#3)

    Oils—^{TA}Calamus, ^{TA}cardamom, ^{TA}carrot seed, ^{TA}cedarwood, ^{TA}cinnamon bark, ^{TA}citronella, ^{TA}fennel, ^{TA}ginger, ^{TA}juniper, ^{TA}lemon, ^{TA}lemongrass, ^{TA}melissa, ^{TA}pepper (black), ^{TA}peppermint, ^{TA}rosemary, ^{TA}spikenard, ^{TA}thymes (all chemotypes), ^{TA}valerian, ^{TA}vetiver, ^{TA}ylang ylang.

  –OPEN

    Oils—^{TA}<u>Harmony</u>.

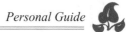

—Sacral Chakra (Sex/Navel -#2)

Oils—^TA^Cassia, ^TA^cinnamon bark, ^TA^clary sage, ^TA^coriander, ^TA^cypress, ^TA^geranium, ^TA^rose geranium, ^TA^jasmine, ^TA^myrrh, ^TA^niaouli, ^TA^patchouli, ^TA^petitgrain, ^TA^pine, ^TA^rose, ^TA^sandalwood, ^TA^tangerine, ^TA^vetiver, ^TA^ylang ylang.

–Balance

Oils—^TA^<u>Acceptance</u> (balances Sacral Chakra which stores denial and sexual abuse), ^TA^sage.

–Open

Oils—^TA^<u>Harmony</u>.

—Base Chakra (Root -#1)

Oils—^TA^Cardamom, ^TA^carrot seed, ^TA^cedar leaf (western red cedar), ^TA^cedarwood, ^TA^clove, ^TA^frankincense, ^TA^ginger, ^TA^laurel, ^TA^myrrh, ^TA^onycha, ^TA^patchouli, ^TA^pepper (black), ^TA^peppermint, ^TA^sandalwood, ^TA^vetiver.

–Open

Oils—^TA^<u>Harmony</u>.

T—Dilute as necessary, and apply on chakras or as indicated. Dilute with V-6 Oil, and massage on chakras.

A—Inhale directly. Diffuse into the air.

Change (Personal): *See also Emotions.*

Oils—^AT^<u>Forgiveness</u>, ^AT^<u>Into the Future</u>, ^AT^<u>Joy</u>, ^AT^<u>Magnify Your Purpose</u>, ^AT^<u>Sacred Mountain</u>, ^AT^<u>3 Wise Men</u>, ^AT^<u>Transformation</u>.

A—Diffuse into the air. Inhale directly or applied to hands, tissue, or a cotton wick.

T—Apply to auricular emotional points.

Charley Horse: *See also Muscles: Spasms.*

Oils—^T^<u>Aroma Siez</u>, ^T^basil, ^T^<u>Deep Relief</u> (roll-on).

T—Dilute as necessary, and apply on location. Dilute with V-6 Oil, and massage on location.

Personal Care—Prenolone/Prenolone+, Progessence/Progessence Plus.

Cheeks:

Oils—^T^Jasmine.

T—Dilute as necessary, and apply on location. Dilute with V-6 Oil, and massage on location

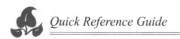

Blend #1—5 drops <u>Aroma Siez</u>, 3 drops wintergreen, and 3 drops spruce. Work oils between hands in a clockwise motion, and pat on cheeks. Cup hands over nose and inhale.

Personal Care—A·R·T Skin Care System, A·R·T Purifying Toner, A·R·T Beauty Masque.

Chelation: *See also Detoxification:* METALS.

Oils—^{TA}Helichrysum, ^{TA}<u>Aroma Life</u>, ^{TA}cardamom, (powerful chelator and anticoagulant).

T—Dilute as necessary, and apply on feet and on liver area.

A—Diffuse into the air. Inhale directly.

*****Comments**—Drink lots of distilled water.

> *Traditional intravenous chelation therapy can cause scar tissue on the vascular walls. These oils, supplements, and tinctures provide a more natural approach to chelation. They may take longer to achieve the same results but with minimal side effects.*

Personal Care—Cel-Lite Magic.

Supplements—Cleansing Trio (ComforTone, Essentialzyme, and ICP), MultiGreens (use with cardamom), Rehemogen Tincture.

*****Comments**—The apple pectin that is contained in ICP helps remove unwanted metals and toxins from the body.

Chemicals: *See Metals.*

Oils—^T_FHelichrysum.

T—Dilute as necessary, and apply on feet and on liver area.

Chicken Pox: *See Childhood Diseases.*

Chiggers: *See Insect.*

Childbirth: *See Pregnancy/Motherhood.*

Childhood Diseases:

—CHICKEN POX (2 WEEKS)—SLEEP IS VERY GOOD. *See also Antiviral, Shingles.*

 ⯈⯈ *Chickenpox is a common childhood illness caused by the virus Varicella zoster (which is also responsible for shingles). Symptoms of chickenpox include mild fever, weakness, and a rash. The rash appears as red spots that form into blisters that eventually burst and then crust over. Chickenpox is highly contagious and can be contracted by anyone, but it is most common in children under the age of 15.*

 Oils—^TLavender, ^{TA}tea tree, ^T<u>Australian Blue</u>, ^Abergamot, ^Teucalyptus, ^TRoman chamomile, ^Tsage lavender.

Bath—(relieves the itching) 2 drops lavender, 1 cup bicarbonate of soda, and 1 cup soda in bath; soak.

Blend #1—5 to 10 drops each of German chamomile and lavender to 1 ounce Calamine lotion. Mix and apply twice a day all over body.

Blend #2—10 drops lavender, 10 drops Roman chamomile, and 4 oz. Calamine lotion. Mix and apply twice a day all over body.

Blend #3—Add enough ravintsara to some green clay (from health food store) to form a paste that can be dabbed on the pox to relieve itching.

Diffuse—an antiviral oil (such as lemon), and apply the same oil all over the body twice a day.

—Measles

>> *Measles is a viral infection of the respiratory system that causes coughing, runny nose, red eyes, fever, and a rash on the skin.*

Oils—**AT**_FEucalyptus, **AT**tea tree, **AT**German chamomile, **AT**lavender.

–German (3 Day)—use antiviral oils. *See Antiviral.*

–Rubella

Recipe #1—Sponge down with one of these oils: chamomile (Roman or German), lavender, tea tree.

—Mumps

>> *Mumps is a viral infection that causes fever, chills, headache, and painful swelling of the saliva glands.*

Oils—**TA**Tea tree, **TA**lemon, **TA**lavender, **TA**eucalyptus radiata[197].

—Whooping Cough

>> *Whooping cough, or pertussis, is a bacterial infection that causes cold-like symptoms, followed by severe coughing fits.*

Oils—**AT**_FOregano, **AT**basil, **AT**cinnamon bark (diffuse, or dilute well; avoid for children), **AT**clary sage, **AT**cypress, **AT**grapefruit, **AT**hyssop, **AT**lavender, **AT**thyme.

Diffuse—Basil, eucalyptus, lavender, tea tree, peppermint, Roman chamomile, rose, thyme.

T—Dilute as necessary, and apply on location or on chest, throat, and Vita Flex points. Use a hot compress for deeper penetration. Add 1–2 drops to 1 quart warm water, and use water for a sponge bath.

A—Diffuse into the air.

Children/Infants: *See also Childhood Diseases, Hyperactive.*

Oils—[TA]Bite Buster, [AT]GeneYus, [TA]Owie, [AT]SleepyIze, [AT]SniffleEase, [AT]TummyGize.

Personal Care—KidScents Bath Gel, KidScents Lotion, KidScents Shampoo, KidScents Tender Tush, KidScents Toothpaste.

Supplements—KidScents MightyVites (chewable vitamin tablets), Life 5 (probiotic; for older children), NingXia Red.

—BONDING

> Oils—[T]Gentle Baby

> **T**—One drop gently rubbed on baby's feet and another drop or two brushed on mom's hair and aura—open palms skimming body surface, head to foot).

—COLIC

>> *Colic is any extended period of crying and fussiness that occurs frequently in an infant. While the exact cause is not known, it has been speculated that the cause may be from indigestion, the build-up of gas, lactose intolerance, or a lack of needed probiotic bacteria in the intestines.*

> Oils— [AT]TummyGize [T]Fennel[198], [T]German chamomile[199], [T]melissa[199], [T,F]marjoram, [T]angelica, [T]bergamot, [T]cardamom, [T]carrot (with fennel), [T]coriander, [T]cumin, [T]dill, [T]ginger, [T]orange, [T]peppermint, [T]Roman chamomile, [T]rosemary, [T]spearmint, [T]ylang ylang.

When using essential oils on babies and children, it is always best to dilute 1–2 drops of pure essential oil with ½–1 tsp. V-6 Oil. If the oils are used in the bath, always use a bath gel base as a dispersing agent for the oils.

Keep the oils out of children's reach. *If an oil is ever ingested, give the child an oil-soluble liquid such as milk, cream, or half & half. Then call your local poison control center or seek emergency medical attention. A few drops of pure essential oil shouldn't be life-threatening, but for your protection, it is best to take these precautions.*

In Shirley Price's book, Aromatherapy for Babies and Children, she mentions twenty oils that are safe for children. Nineteen of them are oils with the same botanical names as those mentioned in this book. These oils are:

Bergamot (Citrus bergamia)*
Cedarwood (Cedrus atlantica)**
Chamomile, Roman (Chamaemelum nobile),
Cypress (Cupressus sempervirens)
Frankincense (Boswellia carterii)
Geranium (Pelargonium graveolens)
Ginger (Zingiber officinale)
Lavender (Lavandula angustifolia)
Lemon (Citrus limon)*
Mandarin (Citrus reticulata)*
Marjoram (Origanum marjorana)
Melaleuca–Tea Tree (Melaleuca alternifolia)
Orange (Citrus aurantium)*
Rose Otto (Rosa damascena)
Rosemary (Rosmarinus officinalis)**
Rosewood (Aniba rosaeodora)
Sandalwood (Santalum album)
Thyme (Thymus vulgaris CT linalol)
Ylang Ylang (Cananga odorata)

*These oils are photosensitive; always dilute. To prevent a rash or pigmentation of the skin, do not use citrus oils when exposed to direct sunlight.

**These oils should never be used undiluted on babies and children.

Caution: *Do not use synthetic or adulterated oils. Do not use oils with different botanical names until the safety data has been thoroughly reviewed.*

T—Dilute 1–2 drops in 2 Tbs. V-6 Oil, and massage a small amount of this blend gently on stomach and back.

Blend #1—Combine 2 Tbs. almond oil with 1 drop Roman chamomile, 1 drop lavender, and 1 drop geranium. Mix and apply to stomach and back.

***Comments**—*Burping the baby and keeping the abdomen warm with a warm water bottle will often bring relief.*

—COMMON COLD

Oils—^{AT}<u>SniffleEase</u>, ^{AT}Thyme, ^{AT}lemon, ^{AT}cedarwood, ^{AT}Tea tree ericifolia, ^{AT}rosemary, ^{AT}rose, ^{AT}sandalwood.

A—Diffuse into the air.

T—Dilute 1–2 drops of oil in 2 Tbs. V-6 Oil, and massage a little on neck and chest.

Blend #2—Combine 2 Tbs. V-6 Oil with 2 drops tea tree (tea tree), 1 drop lemon, and 1 drop rose otto. Massage a little of the blend on the neck and chest.

—CONSTIPATION

Oils— ^{AT}<u>TummyGize</u> ^TRosemary²⁰⁰, ^Tginger, ^Tmandarin, ^Torange.

T—Dilute one of the oils in V-6 Oil, and massage stomach and feet.

—CRADLE CAP REMEDY

➤➤ *Cradle cap is a yellowish scaling of the skin on the head that commonly occurs in young infants. The scaling is yellowish in color and often disappears by the time the infant is a few months old.*

Blend #3—Combine 2 Tbs. almond oil with 1 drop lemon and 1 drop geranium or with 1 drop cedarwood and 1 drop sandalwood. Mix and apply a small amount on head.

—CROUP

➤➤ *Croup is a viral respiratory infection that causes inflammation of the area around the larynx (voice box) and a distinctive-sounding cough. Often, taking an infant or child outside to breath cool night air can help open the restricted airways, as can humidity.*

Oils—^{AT}<u>SniffleEase</u>, ^{AT}Marjoram, ^{AT}thyme, ^{AT}ravintsara, ^{AT}rosewood, ^{AT}sandalwood.

A—Diffuse into the air.

T—Dilute 1–2 drops in 2 Tbs. V-6 Oil. Massage.

—CRYING

Oils—^{AT}<u>SleepyIze</u>, ^{AT}Ylang ylang, ^{AT}lavender, ^{AT}Roman chamomile, ^{AT}cypress, ^{AT}frankincense, ^{AT}geranium,^{AT} rose otto.

A—Diffuse into the air.

T—Dilute 1–2 drops in 2 Tbs. V-6 Oil. Massage.

—Cuts/Scrapes

Oils—**ᵀᴬ**<u>Owie</u>.

T—Apply around location.

—Diaper Rash

≫ *Diaper rash is a red rash of the skin in the diaper area caused by prolonged skin exposure to the moisture and different pH of urine and feces. Often, more frequent bathing of the area and more frequent diaper changes will help alleviate the rash.*

Oils—**ᵀᴬ**<u>Owie</u>, **ᵀ**ₓLavender.

T—Dilute 1–2 drops in 2 Tbs. V-6 Oil, and apply a small amount on location.

Blend #4—Combine 1 drop Roman chamomile and 1 drop lavender with V-6 Oil or Genesis Hand & Body Lotion. Apply.

Personal Care—KidScents Tender Tush (formulated specifically for diaper rash), Rose Ointment.

—Digestion (sluggish)

Oils— **ᴬᵀ**<u>TummyGize</u>, **ᵀ**Lemon, **ᵀ**orange.

T—Dilute 1–2 drops in 2 Tbs. V-6 Oil. Massage on feet and stomach.

—Dry Skin

Oils—**ᵀᴬ**<u>Owie</u>, **ᵀ**Rosewood, **ᵀ**sandalwood.

T—Dilute 1–2 drops in 2 Tbs. V-6 Oil, and apply a small amount on location.

—Earache

Oils—**ᵀ**Tea tree, **ᵀ**lavender, **ᵀ**Tea tree ericifolia, **ᵀ**Roman chamomile, **ᵀ**thyme (sweet).

T—Put a diluted drop of oil on a cotton ball, and place the cotton ball in the ear; rub a little bit of diluted oil behind the ear.

Blend #5—Combine 2 Tbs. V-6 Oil with 2 drops lavender, 1 drop Roman chamomile, and 1 drop tea tree. Put a drop on a cotton ball, and put cotton ball in ear; rub oil behind the ear and on the ear Vita Flex feet points.

Other—Garlic oil works great too, but it is stinky!

—Fever

Oils—**ᴬᵀ**<u>SniffleEase</u>, **ᵀ**Lavender, **ᴬ**peppermint.

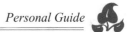

    T—Dilute in V-6 Oil, and massage baby (back of neck, feet, behind ears, etc.).

    A—Diffuse into the air.

—FLU

    » *Flu, or influenza, is a viral infection that affects the respiratory system. Symptoms may include coughing, sneezing, fever, runny nose, congestion, muscle aches, nausea, and vomiting.*

    Oils—^{AT}SniffleEase

    Recipe #1—Cypress, lemon, *Tea tree ericifolia*. Dilute 1 drop of each in 1 Tbs. bath gel for a bath; diffuse.

—HICCOUGHS/HICCUPS

    Oils—^{AT}TummyGize, ^AMandarin.

    A—Diffuse into the air.

—HYPERACTIVE

    Oils—^{AT}GeneYus, ^APeace & Calming, ^ACitrus Fresh, ^ATrauma Life.

    A—Diffuse into the air.

—INSECT REPELLENT

    Oils—^{TA}Bite Buster.

    A—Diffuse into the air.

    T—Apply a small amount on skin and on clothing.

—JAUNDICE

    » *Jaundice is a condition where the liver cannot clear the pigment bilirubin quickly enough from the blood, causing the blood to deposit the bilirubin into the skin and whites of the eyes, turning them a yellowish color.*

    Oils—^TGeranium, ^Tlemon, ^Tlime, ^Tmandarin, ^Trosemary.

    T—Dilute, and apply on the liver area and on the liver Vita Flex feet points.

—PREMATURE

    Oils—Since premature babies have very thin and sensitive skin, it is best to avoid the use of essential oils.

—RASHES

    Oils—^{TA}Owie, ^TLavender, ^TRoman chamomile, ^Trose, ^Tsandalwood.

    T—Dilute in V-6 Oil, and apply a small amount on location.

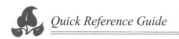

—S**LEEP**

    Oils—^AT^<u>SleepyIze</u>, ^TA^<u>Peace & Calming</u>.

    A—Diffuse into the air or mist on bedding.

    T—Dilute, and apply a small amount to feet.

—T**EETH** G**RINDING**

    Oils—^AT^<u>GeneYus</u>, ^T^Lavender, ^AT^<u>SleepyIze</u>, ^TA^<u>Peace & Calming</u>.

    T—Dilute, and apply a small amount to feet.

    A—Diffuse into the air.

—T**EETHING**

    Oils—^T^Lavender, ^T^German chamomile, ^T^ginger, ^T^marjoram, ^T^tea tree.

    T—Dilute, and apply a small amount to feet.

—T**ONSILLITIS**

    »» *Tonsillitis is inflammation of the tonsils, two lymph-filled tissues located at the back of the mouth that help provide immune support. These may become inflamed due to a bacterial or viral infection.*

    Oils—^AT^<u>SniffleEase</u>, ^T^Tea tree, ^T^lemon, ^T^ginger, ^T^lavender, ^T^Roman chamomile.

    T—Dilute 1–2 drops in 2 Tbs. V-6 Oil, and apply a small amount to tonsils and to lymph nodes.

—T**HRUSH** *See also Antifungal*

    »» *Thrush is an oral fungal infection caused by Candida albicans. It causes painful white-colored areas to appear in the mouth.*

    Oils—^T^Tea tree[201], ^T^lavender[202], ^T^thyme[203], ^TA^<u>Owie</u>, ^T^geranium, ^T^lemon, ^T^Tea tree ericifolia, ^T^rosewood.

    T—Dilute 1–2 drops essential oil in 2 Tbs. V-6 Oil, and apply a small amount on location.

    Blend #3—2 Tbs. garlic oil, 8 drops lavender, 8 drops *Tea tree ericifolia*, 1 ml (1 softgel) vitamin E oil. Apply to nipples just before nursing, or apply with a clean finger into baby's mouth. Also try Animal Scents Pet Ointment.

*****Comments**—Besides <u>Gentle Baby</u> listed under Bonding, no other commercial blends are listed in this section because many of them contain oils that are not recommended for babies. The author's admit that they have used many of the commercial blends mentioned in this book on their babies and children with great success and no side effects. We are careful, however, to use only a couple drops at a time, diluted in V-6 Oil, and only for external application. Also, we do not continue applications for any extended period of time.

Chills:

Oils—ᵀGinger, ᵀonycha (benzoin), ᵀsage lavender.

T—Dilute as necessary, and apply to bottoms of feet and to solar plexus.

C

Chlorophyll:

Supplements—MultiGreens.

Cholera: *See also Antibacterial.*

⟫ *Cholera is a potentially severe bacterial infection of the intestines by the Vibrio cholerae bacteria. This infection can cause severe diarrhea, leading to dehydration that can cause low blood pressure, shock, or death. Rehydration with an oral rehydration solution is the most effective way to prevent dehydration. If no commercially prepared oral rehydration solution is available, a solution made from 1 tsp. salt, 8 tsp. sugar, and 1 liter clean water (with some mashed fresh banana, if available, to add potassium) can work in an emergency.*

Oils—ᵀᴬ_F_Ravintsara, ᵀᴬ_F_rosemary, ᵀᴬclove.

T—Dilute as necessary, and massage gently over stomach and kidney area.

A—Diffuse into the air. Inhale directly.

Cholesterol:

⟫ *Cholesterol is an important lipid that comprises part of the cell membrane and myelin sheath and that plays a role in nerve cell function. It is created by the body and can be found in many foods we eat. An imbalance of certain types of cholesterol in the blood has been theorized to play a role in the formation of plaques in the arteries (atherosclerosis).*

Oils—ᵀᴵLemongrass (clinically shown to help lower cholesterol)[204], ᵀ_F_clary sage, ᵀ_F_helichrysum (regulates), ᴬᵀlavender[205], ᵀᴵdill[206].

Supplements—MultiGreens, Master Formula.

T—Apply on Vita Flex points, over heart, and along arms.

I—Add 3–5 drops to an empty capsule, and swallow.

A—Diffuse into the air. Inhale directly.

Chorea: *See Saint Vitus' Dance.*

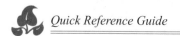

Chronic Fatigue: *See also Acidosis, Hormonal Imbalance.*

▸▸ *Chronic fatigue syndrome refers to a set of debilitating symptoms that may include prolonged periods of fatigue that are not alleviated by rest, difficulty concentrating, muscle and joint pain, headaches, and sore throats that cannot be explained by any other known medical condition. While the exact cause of chronic fatigue syndrome is not known, some have theorized that it is caused by a virus (such as the Epstein-Barr virus) left in the body after an illness.*

> *Chronic Fatigue is often caused by the Epstein-Barr virus. It may also be a result of chemical and metal toxicity or of conditions of high acidity.*
>
> *Women who are pregnant seldom have Chronic Fatigue Syndrome because of the higher amounts of natural progesterone being produced.*

Oils—TAThieves, TAbasil, TApeppermint, TAClarity, TADi-Gize, TAImmuPower, TAlavender, TAlemongrass, TArosemary, TATransformation.

T—Dilute as necessary, and apply to sore muscles or joints, to the back, or to the feet. Add 1–2 drops to warm bathwater, and bathe. Combine any of these oils with the Raindrop Technique.

A—Diffuse into the air. Inhale directly or applied to hands, tissue, or to a cotton wick.

***Comments—Basil and peppermint are a good combination together.

Supplements—NingXia Red, AlkaLime (acid-neutralizing mineral), Balance Complete *(refer to the 5-Day Nutritive Cleanse program listed under Balance Complete in the Supplements section of the Reference Guide for Essential Oils. This program also uses Digest + Cleanse and NingXia Red to help enhance detoxification while maintaining/increasing energy levels)*, Cleansing Trio (ComforTone, Essentialzyme, and ICP), Digest + Cleanse, ImmuPro, Inner Defense, Life 5 (probiotic), Longevity Capsules, Master Formula, Mineral Essence, MultiGreens, Power Meal, and Super Cal.

Personal Care—Prenolone/Prenolone+, Progessence/Progessence Plus.

Dr. Friedmann uses the following recipe on his patients:

Recipe #1—1) Use the Cleansing Trio (ComforTone, Essentialzyme, and ICP) to detoxify. 2) Build the body and tissues with Mineral Essence and Master Formula. 3) Build the immune system with ImmuPower and ImmuPro.

Cigarettes: *See Smoking.*

Circulation: *See Cardiovascular System: CIRCULATION.*

Circulatory System: *See Cardiovascular System.*

Cirrhosis: *See Liver.*

Clarity of Thoughts:

Oils—^AClarity, ^Arosemary, ^ATransformation.

A—Diffuse into the air. Inhale directly or applied to hands.

Cleansing: *See also Housecleaning.*

Oils—^TADi-Gize (when cramping), ^TAfennel, ^TAhyssop, ^TAjuniper, ^Atea tree, ^TAMelrose, ^TRelease (over liver),^TA 3 Wise Men (when trauma—put on liver to let emotions go).

> *Cleansing may help to prevent disease, improve immune function, and make the body stronger. It may also cause an emotional cleansing. DRINK LOTS OF WATER! A child of any age can go on a cleanse. Gary Young suggests that you spend two days cleansing for every year old you are. He recommends that you take ICP and Essentialzyme five days a week and fast once a week on distilled water and lemon juice.*

C

T—Dilute as necessary, and apply on location.
Apply over liver area.

A—Diffuse into the air. Inhale directly or applied to hands, tissue, or a cotton wick.

—BODY CLEANSE

Supplements—**Balance Complete** (*refer to the 5-Day Nutritive Cleanse program listed under Balance Complete in the Supplements section of the Reference Guide for Essential Oils. This program also uses Digest + Cleanse and NingXia Red to help enhance detoxification while maintaining energy levels*), **Cleansing Trio (ComforTone, Essentialzyme, and ICP), Digest + Cleanse.** The oils contained in the Cleansing Trio will push heavy metals into the system; use Sacred Mountain and Peace & Calming to balance the system. If colon is blocked, start with ComforTone to open it. JuvaTone is the final stage of cleansing and can be taken as often as four times a day. **Rehemogen Tincture** supports the body during a cleanse.

—CUTS

Oils—^TElemi, ^Tlavender, ^TMelrose.

T—Dilute as necessary, and apply on location.

—MASTER CLEANSER OR LEMONADE DIET

2 Tbs. fresh lemon or lime juice (approx. ½ lemon), 2 Tbs. of grade B maple syrup (grade A is not as rich in nutrients but can be used if grade B is not available). 1/10 tsp. cayenne pepper or to taste (cayenne is a thermal warmer and dilates

> *Lemon converts to alkaline in the body. Lemons can be harmful to teeth only when in water that is not distilled because there can be a reaction with the minerals in the water. Toxins are eliminated from the bowels and bladder. Drink 6 to 12 glasses of the lemonade drink daily. When you get hungry, just drink another glass of lemonade. No other food or vitamins should be taken; the lemonade is already a food in liquid form. An herbal laxative tea may be used to help elimination. More details can be found in the book by Tom Woloshyn, The Complete Master Cleanse. It will take 30 days on lemon to change the chemistry in the body. We have to change the DNA and RNA (memory or belief system) to change a habit. Then, do 30 days on carrot juice.*

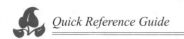
the blood vessels; also has vitamin A). Combine above ingredients in a 10 oz. glass of distilled water. No substitute sugars. In the case of diabetes, use black strap molasses instead of the maple syrup. Drink between three quarts and a gallon of this lemonade each day with an herbal laxative tea first thing in the morning and just before retiring for the night. Refer to the book *The Complete Master Cleanse* for more specific details including suggestions and specific instructions for coming off the cleanse.

Closed Minded:

Oils—^{AT}Awaken, ^{AT}Inspiration.

A—Diffuse into the air. Inhale directly or applied to hands, tissue, or a cotton wick.

T—Apply to auricular emotional points. Dilute with V-6 Oil, and massage into skin.

Clothes:

Recipe #1—Western red cedar. Place a few drops on a cotton ball, and put it in a plastic sack. Leave the sack open so the odor of the oil can do its work without it staining any clothes. Place the bag in a closet or storage box.

Cockroaches: *See Insects:* Cockroaches.

Coffee (Stop Drinking): *See also Addictions. (See the case study on the body's frequency reaction to coffee in the Science and Application section of the Reference Guide for Essential Oils).*

Oils—^APeace & Calming, ^APurification.

A—Inhale directly or applied to the hands. Diffuse into the air.

Supplements—JuvaTone.

Colds: *See also Antiviral, Coughs, Congestion.*

Oils—^{AT}_FTea tree, ^{AT}_Flemon, ^{AT-}Thieves, ^{AT}_Frosemary, ^{AT}thyme, ^{AT}Raven, ^{AT}ravintsara, ^{AT}RC (put a few drops in a box of tissue), ^Ahinoki, ^{AT}angelica, ^{AT}Australian Blue, ^{AT}basil, ^{AT}blue cypress (aches and pains), ^{AT}cajeput, ^{AT}copaiba, ^{AT}eucalyptus (in hot water, breathe deep), ^{AT}Exodus II, ^{AT}fir (aches and pains),

> *It seems that because we live in the South there are a lot of "stuffy noses" in the spring and fall. When I have a client in my business complaining of these types of symptoms, I offer them some oils to sniff for relief. I offer a drop of peppermint first and then a drop of RC blend. Then, if they have used the word "infection," I offer a drop of Thieves blend. I offer one drop of each in the palm of their hand, one at a time. Then I show them how to stir 3 times and cup their hands over the nose and deeply inhale each oil. They are always amazed at the immediate relief.*
>
> *–Submitted by Pam Jones*
> *Benton, Arkansas (July 2004)*

^AT^ginger, ^AT^Idaho tansy, ^AT^lavender, ^AT^ledum, ^AT^myrtle, ^AT^onycha (benzoin), ^AT^orange, ^AT^oregano, ^AT^peppermint (relieves nasal congestion), ^AT^pine, ^AT^sage lavender.

A—Diffuse into the air. Place 1–2 drops in a bowl of hot water, and inhale the vapors. Inhale directly or applied to the hands, tissue, or a cotton wick.

T—Dilute as necessary, and apply 1–2 drops to the throat, temples, forehead, back of neck, sinus area, below the nose, to chest, or to the Vita Flex Points on the feet.

Recipe #1—Apply <u>Raven</u> to the back and <u>RC</u> to the chest with <u>Thieves</u> on the feet. For the next application, rotate <u>Raven</u> and <u>RC</u>. Other oils can be diffused or applied to the forehead, temples, back of neck, and chest. *Refer to the chapter entitled "How to Use—The Personal Usage Reference" in the <u>Essential Oils Desk Reference</u> under "Colds and Flu" for some excellent recipes and supplement recommendations. Also, refer to Comments under Asthma in this book for a discussion on using* **plastic nasal inhalers**.

Blend #1—Mix 6 drops <u>RC</u> and 2 drops ravintsara. Apply to the chest, neck, throat, and sinus area. Diffuse, or put 4 drops in a half cup of hot water; then place nose and mouth over the opening of the cup (not in the water) and breathe deeply.

Supplements—Thieves Lozenges.

***Comments—Dr. Pénoël recommends applying a trace of *Melaleuca alternifolia* to the tip of the tongue and swallowing. This works best when done immediately upon noticing a sore throat. Repeat every minute until the throat feels better. Then apply it behind the ears and down under the jaw line. After repeating this a few times (every 5–10 minutes), massage a couple drops on the back of the neck to relieve any blockage.

Cold Sores: *See also Herpes Simplex.*

Oils—^T^<u>Australian Blue</u>, ^T^tea tree, ^T^melissa, ^T^peppermint, ^T^bergamot, ^T^blue cypress, ^T^geranium, ^T^lavender, ^T^lemon, ^T^<u>Melrose</u> (fights infection), ^T^<u>RC</u>, ^T^Roman chamomile, ^T^<u>Thieves</u>.

Colic: *See Children/Infants: Colic.*

Colitis: *See Colon: Colitis.*

Colon: *See also Diverticulitis.*

≫ *The colon, or large intestine, is the last part of the digestive system. Its function is to extract water and vitamins created by friendly bacterial flora from the material moving through the digestive system.*

Oils—^IT^<u>Di-Gize</u>, ^IT^peppermint, ^T^calamus (may help reduce inflammation), ^T^<u>Release</u>.

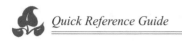
Supplements—Balance Complete (*refer to the 5-Day Nutritive Cleanse program listed under Balance Complete in the Supplements section of the <u>Reference Guide for Essential Oils</u>. This program also uses Digest + Cleanse and NingXia Red to help enhance detoxification while maintaining energy levels.*), Cleansing Trio (ComforTone, Essentialzyme, and ICP), Digest + Cleanse, JuvaPower/JuvaSpice, Life 5 (probiotic). *Refer to the Supplements section of the <u>Reference Guide for Essential Oils</u> for specific usages.*

—COLITIS

➤➤ *Colitis is inflammation of the large intestine or colon. The exact cause is not known, but it may involve an autoimmune response. Symptoms can include abdominal pain, tenderness, frequent need to expel stools, diarrhea, and possibly bloody stools and fever in the case of ulcerative colitis.*

Oils—[TA]FHelichrysum (viral), [TA]Ftarragon, [TA]Fthyme (when there is infection)[207], [I]oregano[207], [I]rosemary[208], [TA]anise, [TA]calamus (viral), [TA]clove (bacterial). Redmond clay (from Redmond Minerals 1-800-367-7258) helps clean fecal matter out of pockets in the colon.

Supplements—AlkaLime, Balance Complete (uses 5 different fibers for optimal absorption and cleansing action), Cleansing Trio (ComforTone, Essentialzyme, and ICP), Digest + Cleanse.

—DIVERTICULITIS

➤➤ *Diverticula, sac-like herniations through the muscular wall of the large intestine (colon), are caused by increased pressure in the bowel from constipation. The existence of these sacs that are filled with trapped fecal sludge is called diverticulosis. When they become infected, the rotting feces erodes the surrounding mucosa and blood vessels, and bleeding, rupturing, and infection begins. This is known as diverticulitis.*

Recipe #1—Use Redmond clay (1-800-367-7258) to help remove fecal matter from the pockets. Rub abdomen with cinnamon bark and V-6 Oil. Anise or lavender may also help. Calamus may help with earlier stages of diverticulitis.

Supplements—Balance Complete (*refer to the 5-Day Nutritive Cleanse program listed under Balance Complete in the Supplements section of the <u>Reference Guide for Essential Oils</u>. This program also uses Digest + Cleanse and NingXia Red to help enhance detoxification while maintaining energy levels*), ComforTone to open blocked colon (use daily, increasing dosage by one until bowels are eliminating waste 2–4 times per day), then ICP (fiber beverage) to cleanse colon, and Essentialzyme or Essentialzymes-4, for digestive enzyme support. Digest + Cleanse and JuvaPower/JuvaSpice may also help.

—Polyps *See also Polyps.*

>> *Colon polyps are tumors that arise from the bowel surface and protrude into the inside of the colon. Most polyps eventually transform into malignant cancer tumors.*

   *****Comments**—Cleanse the colon! Stanley Burroughs' Master Cleanse is an ideal cleansing program which affects the entire body. However, if fecal matter is not being eliminated from the colon 2–3 times per day, it may be necessary to start with ComforTone first until bowel movements are more frequent. Then toxins released during the Master Cleanse can be quickly eliminated from the body. (See MASTER CLEANSER under Cleansing)

   Supplements—Cleansing Trio (ComforTone, Essentialzyme, and ICP). *Refer to the Supplements section of the Reference Guide for Essential Oils.*

—Prolapsed Colon—not assimilating

   Supplements—Essentialzyme, Essentialzymes-4.

   *****Comments**—*Stanley Burroughs recommends performing a colon lift and describes the procedure for doing so in his book* Healing for the Age of Enlightenment *on pages 55 to 59.*

—Spastic (has no peristaltic action)

   Supplements—Balance Complete, ComforTone then ICP (fiber beverage).

T—Apply topically with a compress. Dilute as necessary, and apply 1–2 drops on lower abdomen or on Vita Flex points on the feet. Use 1–2 drops in warm bathwater for a bath.

I—Take 2 drops of each in distilled water 1–2 times per day. Use Redmond clay (from Redmond Minerals 1-800-367-7258) to remove fecal matter from pockets in the colon.

A—Diffuse into the air. Inhale directly or applied to the hands, tissue, or a cotton wick.

Coma:

Oils—^TAwaken, ^Tfrankincense,^Tsandalwood, ^TValor, ^Tblack pepper, ^Tcypress, ^THope, ^Tpeppermint, ^TSurrender, ^TTrauma Life.

T—Dilute as necessary, and massage on brain stem area, mastoids (behind ears), temples, and bottoms of feet.

Supplements—Mineral Essence, Ultra Young+.

Comforting:

Oils—^{AT}Gentle Baby.

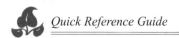

A—Diffuse into the air. Inhale directly or applied to hands, tissue, or a cotton wick.

T—Apply to auricular emotional points. Dilute with V-6 Oil, and massage into skin.

Compassion:

Oils—^{AT}Helichrysum.

A—Diffuse into the air. Inhale directly or applied to hands, tissue, or a cotton wick.

T—Apply to auricular emotional points. Dilute with V-6 Oil, and massage into skin.

Complexion: *See Skin:* COMPLEXION.

Concentration (Poor):

Oils—^ALavender[209], ^Alemon[210], ^Apeppermint, ^A<u>Brain Power</u>, ^A<u>Awaken</u>, ^Abasil, ^Acedarwood, ^A<u>Clarity</u>, ^Acypress, ^A<u>Dream Catcher</u>, ^Aeucalyptus, ^A<u>Gathering</u>, ^Ajuniper, ^Amyrrh, ^Aorange, ^Arosemary, ^Asandalwood, ^A<u>3 Wise Men</u>, ^Aylang ylang.

Supplements— MindWise, Omega Blue, OmegaGize³

Concussion: *See also Brain.*

≫ *A Concussion is a traumatic brain injury that most commonly occurs as a result of a blow to the head. Concussion symptoms include headaches, dizziness, blurred vision, vomiting, disorientation, difficulty focusing attention, ringing in the ears, selective memory loss, etc.*

Oils—^TFrankincense[211], ^Tcypress.

T—Dilute as necessary, and rub on brain stem and bottoms of feet.

*****Comments**—One woman had a concussion with headaches and hallucinations. By applying cypress over her brain stem, her headaches left for good.

Confidence:

Oils—^{AT}Jasmine, ^{AT}<u>Live with Passion</u>, ^{AT}sandalwood (self), ^{AT}<u>Transformation</u>, ^{AT}<u>Valor,</u> ^{AT}<u>Shutran,</u>
^{AT}<u>Oola Friends</u>, ^{TA}<u>Build Your Dream</u>.

A—Diffuse into the air. Inhale directly or applied to hands, tissue, or a cotton wick.

T—Apply to auricular emotional points. Dilute with V-6 Oil, and massage into skin.

Confusion:

Oils—^{AT}<u>Awaken</u>, ^{AT}basil, ^{AT}<u>Brain Power</u>, ^{AT}cedarwood, ^{AT}<u>Clarity</u>, ^{AT}cypress, ^{AT}fir, ^{AT}frankincense, ^{AT}<u>Gathering</u>, ^{AT}geranium, ^{AT}ginger, ^{AT}<u>Harmony</u>, ^{AT}jasmine, ^{AT}juniper, ^{AT}marjoram, ^{AT}peppermint, ^{AT}<u>Present Time</u>, ^{AT}rose, ^{AT}rosemary, ^{AT}rosewood, ^{AT}sandalwood, ^{AT}spruce, ^{AT}thyme, ^{AT}<u>Transformation</u>, ^{AT}<u>Valor</u>, ^{AT}ylang ylang.

A—Diffuse into the air. Inhale directly or applied to hands, tissue, a or a cotton wick.

T—Apply to auricular emotional points. Dilute with V-6 Oil, and massage into skin.

Congestion: *See also Anticatarrhal.*

Oils—^{AT}Eucalyptus[212], ^{AT}Eucalyptus radiata, ^{AT}<u>RC</u>, ^{AT}<u>Di-Gize</u>, ^T<u>Breathe Again</u>, ^{AT}cedarwood, ^{AT}coriander, ^{AT}cypress, ^{AT}<u>Exodus II</u>, ^{AT}fennel, ^{AT}ginger, ^{AT}myrtle (excellent for children), ^{AT}<u>Raven</u>, ^{AT}rosemary.

Personal Care—Cel-Lite Magic.

Supplements—Cleansing Trio (ComforTone, ICP, Essentialzyme), Digest + Cleanse.

—DECONGESTANT

Oils—^{AT}_FCypress, ^{AT}_FGerman chamomile, ^{AT}any of the citrus oils, ^{AT}juniper, ^{AT}tea tree, ^{AT}patchouli.

—EXPECTORANT

Oils—^{AT}Eucalyptus[212], ^{AT}_Fmarjoram, ^{AT}_Fravintsara, ^{AT}black pepper, ^{AT}elemi, ^{AT}frankincense, ^{AT}helichrysum, ^{AT}mugwort, ^{AT}pine.

—MUCUS

Oils—^{AT}Eucalyptus[212], ^{AT}_Fcypress, ^{AT}_Frosemary, ^{AT}helichrysum (discharge), ^{AT}goldenrod (discharges respiratory mucus), ^{AT}hyssop (opens respiratory system and discharges toxins and mucus), ^{AT}mugwort (expels), ^{AT}onycha (benzoin), ^{AT}<u>Thieves</u> (dissolves excess mucus).

T—To help discharge mucus, rub oil(s) on chest, neck, back, feet, throat, or lungs.

A—Diffuse oils into the air. Inhale directly or applied to tissue or a cotton wick.

Conjunctivitis: *See Eyes: Conjunctivitis.*

Consciousness:

Oils—^{AT}Lavender.

—OPEN

Oils—^{AT}Rosemary.

—PURIFYING

Oils—^{AT}Peppermint.

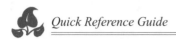

—STIMULATING

  Oils—^{AT}Peppermint, ^{AT}<u>Transformation</u>.

A—Diffuse into the air. Inhale directly or applied to hands, tissue, or a cotton wick.

T—Apply to auricular emotional points. Dilute with V-6 Oil, and massage into skin.

Constipation: *See Digestive System.*

Contagious Diseases:

Oils—^{AT}_FGinger.

A—Diffuse into the air. Inhale directly or applied to hands, tissue, or a cotton wick.

T—Dilute as necessary, and apply to Vita Flex points on the feet, or over lymph nodes.

Control:

—OF YOUR LIFE

  Oils—^{AT}Cedarwood, ^{AT}<u>Dream Catcher</u>, ^{AT}<u>Envision</u>.

—SELF

  Oils—^{AT}<u>Motivation</u>, ^ARoman chamomile.

A—Diffuse into the air. Inhale directly or applied to hands, tissue, or a cotton wick.

T—Apply to auricular emotional points.

Convulsions: *See Seizure:* CONVULSIONS.

Cooling Oils: *See also Temperature:* LOWER.

Oils—^{TA}Angelica, ^{TA}citrus oils, ^{TA}eucalyptus, ^{TA}lavender, ^{TA}tea tree, ^{TA}mountain savory, ^{TA}peppermint, ^{TA}Roman chamomile, ^{TA}spruce. Other oils that are high in aldehydes and esters can produce a cooling effect.

T—Dilute as necessary, and apply to the skin. Dilute with V-6 Oil to create massage oil, and massage into skin.

A—Diffuse into the air.

Corns: *See Feet:* CORNS. *See also Warts.*

Cortisone:

  ≫ *Cortisone is a type of steroid hormone. It suppresses the immune system and reduces inflammation.*

Oils—ᵀꜰSpruce (is like cortisone), ᵀ<u>EndoFlex</u>, ᵀlavender, ᵀ<u>Relieve It</u>, ᵀRoman chamomile, ᵀwintergreen.

T—Dilute as necessary, and apply on skin.

Blend #1—Combine 3 drops Roman chamomile, 3 drops lavender, 5 drops spruce, and 1 drop wintergreen, and apply as a natural cortisone.

Supplements— Prostate Health and Thyromin, together with <u>EndoFlex</u> are beneficial for both men and women. The three items together may also help the body produce its own cortisone. Can also try EndoGize.

Coughs:

Oils—ᴬᵀ<u>RC</u>, ᴬᵀfrankincense, ᴬᵀꜰeucalyptus, ᴬᵀꜰtea tree, ᴬᵀꜰmyrtle (helps remove mucus from lungs), ᴬᵀcedarwood, ᴬᵀangelica, ᴬᵀcajeput, ᴬᵀcardamom, ᴬᵀelemi (unproductive), ᴬᵀfir, ᴬᵀginger, ᴬᵀhinoki, ᴬᵀjasmine, ᴬᵀjuniper, ᴬᵀmyrrh, ᴬᵀonycha (benzoin), ᴬᵀpeppermint, ᴬᵀpine, ᴬᵀmyrrh, ᴬᵀravintsara, ᴬᵀRoman chamomile, ᴬᵀsage lavender, ᴬᵀsandalwood, ᴬᵀ<u>Thieves</u> (dissolves excess mucus and reduces inflammation), ᴬᵀthyme.

Supplements—Thieves Lozenges.

—Allergy

Oils—ᴬ<u>Purification</u>.

—Severe

Oils—ᴬᵀElemi, ᴬᵀfrankincense.

Blend #1—3 drops fir, 3 drops lemon, 2 drops ravintsara, and 1 drop thyme.

Blend #2—15 drops <u>Raven</u>, 15 drops <u>RC</u>, 5 drops lemon, and 10 drops <u>Peace & Calming</u>. Rub on chest, throat, and neck. Can also be diffused.

—Smokers

Oils—ᴬᵀMyrtle.

A—Diffuse into the air. Place 1–2 drops in bowl of hot water, and inhale vapors.

T—Dilute as necessary, and apply to throat and chest area.

Courage:

Oils—ᴬClove, ᴬfennel, ᴬᵀginger, ᴬᵀ<u>Live with Passion</u>, ᴬᵀ<u>Valor</u> (gives).

A—Diffuse into the air. Inhale directly or applied to hands, tissue, or a cotton wick.

T—Apply to auricular emotional points. Dilute with V-6 Oil and massage into skin.

Cradle Cap: *See Children/Infants: Cradle Cap.*

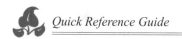
Cramps: See also Digestive System, Hormonal Imbalance, Menstruation, Muscles, PMS.

>> *Cramps are sudden, involuntary muscle contractions that often cause severe pain. Abdominal cramps are commonly caused by stress, menstruation, mild food poisoning, and Irritable Bowel Syndrome.*

Oils—^T_FCypress, ^T_Fmarjoram, ^T<u>Aroma Siez</u>, ^T_Flavender, ^Twintergreen, ^Tbasil, ^Tblue cypress (abdominal), ^Tclary sage, ^T<u>Exodus II</u>, ^Tgalbanum, ^Tginger, ^Trosemary.

Personal Care—Relaxation Massage Oil.

Supplements—Digest + Cleanse (contains oils proven to soothe gastrointestinal upset).

—LEG CRAMPS

Oils—^T<u>Aroma Siez</u>, ^Tmarjoram, ^Tbasil, ^TGerman chamomile, ^Tlavender, ^Trosemary, ^Tvetiver.

Personal Care—Ortho Ease, Ortho Sport, or Relaxation Massage Oils, Prenolone/Prenolone+, Progessence/Progessence Plus.

Supplements—BLM, Mineral Essence, Super Cal.

—MENSTRUAL CRAMPS *See Dysmenorrhea.*

Personal Care—Prenolone/Prenolone+, Progessence/Progessence Plus.

Supplements—FemiGen.

Recipe #1—Take 2 FemiGen three times a day, 10 days before period. Start again two days after cycle. May take up to 6 tablets three times a day.

—STOMACH CRAMPS

Recipe #2—Add 3 drops basil in a capsule with <u>Di-Gize</u>; swallow.

T—Dilute as necessary, and apply on location. Dilute with V-6 Oil to create a massage oil; massage on location. Apply as a warm compress.

Creates Sacred Space:

Oils—^{AT}<u>Sacred Mountain</u>.

A—Diffuse into the air. Inhale directly or applied to hands, tissue, or a cotton wick.

T—Apply to auricular emotional points. Dilute with V-6 Oil, and massage into skin.

Crohn's Disease:

>> *Crohn's disease is a chronic inflammation of part of the intestinal wall that is thought to be caused by an over-active immune response. It can cause abdominal pain, diarrhea, nausea, and loss of appetite.*

Oils—[IT]**Peppermint,** [IT]<u>Di-Gize</u>, [IT]basil, [T]calamus, [I]caraway[213].

Recipe #1—Do Raindrop Technique on spine with <u>ImmuPower</u>.

Supplements—**Sulfurzyme,** AlkaLime, Balance Complete, Cleansing Trio (ComforTone, ICP, and Essentialzyme), Digest + Cleanse, Life 5 (probiotic), Mineral Essence, Multi-Greens, Power Meal.

***Comments—*Refer to the chapter entitled "How to Use—The Personal Usage Reference" in the* <u>Essential Oils Desk Reference</u> *under "Crohn's Disease" for a specific regimen of supplements.*

I—Add 2–5 drops to an empty capsule with 2–5 drops of V-6 Oil; swallow.

T—Dilute as necessary, and apply on abdomen or on Vita Flex points on the feet. Dilute with V-6 Oil to create massage oil, and massage over abdomen and on feet.

Crown Chakra: *See Chakras*

Cushing's Disease: *See Adrenal Glands: Cushing's Disease.*

Cuts: *See also Tissue, Wounds.*

Oils—[T]**Helichrysum,** [T]lavender, [T]tea tree, [T]basil[214], [T]hinoki, [T]cypress, [T]elemi (infected), [T]<u>Melrose</u> (rejuvenates tissue), [T]onycha (benzoin), [T]pine, [T]ravintsara, [T]<u>Relieve It</u>, [T]Roman chamomile (healing), [T]rosewood, [T]sage lavender, [T]<u>Thieves</u>.

T—Dilute as necessary, and apply on location.

Cystic Fibrosis:

▸▸ *Cystic Fibrosis is an hereditary disease where thick, sticky mucus builds up in the lungs and in the digestive track. Cystic Fibrosis is life-threatening and can result in respiratory failure.*

Oils—[TI]Bergamot[215].

Recipe #1—Alternate with <u>Thieves</u>, <u>RC</u>, lavender, and myrtle. Apply to brain stem area (back of neck), temples, chest, bottoms of feet. Diffuse. <u>Raven</u> is stronger and can replace myrtle for helping to remove mucus accumulation in the lungs. <u>EndoFlex</u> and helichrysum can also be used with benefit.

Recipe #2—(*Staphylococcus*) Oregano, thyme, and <u>Melrose</u> (up the spine using the Raindrop Technique), then 10 drops lemon, 5 drops tea tree, and 3 drops frankincense (rub on feet and chest, and diffuse) **or** 10 drops <u>Raven</u> and 5 drops hyssop.

Supplements—EndoGize, Essentialzyme, Essentialzymes-4, Master Formula, Multi-Greens, all vitamins.

Cystitis (Bladder Infection): *See Bladder: Infection.*

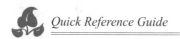

Dandruff: *See Hair: DANDRUFF.*

Day Dreaming:

Oils—^{AT}Awaken, ^{AT}cedarwood, ^{AT}Clarity, ^{AT}Dream Catcher, ^{AT}eucalyptus, ^{AT}Gathering, ^{AT}ginger, ^{AT}Harmony, ^{AT}helichrysum, ^{AT}Highest Potential, ^{AT}lavender, ^{AT}lemon, ^{AT}myrrh, ^{AT}peppermint, ^{AT}Present Time, ^{AT}rose, ^{AT}rosemary, ^{AT}rosewood, ^{AT}Sacred Mountain, ^{AT}sandalwood, ^{AT}spruce, ^{AT}3 Wise Men, ^{AT}thyme, ^{AT}Valor, ^{AT}ylang ylang.

A—Diffuse into the air. Inhale directly or applied to hands, tissue, or a cotton wick.

T—Apply to auricular emotional points. Dilute with V-6 Oil, and massage into skin.

Death (of Loved One): *See Emotions: LOSS.*

Oils—^{AT}Trauma Life.

A—Diffuse into the air. Inhale directly or applied to hands, tissue, or a cotton wick.

T—Apply to auricular emotional points. Dilute with V-6 Oil, and massage into skin.

Debility:

Oils—^{AT}_FNutmeg, ^{AT}cardamom, ^{AT}cumin (nervous), ^{AT}sage lavender.

A—Diffuse into the air. Inhale directly or applied to hands, tissue, or a cotton wick.

T—Dilute with V-6 Oil, and massage into skin.

Decongestant: *See Congestion: DECONGESTANT.*

Defeated: *See Emotions: Defeated.*

Degenerative Disease: *See pH Balance.*

›› *A degenerative disease is a disease where the affected tissues or organs are damaged due to internal mechanisms, and not due to infection. Quite a few different diseases can be categorized as degenerative diseases, including Alzheimer's disease, cancer, Parkinson's disease, atherosclerosis, diabetes, osteoporosis, rheumatoid arthritis, and many others. Support the cells and tissues through proper nutrition, reducing stress, exercising regularly, and eliminating toxins. See specific conditions in this guide for lists of oils and other products that can support the body for each condition.*

Oils—^ACitrus Fresh, ^AExodus II, ^Afrankincense, ^Alavender, ^Alemon, ^Aorange, ^APurification, ^Atangerine, ^ATransformation.

A—These oils are excellent to diffuse in the room. Not only do they purify the air, but they also help deliver needed oxygen to the starving cells. All other essential oils and supplements are beneficial for providing oxygen and nutrients to the cells of the body. *See specific ailments.*

Supplements—NingXia Red (provides a full range of nutrients), Power Meal, Master Formula.

*****Comments**—A lack of nutrients at the cellular level causes degenerative disease. The general health condition of the body will improve if the necessary nutrients are received by the body at the cellular level. Toxins change the pH of the cell wall, which change significantly reduces the ability of the cell to assimilate nutrients and oxygen. This process is the beginning of cellular starvation, which leads to degenerative disease. We then become hosts to viral and bacterial invasions due to our weakened or compromised immune system. Essential oils are antimicrobial and help our immune systems fight off the ravages of disease. They also have the ability to deliver nutrients to our nutritionally depleted cells. When essential oils are blended with the proper nutrients that the body requires, the essential oils act as the delivery system to take the nutrients directly into the cell and through the compromised cell wall, which has had the pH altered due to chemical toxins in the body. This process allows the body to rebuild and regain its healthful condition and allows the body's immune system to normalize. In addition, essential oils have the highest oxygenating molecules of any known substance. So they deliver oxygen to the cells, which helps in the regeneration process. (Young Living Essential Edge Newsletter —July 1996).

D

Dehydration:

›› *Rehydration with an oral rehydration solution is the most effective way to prevent dehydration. If no commercially prepared oral rehydration solution is available, a solution made from 1 tsp. salt, 8 tsp. sugar, and 1 liter clean water (with some mashed fresh banana, if available, to add potassium) can work in an emergency.*

Supplements—Mineral Essence.

Delivery: *See Pregnancy: Delivery.*

Denial:

Oils—^{AT}Roman chamomile, ^{AT}sage.

—OVERCOME

Oils—^{AT}<u>Abundance</u>,^{AT}<u>Acceptance</u>, ^{AT}<u>Awaken</u>, ^{AT}<u>Transformation</u>.

A—Diffuse into the air. Inhale directly or applied to hands, tissue, a or a cotton wick.

T—Apply to auricular emotional points. Dilute with V-6 Oil, and massage into skin.

Dental Infection: *See Oral Conditions: INFECTION.*

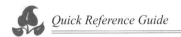

Deodorant:

Oils—ᵀ<u>Acceptance</u>, ᵀ<u>Aroma Siez</u>, ᵀbergamot, ᵀcitronella, ᵀcypress, ᵀ<u>Dragon Time</u>, ᵀ<u>Dream Catcher</u>, ᵀ<u>EndoFlex</u>, ᵀeucalyptus, ᵀgeranium, ᵀ<u>Harmony</u>, ᵀ<u>Joy</u>, ᵀlavender, ᵀtea tree, ᵀ<u>Mister</u>, ᵀmyrtle, ᵀ<u>Peace & Calming</u>, ᵀ<u>RC</u>, ᵀ<u>Release</u>, ᵀ<u>White Angelica</u>.

T—Apply oils neat to the skin, or dilute with some V-6 Oil for application under the arms. Also, 2–3 drops of an oil can be added to 4 oz. of unscented talcum powder and 2 oz. of baking soda. Mix this well, and apply under the arms, on the feet, or on other areas of the body.

Personal Care—AromaGuard Deodorants, Dragon Time Bath & Shower Gel, Dragon Time Massage Oil, Evening Peace Bath & Shower Gel, Morning Start Bath & Shower Gel, Relaxation Massage Oil, Lavender Hand & Body Lotion, Sandalwood Moisture Cream. Add a couple drops of one of the oils listed above for additional fragrance.

Deodorizing:

Oils—ᴬ_F_Myrtle, ᴬ<u>Purification</u>, ᴬclary sage, ᴬmyrrh, ᴬpeppermint, ᴬsage, ᴬthyme.

A—Diffuse into the air. Add 8–10 drops in 1 tsp. perfumers or grain alcohol (such as vodka), and combine with distilled water in a 1 oz. spray bottle. Spray into the air or on affected surface.

Depletion:

Oils—ᴬᵀCypress.

A—Diffuse into the air. Inhale directly or applied to tissue or a cotton wick.

T—Dilute with V-6 Oil to create a massage oil, and massage onto the skin.

Depression: *See Diet.*

>> *Depression is a disorder marked by excessive sadness, energy loss, feelings of worthlessness, irritableness, sudden weight loss or gain, trouble sleeping, and loss of interest in activities normally enjoyed. These symptoms can continue for weeks or months if not treated and can destroy an individual's quality of life.*

Oils—ᴬᵀLemon[216], ᴬᵀ_F_frankincense[217], ᴬlavender[218], ᴬᵀJoy (5 drops in palm of non-dominant hand, stir clockwise three times with dominant hand, then apply over heart and breathe in deeply), ᴬ_F_bergamot[219], ᴬᵀ<u>Valor</u> (helps balance energies), ᴬᵀ_F_ylang ylang[220], ᴬᵀ_F_rosemary (nervous)[221], ᴬᵀ_F_rose-

> *Depression can be caused by a calcium deficiency. Stay away from carbonated soft drinks, specifically cola drinks that are high in phosphorus; they leech calcium from the body. Eating heavy protein at night does not give the body enough time to digest the food before going to sleep. The undigested food then ferments, which robs the system of needed oxygen and heightens the sense of depression.*

wood, **AT**tangerine[219], **AT**grapefruit[219], **AT**mastrante, **AT**<u>Hope</u> (on ears, especially for emotional clearing), **AT**jasmine, **AT**neroli, **AT**sage (relieves depression), **AT**<u>Sensation</u>, **AT**<u>Acceptance</u>, **AT**basil, **AT**calamus, **AT**clary sage[222], **AT**<u>EndoFlex</u> (apply often while taking Mineral Essence and Thyromin supplements), **AT**<u>Gathering</u>, **AT**<u>Gentle Baby</u> (on solar plexus), **AT**geranium, **AT**ginger, **AT**<u>Harmony</u>, **AT**<u>Highest Potential</u>, **AT**<u>Inspiration</u>, **AT**juniper (over heart), **AT**<u>M-Grain</u>, **AT**onycha (benzoin), **AT**<u>PanAway</u>, **AT**<u>Live with Passion</u>, **AT**patchouli, **AT**<u>Peace & Calming</u> (back of neck), **AT**pepper (on crown for spirit protection), **AT**ravintsara (lifts emotions), **AT**<u>Release</u>, **AT**Roman chamomile, **AT**sandalwood, **AT**<u>Trauma Life</u>.

A—Diffuse into the air. Inhale directly or applied to hands, tissue, or a cotton wick. *See Comments under Asthma for a discussion on using* **plastic nasal inhalers**.

D

T—Dilute with V-6 Oil to create a massage oil, and massage[115] onto the skin. Apply to auricular emotion points.

Personal Care—**Sensation Massage Oil,** Lemon Sandalwood or Thieves Cleansing Soaps, Prenolone/Prenolone+, Progessence/Progessence Plus, Sensation Bath & Shower Gel.

Supplements—**Mineral Essence, NingXia Red** (helps raise energy levels), **Omega Blue, OmegaGize**[3], EndoGize, PD 80/20, Thyromin, Master Formula, Ultra Young+ (helps lift depression).

Blend #1—Combine 1–2 drops each of frankincense, <u>3 Wise Men</u>, and <u>Hope</u> in the palm of your hand; rub hands together clockwise, cup hands over nose and mouth, and breathe deeply.

—Antidepressant

Oils—**AT**Lemon[219], **AT**bergamot[219], **AT**orange[219], **AT**₍F₎frankincense[217], **AT**lavender[218], **AT**Joy, **AT**<u>Abundance</u>, **AT**<u>Awaken</u>, **AT**<u>Christmas Spirit</u>, **AT**<u>Citrus Fresh</u>, **AT**<u>Dream Catcher</u>, **AT**elemi, **AT**geranium, **AT**jasmine, **AT**melissa, **AT**<u>Motivation</u>, **AT**neroli, **AT**onycha (benzoin) (combine with rose for massage), **AT**<u>Peace & Calming</u>, **AT**ravintsara, **AT**Roman chamomile, **AT**rose, **AT**<u>Sacred Mountain</u>, **AT**sandalwood, **AT**<u>3 Wise Men</u>, **AT**<u>Valor</u>.

T—Dilute as necessary, and apply to bottoms of feet and over heart.

A—Diffuse into the air.

Supplements—Omega Blue, OmegaGize[3]

***Comments—See the "Single Oil Property Chart" in the Appendix of this book for additional antidepressant oils and their strengths.

–Recovery from Commercial Antidepressants like Prozac

Recipe #1—<u>Brain Power</u>, <u>Clarity</u>, <u>Joy</u>, <u>Peace & Calming</u>, and <u>Valor</u> all help repair brain damage from the commercial drugs that inhibit serotonin metabolism. They also stimulate the pineal gland which normally metabolizes 50% of the serotonin in the body. The liver and pancreas are extremely toxic. Cleanse with <u>GLF</u>, JuvaPower, <u>Juva Cleanse</u>, and/or <u>JuvaFlex</u>. Coriander, dill and <u>Thieves</u> help regulate the blood sugar. Frankincense helps prevent cancer (risk of breast cancer increases by 7x with the use of Paxil). Balsam fir helps to decrease the cortisol levels. Also focus on strengthening the smooth muscle tissues (especially heart and intestines) as they are contracted by the drugs.

Supplements— CortiStop (Women's), Digest + Cleanse, JuvaPower/JuvaSpice, Omega Blue, OmegaGize[3,] Power Meal.

—**IMMUNE DEPRESSION**

Oils—[TA]$_F$Spruce.

T—Dilute with V-6 Oil to create a massage oil, and massage onto the skin.

A—Diffuse into the air.

Personal Care Products—Morning Start Bath & Shower Gel, Thieves Cleansing Soap.

Blend #2—5 drops bergamot, 5 drops lavender; diffuse.

Supplements—ImmuPro, Inner Defense, Master Formula.

—**POSTPARTUM DEPRESSION (BABY BLUES)** *See Pregnancy/Childbirth: POSTPARTUM DEPRESSION*

—**SEDATIVES** *SEE ALSO CALMING*

Oils—[AT]Lavender[223], [TA]ylang ylang[224], [AT]melissa[225], [AT]tarragon[226], [AT]<u>RutaVaLa</u> (roll-on), [AT]<u>Peace & Calming</u>, [TA]valerian, [T]<u>Tranquil</u> (roll-on), [AT]bergamot, [AT]cedarwood, [AT]clary sage, [AT]cypress, [AT]frankincense, [AT]geranium, [AT]hyssop, [AT]jasmine, [AT]juniper, [AT]marjoram, [AT]Tea tree ericifolia, [AT]melissa, [AT]neroli, [AT]onycha (benzoin), [AT]patchouli, [AT]Roman chamomile, [AT]rose, [AT]sandalwood, [T]<u>Stress Away</u>. Use intuition as to which one may be best for the given situation. In addition, check the safety data for each of the oils in the Appendix of this book.

A—Diffuse into the air. Inhale directly or applied to hands, tissue, or a cotton wick. *See Comments under Asthma for a discussion on using* **plastic nasal inhalers**.

T—Dilute with V-6 Oil to create a massage oil, and massage onto the skin. Apply to auricular emotion point.

—**SUICIDAL DEPRESSION**

Recipe #1—Put <u>Valor</u> and then <u>Inspiration</u> on feet, and hold feet for a few minutes until relaxed; this may start to release a past negative memory, which could lead to crying, etc. If not, rub <u>Present Time</u> over thymus and then a drop of <u>Inner Child</u> on their thumb, and have them suck the thumb, pushing the pad of the thumb to the roof of the mouth. Once the emotional release starts, put <u>Grounding</u> on the back of the neck and sternum, and then put <u>Release</u> on the crown of the head; wait for a while, allowing then to deal with the release. After the emotional release has subsided, rub <u>Joy</u> over the heart and <u>Hope</u> on the ears. After they wake up the next morning, apply a couple drops of <u>Gentle Baby</u> on solar plexus and over the heart. <u>Magnify Your Purpose</u> may also be helpful to wear as a perfume/cologne.

Supplements—Thyromin.

—Cleansing the Flesh and Blood of Evil Deities

Oils—^{AT}Cedarwood, ^{AT}myrrh.

A—Diffuse into the air.

T—Dilute with V-6 Oil to create a massage oil, and massage onto the skin. Apply to auricular emotion points.

–History

"Breaking the lineage of iniquity." The ancient Egyptians believed that if they didn't clear the body and mind of negative influences before dying, they could not progress into the next life and return to this world to take up the body they had left in the tomb (resurrection).

Deprogramming:

Oils—^{AT}<u>Forgiveness</u>, ^{AT}<u>Inner Child</u>, ^{AT}<u>Release</u>, ^{AT}<u>SARA</u>, ^{AT}<u>Trauma Life</u>.

A—Diffuse into the air. Inhale directly or applied to tissue or a cotton wick.

T—Apply to chakras. Dilute with V-6 Oil to create a massage oil, and massage onto the skin.

Dermatitis: *See Skin:* Dermatitis.

Despair:

Oils—^{AT}Lemon, ^{AT}lavender, ^{AT}Joy, ^{AT}<u>Acceptance</u>, ^{AT}<u>Believe</u>, ^{AT}cedarwood, ^{AT}clary sage, ^{AT}fir, ^{AT}<u>Forgiveness</u>, ^{AT}frankincense, ^{AT}<u>Gathering</u>, ^{AT}geranium, ^{AT}<u>Gratitude</u>, ^{AT}<u>Grounding</u>, ^{AT}<u>Harmony</u>, ^{AT}<u>Hope</u>, ^{AT}lemongrass, ^{AT}orange, ^{AT}peppermint, ^{AT}rosemary, ^{AT}sandalwood, ^{AT}spearmint, ^{AT}spruce, ^{AT}thyme, ^{AT}<u>Transformation</u>, ^{AT}<u>Valor</u>, ^{AT}ylang ylang.

A—Diffuse into the air. Inhale directly or applied to tissue or a cotton wick.

T—Apply to auricular emotion points. Dilute with V-6 Oil to create a massage oil, and massage onto the skin.

Despondency:

Oils—^{AT}Bergamot, ^{AT}clary sage, ^{AT}cypress, ^{AT}Gathering, ^{AT}geranium, ^{AT}ginger, ^{AT}Harmony, ^{AT}Hope, ^{AT}Inner Child, ^{AT}Inspiration, ^{AT}Joy, ^{AT}orange, ^{AT}Peace & Calming, ^{AT}Present Time, ^{AT}rose, ^{AT}rosewood, ^{AT}sandalwood, ^{AT}Transformation, ^{AT}Trauma Life, ^{AT}Valor, ^{AT}ylang ylang.

A—Diffuse into the air. Inhale directly or applied to tissue or a cotton wick.

T—Apply to auricular emotion points. Dilute with V-6 Oil to create a massage oil, and massage onto the skin.

Detoxification: *See also Chelation, Cleansing, Housecleaning.*

Oils—^T_FHelichrysum, ^T_Ijuniper (detoxifier), ^TGLF, ^Trosemary[227], ^Tdill[228], ^TJuvaFlex, ^Tcoriander[229].

T—Apply oils to liver area, intestines, and Vita Flex points on feet.

Supplements—Balance Complete (*refer to the 5-Day Nutritive Cleanse program listed under Balance Complete in the Supplements section of the Reference Guide for Essential Oils. This program also uses Digest + Cleanse and NingXia Red to help enhance detoxification while maintaining energy levels*), Cleansing Trio (ComforTone, Essentialzyme, and ICP), Digest + Cleanse, JuvaTone.

—Metals *See also Chelation*

Oils—^{TA}Helichrysum, ^{TA}clove (chelates metal ions), ^{TA}Juva Cleanse (helps to remove metals from the body), ^{TA}Peace & Calming, ^{TA}Sacred Mountain, ^{TA}Valor.

> *Heavy metals in the system give off toxic gases and can create allergic symptoms and hormonal imbalances. For example, cadmium can create hyperactivity and learning disabilities in children. Cigarette smoke and caffeine all contain cadmium. Ridding the body of heavy metals is extremely important for proper immune function. Cast iron cookware leaves heavy iron deposits in the body. Aluminum cookware leaves aluminum deposits in the body. Glass or Stainless Steel cookware is best.*

T—Dilute as necessary, and apply on feet and on liver area.

A—Diffuse into the air. Inhale directly.

Supplements— Cleansing Trio (ComforTone, Essentialzyme, and ICP), JuvaTone, Longevity Capsules.

–Pull Out

Recipe #1—Drink distilled water. The absence of minerals in distilled water creates a vacuum-like action that pulls metals and toxins from the body.

Blend #1—Combine 10 drops cypress, 10 drops juniper, and 10 drops lemongrass with 1 oz. V-6 Oil, and massage under arms, over kidneys, and on bottoms of feet.

Blend #2—Add 2–4 drops <u>Thieves</u> and 1–3 drops helichrysum to a rolled gauze, and place between cheek and gums to pull out dental mercury. Leave in one place during the night, and throw away the gauze roll in the morning. The next night, place a new gauze roll with oil in a different place. Continue in a like manner until all areas have been affected. **Note:** *Dilute with V-6 Oil for use on very sensitive gums or on children.*

—TOXINS

Oils—[TA]Hyssop (opens respiratory system and discharges toxins and mucus), [T]lemongrass (helps increase lymphatic circulation for enhanced toxin removal), [T]patchouli (digests toxic wastes), [TA]fennel, [TA]fir.

T—Dilute as necessary, and apply on feet and on liver area.

A—Diffuse into the air. Inhale directly.

Supplements—Balance Complete, Cleansing Trio (ComforTone, Essentialzyme, and ICP), Digest + Cleanse. These cleansing products may help remove toxic by-products from the body. Also, take Detoxzyme between meals to break down toxins.

***Comments—Another way to help remove toxins through the skin is to add 2 cups of apple cider vinegar to warm bathwater, and soak in the tub for 25 minutes.

Diabetes:

>> *Diabetes is a disease characterized by the body's inability to properly produce or use the hormone insulin. Insulin, produced in the pancreas, helps regulate the level of sugars in the blood, as well as the conversion of starches and sugar into the energy necessary for life. Common diabetes symptoms include a frequent need to drink and urinate, blurred vision, mental fatigue, and possibly weight loss (depending on the type). Over time, diabetes can lead to additional complications, such as strokes, heart disease, kidney failure, and even the necessity of removing a limb.*

Oils—[IA]Cinnamon bark[230], [TA_F]rosemary[231], [TA]sage[232], [TA]cumin[233], [TA_F]eucalyptus, [TA_F]geranium, [IAT]basil[234],

> *Caution: Diabetics should not use angelica. Watch insulin intake carefully; you may have to cut down. Keep your physician informed!*

[TA_F]pine, [TA_F]ylang ylang, [TA]coriander (normalizes glucose levels), [TA]cypress, [TA]dill (helps lower glucose levels by normalizing insulin levels and supporting pancreas function)[235], [TI]cassia[236], [TA]fennel, [TA]ginger, [TA]hyssop, [TA]juniper, [TA]lavender, [TA]<u>Thieves</u>.

Blend #1—8 drops clove, 8 drops cinnamon bark, 15 drops rosemary, and 10 drops thyme in 2 oz. of V-6 Oil. Put on feet and over pancreas.

Blend #2—5 drops cinnamon bark and 5 drops cypress. Rub on feet and on pancreas.

Supplements—Balance Complete (contains a blend of fibers to help maintain stable blood sugar levels), Cleansing Trio (ComforTone, Essentialzyme, and ICP), Digest +

A=Aromatic   **T**=Topical   **I**=Internal | 155

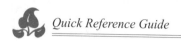
Cleanse, ImmuPro, Inner Defense, Majestic Essence Chocolates (low glycemic choco-
late), Mineral Essence, MultiGreens, Power Meal, Pure Protein Complete (contains
a blend of proteins and fibers to help reduce spikes and maintain stable blood sugar
levels), Stevia, Sulfurzyme (take in morning with vitamin C before breakfast and at bed
time), Master Formula, Yacon Syrup.

***Comments**—A seven-year-old girl took 6 MultiGreens a day (balances blood sugar),
Bodygize three times a day, and ImmuneTune.

—PANCREAS SUPPORT

Oils—^{TA}Cinnamon bark[237], ^{TA}fennel, ^{TA}geranium.

—SORES (DIABETIC)

Recipe #1—Do the Raindrop Technique, and put <u>Valor</u> on the Vita Flex points. Also
lavender and <u>Melrose</u>.

T—Dilute as necessary, and apply on back, chest, feet, and over pancreas.

A—Diffuse into the air.

Diaper Rash: *See Children/Infants: DIAPER RASH.*

Diarrhea: *See Digestive System: DIARRHEA.*

Diet: *See Blood, Fasting, Food, and Cleansing.*

›› *Diet is extremely important when trying to correct cancer, hypoglycemia, candida, etc. First,
cleanse the body: drink a lot of distilled water; stay away from sugars and meats; eat vegetable
protein in the mornings, carbohydrates and starches for lunch, and fruit in the evening. Hydro-
chloric acid and pepsin are secreted in the morning to help digest protein.*

Supplements—Enzyme products: **Allerzyme** (aids the digestion of sugars, starches, fats,
and proteins), **Detoxzyme** (helps maintain and support a healthy intestinal environment), **Digest + Cleanse**.

—POST-DIET SAGGY SKIN

Recipe #1—Combine 8 drops each of sage, pine, lemongrass, and 1 oz. of V-6 Oil. Rub
on saggy areas.

Digestive System: *See also Bowel, Colon, Giardia, Hiccoughs/Hiccups, Stomach,
Ulcers.*

›› *The human digestive system is the series of organs and glands that process food. The digestive
system breaks down food, absorbs nutrients for the body to use as fuel, and excretes as bowel movements the part that cannot be broken down.*

Oils—[IT]_FPeppermint[238], [IT]caraway[239], [TI]Di-Gize (acid stomach; aids the secretion of digestive enzymes), [TI]_Ffennel[240] (sluggish), [T]_Flemongrass[241] (purifier), [AT]AromaEase, [TI]ginger[242], [TI]_Fclary sage (weak), [TI]_Fmarjoram (stimulates), [T]_Fnutmeg (for sluggish digestion; eases), [T]_Fpatchouli (stimulant), [TI]_Fgrapefruit, [TI]_Fsage (sluggish), [TI]angelica[243], [TI]anise (accelerates), [TI]basil, [TI]bergamot, [TI]black pepper, [TI]cardamom (nervous), [T]cinnamon bark, [TI]clove, [TI]coriander (spasms), [TI]cumin (spasms and indigestion), [T]GLF, [T]juniper, [TI]JuvaFlex (supports and detoxifies), [TI]laurel, [IT]lemon (indigestion), [TI]mandarin (tonic), [T]myrrh, [T]myrtle, [T]neroli, [TI]ocotea, [TI]orange (indigestion), [TI]oregano[244], [TI]rosemary[245], [TI]spearmint, [TI]tangerine (nervous and sluggish), [TI]tarragon (nervous and sluggish).

I—Add the oil(s) to your food. Add 1–5 drops of oil to an empty capsule with 1–5 drops of V-6 Oil; swallow.

> *Digestive problems may indicate a mineral deficiency. Use Mineral Essence. Life 5 (probiotic) is necessary when you are detoxifying or on any type of prescription drug; you must feed the intestinal tract. If you have digestion problems, take Life 5 to stop the fermentation process.*

T—Dilute as necessary, and rub on stomach or apply as a compress over abdomen.

Diffusion—See Negative Ions for oils that produce negative ions when diffused to help stimulate the digestive system.

Supplements—AlkaLime (combats yeast and fungus overgrowth and preserves the body's proper pH balance), Balance Complete, ComforTone, Digest + Cleanse (contains oils proven to soothe gastrointestinal upset and promote healthy digestion), Essentialzyme, Essentialzymes-4 (enzymes help build the digestive system; take before meals for acid stomach), ICP (helps speed food through digestive system; lower incidence of fermentation), Life 5 (probiotic), Master Formula, Mineral Essence, MultiGreens, NingXia Red, ParaFree, Sulfurzyme. Other enzyme products include: Allerzyme (aids the digestion of sugars, starches, fats, and proteins), Detoxzyme (helps maintain and support a healthy intestinal environment).

—**BLOATING**

Oils—[TA]Di-Gize.

T—Apply to stomach and to Vita Flex points

A—Diffuse into the air.

Supplements—ComforTone.

—**CONSTIPATION**

> *Poor bowel function may be caused by enzyme deficiency, low fiber, poor bowel tone, not enough liquid in diet, stress, incorrect pH balance, and/or bad diet.*

≫ *Constipation is a condition characterized by infrequent or difficult bowel movements. A person is considered constipated if he or she has fewer than three bowel movements a week or if the stools are hard and difficult to expel. Common causes of consti-*

A=Aromatic **T**=Topical **I**=Internal

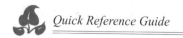

pation include a lack of fiber, dehydration, ignoring the urge to have a bowel movement, depression, medications, large dairy intake, stress, and abuse of laxatives.

Oils—[T]F Orange, [T]rosemary[245], [T]lemon[245], [T]peppermint[245], [T]F marjoram, [T]<u>Di-Gize</u>, [T]anise, [T]black pepper, [T]copaiba, [T]fennel, [T]ginger, [T]juniper, [T]patchouli, [T]rose, [T]sandalwood, [T]tangerine, [T]tarragon.

T—Dilute as necessary, and massage clockwise around abdomen and on Vita Flex points (feet & shins).

Supplements—**ComforTone**, **ICP** (fiber beverage), AlkaLime, Essentialzymes-4, Essentialzyme, Sulfurzyme, and lots of **water**. If there is a chronic history of constipation, use **ComforTone** until the system is open, and then start **ICP**.

Blend #1—Mix together 6 drops each of orange, tangerine, and spearmint, and rub on lower stomach and colon.

Blend #2—15 drops cedarwood, 10 drops lemon, 5 drops peppermint, and 2 oz. V-6 Oil. Massage clockwise over lower abdomen three times a day, and take supplements.

–CHILDREN

> **Oils**—Fruit juices or lots of water. Geranium, patchouli, Roman chamomile, rosemary, tangerine.

—CRAMPS *SEE CRAMPS*

—DIARRHEA *SEE ALSO ACIDOSIS*

>> *Diarrhea is an abnormal increase in the frequency of bowel movements, marked by loose, watery stools. Diarrhea is defined as more than three bowel movements a day. Cases of Diarrhea that last more than two days can become a serious problem and can cause dehydration.*

Oils—[IT]F Peppermint[246], [IT]F ginger, [IT]F geranium, [T]F tea tree, [T]myrrh, [T]F sandalwood (obstinate), [T]cardamom, [T]cistus, [T]cumin, [T]myrtle, [T]ocotea, [T]spearmint (not for babies).

Supplements—AlkaLime, Essentialzyme, Essentialzymes-4, Life 5 (probiotic).

–ANTISPASMODIC

> **Oils**—[IT]Peppermint[247], [T]galbanum[248], [T]cypress, [T]eucalyptus, [T]Roman chamomile.

–CHILDREN

> **Oils**—[T]Geranium, [T]ginger, [T]Roman chamomile, [T]sandalwood.

–CHRONIC

> **Oils**—[T]F Nutmeg, [T]F orange, [T]<u>Di-Gize</u> (apply over stomach, colon, and VF points), [T]neroli.

-STRESS-INDUCED

Oils—[T]Lavender[249].

I—Place 1–3 drops in an empty capsule; swallow.

T—Dilute as necessary, and apply 1–2 drops on stomach, abdomen, or Vita Flex points on the feet.

—GAS/FLATULENCE

Oils—[TF]Ginger, [TF]lavender, [TF]tarragon, [T]peppermint, [AT]AromaEase, [T]fennel, [T]angelica, [T]anise, [T]bergamot, [T]cardamom, [T]coriander, [T]copaiba, [T]cumin, [T]eucalyptus, [T]juniper, [T]myrrh, [T]nutmeg, [T]onycha (benzoin), [T]Roman chamomile, [T]rosemary, [T]spearmint (not for babies).

T—Dilute as necessary, and apply to large intestine, stomach, abdomen, and Vita Flex points of feet.

—GASTRITIS *SEE ALSO ANTI-INFLAMMATORY*

>> *Gastritis is inflammation of the stomach lining.*

Oils—[TI]Di-Gize, [TI]peppermint, [TI]fennel, [I]lemongrass[241], [T]calamus, [T]laurel, [T]pine, [TI]sage, [T]spikenard, [TI]tarragon, [T]yarrow.

T—Apply over stomach area with hot compress.

I—One drop of oil in rice or almond milk taken as a dietary supplement. Place 1–2 drops in an empty capsule; swallow.

Supplements—AlkaLime, Balance Complete, Cleansing Trio (ComforTone, Essentialzyme, and ICP), Digest + Cleanse, Life 5 (probiotic), Mineral Essence.

—HEARTBURN

>> *Heartburn is a painful burning sensation in the chest or throat. It occurs as a result of backed up stomach acid in the esophagus. Heartburn can be triggered by certain foods, medication, pregnancy, and alcohol.*

Oils—[TF]Lemon, [TF]peppermint, [T]Di-Gize (over stomach and colon), [T]cardamom, [T]Gentle Baby (over thymus).

T—Dilute as necessary, and apply 1–2 drops to chest or to area indicated.

Blend #1—2 drops lemon, 2 drops peppermint, 3 drops sandalwood, and ½ oz. V-6 Oil. Apply to breast bone. Using palm of hand, massage in a clockwise motion—applying pressure. Do Vita Flex on feet.

Supplements—AlkaLime, Essentialzyme, Essentialzymes-4, JuvaPower/JuvaSpice.

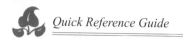

—INDIGESTION

Oils—[T][F]Peppermint, [T]ginger, [T][F]lavender, [T][F]thyme, [AT]AromaEase, [T][F]grapefruit, [T][F]orange (nervous), [T]angelica, [T]cardamom, [T]copaiba, [T]coriander, [T]cumin, [T]GLF, [T]goldenrod, [T]JuvaFlex, [T]laurel, [T]myrrh, [T]nutmeg, [T]tarragon, [T]valerian (nervous indigestion).

T—Dilute as necessary, and apply to stomach, intestines, and Vita Flex points on feet.

Supplements—AlkaLime, Balance Complete, Cleansing Trio (ComforTone, Essentialzyme, and ICP), Digest + Cleanse (contains oils proven to soothe gastrointestinal upset and to promote healthy digestion).

—INTESTINAL PROBLEMS *See also Colon*

Oils—[TI][F]Basil, [TI][F]marjoram, [TI]ginger, [TI]rose[250], [TI]rosemary, [T]cajeput, [T]calamus (reduces inflammation and detoxifies), [T]patchouli (aids in the digestion of toxic waste), [T]tarragon.

Supplements—Digest + Cleanse (helps soothe gastrointestinal upset), Life 5 (probiotic), AlkaLime, Balance Complete, Cleansing Trio (ComforTone, Essentialzyme, and ICP), ParaFree, JuvaTone.

–ANTISEPTIC

Oils—[T]Nutmeg.

–CRAMPS

Oils—[TI][F]Clary sage, [IT]Di-Gize (add 3 drops basil in capsule with Di-Gize), [T]blue cypress.

–FLORA

Recipe #1—Take kefir with Life 5 (probiotic) first thing in the morning on an empty stomach to help implant good bacteria in the intestines (yogurt will help maintain good bacteria but not implant it).

Supplements—Life 5 (probiotic), Balance Complete (contains inulin, which helps build intestinal flora).

–PARASITES

Oils—[IT]Oregano[251], [T]palmarosa[252], [IT]lavender[253], [IT][F]bergamot, [IT][F]clove, [IT]Di-Gize, [IT][F]fennel, [IT][F]lemon, [IT][F]Roman chamomile, [IT]ginger (helps to create an unfriendly environment for parasites), [IT]peppermint, [IT]ravintsara.

Supplements—AlkaLime, Cleansing Trio (ComforTone, Essentialzyme, and ICP), Digest + Cleanse (contains oils that create an unfriendly environment

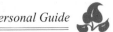

for parasites), and ParaFree assist in cleansing the intestinal tract of toxic debris and parasites, which are hosts for many diseases.

–Soothe

　Oils—[T]Spearmint.

–Spasm

　Oils—[T][F]Tarragon, [T][F]fennel.

T—Dilute as necessary, and apply to stomach, intestines, and Vita Flex points on feet.

I—Place 1–2 drops of oil in an empty capsule, and swallow. Add 1–2 drops of oil to 16 oz. of water, or to 8 oz. rice or almond milk, and drink. Add oils as flavoring to food.

—**Irritable Bowel Syndrome**

　Oils—[IT]Peppermint[254], [IT]caraway[255], [IT]<u>Di-Gize</u>, [IT]calamus, [T]Idaho tansy, [T]anise, [I]<u>Juva Cleanse</u>.

　I—Place 1–2 drops of oil in an empty capsule, and swallow. Add 1–2 drops of oil to 16 oz. of water, or to 8 oz. rice or almond milk, and drink. Add oils as flavoring to food

　T—Dilute 1–2 drops with V-6 Oil, and apply over abdomen with a hot compress

　Recipe #1—Take 2 drops each of calamus, caraway, <u>Di-Gize</u>, and peppermint in distilled water 1–2 times per day.

　Blend #1—10–15 drops <u>Di-Gize</u>, 5–6 drops ledum, and 1 drop peppermint in a capsule; take internally. *Abundant Health offers capsules that work well with the oils.*

　Supplements—Balance Complete, ComforTone, Digest + Cleanse, (enteric-coated to release in the bowels) ICP (fiber beverage), JuvaPower/JuvaSpice, JuvaTone, Life 5 (probiotic), Majestic Essence Chocolates (contain boswellic acid that can help alleviate IBS), NingXia Red.

—**Normal Function Of Bowels (Intestines)**

　Supplements—Balance Complete (utilizes five different fibers for optimal cleansing power), ComforTone, Digest + Cleanse, ICP (fiber beverage for normal function of bowels).

—**Paralysis of Bowels (Intestines)**

　Supplements—ComforTone, Digest + Cleanse.

　***Comments—*One women was paralyzed by surgery and had to have 2 colonics a day. She took ComforTone and then she was able to have natural bowel movements.*

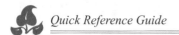

Diphtheria:

>> *Diphtheria is an infectious bacterial (Corynebacterium diphtheriae) disease that causes fever, sore throat, swollen glands, bluish coloration of the skin, bloody liquid drainage from the nose, and a gray covering in the back of the throat that blocks the airways and makes it difficult to breath.*

Oils—[TA]Frankincense, [TA]goldenrod.

T—Dilute as necessary, and apply 1–2 drops on throat, sinuses, or Vita Flex points on the feet.

A—Diffuse into the air. Inhale directly or applied to hands.

Disappointment:

Oils—[AT]Clary sage, [AT]Dream Catcher, [AT]eucalyptus, [AT]fir, [AT]frankincense, [AT]Gathering, [AT]geranium, [AT]ginger, [AT]Grounding, [AT]Harmony, [AT]Hope, [AT]Joy, [AT]juniper, [AT]lavender, [AT]orange, [AT]Present Time, [AT]spruce, [AT]thyme, [AT]Valor, [AT]ylang ylang.

A—Diffuse into the air. Inhale directly or applied to tissue or a cotton wick.

T—Apply to auricular emotion points. Dilute with V-6 Oil to create a massage oil, and massage onto the skin.

Discouragement:

Oils—[AT]Bergamot, [AT]cedarwood, [AT]Dream Catcher, [AT]frankincense, [AT]geranium, [AT]Hope, [AT]Joy, [AT]juniper, [AT]lavender, [AT]lemon, [AT]orange, [AT]rosewood, [AT]Sacred Mountain, [AT]sandalwood, [AT]spruce, [AT]Valor.

A—Diffuse into the air. Inhale directly or applied to tissue or a cotton wick.

T—Apply to auricular emotion points. Dilute with V-6 Oil to create a massage oil, and massage onto the skin.

Disinfectant: *See also Antibacterial, Antifungal, Antiviral.*

Oils—[T][F]Lemon, [T]Purification, [T][F]sage, [T]ocotea, [T]grapefruit.

T—Add —2 drops of oil to a wet cloth, and use the cloth to wipe down counters and other surfaces.

A—Diffuse into the air.

Blend #1—Add the following number of drops to a bowl of water (numbers in parenthesis indicate portions for a smaller batch): 10 lavender (2), 20 thyme (4), 5 eucalyptus (1), 5 oregano (1). If using the larger portions, add to a large bowl of water. If using the numbers in the parentheses, add the oils to a small bowl of water. Use blend to disinfect small areas.

Diuretic:

>> *A diuretic is a substance that causes the body to increase the rate of urination and fluid elimination.*

Oils—^T_FLemongrass, ^T_Frosemary, ^T_Fsage, ^T_Fcedarwood, ^T_Flavender, ^{T}tangerine, ^{T}cardamom, ^{T}cypress, ^{T}<u>EndoFlex</u>, ^{T}fennel, ^{T}grapefruit (all citrus oils), ^{T}juniper, ^{T}lemon, ^{T}marjoram, ^{T}mugwort, ^{T}onycha (benzoin), ^{T}orange, ^{T}oregano, ^{T}valerian.

—**ALLEVIATES FLUIDS**

Oils—^{T}Tangerine, ^{T}cypress, ^{T}fennel.

Blend #1—1 drop fennel, 2 drops cypress, 5 drops tangerine; apply from the top of the foot to the knee.

T—Dilute as necessary, and apply oil(s) to kidney area on back, to bottoms of feet, and on location.

Diverticulitis: *See Colon: Diverticulitis.*

Dizziness:

Oils—^{A}Tangerine.

A—Inhale directly or applied to hands.

DNA:

>> *DNA is the genetic material of the cell. DNA contains all of the codes that enable the cell to build the materials needed for proper cell structure and function. Mutation of DNA can lead to cell death or to cancer.*

Oils—^{AT}Chamomile (strengthens positive imprinting in DNA).

—**UNLOCK EMOTIONAL TRAUMA IN DNA**

Oils—^{AT}<u>Acceptance</u>, ^{AT}<u>3 Wise Men</u> (instructs DNA to open for discharge of negative trauma), ^{AT}sandalwood (unlocks negative programing in DNA and enhances the positive programming in the DNA cell to create a feeling of security and protection).

A—Diffuse into the air. Inhale directly or applied to tissue or a cotton wick.

T—Dilute with V-6 Oil to create a massage oil, and massage onto the skin. Apply to Vita Flex points.

Down Syndrome:

>> *Down syndrome is a genetic disorder that typically results in slower physical and mental development and in distinct facial features. Down syndrome is the single most common human birth defect.*

A=Aromatic **T**=Topical **I**=Internal

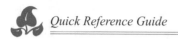

Oils—^{TA}<u>Clarity</u>, ^{TA}<u>Valor</u>.

T—Apply to bottoms of feet.

A—Diffuse into the air.

Supplements— Master Formula, Mineral Essence.

Dream State:

Recipe #1—^{AT}<u>Dream Catcher</u> dissipates negative thoughts and helps one hold onto dreams until they become reality. To help enhance the vividness of dreams, try applying cedarwood and valerian to the back of the neck (from the top of the shoulders to the base of the skull), and work the oils in with the Vita Flex technique. *For help with getting to a deep sleep, see Blend #3 under Insomnia.*

—INFLUENCES

    Oils—^{AT}Clary sage (enhances vivid dream recall). ^{AT}<u>Transformation</u>.

—PROTECTION FROM NEGATIVE DREAMS (THAT MIGHT STEAL YOUR VISION)

    Oils—^{AT}<u>Dream Catcher</u> (helps one achieve dreams).

A—Diffuse into the air. Inhale directly or applied to tissue or a cotton wick.

T—Apply to auricular emotion points or to back of neck. Dilute with V-6 Oil to create a massage oil, and massage onto the skin.

Drowning in Own Negativity:

Oils—^{AT}Grapefruit (prevent), ^{AT}<u>Transformation</u>.

A—Diffuse into the air. Inhale directly or applied to tissue or a cotton wick.

T—Apply to auricular emotion points. Dilute with V-6 Oil to create a massage oil, and massage onto the skin.

Drugs: *See Addictions; Drugs.*

Dying:

Oils—^{AT}<u>Awaken</u>, ^{AT}<u>Transformation</u>.

Recipe #1—The following combinations have also been used to help individuals pass on more peacefully into the next life: Frankincense (under the nose) and rose (over the heart), **or** <u>3 Wise Men</u> (under the nose) and <u>Joy</u> (over the heart).

A—Diffuse into the air. Inhale directly or applied to tissue or a cotton wick.

T—Apply to auricular emotion points. Dilute with V-6 Oil to create a massage oil, and massage onto the skin.

Dysentery: *See also Digestive System: DIARRHEA.*

▸▸ *Dysentery is severe, frequent diarrhea, often with blood or mucus, that occurs because of infection by bacteria or amoeba. Dysentery can be fatal, due to dehydration, if left untreated.*

Oils—T_FMyrrh, Teucalyptus, Tlemon, TRoman chamomile, Tblack pepper, Tcajeput, Tcistus, Tclove (amoebic), Tcypress, Tmelissa.

T—Dilute as necessary, and apply on abdomen and on bottoms of feet.

Supplements—JuvaPower/JuvaSpice

Dyspepsia: *See Digestive System: INDIGESTION.*

Ears:

Oils—TAHelichrysum (improves certain hearing losses), TAPurification, TAeucalyptus, TAMelrose (fights infection and earache), TAcumin (deafness following a bad viral flu infection), TAelemi, TAgeranium, TAIdaho tansy, TAjuniper, TAmarjoram, TAvalerian (combine with helichrysum for added pain relief), TAValor, TAvitex.

Instructions to increase and restore hearing—

1. Rub **Valor** on bottoms of feet, especially on the 2 smallest toes, and on the smallest fingers of the hand.

2. For each ear, layer 2 drops of **helichrysum**, **Purification**, **juniper**, and **peppermint** (in that order) around the inside (not deep) and back of ear, on the mastoid bone (behind ear), along the bottom of the skull around to the back of the head, and down the brain stem area.

3. Then do the following ear adjustment:

   1. Pull one ear **up** and then the other ear up—10 times each side; 20 times total.

   2. Pull one ear **back** and then the other back—5 times each side; 10 times total.

   3. Pull one ear **down** and then the other down—5 times each side; 10 times total.

   4. Pull one ear **forward** and then the other forward—5 times each side; 10 times total.

   5. Then make one quick pull with fingers in each direction (up/back/down/forward).

4. Rub **geranium** all around back and front of ear.

5. (Optional) Rub 2 drops **ravintsara** around base of both ears.

A=Aromatic   **T**=Topical   **I**=Internal

—EARACHE

> **Recipe #1**—1 drop of either basil, <u>Melrose</u>, or <u>ImmuPower</u>. Can also try 1 drop each of helichrysum and valerian together. Put the drop in your hand, and soak a small piece of cotton (small enough to fit snugly in the ear) in the oil. Place the piece of cotton in the ear, and apply the leftover oil on both the front and back of the ear with a finger.
>
> **Supplements**—JuvaPower/JuvaSpice.

—EARACHE IN ANIMALS

> **Recipe #1**—(Not cats) 1 drop <u>Melrose</u> on cotton swab, and then swab around in well of ear.
>
> **<u>Do not put oils directly into ear canal</u>**.

—HEARING IN A TUNNEL

> **Oils**—^{TA}<u>Purification</u>, ^{TA}ravintsara.

—INFECTION

> **Recipe #2**—<u>ImmuPower</u>, tea tree, <u>Melrose</u> (inside well of ear; down and around ear on the outside and under chin). <u>Purification</u> (inside well of ear), *Tea tree ericifolia* and lavender (all around outside of ear). Can also try myrrh and rosemary cineol together.

> *Ear infections can be caused by food allergies!*
>
> *Caution: When working on the ears, <u>do not put the oils directly into the ear canal</u>. Apply only 1–2 drops of oil to the ear by rubbing on the inside, outside, and on the mastoid bone directly behind the ear.*

—INFLAMMATION

> **Oils**—^{TA}Eucalyptus, ^{TA}palo santo.

—PIMPLES (IN EARS)

> **Oils**—^{TA}<u>ImmuPower</u>.

—TINNITUS

>> *Tinnitus is a ringing or other audible noise in the ears caused by ear infection, wax buildup, or a block in the Eustachian tube.*

> **Oils**—^{TA}Helichrysum (rub on inside and outside of ears, along mastoid bone behind ear), ^{TA}juniper.

T—Dilute as necessary, and apply on surface of the ear (not inside the ear canal) and behind the ear on the mastoid bone. Place 1 drop of oil on a cotton swab, and swab around the ear canal.

A—Diffuse into the air.

Eating Disorders:

—ANOREXIA

>> *Anorexia is a psychological disorder where a person becomes obsessed with body size and weight, often depriving him or herself of food to avoid gaining weight.*

Oils—^{TA}F Tarragon, ^{TA}grapefruit, ^{TA}Citrus Fresh, ^{TA}angelica, ^{TA}Christmas Spirit, ^{TA}coriander, ^{TA}Purification, ^{TA}Melrose, ^{TA}Valor.

T—Dilute as necessary, and apply to stomach and bottoms of feet.

A—Diffuse into the air. It may also help to diffuse antidepressant oils.

***Comments**—*Some studies have shown that people suffering from anorexia have a tendency to have lower levels of zinc.*

Supplements—Mineral Essence.

–ANTIDEPRESSANTS

Oils—^{AT}Lemon[216], ^{AT}lavender[218], ^{AT}bergamot[219], ^{AT}Citrus Fresh[219], ^{AT}Acceptance, ^{AT}basil, ^{AT}clary sage, ^{AT}neroli, ^{AT}Roman chamomile, ^{AT}ylang ylang ^{AT}coriander, ^{AT}grapefruit.

A—Diffuse into the air.

T—Dilute with V-6 Oil to create a massage oil, and massage onto skin.

—BULIMIA

>> *Bulimia is a disorder categorized by periods of overeating, or binging, followed by periods of self-induced vomiting, fasting, or abuse of laxatives and diuretics to purge the body of the food or to compensate for the overeating.*

Oils—^TCitrus Fresh, ^Tgrapefruit.

T—Apply to stomach and bottoms of feet.

—OVEREATING

>> *Overeating is eating too much food for the body. It can include binging (eating so much at one time that the stomach is overly filled and uncomfortable or painful), or chronic overeating (eating more than the body needs over a long period of time). Consistently overeating can lead to obesity and other health problems.*

Oils—^AGrapefruit[256], ^Alemon[256], ^Aginger, ^Apeppermint, ^Aspearmint.

A—Diffuse into the air. Inhale directly or applied to hands, tissue, or a cotton wick.

Eczema: *See Skin: ECZEMA.*

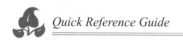

Edema: *See also Hormonal Imbalance, Inflammation.*

▸▸ *Edema is swelling caused by the abnormal accumulation of fluids in a tissue or body cavity. This can be caused by an allergic reaction, inflammation, injury, or as a signal of problems with the heart, liver, or kidneys.*

Oils—$^{TI}_F$Grapefruit, ^T_Fcypress (alleviates fluids), ^T_Flemongrass, tangerine (alleviates fluids), ^{T}fennel (breaks up fluids), ^{T}juniper, ^{T}geranium, ^{T}ledum, ^{T}rosemary.

Blend #1—1 drop fennel, 2 drops cypress, 5 drops tangerine. Apply from the top of the foot to the knee.

—**Ankles**

Blend #2—5 drops cypress, 3 drops juniper, and 10 drops tangerine, or use equal parts of cypress and tangerine. Apply from ankles to knees and on Vita Flex bladder points on feet.

—**Diuretic** *See Diuretic*

Oils—^T_FLemongrass, ^T_Frosemary, ^T_Fsage, ^T_Fcedarwood, ^T_Flavender, ^{T}tangerine, ^{T}cardamom, ^{T}cypress, ^{T}EndoFlex, ^{T}fennel, ^{T}grapefruit (all citrus oils), ^{T}juniper, ^{T}lemon, ^{T}marjoram, ^{T}mugwort, ^{T}onycha (benzoin), ^{T}orange, ^{T}oregano, ^{T}valerian.

***Comments—For water retention in the legs, Dr. Friedmann would rub tangerine, cypress, and juniper on inside of ankle(s) and leg(s) and on the kidney and heart Vita Flex points. He also had his patients inhale the oils as they were rubbed on.

T—Dilute as necessary, and apply 1–2 drops on location.

I—Add 1–2 drops to 8 oz. of water; drink every 3 hours.

Elbow: *See Tennis Elbow.*

Electrical Problems in the Body: *See Balance for methods of balancing the electrical energies of the body.*

Oils—^{TA}Valor, ^{TA}frankincense, ^{TA}Harmony.

T—Dilute as necessary, and apply to back and to bottoms of feet.

A—Diffuse into the air. Inhale directly or applied to hands.

Electrolytes:

▸▸ *Electrolytes are chemicals in the body, such as salts and minerals, needed for proper body functioning.*

—**Balancing**

Oils—^{I}Citrus Fresh (increases absorption of vitamin C).

I—Add 1–2 drops to empty capsule; swallow.

Supplements—Super C / Super C Chewable, Mineral Essence.

Emergency Oils:

Oils—**Start with the Everyday Oils collection** (frankincense, lemon, lavender, peppermint, <u>Purification</u>, <u>PanAway</u>, <u>Peace & Calming</u>, <u>Thieves</u>, and <u>Valor</u>), then add to that **cistus** and **helichrysum** (for bleeding and tissue repair), then **oregano, balsam fir**, and **sandalwood** (for DNA repair and any tissue damage).

The following oils are recommended by Dr. Daniel Pénoël as ones that everyone should have with them for any emergency:

Tea tree (*alternifolia*)—Colds, coughs, cuts, sore throat, sunburn, wounds.

Ravintsara—Powerful antiviral and antiseptic. Respiratory problems, viral infections, wounds.

Peppermint—Analgesic (topical pain reliever) for bumps and bruises. Also for fever, headache, indigestion, motion sickness, nausea, nerve problems, spastic colon, vomiting.

Basil—Earache, fainting, headaches, spasms (can substitute fennel), poisonous insect or snake bites, malaria.

Lavender—Burns (mix with tea tree), leg cramps, herpes, heart irregularities, hives, insect bites and bee stings, sprains, sunstroke. *If in doubt, use lavender!*

Geranium—Bleeding (increases to eliminate toxins, then stops; can substitute cistus), diarrhea, liver, regenerates tissue and nerves, shingles.

Helichrysum—Bruises, bleeding (stops on contact), hearing, pain, reduce scarring, regenerate tissue.

*****Comments**—*Dr. Pénoël also recommends including Tea tree ericifolia because it is more suited to children then Melaleuca alternifolia, and also elemi because it has similar properties to frankincense and myrrh but is less expensive.*

Emotions: *See Emotional Release in the Science and Application section at the beginning of the Reference Guide for Essential Oils. Also, refer to the Auricular Emotional Therapy chart in that same section for points on the ears where the oils can be applied.*

Oils—^{AT}<u>Acceptance</u>, ^{AT}<u>Aroma Siez</u>, ^{AT}<u>Awaken</u> (supports spiritual

> *For **Emotions**, see other topics such as: Abuse, Agitation, Anger, Anxiety, Apathy, Argumentative, Boredom, Concentration (Poor)Confusion, Daydreaming, Despair, Despondency, Disappointment, Discouragement, Fear, Frustration, Grief/Sorrow, Guilt, Irritability, Jealously, Mood Swings, Obsessiveness, Resentment, Restlessness, and Shock.*
>
> *For more information on using essential oils to help release stored emotions, read <u>Releasing Emotional Patterns using Essential Oils</u> by Carolyn Mein.*
>
> *For some exciting information about how emotions and feelings affect one's physical health, you may want to read Karol K. Truman's books, <u>Feelings Buried Alive Never Die …</u> and <u>Healing Feeling from Your Heart</u>.*

A=Aromatic   **T**=Topical   **I**=Internal | 169

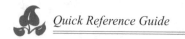

emotions), ^{AT}<u>Citrus Fresh</u> and ^{TA}spruce (on the chest and breathe in <u>Sacred Mountain</u>), ^Acypress (healing), ^{AT}<u>Envision</u> (support and balance), ^{AT}balsam fir (balancing), ^{AT}<u>Freedom</u>, ^{AT}<u>AromaSleep</u>, ^{AT}<u>Inner Harmony</u>, ^{AT}<u>Divine Release</u>, ^{AT}<u>T.R. Care</u>, ^{AT}<u>Gathering</u> (to help with feelings and thoughts), ^{AT}geranium (women), ^{AT}German chamomile (stability), ^{AT}goldenrod (relaxing and calming), ^{AT}<u>Gratitude</u>, ^{AT}<u>Humility</u>, and ^{AT}<u>Forgiveness</u> (to help with forgiveness), ^{AT}lavender (men), ^{AT}melissa (supports mind and body), ^{AT}<u>Live with Passion</u> (balancing, uplifting, strengthening, and stabilizing), ^{AT}palo santo, ^{AT}ravintsara (lifts emotions), ^{AT}<u>Release</u> (soothing), ^{AT}rose (brings balance and harmony to the body), ^{AT}sage lavender (improves mood), ^{AT}<u>Surrender</u> (calming and balancing), ^{AT}<u>3 Wise Men</u>, ^{AT}<u>Transformation</u>, ^{AT}<u>Trauma Life</u>, ^{AT}valerian (helps replace emotions), ^{AT}<u>White Angelica</u> (balances and protects), ^{AT}white lotus.

Blend #1—Layer the oils listed below. Wait 10 minutes between each oil to allow the emotions to be released more gently. The individual releasing the emotions should shut their eyes and should have no sounds, music, or candles in the room to distract them. They need to shut down their senses to get into their subconscious deep seated emotions. Breathe synergistically with their breathing.

1. Rub <u>Valor</u> on feet. If there are 2 helpers, have one person hold the individual's feet (your right hand to their right foot, left to left; cross arms if necessary) during the entire procedure. Be sure not to break the energy.

2. Rub <u>Peace & Calming</u> on navel, feet, and on the forehead (from left to right).

3. Put <u>Harmony</u> on each chakra in clockwise direction, on wrists, on shoulders, and on inside ankles.

4. Put <u>3 Wise Men</u> on crown.

Personal Care—Evening Peace or Sensation Bath & Shower Gel; Relaxation or Sensation Massage Oil; Sacred Mountain, Lavender Rosewood, or Peppermint Cedarwood Moisturizing Soaps; Prenolone/Prenolone+, Progessence/Progessence Plus, Sensation Hand & Body Lotion.

—ACCEPTANCE (SELF-ACCEPTANCE)

    Oils—^{AT}<u>Acceptance</u>, ^{AT}<u>Forgiveness</u>, ^{AT}<u>Joy</u>, and ^{AT}<u>Transformation</u>.

—ANGER AND HATE

    Oils—^T<u>Joy</u> (apply to pituitary Vita Flex points on feet and hands), ^T<u>Release</u>, and ^T<u>Valor</u> (layer these three oils on the

> *The emotions of the mind are the most elusive part of the human body. People are extremely handicapped emotionally and are continually looking for ways to clear these negative emotions. Many of the emotional blends referred to in this book were created from the research of the ancient Egyptian rituals of clearing emotions. They were created with the intent of helping people overcome the trauma of emotional and physical abuse enabling them to progress and achieve their goals and dreams. The Egyptians took three days and three nights to clear emotions. In order to create a very peaceful setting, they would put the person in a room with 10–12 inch thick walls of solid cement and close the door so there would be no sight or sound.*

anger or hate auricular ear point). ^{AT}<u>Acceptance</u>, ^{AT}<u>Forgiveness</u>, ^{AT}helichrysum (with deep-seated anger for strength to forgive), ^{AT}<u>Humility</u>.

—BALANCE

Oils—^{AT}<u>Australian Blue</u>, ^{AT}balsam fir, ^{AT}<u>Forgiveness</u>, ^{AT}frankincense, ^{AT}geranium, ^{AT}<u>Grounding</u>, ^{AT}<u>Harmony</u>, ^{AT}<u>Hope</u>, ^{AT}<u>Inner Child</u>, ^{AT}<u>Joy</u>, ^{AT}juniper, ^{AT}lavender, ^{AT}onycha (combine with rose for massage), ^{AT}orange, ^{AT}<u>Present Time</u>, ^{AT}<u>Release</u>, ^{AT}Roman chamomile, ^{AT}sage lavender, ^{AT}sandalwood, ^{AT}<u>SARA</u>, ^T<u>Stress Away</u>, ^{AT}<u>3 Wise Men</u>, ^{AT}<u>Transformation</u>, ^{AT}<u>Trauma Life</u>, ^{AT}<u>Valor</u>, ^{AT}vetiver, ^{AT}<u>White Angelica</u>.

Personal Care—Prenolone/Prenolone+, Progessence/Progessence Plus.

—BLOCKS

Oils—^{AT}Cypress, ^{AT}frankincense, ^{AT}<u>Harmony</u>, ^{AT}helichrysum, ^{AT}<u>Release</u> (over liver), ^{AT}sandalwood, ^{AT}spearmint, ^{AT}spikenard, ^{AT}spruce, ^{AT}<u>3 Wise Men</u>, ^{AT}<u>Trauma Life</u>, and ^{AT}<u>Valor</u> (help to release emotional blocks). ^{AT}<u>Acceptance</u> (can help one accept the change).

—BURDENED (BEARING BURDENS OF THE WORLD)

Oils—^T<u>Release</u> and ^T<u>Valor</u> (layer these two oils on the specific ear point). ^{AT}<u>Acceptance</u>.

—CHILDHOOD ISSUES

Oils—^T<u>SARA</u> (apply to the heart point on the ears).

–FEAR (relating to Childhood Issues)

Oils—^T<u>Gentle Baby</u>, ^T<u>Highest Potential</u>, ^T<u>Inner Child</u>, ^T<u>SARA</u>.

–FATHER OR MOTHER

Oils—^T<u>Gentle Baby</u> and/or ^T<u>Inner Child</u>.

—CLEARING

Oils——^{AT}<u>Forgiveness</u>, ^{AT}<u>Grounding</u>, ^{AT}<u>Harmony</u> (use <u>Hope</u> when emotional clearing), ^{AT}<u>Inner Child</u>, ^{AT}<u>Joy</u>, ^{AT}juniper, ^{AT}<u>Present Time</u>, ^{AT}<u>Release</u> (massage a couple drops on both ears for a general clearing), ^{AT}<u>SARA</u>, ^{AT}<u>3 Wise Men</u>, ^{AT}<u>Valor</u>, ^{AT}<u>White Angelica</u>.

***Comments—For some simple instructions on how to do emotional clearing, refer to the page on Emotional Release in the Science and Application section of the Reference Guide for Essential Oils. Another good reference for information on clearing negative emotions is the book, <u>Releasing Emotional Patterns</u> by Carolyn L. Mein, D.C.

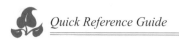

—**Coldness (emotional)**

　　Oils—ᴬᵀMyrrh, ᴬᵀylang ylang.

—**Confidence**

　　Oils—ᴬᵀEnvision, ᴬᵀHighest Potential, ᴬᵀjasmine (euphoria), ᴬᵀLive with Passion.

—**Defeated**

　　Oils—ᴬᵀAcceptance, ᴬᵀcypress, ᴬᵀfir, ᴬᵀForgiveness, ᴬᵀInspiration, ᴬᵀJoy, ᴬᵀjuniper,
　　　　ᴬᵀspruce,
　　　　ᴬᵀ3 Wise Men, ᴬᵀValor.

—**Depression** *See also Depression*

　　Oils—Most of the single oils and blends help with depression as they tend to lift
　　　　by raising one's frequency. Some of the best include ᴬᵀChristmas Spirit, ᴬᵀCitrus
　　　　Fresh, ᴬᵀGentle Baby, ᴬᵀHighest Potential, ᴬᵀHope, ᴬᵀJoy, ᴬᵀPeace & Calm-
　　　　ing, ᴬᵀValor, and ᴬᵀWhite Angelica. Use whichever blend(s) work best for you.
　　　　Other oils that may be good to use include ᴬᵀHumility, ᴬᵀInner Child, ᴬᵀlavender,
　　　　ᴬᵀSARA, and ᴬᵀTransformation.

　　Supplements—Omega Blue, OmegaGize^3.

—**Emotional Trauma**

　　Oils—ᴬᵀSandalwood, ᴬᵀFreedom, ᴬᵀAromaSleep, ᴬᵀInner Harmony, ᴬᵀDivine
　　　　Release, ᴬᵀT.R. Care, ᴬᵀTrauma Life.

—**Expression (self-expression)**

　　Oils—ᵀMotivation and ᵀValor (for courage to speak out—ᵀJoy may be added to
　　　　encourage enjoying life to its fullest). Take deep breaths to help express oneself.

—**Excessive**

　　Oils—ᵀSurrender (apply to the **self-expression** point on the ears).

—**Focused**

　　Oils—ᵀRelease, then ᵀAcceptance or ᵀGathering (layer oils on the **self-expression**
　　　　point on the ears).

—**Lost Identity**

　　Oils—ᵀᴬInner Child (apply to the **self-expression** point on the ears).

—**Eyes** *See Eyes for oils that help with eyesight.*

—**Vision of Goals**

　　Oils—ᵀBelieve, ᵀDream Catcher, ᵀAcceptance, ᴬᵀ3 Wise Men (layer on the **eyes &
　　　　vision** point on the ears). ᴬᵀEnvision, ᴬᵀInto the Future.

—FATHER

> **Oils—**^{TA}Lavender. Another oil that may be helpful to layer on top of lavender is ^Thelichrysum, especially when deep-seated anger is present.

> **–CHILDHOOD ISSUES**

>> **Oils—**^{TA}Gentle Baby, ^{TA}Inner Child.

> **–Male Abuse**

>> **Oils—**^THelichrysum and ^{TA}lavender (layer oils on the father point on the ears).

> **–SEXUAL ABUSE**

>> **Oils—**^TLavender, ^TRelease, and ^Tylang ylang (layer oils on the father point on the ears). ^{TA}SARA.

—FEAR

> **Oils—**^TValor, ^TRelease, and ^TJoy (layer on the fear point on the ears). ^{TA}Acceptance, ^{TA}Harmony, ^{TA}Highest Potential.

> **–CHILDHOOD ISSUES**

>> **Oils—**^{TA}Gentle Baby, ^{TA}Inner Child, ^{TA}SARA.

> **–FUTURE**

>> **Oils—**^{TA}Into the Future.

—FEMALE ISSUES *See MOTHER, below.*

—GRIEF

> **Oils—**^{TA}Bergamot (apply to the heart point on the ears), ^Atangerine (increases optimism and releases emotional stress).

—HEART (BROKEN OR HEAVY HEART): *Refer to both GRIEF and LOSS as well.*

> **Oils—**^TAcceptance, ^TForgiveness, and ^TJoy (layer oils on the heart point on the ears). ^{TA}Release, ^{TA}Transformation, ^{TA}Valor.

—LOSS (EASES THE FEELING)

> **Oils—**^{TA}Joy, ^{TA}Sensation, ^{TA}tangerine (stability).

—MALE ISSUES: *See FATHER, above.*

—MIND (OPEN)

> **Oils—**^T3 Wise Men (apply to the open the mind point on the ears as well as to the crown of the head and the navel). ^{TA}Acceptance, ^{TA}Believe, ^{TA}Clarity, ^{TA}frankincense, ^{TA}Gathering, ^{TA}Magnify Your Purpose, ^{TA}Motivation, ^{TA}Release, ^{TA}sandalwood, ^{TA}Transformation.

A=Aromatic　**T**=Topical　**I**=Internal

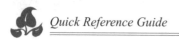

—Mood Elevation Protocol

> **Recipe #1**—<u>Valor</u> (one drop on each wrist; hold wrists together), <u>Harmony</u> (one drop on solar plexus), <u>Joy</u> (one drop over the heart), <u>White Angelica</u> (one drop on hands—rub hands together; then brush through hair, over the face, shoulders, and chest, and down the legs).

—Mother

> **Oils**—ᵀGeranium (apply to the **mother** point on the ears), ᵀᴬ<u>Inner Child</u>, ᵀᴬ<u>SARA</u>.

> –Abandonment

>> **Oils**—ᵀGeranium, ᵀ<u>Acceptance</u>, and ᵀ<u>Forgiveness</u> (layer oils on the **mother** point on the ears).

> –Sexual Abuse

>> **Oils**—ᵀGeranium and ᵀylang ylang (layer oils on the **mother** point on the ears).

—Overwhelmed

> **Oils**—ᵀ<u>Acceptance</u> and ᵀ<u>Hope</u> (layer on the **overwhelmed** point on the ears), ᵀᴬ<u>Grounding</u>, ᵀᴬ<u>Valor</u>.

—Pity (self-pity)

> **Oils**—ᵀ<u>Acceptance</u> (apply to the **self-pity** point on the ears). ᵀᴬ<u>Forgiveness</u>, ᵀᴬ<u>Joy</u>.

> –Courage (to move beyond feeling)

>> **Oils**—ᵀ<u>Release</u> then ᵀ<u>Valor</u> (layer on the **self-pity** point on the ears).

> –Painful (Can feel like heaviness in the chest)

>> **Oils**—ᵀ<u>PanAway</u> (apply to the **self-pity** point on the ears).

—Protection From Negative Emotions

> **Oils**—ᵀ<u>Magnify Your Purpose</u> (empowering and uplifting), ᵀgrapefruit, ᵀ<u>Highest Potential</u>, ᵀpalo santo, ᵀ<u>3 Wise Men</u> (release), ᵀ<u>White Angelica</u>. Apply oils to the forehead and over the heart.

—Rejection

> **Oils**—ᵀ<u>Forgiveness</u> and ᵀ<u>Acceptance</u> (layer on the rejection point on the ears). ᵀᴬ<u>Grounding</u>, ᵀᴬ<u>Valor</u>.

> –From Father

>> **Recipe #2**—Use lavender first then <u>Forgiveness</u> and <u>Acceptance</u>. Layer on the **rejection** point on the ears.

–FROM MOTHER

> **Recipe #3**—Use geranium first then <u>Forgiveness</u> and <u>Acceptance</u>. Layer on the **rejection** point on the ears.

—RELEASE

Oils— ^{AT}<u>Freedom</u>, ^{AT}<u>AromaSleep</u>, ^{AT}<u>Inner Harmony</u>, ^{AT}<u>Divine Release</u>, ^{AT}<u>T.R. Care</u>, ^{TA}_FRoman chamomile.

—STRESS *See also Anxiety*

Oils—^{TA}<u>Believe</u>, ^{TA}clary sage, ^{TA}<u>Evergreen Essence</u>, ^{TA}<u>Live with Passion</u>, ^{TA}<u>Surrender</u>.

—SUICIDAL

Oils—^{TA}<u>Gathering</u>, ^{TA}<u>Hope</u>, ^{TA}<u>Joy</u>, ^{TA}<u>Live with Passion</u>, ^{TA}<u>Release</u>, ^{TA}<u>Trauma Life</u>.

—SYMPATHY & GUILT

Oils—^T<u>Joy</u> and ^T<u>Inspiration</u> (layer on the **sympathy & guilt** point on the ears). ^{TA}<u>Release</u>, ^{TA}<u>PanAway</u>, ^{TA}<u>Acceptance</u>.

—UPLIFTING

Oils—^{TA}<u>Valor</u> (on feet), ^{TA}<u>Dream Catcher</u>, ^{TA}<u>En-R-Gee</u>, ^{TA}<u>Gratitude</u>, ^{TA}<u>Highest Potential</u>, ^{TA}lemon, ^{TA}orange, ^{TA}<u>Transformation</u>, ^{TA}wintergreen.

—VISION *See Eyes.*

A—Diffuse into the air. Wear as a perfume or cologne. Inhale directly or applied to hands, tissue, or a cotton wick. *See Comments under Asthma for a discussion on using* **plastic nasal inhalers**.

T—Apply to the specific auricular emotion points (*See Auricular Emotion Chart in the Science and Application chapter of this book for point locations*), or to area(s) indicated above. Apply behind ears and across forehead. Dilute with V-6 Oil to create a massage oil, and massage onto the skin.

Emphysema: *See also Blend #5 under Respiratory System.*

>> *Emphysema is a chronic pulmonary disease where airflow is restricted through the lungs due to destruction (typically caused by airborne toxins such as those in cigarette smoke) of the wall of the alveoli (small air sacs in the lungs where oxygen and carbon dioxide is exchanged with the blood). This destruction of the alveolar wall causes the alveoli to collapse when air is expelled from the lungs, trapping air inside.*

Oils—^{AT}Eucalyptus, ^{TA}<u>Raven</u> (hot compress on chest), ^{AT}Eucalyptus radiata, ^{AT}<u>Exodus II</u>.

Recipe #1—May use <u>Raven</u> rectally; <u>RC</u> on chest and back. Reverse each night. <u>Thieves</u> on feet; <u>ImmuPower</u> on spine.

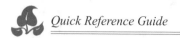
Blend #1—Equal parts rosemary cineol, lemon, and peppermint. Diffuse.

A—Diffuse into the air.

T—Dilute as necessary, and apply to chest and back. Apply as a warm compress on chest.

Empowerment:

Oils—^{AT}<u>Magnify Your Purpose</u>, ^{AT}<u>Sacred Mountain</u>, ^{AT}<u>Transformation</u>, ^{TA}<u>Oola Grow</u>, ^{TA}<u>Build Your Dream</u>.

A—Diffuse into the air. Inhale directly or applied to tissue or a cotton wick.

T—Apply to auricular emotion points. Dilute with V-6 Oil to create a massage oil, and massage onto the skin.

Endocrine System: *See Adrenal Glands, Thyroid, Pituitary Gland, Lupus, etc.*

>> *The adrenal glands, pituitary gland, thyroid gland, parathyroid glands, thymus gland, pineal gland, pancreas, ovaries, and testes are all a part of the endocrine system. The endocrine glands secrete hormones, transmitted via the bloodstream, which are responsible for regulating growth, metabolism, enzyme activity, and reproduction. Essential oils may either act as hormones or stimulate the endocrine glands to produce hormones. This production of hormones has a regulating effect on the body.*

Oils—^{AT}ᵣRosemary, ^{AT}cinnamon bark, ^{AT}black pepper, ^{AT}dill, ^{AT}<u>EndoFlex</u>, ^{AT}sage lavender.

A—Diffuse into the air. Inhale directly or applied to tissue or a cotton wick.

T—Dilute as necessary, and apply 1–2 drops on the reflex points on the feet, lower back, thyroid, liver, kidneys, gland areas, the center of the body, or both sides of the spine and clavicle area. Dilute with V-6 Oil to create a massage oil, and massage onto skin.

Personal Care—Prenolone/ Prenolone+, Progessence/Progessence Plus.

Supplements— **EndoGize,** Thyromin and FemiGen (women) or Prostate Health (men), Power Meal (pre-digested protein).

Endometriosis: *See Hormonal Imbalance.*

>> *Endometriosis is the growth of endometrial tissue in abnormal locations, such as on the ovaries or in the peritoneal (abdominal) cavity.*

Oils—^TGeranium, ^Tcypress, ^Tclary sage, ^Teucalyptus, ^T<u>Melrose</u> (hot compress on abdomen), ^Tnutmeg, ^T<u>Thieves</u> (on feet).

T—Dilute as necessary, and apply on lower abdomen or on feet. Apply as a warm compress. Place 1–2 drops in warm bathwater, and bathe.

Personal Care—Prenolone/ Prenolone+, Progessence/Progessence Plus, ClaraDerm (spray).

Supplements—Cleansing Trio (ComforTone, Essentialzyme, and ICP), Digest + Cleanse, Super C / Super C Chewable, FemiGen.

Recipe #1—Combine bergamot, lavender, and clary sage, and use with a hot compress over the abdomen or add 2 drops of each to 1 Tbs. V-6 Oil, and insert into the vagina; use a tampon to retain overnight. This may help rebuild the normal tissue.

Endurance:

—Physical

Oils—^ABalsam fir (inhale from hands), ^TEn-R-Gee (on feet), ^{AT}peppermint (cooling)[257].

A—Inhale directly or applied to hands, tissue, or a cotton wick. *See Comments under Asthma for a discussion on using plastic nasal inhalers.*

T—Dilute as necessary, and apply on skin.

Supplements— NingXia Nitro, Power Meal, Pure Protein Complete.

Energy:

Oils—^{AT}Fir, ^{AT}En-R-Gee, ^{AT}Valor (balances), ^{AT}peppermint, ^{AT}Oola Fitness, ^{AT}Abundance, ^{AT}Awaken, ^{AT}basil (when squandering energy), ^{AT}black pepper, ^{AT}Clarity, ^{AT}cypress, ^{AT}Envision (balances), ^{AT}eucalyptus (builds), ^{AT}Hope, ^{AT}Joy, ^{AT}juniper, ^{AT}lemon, ^{AT}lemongrass, ^{AT}Motivation, ^{AT}myrtle (supports adrenal glands to increase energy), ^{AT}nutmeg (increases), ^Aorange, ^{AT}Shutran, ^{AT}palo santo, ^{AT}rosemary, ^Athyme (gives energy in times of physical weakness and stress), ^{AT}White Angelica.

Personal Care—Morning Start Bath & Shower Gel or Lemon Sandalwood Cleansing Soap gives you a fresh start with a surge of energy.

Supplements—NingXia Red, NingXia Nitro, MultiGreens (gives energy), Master Formula (Multi-Vitamin), Mineral Essence, Thyromin, Super B.

—Electrical Energy (frequency)

Oils—^{AT}Forgiveness (high frequency), ^{AT}rose.

—Increase

Oils—^{AT}En-R-Gee, ^{AT}peppermint, ^{AT}Oola Fitness, ^{AT}Oola Fun, ^{AT}Brain Power, ^{AT}Clarity, ^{AT}eucalyptus, ^{AT}grapefruit, ^{AT}palo santo, ^{AT}rosemary.

Diffusion—*See Positive Ions for oils that produce positive ions when diffused to help increase energy.*

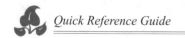

Supplements—Ultra Young+.

—INTEGRATES ENERGY FOR EQUAL DISTRIBUTION

Oils—**^{AT}**Patchouli.

—MAGNETIC

Oils—**^{AT}**<u>Abundance</u>, **^{AT}**<u>Joy</u> (enhances and attracts magnetic energy of prosperity and joy around
the body).

—NEGATIVE

Oils—**^{AT}**<u>White Angelica</u> (frequency protects against bombardment of), **^{AT}**ginger, **^{AT}**juniper (clears negative energy), **^{AT}**palo santo (clears).

—PHYSICAL

Oils—**^A**Cinnamon bark, **^A**lemon, **^{AT}**bergamot, **^A**patchouli.

—SEXUAL

Oils—**^{AT}**<u>Lady Sclareol</u>, **^A**ylang ylang (influences).

A—Inhale directly or applied to hands. Diffuse into the air.

T—Dilute with V-6 Oil to create massage oil, and massage into muscles. Place 1–2 drops in warm bathwater, and bathe. Dilute as necessary, and apply 1–2 drops on temples, back of neck, liver area, or feet.

Energy Centers: *See Chakras.*

Enlightening:

Oils—**^A**Helichrysum.

A—Diffuse into the air. Inhale directly or applied to hands, tissue, or a cotton wick.

Enteritis:

▸▸ *Enteritis is inflammation of the small intestine, usually caused by consuming food or drink contaminated with bacteria or a virus. Symptoms include abdominal pain, severe diarrhea, and loss of appetite.*

Oils—**^T**Cajeput.

T—Apply on abdomen or on Vita Flex points on the feet.

Enzymes:

▸▸ *Enzymes are proteins that facilitate the acceleration of natural chemical processes within the body.*

Recipe #1—Fresh carrot juice has one of the largest concentrations of enzymes. Drink 8 oz. per day. Add apple and lemon to help with detoxification.

Supplements—Enzyme products: **Allerzyme** (aids the digestion of sugars, starches, fats, and proteins), **Detoxzyme** (helps maintain and support a healthy intestinal environment).

Epilepsy: *See Seizure: EPILEPSY.*

Epstein-Barr: *See also Antiviral, Chronic Fatigue, Hypoglycemia, Mononucleosis.*

Oils—^{TA}ImmuPower, ^{TA}Thieves, ^{TA}eucalyptus.

Recipe #1—Do **Raindrop Technique** on spine with the addition of ImmuPower.

Supplements—AlkaLime, ComforTone, Essentialzyme, Essentialzymes-4, ICP, Immu-Pro, Inner Defense, JuvaPower/JuvaSpice, JuvaTone, Mineral Essence, MultiGreens, Super C / Super C Chewable, Thyromin, Master Formula.

E

Equilibrium:

Oils—^{AT}Surrender (emotional), ^{AT}ylang ylang.

—NERVE

Oils—^{AT}Petitgrain.

A—Diffuse into the air. Inhale directly or applied to tissue or a cotton wick.

T—Dilute as necessary, and apply on location. Dilute with V-6 Oil to create a massage oil, and massage onto the skin.

Essential Oils:

Essential oils function as a **catalyst** to deliver nutrients to starving cells.

—SENSITIVE TO SKIN (CAUSTIC, HIGH IN PHENOLS, MAY NEED TO DILUTE)

Oils—Cinnamon bark, clove, fennel, grapefruit, lemon, nutmeg, orange, oregano, peppermint. Test the oil first in a small, sensitive area. If irritation occurs, dilute with 1 drop of above oil to 20 drops lavender, or mix 1:4 with V-6 Oil.

Estrogen:

>> *Estrogens are hormones produced by the ovaries that regulate the development of female characteristics and the menstrual cycle in females.*

Oils—^{TA}Clary sage, ^{TA}SclarEssence, and ^{TA}Mister help the body produce estrogen. ^{TA}Anise (increases).

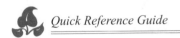

T—Dilute as necessary, and apply on the lower abdomen. Dilute in V-6 Oil, and use as massage oil.

A—Diffuse into the air. Inhale directly or applied to hands, tissue, or a cotton wick.

*****Comments**—Some sugar sweeteners block estrogen. Honey goes into the bloodstream quickly, which affects the pancreas and the production of estrogen.

Personal Care—**Prenolone/Prenolone+** (pregnenolone is the master hormone; it is used to balance estrogen and progesterone, whichever is needed).

Supplements—2 **FemiGen** three times a day, ten days before period. Start again two days after cycle. May take up to 6 tablets three times a day. **CortiStop** (Women's) can also help increase estrogen levels by lowering cortisol levels. 1 dropper of **Estro Tincture** three times a day in water

Euphoria:

Oils—^AClary sage, ^Ajasmine, ^{AT}Oola Fun.

A—Inhale directly or applied to hands, tissue, or a cotton wick. Diffuse into the air.

Exhaustion: *See also Energy.*

Recipe #1—First, work with one or more of the following nervous system oils to calm and relax: Bergamot, clary sage, coriander, cumin, elemi, frankincense, lavender, pine, sage lavender. Secondly, use basil, ginger, grapefruit, lavender, lemon, Roman chamomile, rosemary, sandalwood, or Transformation.

Expectorant: *See Congestion: EXPECTORANT.*

Expression (Self Expression):

Oils—^{AT}Helichrysum, ^{AT}Into the Future, ^{AT}Joy (when unable to express physically), ^{AT}Motivation, ^{AT}Raven, ^{AT}RC, ^{AT}Transformation, ^{AT}Valor.

A—Diffuse into the air. Inhale directly or applied to tissue or a cotton wick.

T—Apply to self expression auricular emotion point. Dilute with V-6 Oil to create a massage oil, and massage onto the skin.

Eyes:

Oils—^TCarrot (is good around eye area), ^Tlemongrass (improves eyesight), ^Tcypress (also helps

> ### *NEVER PUT OILS DIRECTLY IN THE EYES!*
> *Be careful when applying oils near the eyes. Be sure to have some V-6 Mixing Oil handy for additional dilution if irritation occurs. Never use water to wash off an oil that irritates.*

circulation), ᵀlemon, ᵀEucalyptus radiata, ᵀfennel, ᵀfrankincense, ᵀGerman chamomile, ᵀlavender, ᵀsandalwood.

Recipe #1—<u>Thieves</u> on feet (especially 2 big toes), <u>M-Grain</u> on thumb prints, layer <u>Mister</u>, <u>Dragon Time</u>, and <u>EndoFlex</u> on Vita Flex points, ankles, and pelvis.

Base Oils (good blends of)—Almond or hazelnut.

Supplements—**NingXia Red** (provides a significant amount of minerals and carotenoids that protect against eyesight deterioration. *See Comments below*), Power Meal, Sulfurzyme, Master Formula, Wolfberry Crisp Bars.

***Comments—According to the book <u>Discovery of the Ultimate Superfood</u>, "The Ningxia wolfberry is rich in two eye-protecting carotenoids—zeaxanthin and lutein—that are absolutely essential for protecting vision from the free radical damage, protein destruction, and blindness that occur with age."

E

Eye Drop Recipe—Combine 5 parts distilled water, 2 parts honey, and 1 part apple cider vinegar (do not use white vinegar). Mix together, and store in a bottle. Does not need to be refrigerated. This special eye drop formula is found in Stanley Burroughs' book, *Healing for the Age of Enlightenment* and has proven over the years to be superior to most commercial eye drops. These drops have been successful for helping to clear glaucoma, cataracts, spots, film, and growths of various kinds. Apply drops one at a time to each eye several times a day until condition has cleared.

—CATARACTS

>> *A cataract is a clouding of the normally transparent lens of the eye. This clouding results in blurry vision, seemingly faded colors, double vision, glare, and difficulty seeing at night. Over time, the clouding can increase and lead to severe vision problems.*

Blend #1—8 drops lemongrass, 6 drops cypress, and 3 drops eucalyptus. Apply around the eye area two times a day. Don't get in the eyes.

—DRY-ITCHY

Oils—ᴬTea tree (in humidifier).

—CONJUNCTIVITIS (PINK EYE)

>> *Conjunctivitis is an inflammation or infection of the membranes covering the whites of the eyes (conjunctiva) and the inner part of the eyelids. Swelling, redness, itching, discharge, and burning of the eyes are common symptoms. Frequent causes include allergies, bacterial or viral infection, contact lenses, and eye drops.*

Oils—ᴬᵀEucalyptus radiata, ᴬᵀjasmine.

A—Diffuse oils into the air.

A=Aromatic   **T**=Topical   **I**=Internal

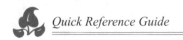

T—Dilute as necessary, and apply oils to Vita Flex points on the feet or to temples.

—EYE LID DROP (OR DROOPING EYELIDS)

›› *A drooping eyelid is characterized by an excessive sagging of the upper eyelid. Drooping can be present at birth as a result of underdeveloped eyelid muscles, or it can occur with aging. Drooping eyelids can cause visual impairment if they droop enough to partially cover the eye.*

Blend #2—1 drop <u>Aroma Life</u>, 1 drop helichrysum, 5 drops lavender.

Blend #3—Helichrysum and peppermint (don't get in the eyes).

Personal Care—**Cel-Lite Magic** (around eyes).

Supplements—3 MultiGreens four times a day. After massaging Vita Flex points, eat two whole oranges a day with the white still on the orange. It is very important to eat all the white you can plus Super C / Super C Chewable, ComforTone, and ICP (fiber beverage) after meals.

Vita Flex Points—Fingers, toes, and around the eyes.

> *I have had glaucoma for several years and have had my eye drop prescription changed numerous times because of rising pressure. I used a mixture of one third clove, one third lemon, and one third olive oil and rubbed it on my face above and below my eyes. The last time I was at the doctor, my pressure was 14. It was the lowest pressure I have had since I was diagnosed.*
> *–Submitted by K. Ernst (July 2004)*

—GLAUCOMA

Supplements—**Essentialzyme /Essentialzymes-4** (to help relieve stress on the pancreas, if congested), **Sulfurzyme** (to help regulate the fluid pressure in the eye), Super C / Super C Chewable, Super B, Master Formula.

—IMPROVE VISION

Oils—ᵀFrankincense, ᵀjuniper, ᵀlemongrass, ᵀ<u>Dragon Time</u>, ᵀ<u>EndoFlex</u>, ᵀ<u>Mister</u>, ᵀ<u>M-Grain</u>, ᵀsandalwood, ᵀ<u>Thieves</u>.

***Comments—According to Dr. Mercola, just about any oil can be used if it is consistently rubbed around each eye for several minutes twice a day. This must be continued for at least 3 weeks before any improvement can be seen. He recommends using frankincense and lavender.

Blend #4—10 drops lemongrass, 5 drops cypress, and 3 drops *Eucalyptus radiata* in 1 oz. V-6 Oil. Apply around eyes morning and night to improve eyesight. Can also be applied to Vita Flex eye points on fingers and toes and also on the ears *(refer to the Auricular Emotional Therapy chart in the Science & Application section of this book for the Eyes and Vision point on the ears).*

Blend #5—5 drops lemongrass, 3 drops cypress, and 2 drops eucalyptus in 1 oz. of V-6 Oil. Apply as a blend, or layer the oils on the eye area (not in eyes).

*****Comments**—*One individual who was not able to see color and who had no peripheral vision rubbed frankincense on his eyelids and just above his eyebrows. Soon thereafter he was able to see color, and his peripheral vision returned.*

—IRIS, INFLAMMATION OF

    ▸▸ *The iris is the colored part of the eye that regulates the amount of light entering the eye through the pupil. When the iris becomes inflamed, it results in a condition called iritis. Iritis is normally related to a disease or infection in another part of the body, but it can also be caused by injury to the eye. Symptoms of iritis include blurred vision, pain, tearing, light sensitivity, red eye, and a small pupil size.*

    Oils—ᵀEucalyptus.

—RETINA (BLEEDING)

    Blend #6—5 drops tangerine, 5 drops orange, and 5 drops grapefruit. Mix, and apply 2 drops on fingers and toes. Massage Vita Flex points two times a day or more. Diffuse, and let vapor mist around eye. Rub Cel-Lite Magic around the eyes too. Then eat two whole oranges a day with the white still on the orange. Eat all of the white you can.

    Supplements—Super C / Super C Chewable.

—RETINA (STRENGTHEN)

    ▸▸ *The retina is a layer of nerves lining the back of the eye. The retina is responsible for sensing light and then sending impulses (via the optic nerve) back to the brain so that visual images can be formed.*

    Oils—ᵀCypress, ᵀlemongrass, ᵀhelichrysum, ᵀjuniper, ᵀlavender, ᵀpeppermint, ᵀsandalwood.

    Blend #7—5 drops juniper, 3 drops lemongrass, 3 drops cypress. Rub on brain stem twice a day.

—SPIRITUAL EYES (3RD EYE, BROW CHAKRA) *See also Chakras*

    Oils—ᵀAcceptance, ᵀAwaken, ᵀDream Catcher.

    T—Rub oil on earlobe to increase both physical and spiritual vision.

—SWOLLEN EYES

    Blend #1—Cypress and helichrysum. Lavender (antiseptic) is also safe around eyes. If swollen eyes are due to allergies, try putting peppermint on the back of the neck.

T—Caution: Never put essential oils directly in the eyes! Be careful when applying oils near the eyes. Be sure to have some V-6 Oil handy for additional dilution if irritation

---

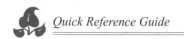
occurs. Dilute as necessary, and apply oils to feet, Vita Flex eye points, thumbs, ankles, pelvis, eye area (not in eyes), and eyebrows.

A—Diffuse into the air.

Facial Oils: *See also Skin.*

Oils—ᵀMyrrh, ᵀpatchouli, ᵀsandalwood, ᵀvetiver. *Refer to the Personal Care Products section of the <u>Reference Guide for Essential Oils</u> for many other beneficial skin care products.*

Personal Care—Essential Beauty Serums (Dry & Acne-Prone Skin Blends).

—BROKEN CAPILLARIES

    Oils—ᵀCypress, ᵀgeranium, ᵀhyssop, ᵀRoman chamomile.

—DEHYDRATED

    Oils—ᵀGeranium, ᵀlavender.

—DISTURBED

    Oils—ᵀGeranium, ᵀlavender, ᵀRoman chamomile, ᵀclary sage, ᵀhyssop, ᵀjuniper, ᵀlemon, ᵀpatchouli, ᵀsandalwood.

—DRY

    Oils—ᵀGeranium, ᵀGerman chamomile, ᵀrosemary, ᵀhyssop, ᵀlemon, ᵀpatchouli, ᵀsandalwood.

—ENERGIZING

    Oils—ᵀBergamot, ᵀlemon.

—HYDRATING

    Oils—ᵀGeranium, ᵀlavender, ᵀcypress, ᵀfennel, ᵀhyssop, ᵀlemon, ᵀpatchouli, ᵀsandalwood.

—NORMAL

    Oils—ᵀGeranium, ᵀlavender, ᵀlemon, ᵀRoman chamomile, ᵀsandalwood.

—OILY

    Oils—ᵀLemon, ᵀorange, ᵀcypress, ᵀfrankincense, ᵀgeranium, ᵀjasmine, ᵀjuniper, ᵀlavender, ᵀmarjoram, ᵀpatchouli, ᵀRoman chamomile, ᵀrosemary.

—REVITALIZING

    Oils—ᵀCypress, ᵀfennel, ᵀlemon.

—SENSITIVE

    Oils—ᵀGeranium, ᵀGerman ᵀchamomile, ᵀlavender.

T—Dilute as necessary, and apply to face (avoiding eyes), back of neck, behind ears, or Vita Flex points on the feet.

Fainting: *See also Shock.*

» *Fainting is a temporary loss of consciousness caused by a momentary disruption of blood flow to the brain. Fainting can result from standing in one place too long, coughing very hard, fear, emotional trauma, heavy bleeding, or severe dehydration. Fainting can sometimes be a symptom of a more serious condition.*

Oils—ᴬPeppermint, ᴬrosemary, ᴬTrauma Life, ᴬblack pepper[258], ᴬnutmeg, ᴬbasil, ᴬBrain Power, ᴬClarity, ᴬlavender, ᴬneroli, ᴬspearmint.

A—Inhale directly.

Faith:

Oils—ᴬᵀHope (increases), ᴬᵀTransformation (for anchoring and stabilizing new-found faith).

A—Diffuse into the air. Inhale directly or applied to tissue or a cotton wick.

T—Apply to crown chakra or to auricular emotion point. Dilute with V-6 Oil to create a massage oil, and massage onto the skin.

Fasting:

» *Fasting is the avoidance of solid foods altogether, while liquid consumption ranges between nothing (complete avoidance of all liquids as well) and fresh juices, with just water being somewhere in the middle. **Complete avoidance fasting (no food or liquid) should only be done when you are feeling good**, while fasting on fresh juices can be very healing when sick. The Master Cleanser lemonade fast (see Cleansing) is one of the most beneficial juice fasts. While it takes 30 days on this cleanse to change the chemistry in the body (such as eliminating the need or desire for animal proteins), very effective health results can be achieved after only 10 days. To enhance the effectiveness of the change in body chemistry, the 30 day lemon juice fast can be followed by a carrot juice fast for another 30 days. MultiGreens may be taken two times a day for two weeks but should then be stopped so changes can be made at the cellular level; protein prevents this change. When a mother fasts, the breast-fed baby gets the benefits as well (the mammary glands filter the toxins so they are not harmful to the baby).*

Fat: *See also Cellulite, Diet, and Weight.*

Bath (**attack fat**)—Add 6 drops of the following blend to the bathwater, and soak in tub.

> *Ultra Young+ may help stimulate the pituitary for increased production of the human growth hormone. This hormone is one of the most powerful side effect–free agents for rejuvenating the body, restoring lean body mass, and reducing fat.*

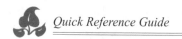

Blend #1—8 drops grapefruit, 5 drops cypress, 4 drops lavender, 4 drops basil, and 3 drops juniper.

Supplements—Allerzyme (aids the digestion of sugars, starches, fats, and proteins), Balance Complete, Digest + Cleanse, Power Meal (eat for breakfast as a meal replacement), Ultra Young+ (improves fat-to-lean ratios by stimulating production of the human growth hormone).

***Comments—Eat more grapefruit to dissolve fat faster. Also, trans fats replace essential fatty acids in the brain and are highly acidic. Remove trans fats from diet!

Father (Problems With):

Oils—^{TA}Acceptance, ^{TA}lavender, ^{TA}Valor.

T—Apply to father auricular emotion point. Dilute with V-6 Oil to create a massage oil, and massage onto the skin.

A—Diffuse into the air. Inhale directly or applied to tissue or a cotton wick.

Fatigue: *See also Energy.*

Oils—^{TA}_FRavintsara (muscle), ^{TA}_Frosemary (nervous), ^{TA}_Fthyme (general) ^{TA}En-R-Gee, ^{TA}clove, ^{TA}pine.

Supplements—NingXia Red.

—MENTAL

Oils—^{TA}Basil, ^{TA}lemongrass, ^{TA}Clarity, ^{TA}Peace & Calming.

Blend #1—Basil and lemongrass together are a good combination. Apply on temples, back of neck, and feet. Diffuse.

—OVERCOMING

Recipe #1—Thyme or En-R-Gee on spine, wait a few minutes, then Awaken all over the back and spine; **or** En-R-Gee on feet and Awaken on temples and cheeks.

—PHYSICAL *See Energy*

Oils—^{TA}Clarity, ^{TA}Peace & Calming.

Supplements—AlkaLime (acid-neutralizing mineral formulation), MultiGreens, Omega Blue, OmegaGize³, Power Meal, Sulfurzyme, Thyromin, Wolfberry Crisp Bars.

T—Dilute as necessary, and apply on liver or on feet. Dilute with V-6 Oil, and apply as a body massage.

A—Diffuse into the air. Inhale directly or applied to hands.

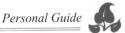
Fatty Deposits: *See also Cellulite, Fat, Weight.*

—Dissolve

> **Supplements**— Allerzyme (aids the digestion of sugars, starches, fats, and proteins), Balance Complete (contains a mix of 5 different kinds of fibers to help cleanse the digestive system), Digest + Cleanse, Master Formula, MultiGreens, Power Meal.

Fear: *See also Anxiety, Calming.*

> Oils—^{AT}Bergamot, ^{AT}clary sage, ^{AT}cypress, ^{AT}fir, ^{AT}geranium,

> *Fear causes the blood vessels to tighten, restricting the amount of oxygen and nutrients that can reach the cells.*

> ^{AT}<u>Highest Potential</u>, ^{AT}<u>Hope</u>, ^{AT}juniper, ^{AT}marjoram, ^{AT}<u>Motivation</u> (releases emotional and physical fears), ^{AT}myrrh, ^{AT}orange, ^{AT}<u>Present Time</u>, ^{AT}Roman chamomile, ^{AT}rose, ^{AT}sandalwood, ^{AT}spruce, ^{AT}<u>Valor</u>, ^{AT}<u>White Angelica</u>, ^{AT}ylang ylang.

A—Diffuse into the air. Inhale directly or applied to tissue or a cotton wick.

T—Apply to auricular emotion points. Dilute with V-6 Oil for massage onto the skin.

Feet:

> Oils—^TLemon, ^Tlavender, ^TRoman chamomile, ^Tfennel, ^Tpine (excessive sweating).

—Calluses

> Oils—^T<u>Melrose</u>, ^Toregano

—Club Foot

> Oils—^TGinger (see below), ^Trosemary (see below), ^Tlavender, ^TRoman chamomile.

> ***Comments—Do not use ginger or rosemary on babies *except* for treating for club foot.

—Corns

> Oils—^TClove, ^Tcarrot, ^T<u>Citrus Fresh</u>, ^Tgrapefruit, ^Tlemon, ^Tmyrrh, ^Tpeppermint, ^TRoman chamomile, ^Ttangerine.

> *Stanley Burroughs touts clove oil as being wonderful for corns, skin cancer, and warts. He suggests using your finger to apply a small amount of clove oil directly on warts or corns. After a short time, use an emery stick to scrape off the top of the wart or corn and apply the oil again. Repeat several times daily until wart or corn disappears. The same technique can be used for skin cancer. (Healing for the Age of Enlightenment, p. 104.)*

> **T**—Apply 1 drop of oil directly on corn.

—Odor

> **Recipe #1**—Mix 1 Tbs. baking powder with 2 drops of sage, and put in a plastic bag. Shake and eliminate lumps with a rolling pin and put in shoes. Rub calamus on feet.

T—Dilute as necessary, and apply on location. Dilute with V-6 Oil, and massage on location.

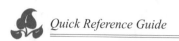

Female Specific Conditions: *See also Hormonal Imbalance, Infertility, Ovaries, Pregnancy/Motherhood, Uterus.*

Oils—^{TA}<u>Mister</u> (during time of month when you are out of sorts), ^{TA}clary sage, ^{TA}anise, ^{TA}<u>Sacred Mountain</u> (female balance).

Supplements— Master Formula, MultiGreens, FemiGen, Prenolone/Prenolone+, Progessence/Progessence Plus.

—ABNORMAL PAP SMEARS

Recipe #1—Add 10 drops <u>ImmuPower</u> and 5 drops frankincense to 1 Tbs. V-6 Oil, and insert into vagina. Use tampon to retain overnight. Take Master Formula to support nutrient level. May continue daily for as long as necessary.

—BALANCE FEMALE HORMONES

Oils—^{TA}Ylang ylang, ^{TA}bergamot, ^{TA}sage lavender.

Personal Care—Dragon Time Bath & Shower Gel for that time of month that leaves women with lower back pain, stress, and sleeping difficulties. Pour between 1 tsp. and 1 oz. of the gel in water while filling your tub.

Supplements—One week after the cycle, take Master Formula four times a day and 6 MultiGreens a day. CortiStop (Women's) can also help reduce cortisol levels and balance hormones.

—HEMORRHAGING *See also Hemorrhaging.*

Recipe #2—Combine 10 drops helichrysum with 1 tsp. V-6 Oil, and massage on ankles, lower back, and stomach.

—HOT FLASHES

» *A hot flash is a sudden, intense feeling of heat in the face and upper body, often accompanied by an increased heart rate, sweating, dizziness, headache, weakness, or anxiety. Hot flashes are generally associated with the symptoms of menopause and premenopause.*

Oils—^T_FPeppermint, ^Tclary sage (estrogen),^T<u>EndoFlex</u>, ^Tbergamot (estrogen), ^Tfennel, ^T<u>Dragon Time</u>, ^T<u>Mister</u> (estrogen—works for women in Canada).

T—Apply these oils on the ankles at the ovary and uterus Vita Flex points.

Blend #1—If hypoglycemic, use <u>Aroma Siez</u> with <u>M-Grain</u>. Apply over ovaries, pelvis, ankles, bottoms of feet.

***Comments—Some women have had success using a drop of <u>EndoFlex</u> under their tongue three times a day. Be cautious as it contains nutmeg and an overdose could cause problems.

Personal Care—Prenolone/Prenolone+, Progessence/Progessence Plus.

Supplements—CortiStop (Women's), EndoGize, FemiGen, Mineral Essence.

—INFECTION

    Oils—^{TA}_FBergamot (general), ^{TA}<u>Melrose</u>, ^{TA}frankincense

    ***Comments—You may mix the oils listed above and insert in vagina at night; may alternate with the blend below.

    Blend #2—8 drops juniper, 8 drops tea tree, and 8 drops <u>Purification</u>. Put in water and douche **or** add 3 drops of each to 1 tsp. V-6 Oil, and insert at night using a tampon to retain.

    Blend #3—8 drops juniper, 8 drops lavender, and 8 drops <u>Melrose</u>. Alternate with Blend #1, and follow same instructions.

—INFERTILITY (FEMALE) *See also Fertility.*

    Oils—^TClary sage, ^T<u>Sclar-Essence</u>, ^Tcypress, ^Tfennel, ^Tgeranium, ^Tmelissa, ^Tnutmeg, ^TRoman chamomile, ^Tthyme.

    Recipe #3—Before the cycle, rub 10 drops <u>Dragon Time</u> around ankles, lower back, and lower stomach. During the cycle, rub 4 drops basil in the same places as before.

    Personal Care—Prenolone/Prenolone+, Progessence/Progessence Plus.

    Supplements—FemiGen, Master Formula.

—MENOPAUSE *See also Hormonal Imbalance*

   ▸▸ *Menopause is the permanent ending of a female's menstruation and fertility. For most American women, Menopause occurs around age 51 and is often recognized by hot flashes, irregular periods, vaginal dryness, mood swings, difficulty sleeping, thinning hair, abdominal weight gain, and decreased fertility.*

    Oils—^T_FCypress, ^T_Flavender[259], ^T_Forange, ^T_Ffennel[260], ^T_Fsage, ^TRoman chamomile, ^Tangelica, ^Tbasil, ^Tbergamot, ^Tcardamom, ^Tclary sage, ^T<u>Dragon Time</u> (add V-6 Oil and use in douche, enema, or in rectum), ^T<u>EndoFlex</u> (on throat, parathyroid, and thyroid), ^Tgeranium, ^Tjasmine, ^T<u>Mister</u>, ^Tneroli, ^Tnutmeg (balances hormones), ^Trose, ^Trosemary, ^T<u>SclarEssence</u>, ^Tthyme.

    Personal Care—Add between 1 tsp. and 1 oz. of **Dragon Time Bath & Shower Gel** to bath while filling tub with water. Soaking helps relieve lower back pain, stress, and sleeping difficulties that are associated with a woman's cycle. **Dragon Time Massage Oil.**

    Supplements—Progessence/Progessence Plus, CortiStop (Women's), EndoGize, FemiGen, PD 80/20, Prenolone/ Prenolone+.

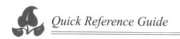

*****Comments**—The possibility for heart attacks in women increases by 5–10% following menopause.

–Pre-Menopause

> Oils—ᵀ_F_Clary sage, ᵀ_F_fennel, ᵀsage lavender (helps raise hormone levels naturally), ᵀ<u>EndoFlex</u>, ᵀlavender, ᵀ<u>Mister</u>, ᵀnutmeg (balances hormones), ᵀ<u>SclarEssence</u>, ᵀtarragon.

—Menstruation *See Also Endometriosis, Hormonal Imbalance*

>> *Menstruation, also known as a woman's "period," is the regular shedding of the uterus lining and vaginal discharge of blood when a woman is not pregnant. A woman's period lasts between two and seven days and reoccurs on an average of every 28 days.*

> *Amenorrhea is the absence of menstruation. The oils listed are those which induce menstrual flow (emmenagogic).*
>
> *Emmenagogue is an agent that induces or hastens menstrual flow. Many of these oils should be avoided during pregnancy. Please see* pregnancy *for safety data.*
>
> *Dysmenorrhea is painful menstruation. Apply one or more of these oils to the abdomen. It may also help to use a hot compress. Each of us has different body chemistries, so if one oil doesn't work, try a different one.*
>
> *Menorrhagia is abnormally heavy or extended menstrual flow. It may also refer to irregular bleeding at any time. This situation may be a sign of a more serious condition, so please see your doctor.*

–Amenorrhea

> Oils—ᵀ_F_Basil, ᵀ<u>Dragon Time</u>, ᵀcarrot, ᵀcistus, ᵀclary sage, ᵀfennel, ᵀhyssop, ᵀjuniper, ᵀlavender, ᵀmarjoram, ᵀmyrrh, ᵀpeppermint, ᵀRoman chamomile, ᵀrose, ᵀrosemary, ᵀsage, ᵀsage lavender.

–Dysmenorrhea

> Oils—ᵀ_F_Tarragon, ᵀclary sage (followed by basil)[261], ᵀlavender[261], ᵀrose[263], ᵀcypress, ᵀpeppermint, ᵀ<u>Dragon Time</u>, ᵀ<u>EndoFlex</u>, ᵀfennel, ᵀjasmine, ᵀjuniper, ᵀmarjoram[262], ᵀRoman chamomile, ᵀrosemary, ᵀsage, ᵀsage lavender, ᵀyarrow.

> Bath & Shower Gels— Add 1 tsp.–1 oz. **Dragon Time Bath & Shower Gel** to bath while filling tub with water. Soaking helps relieve lower back pain, stress, and sleeping difficulties that are associated with a woman's cycle.

> *I have been using Young Living Essential Oils for a little over a year now. Since then, my health has improved somewhat. I decided to stop using birth control pills on Labor Day of 2003, due to being sick from them most of the time and wanting to try something else. I started putting <u>EndoFlex</u> on the bottom of my feet on the endocrine reflex areas. I also continued receiving colonics twice a month and eating cultured vegetables. Between the <u>EndoFlex</u>, colonics, and cultured vegetables, my periods have become more regular and less painful. A friend of mine who's also using <u>EndoFlex</u> on her feet has said that her hot flashes have stopped since she's been using EndoFlex.*
>
> *-Submitted by Christie Krajewski*
> *Batesville, Arkansas (July 2004)*

–GENERAL CARE

> Blend #4—Before and during cycle, combine 10 drops <u>Dragon Time</u> with 4 drops basil, and rub around ankles, lower back, and lower stomach.

> Personal Care—Dragon Time Massage Oil (uncomfortable days and irregularity). PD 80/20, Prenolone/Prenolone+, or Progessence/Progessence Plus may help to regulate the hormones which should alleviate many of the problems associated with menstruation. *See Hormonal Imbalance.*

> Supplements—One week after the cycle, take Master Formula, four times a day and 6 MultiGreens a day. Also EndoGize, FemiGen (for PMS).

–IRREGULAR

> Oils—^T_FSage, ^T_Fpeppermint, ^T_Frosemary, ^Tclary sage, ^Tfennel, ^Tlavender, ^Tmelissa, ^TRoman chamomile, ^Trose.

–MENORRHAGIA

> Oils—^TCypress, ^Tgeranium, ^TRoman chamomile, ^Trose.

–SCANTY

> Oils—^TLavender, ^Tpeppermint, ^Tjasmine, ^Tmelissa. *See also oils listed under Amenorrhea.*

—OVARIES *See Ovaries.*

—PMS (Premenstrual Syndrome) *See also Hormonal Imbalance.*

>> *Premenstrual syndrome (PMS) is a group of symptoms such as irritability, anxiety, moodiness, bloating, breast tenderness, headaches, and cramping that occur in the days or hours before menstruation begins and then disappear once menstruation begins. PMS is thought to be caused by the fluctuation in hormones during this time, or by the way progesterone is broken down by the body. Caffeine intake from beverages or chocolate is also thought to enhance PMS symptoms.*

> Oils—^{TA}_FClary sage, ^{TA}_Ftarragon, ^{TA}fennel[264], ^{TA}angelica, ^{TA}anise, ^{TA}bergamot, ^{TA}<u>Exodus II</u>, ^{TA}geranium, ^{TA}grapefruit, ^{TA}jasmine, ^Alavender, ^{TA}nutmeg, ^{TA}<u>Peace & Calming</u>, ^{TA}Roman chamomile.

> Personal Care—Dragon Time Massage Oil, Progessence/Progessence Plus, Prenolone/Prenolone+.

> Supplements—FemiGen, Master Formula, MultiGreens, Omega Blue, Omega-Gize[3], Wolfberry Crisp Bars.

–Apathetic-Tired-Listless

> Oils—^{TA}Geranium, ^{TA}grapefruit, ^{TA}bergamot, ^{TA}fennel, ^{TA}Roman chamomile.

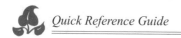

Personal Care—Dragon Time Bath & Shower Gel.

Blend #5—10 drops <u>Dragon Time</u> and 4 drops basil. Rub blend on ankles, lower back, and lower stomach. Use before and during cycle.

–Irritable

Oils—^{TA}Bergamot, ^{TA}clary sage, ^{TA}nutmeg, ^{TA}Roman chamomile.

Blend #5—Before and during cycle, combine 10 drops <u>Dragon Time</u> with 4 drops basil, and rub on ankles, lower back and lower stomach.

Supplements—NingXia Red, Omega Blue, OmegaGize³, PD 80/20, Prenolone/Prenolone+, Progessence/Progessence Plus, Wolfberry Crisp Bars. One week after the cycle, take Master Formula four times a day and 6 Multi-Greens a day. Also FemiGen (for PMS)—take 2 FemiGen three times a day before period, and start again two days after cycle.

–Violent Aggressive

Oils—^{TA}Bergamot, ^{TA}geranium, ^{TA}nutmeg.

Supplements—Omega Blue, OmegaGize³.

–Weeping-Depression

Oils—^{TA}Bergamot, ^{TA}clary sage, ^{TA}geranium, ^{TA}nutmeg.

Supplements—Omega Blue, OmegaGize³.

—Postpartum Depression *See Pregnancy/Motherhood: Postpartum Depression*

—Reproductive System

Supplements—^{TA}FemiGen (may help build and balance the reproductive system and help maintain better hormonal balance for developmental years all the way through menopause).

T—Dilute as necessary, and apply to the abdomen, lower back, groin, shoulders, or Vita Flex points on the feet. Dilute with V-6 Oil for massage oil, and massage on abdomen, lower back, and shoulders. Apply as a warm compress to the abdomen. Add 1–2 drops to 2 tsp. olive oil, insert into vagina, and retain overnight with a tampon.

A—Diffuse into the air. Inhale directly or applied to hands.

Fertility: *See also Female Specific Conditions, Male Specific Conditions.*

Oils—^TClary sage, ^T<u>Mister</u>, ^I<u>SclarEssence</u> (taken as a dietary supplement to help raise estradiol and testosterone levels), ^Tbergamot, ^T<u>Dragon Time</u>, ^Tfennel, ^Tgeranium, ^Tmelissa, ^Tsage, ^T<u>Sensation</u>, ^Tyarrow.

T—Apply on reproductive Vita Flex areas on feet, particularly around front of ankle, in line with ankle bone, on each side of ankle under ankle bone, and up along the Achilles tendon. Women: on lower back and on lower abdomen near pubic bone. Can also dilute with V-6 Oil and use as vaginal retention implant. Men: on lower abdomen near pubic bone, on area between scrotum and rectum, and as a rectal implant (diluted with V-6 Oil).

I—Add 2–4 drops to an empty capsule with 2–4 drops V-6 Oil, and swallow.

Personal Care—Prenolone/Prenolone+, Progessence/Progessence Plus, Protec (as rectal or vaginal implant).

Supplements—AlkaLime, Balance Complete (*refer to the 5-Day Nutritive Cleanse program listed under Balance Complete in the Supplements section of the <u>Reference Guide for Essential Oils</u>. This program also uses Digest + Cleanse and NingXia Red to help enhance detoxification while maintaining energy levels*), Digest + Cleanse, Ultra Young+, MultiGreens. FemiGen (women), Prostate Health (men), Master Formula.

***Comments—An accumulation of petrochemicals in the body can cause sterility in both men and women. Do the **MASTER CLEANSER** (See Cleansing) for 10 to 20 days consecutively. After coming off the cleanse, focus on alkaline-ash foods. When the body is acidic, it can be hard to conceive.

Fever:

» *Fever is an increase of the body's core temperature, typically in response to an infection or injury. A fever is the body's natural response to help enhance the immune system's ability to fight the infection.*

Oils—^{ITA}ₚPeppermint (reduces), ^Iₚlemon or lime (reduces), ^{TA}ₚeucalyptus, ^Iclove, ^{TA}basil, ^{TA}bergamot, ^{TA}fennel (breaks up), ^{TA}fir, ^{TA}ginger, ^T<u>ImmuPower</u> (rub on spine), ^{TA}lavender, ^{TA}ledum, ^{TA}tea tree, ^{TA}rosemary cineol, ^{TA}sage lavender, ^{TA}spearmint (not on babies).

Personal Care—Cinnamint Lip Balm.

Supplements—AlkaLime, MineralEssence, Super C / Super C Chewable.

—To Cool the System

    Oils—^{IA}Clove, ^{ITA}peppermint, ^{TA}bergamot, ^{TA}Eucalyptus radiata.

—To Induce Sweating

    Oils—^{ITA}Peppermint, ^{TA}lavender, ^TRoman chamomile, ^Trosemary, ^Tbasil, ^Tcypress, ^Tfennel, ^Ttea tree.

> *My daughter, Haley, at age 18 was ill one Sunday, and later in the evening she was feeling quite worse. When we checked, she had a fever of 105 degrees. I filled a gel capsule with 10 drops of clove oil and had her take it with some water. In ½ an hour I checked her temperature again, and it was down to 102. I gave her 5 more drops in another capsule, and in another ½ hour her fever was totally gone!*
>
>   *-Submitted by Sally Donahue*
>   *Wilsonville, Oregon (July 2004)*

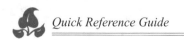

I—Add 1 or 2 drops to 8 oz. rice milk or water, and sip slowly.

T—Dilute as necessary, and apply to bottoms of feet or to spine.

A—Diffuse into the air.

Fiber:

There are two kinds of fiber: soluble fiber is important for absorbing toxins and removing them from the body; insoluble fiber is important for scrubbing the intestines to remove any buildup of waste material. Viscosity is the balance between soluble and insoluble fiber. A blend of different fibers provides for maximum viscosity, which equals optimal absorption and cleansing capabilities. Fiber also helps to slow and balance the absorption of sugars and fats, thereby balancing blood sugar levels. Research has shown that balancing blood sugar levels can extend life expectancy by up to 50%.

Supplements—**Balance Complete** (contains a blend of 5 different fibers for maximum viscosity), **Cleansing Trio (ComforTone, Essentialzyme, and ICP)**.

Fibrocysts: *See Hormonal Imbalance.*

Fibroids: *See also Hormonal Imbalance.*

 ≫ *Fibroids are noncancerous growths of muscle and connective tissue in the uterus. Fibroids can be painful and may affect fertility and pregnancy*

Oils—ᵀ**Frankincense,** ᵀ**helichrysum,** ᵀcistus, ᵀ<u>EndoFlex</u>, ᵀIdaho tansy, ᵀlavender, ᵀoregano, ᵀpine, ᵀ<u>Valor</u>.

T—Put 3 drops of either oil in douche. Also apply to Vita Flex points of feet.

Personal Care—Cel-Lite Magic, Protec.

Supplements—AlkaLime, EndoGize, Essentialzyme, Essentialzymes-4, Power Meal, Thyromin, Ultra Young+, MultiGreens.

Fibromyalgia: *See also Acidosis, Hormonal Imbalance.*

 ≫ *Fibromyalgia is long-term localized or generalized aches, pain, or tenderness in the muscles, ligaments, or other soft tissue that can interfere with normal movement, sleep, or other activities. There is no known cause of fibromyalgia, and many different factors may contribute to the development of this condition. Some have suggested eliminating refined sugar or lowering the body's pH level. Others have recommended stretching, reducing stress, exercises, massage, or better sleep.*

Recipe #1—May need to detoxify the liver. **<u>ImmuPower</u>**; massage with **<u>PanAway</u>**, adding wintergreen & spruce for an additional cortisone response. It may be helpful to use some anti-inflammatory oils like helichrysum, lavender, myrrh, patchouli, rosemary, rosewood, spruce, thyme, or wintergreen.

Blend #1—Combine 2 drops cinnamon bark, 10 drops eucalyptus, 10 drops ginger, 6 drops nutmeg, 10 drops peppermint, and 3 drops rosemary with 2 Tbs. V-6 Oil, and massage chest and back once a day.

Personal Care—**Ortho Ease** or **Ortho Sport** Massage Oils (for full body); do Raindrop Technique.

Supplements—**NingXia Red, Sulfurzyme,** Allerzyme (aids the digestion of sugars, starches, fats, and proteins), AlkaLime (combat yeast and fungus overgrowth and preserve the body's proper pH balance), Balance Complete (high in fiber to absorb toxins and clean the intestinal tract), Digest + Cleanse, JuvaTone, Life 5 (probiotic), Mineral Essence, MultiGreens, PD 80/20, Power Meal, Super C / Super C Chewable, Super Cal (no more than 1 per day, because of the poor ability to utilize minerals), Thyromin, Master Formula.

*****Comments**—Dr. Bernard Jensen suggested that people with fibromyalgia should eliminate all refined sugars from their diet. *Refer to the chapter entitled "How to Use—The Personal Usage Reference" in the* <u>Essential Oils Desk Reference</u> *under "Fibromyalgia" for an excellent supplement regimen.*

Fibrositis: *See Fibromyalgia.*

Finger:

—MASHED

Recipe #1—Geranium (for the bruising), helichrysum (to stop the bleeding), lavender (to help everything), lemongrass (for tissue repair), and PanAway (for the pain). Layer oils on location.

Flatulence: *See Digestive System: GAS/FLATULENCE.*

Flu: *See Influenza.*

Fluids: *See Edema or Diuretic.*

Focus:

Oils—<u>^ABrain Power</u> (during strenuous mental activity), ^Alavender[265], ^A<u>Gathering</u> (for greater focus), ^A<u>Believe,</u> ^A<u>Clarity,</u> ^A<u>Highest Potential,</u> ^AT<u>Reconnect,</u> ^AT<u>InTouch,</u> ^A<u>Surrender</u> (balancing; clears the mind).

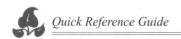
A—Diffuse into the air. Inhale directly or applied to hands.

Supplements— **MindWise, Omega Blue, OmegaGize³,** Sulfurzyme.

Food: *See pH Balance.*

> *The body secretes pepsin, protease, and hydrochloric acid in the morning for the digestion of protein. If you eat fruit in the morning, you have almost instant putrefaction (fermentation). Subacid fruits (like strawberries) are the only fruits that can be eaten with protein.*

　　Oils—Use **basil** for soups and stuffing. Use **cinnamon bark, clove, orange, tangerine,** and **thyme** for flavorings.

*** COMMENTS—According to the <u>Essential Oils Desk Reference</u>, "They are so concentrated that only 12 drops of an essential oil is equivalent to a full 1–2 oz. bottle of dried herbs. For a recipe that serves 6–10 people, add 1–2 drops of an oil, and stir in after cooking and just before serving so that the oil does not evaporate" (EDR-June 2002; Ch. 4; Other Uses; Cooking). Refer to that same section in the <u>Essential Oils Desk Reference</u> for more ideas on cooking with essential oils.

—BREAKFASTS

　　Recipe #1—Proteins (meat, fish, eggs), mixed grains, sunflower seeds, nuts, Power Meal, and Pure Protein Complete. Fruit in the morning will cause candida overgrowth, hypoglycemia, and dysfunction of the thyroid gland. Take Essentialzymes-4 to help with the digestion, especially when animal protein has been eaten. Also, 8 oz. of carrot juice per day with apple and lemon helps detoxify the body and provides necessary enzymes.

—LUNCH

　　Recipe #2—Eat salads and complex carbohydrates like rice, beans, soup, steamed vegetables, bread (Jack Sprout Bread is good) that is toasted (reduces gluten content), baked potatoes, yams, and squash.

> **Buttered Basil Garlic Melt**
>
> 1 loaf cheese bread or any artisan bread,
> 　cut into 1 inch slices
> 1/2 stick butter
> 1/2 teaspoon garlic powder
> 4 drops basil essential oil
> Sliced mozzarella cheese
>
> Melt butter; then add garlic powder, and stir well. Add basil oil; mix well. With a large unused paint brush, brush on butter mixture until saturated. Cover sliced bread with slices of cheese, and bake at 350° until golden brown. Yummmmmie! Even my Baby loved it.
>
> 　　　　　*-Submitted by Jill Burk*
> 　　　　　*Saginaw, Michigan (July 2004)*

—AFTER 3:00 PM

　　Recipe #3—Refrain from eating animal proteins. Power Meal is predigested proteins and can be eaten with fruit. Foods that are easier on the digestive system at night are fruit, soups, lightly steamed vegetables, and salads.

—ASSIMILATION OF

Supplements—Enzyme products: **Allerzyme** (aids the digestion of sugars, starches, fats, and proteins), **Detoxzyme** (helps maintain and support a healthy intestinal environment), **Digest + Cleanse, Essentialzyme/Essentialzymes-4** (multiple enzyme products).

—FIBER

Supplements—Balance Complete, ICP (fiber beverage).

—OIL

Supplements—**V-6 Oil** (six different vegetable oils) is excellent for cooking and for making salad dressings.

—SUGAR SUBSTITUTE

Supplements—**Stevia, Yacon Syrup.**

Food Poisoning:

>> *Food poisoning refers to the effects on the digestive tract of pathogenic organisms—or the toxins they produce—that are ingested into the body in food. Symptoms of food poisoning can include stomach pain, cramps, diarrhea, nausea, and vomiting.*

Oils—ᵀThieves, ᵗtarragon, ᴵExodus II, ᵗpatchouli, ᵗrosemary cineol.

Personal Care—**Thieves Fruit and Veggie Soak and Spray to clean germs and pesticides off produce.**

I—Place 2–5 drops in an empty capsule with 2–5 drops V-6 Oil, and swallow.

Recipe #1—Flavor a cup of water with 6 drops Di-Gize, swish around in mouth, and swallow.

Supplements—Detoxzyme, Essentialzyme, Essentialzymes-4,.

Foot: *See Feet.*

Forehead:

Oils—ᵀJasmine.

T—Apply 1 drop to forehead.

Forgetfulness: *See Memory.*

Forgive (and Forget):

Oils—ᵀᴬAcceptance, ᵀᴬForgiveness, ᵀᴬ3 Wise Men, ᵀᴬTransformation, ᵀᴬValor, ᵀᴬWhite Angelica.

A—Diffuse into the air. Inhale directly or applied to tissue or a cotton wick.

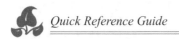

T—Apply to auricular emotion points. Dilute with V-6 Oil to create a massage oil, and massage onto the skin.

*****Comments**—It has been said that "the conscious thought to forgive quells the fear response in the amygdala."

Formaldehyde:

Oils—^TPurification (removes).

T—Dilute as necessary, and apply to feet. Massage into the skin.

Fortifying:

Oils—^{TA}Cypress.

T—Dilute with V-6 Oil to create massage oil, and massage into the skin.

A—Diffuse into the air. Inhale directly or applied to hands.

Freckles:

Oils—^TIdaho tansy.

T—Mix 2–3 drops with lotion, and spread over face. Can be used two or three times per week.

Free Radicals: *See also Antioxidant.*

▸▸ *Free radicals are highly reactive molecules with at least one unpaired electron. The unpaired electron can cause harm to the body as it tries to take electrons from another molecule to make itself more stable, subsequently causing disease formation.*

—ELIMINATE

Oils—^ILongevity

I—Dilute 1 drop in 4 oz. soy or rice milk; drink. Place 2–5 drops in an empty capsule with 2–5 drops V-6 Oil; swallow.

Supplements—**Longevity Capsules** and **NingXia Red** help eliminate and prevent the buildup of free radicals.

Frigidity: *See also Libido, Sex Stimulant.*

Oils—^{TA}_FClary sage, ^{TA}_Fylang ylang (helps balance male/female energies), ^{TA}Lady Sclareol, ^{TA}Chivalry, ^{TA}jasmine, ^{TA}nutmeg (overcome frigidity and impotence), ^{TA}rose.

T—Dilute with V-6 Oil to create massage oil, and massage into the skin.

A—Diffuse into the air. Wear as perfume or cologne. Inhale directly or applied to the hands.

Supplements—Prenolone/Prenolone+, Progessence/Progessence Plus.

Frustration:

Oils—^{TA}<u>Acceptance</u>, ^{TA}clary sage, ^{TA}frankincense, ^{TA}<u>Gathering</u>, ^{TA}ginger, ^{TA}<u>Hope</u>, ^{TA}<u>Humility</u>, ^{TA}juniper, ^{TA}lavender, ^{TA}lemon, ^{TA}orange, ^{TA}peppermint, ^{TA}<u>Present Time</u>, ^{TA}Roman chamomile, ^{TA}spruce, ^{TA}<u>3 Wise Men</u>, ^{TA}thyme, ^{TA}<u>Valor</u>, ^{TA}ylang ylang.

A—Diffuse into the air. Inhale directly or applied to tissue or a cotton wick.

T—Apply to auricular emotion points. Dilute with V-6 Oil to create a massage oil, and massage onto the skin.

Fungus: *See Antifungal: Fungus.*

Gallbladder:

≫ *The gallbladder is a small sac that stores extra bile from the liver until it is needed to help with digestion in the small intestine. The gallbladder is located just below the liver.*

Oils—^T_FGeranium, ^T_FGerman chamomile, ^{TI}<u>JuvaFlex</u> (stimulates), ^{TI}<u>Juva Cleanse</u>, ^T<u>Forgiveness</u>, ^T<u>GLF</u>, ^Tjuniper, ^Tlavender, ^T<u>Release</u>, ^Trosemary (supports), ^T<u>Surrender</u> (over liver & pancreas).

Recipe #1—Take 2 capsules <u>JuvaFlex</u> - AM, 2 <u>Juva Cleanse</u> - PM.

Supplements—Essentialzyme, Essentialzymes-4, Sulfurzyme (aids bile secretion and magnifies effects of vitamins).

—Infection In

Oils—^T_FHelichrysum.

—Stones

≫ *Gallstones are formed by cholesterol that has crystallized from the bile stored in the gallbladder. These stones can sometimes block the duct that comes from the gallbladder or the small opening from the common hepatic duct that allows bile to flow into the small intestine. This can result in pain and can lead to more serious complications, such as infections or jaundice.*

Oils—^T_FNutmeg, ^Tgeranium, ^Tgrapefruit, ^Tjuniper, ^T<u>Juva Cleanse</u>, ^Tlime, ^Trosemary, ^Twintergreen.

T—Dilute as necessary, and apply over gallbladder area (can use a hot compress) and on Vita Flex points on feet.

I—Place 2–5 drops in empty capsule, and swallow.

Gangrene:

>> *Gangrene is the localized decay of body tissue caused by a loss of blood to that area. Gas gangrene is caused by bacteria invading a deep wound that has lessened the blood supply or cut it off entirely. The bacteria create gases and pus in the infected area, causing severe pain and accelerating decay of the tissue.*

Oils—ᵀLavender (used by Dr. Gattefossé to recover from gas gangrene), ᵀThieves, ᵀImmuPower, ᵀcistus, ᵀelemi, ᵀExodus II, ᵀMelrose, ᵀmountain savory, ᵀravintsara, ᵀthyme.

Supplements—ImmuPro, Inner Defense, Super C / Super C Chewable.

Gas: *See Digestive System: Gas/Flatulence.*

Gastritis: *See Digestive System: Gastritis.*

General Tonic:

Oils—ᵀᴬ_FSpruce, ᵀᴬgrapefruit, ᵀᴬlemon, ᵀᴬmountain savory.

T—Dilute with V-6 Oil to create massage oil, and massage onto the skin. Dilute as necessary, and apply to bottoms of feet.

A—Diffuse into the air.

Genitals:

Oils—ᵀ_FClary sage.

T—Apply 1–2 drops on location or on Vita Flex points on the feet.

Gentleness:

Oils—ᴬRosewood.

A—Diffuse into the air. Inhale directly or applied to tissue or a cotton wick.

Germs: *See also Antibacterial, Antifungal, Antiviral.*

—Airborne

Oils—ᴬFir.

—Germicidal

Oils—ᴬᵀ_FLemon, ᴬRC.

A—Diffuse into the air.

T—Dilute as necessary, and apply on location. Add 2–5 drops to a small bowl of water, and use water on a cloth to wipe intended areas.

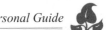
Gingivitis: *See Oral Conditions: Gingivitis.*

Glandular System: *See also Endocrine System.*

    Oils—^T_FSage, ^{T}<u>Egyptian Gold</u>, ^{T}blue cypress (may help stimulate the amygdala, pineal gland, pituitary gland, and hypothalamus), ^{T}spearmint, ^{T}spruce.

    T—Dilute as necessary, and apply on location or on the Vita Flex points on the feet.

    Supplements— **Prostate Health** (male) or **FemiGen** (female) for glandular nutrients.

Glaucoma: *See Eyes: Glaucoma.*

Goiter: *See also Endocrine System, Lymphatic System, Thyroid: HYPERTHYROIDISM.*

    »» *Goiter is a condition where the thyroid gland grows larger than is normal, often causing the neck and larynx to enlarge as well. This enlargement can cause a cough and make it difficult to breathe and to swallow. Goiter is often caused by an iodine deficiency in the body, but it can have other causes as well.*

      Recipe #1—Cleanse the lymphatic system. Balance the endocrine system with <u>EndoFlex</u> and EndoGize.

Gout:

    »» *Gout is the painful inflammation of a joint caused by a buildup of uric acid crystals deposited in the joint. Uric acid is formed during the natural breakdown of dead tissues in the body. An excess of uric acid in the bloodstream can lead to the formation of crystals in the joints or kidneys (kidney stones). Some good ways to prevent the formation of uric acid crystals include maintaining a healthy body weight (which leaves less body tissue to be broken down), exercising, and drinking plenty of water.*

    Oils—^T_FFennel, $^{IT}_F$lemon, ^{T}PanAway, ^{T}wintergreen, ^{T}pine, ^{T}basil, ^{T}calamus, ^{T}geranium, ^{T}hyssop, ^{T}<u>Juva Cleanse</u>, ^{T}<u>JuvaFlex</u>, ^{T}nutmeg, ^{T}onycha (benzoin), ^{T}thyme, ^{T}yarrow.

    T—Dilute as necessary, and apply on location. Dilute with V-6 Oil to create a massage oil, and massage on location.

    I—Add 1–2 drops to 8 oz. water, and drink.

    Recipe #1—Cleanse with the **Master Cleanser** program(*See Cleansing*), and drink lots of fluids (water, juices, etc.).

    Personal Care—**Ortho Ease** and **Ortho Sport Massage Oils**.

    Supplements—Balance Complete, Cleansing Trio (ComforTone, Essentialzyme, and ICP), Digest + Cleanse, JuvaTone, Mineral Essence, MultiGreens, Sulfurzyme, Super C / Super C Chewable, Super Cal, Thyromin.

*****Comments**—Refer to the chapter entitled "How to Use—The Personal Usage Reference" in the <u>Essential Oils Desk Reference</u> under "Gout" for some excellent blend recipes and supplement recommendations.

Grave's Disease: *See also Thyroid: HYPERTHYROIDISM.*

▷▷ *Graves' disease is an autoimmune disease caused by an abnormally-shaped protein stimulating the thyroid to make and secrete more hormones. This can cause an enlargement of the thyroid, bulging eyes, increased heart rate, high blood pressure, and anxiety.*

Oils—^{TA}Lemongrass, ^{TA}blue tansy, ^{TA}<u>EndoFlex</u>, ^{TA}myrrh, ^{TA}spruce.

T—Dilute as recommended, and apply on thyroid area or on reflex points on the feet.

A—Diffuse into the air.

Supplements—EndoGize, ImmuPro, Inner Defense, Mineral Essence, MultiGreens, Sulfurzyme (helps mitigate the effects of autoimmune diseases), Thyromin, Master Formula.

Grief/Sorrow:

Oils—^{AT}Bergamot (turns grief into joy), ^{AT}clary sage, ^{AT}eucalyptus, ^{AT}<u>Forgiveness</u>, ^{TA}<u>Gentle Baby</u> (massage whole body), ^{AT}<u>Hope</u>, ^{TA}<u>Joy</u> (over the heart), ^{AT}juniper, ^{AT}lavender, ^{AT}<u>Present Time</u>, ^{AT}<u>Release</u>, ^{AT}Roman chamomile, ^{TA}<u>Sacred Mountain</u> (back of the neck), ^T<u>3 Wise Men</u> (rub on crown), ^{AT}<u>Transformation</u>, ^{AT}<u>Valor</u> (on the feet), ^{TA}<u>White Angelica</u> (on the forehead or shoulders).

A—Diffuse into the air. Inhale directly or applied to tissue or a cotton wick.

T—Apply to auricular emotion points. Dilute with V-6 Oil to create a massage oil, and massage onto the skin.

Grounding:

Oils—^{AT}<u>Grounding</u>, ^{AT}fir, ^{AT}<u>Hope</u>, ^{AT}<u>Joy</u>, ^{AT}patchouli, ^{AT}spruce, ^{AT}<u>3 Wise Men</u>, ^{AT}mastrante, ^{AT}tsuga.

—FEELING OF

Oils—^ACypress.

A—Diffuse into the air. Inhale directly or applied to tissue or a cotton wick.

T—Apply to auricular emotion points or on sacral chakra. Dilute with V-6 Oil to create a massage oil, and massage onto the skin.

Guilt:

Oils—^{AT}<u>Acceptance</u>, ^{AT}<u>Awaken</u>, ^{AT}cypress, ^{AT}<u>Forgiveness</u>, ^{AT}frankincense, ^{AT}<u>Gathering</u>, ^{AT}geranium, ^{AT}<u>Harmony</u>, ^{AT}<u>Inner Child</u>, ^{AT}<u>Inspiration</u>, ^{AT}juniper, ^{AT}lemon, ^{AT}marjoram, ^{AT}<u>Peace & Calming</u>, ^{AT}<u>Present Time</u>, ^{AT}<u>Release</u>, ^{AT}Roman chamomile, ^{AT}rose, ^{AT}sandalwood, ^{AT}spruce, ^{AT}thyme, ^{AT}<u>Valor</u>, ^{AT}<u>White Angelica</u>.

A—Diffuse into the air. Inhale directly or applied to tissue or a cotton wick.

T—Apply to auricular emotion points. Dilute with V-6 Oil to create a massage oil, and massage onto the skin.

Gulf War Syndrome:

Oils—^{AT}<u>Exodus II</u>.

A—Diffuse into the air.

T—Dilute with V-6 Oil to create a massage oil, and massage onto the skin. Apply to Vita Flex points on the feet.

Gum Disease: *See Oral Conditions: Gum Disease.*

Gums: *See also Oral Conditions: GINGIVITIS, GUM DISEASE.*

Oils—^TMyrrh (infection), ^Tlavender, ^T<u>Melrose</u> (fights infection), ^TRoman chamomile, ^Tsage lavender (infection).

T—Dilute as necessary, and apply 1–2 drops on location with a cotton ball or a cotton swab. Mix 1–2 drops with 4 oz. water, and use as a mouth-rinse.

Personal Care—Thieves Dentarome/Dentarome Plus Toothpaste, Thieves Fresh Essence Plus Mouthwash, KidScents Toothpaste (for children).

—SURGERY ON GUMS

*****Comments**—For one individual, helichrysum was applied with a Q-tip every 15 minutes to kill the pain. No other pain killer was used.

Habits: *See also Addictions.*

Oils—^{AT}<u>Acceptance</u>, ^{AT}lavender, ^{AT}<u>Transformation</u>.

A—Diffuse into the air. Inhale directly or applied to tissue or a cotton wick.

T—Dilute with V-6 Oil to create a massage oil, and massage onto the skin.

*****Comments**—To break bad habits, you need to change the DNA and RNA. Sandalwood and frankincense help with this.

A=Aromatic **T**=Topical **I**=Internal

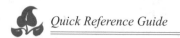

Hair: *Refer to the Personal Care Products section of this book for a list of ingredients and more details on chemical-free shampoos and conditioners.*

*****Comments**—Refer to the chapter entitled "How to Use—The Personal Usage Reference" in the *Essential Oils Desk Reference* under "Hair and Scalp Problems" for some excellent blend recipes.

—Baldness *See also Loss below*

    Recipe #1—Apply 2–3 drops each of cedarwood, lavender, rosemary, and sage oil on location and on bottoms of feet before bedtime and/or in the morning after washing with Lavender Volume products shown below.

    Personal Care—**Lavender Volume Shampoo** and **Lavender Volume Conditioner** together.

    Supplements—Sulfurzyme may help if the hair is falling due to a sulfur deficiency.

—Beard

    Oils—ᵀLemon, ᵀrosemary, ᵀcypress, ᵀlavender, ᵀthyme.

—Body

    Oils—ᵀCedarwood (gives the hair shaft more body, more strength, and more life), ᵀtamanu.

—Children

    Personal Care—**Lavender Volume Shampoo** with **Lavender Volume Conditioner** or **KidScents Shampoo**.

—Color

    Recipe #1—(keep light) Apply 1 drop chamomile, 1 drop lemon, and 1 quart of water. Rinse hair.

—Damaged (perms, color-treated, bleached)

    Oils—ᵀTamanu.

    Personal Care— **KidScents Shampoo**.

—Dandruff *See also Antifungal*

    ▸▸ *Dandruff is a scalp condition characterized by the excessive shedding of dead skin cells. A small amount of flaking on the scalp is normal as old skin cells die off and fall away; but dandruff results when the amount of dead skin cells becomes excessive and visible.*

    Oils—ᵀ_F_Rosemary, ᵀ_F_lavender, ᵀwintergreen, ᵀtea tree, ᵀbasil, ᵀcedarwood, ᵀcypress, ᵀpatchouli, ᵀsage, ᵀsage lavender, ᵀthyme, ᵀvalerian.

Personal Care—KidScents Shampoo, Lavender Volume Shampoo, Lavender Volume Conditioner.

—DRY

Oils—[T]Geranium, [T]sandalwood, [T]lavender, [T]rosemary, [T]wintergreen.

—ESTROGEN BALANCE

» *Estrogen is a steroid hormone that causes the development of female characteristics such as breasts and larger hips, that helps with calcium uptake and balance, and that plays many other important roles. Estrogen also helps hair to grow faster and to stay on the head longer. If estrogen levels fall, hair loss can quickly result.*

Recipe #2—Clary sage in Lavender Volume Shampoo and Lavender Volume Conditioner helps promote estrogen balance in the membrane tissue around the hair follicle. This serves to balance testosterone levels and to prevent the thickening of the tissue around the follicle that results in hair loss.

Blend #1—1 drop lavender and 6 drops patchouli in 2–5 oz. Lavender Volume Shampoo.

Blend #2—Mix together 2 drops cinnamon bark, 4 drops cypress, 4 drops geranium, 2 drops juniper, 5 drops lavender, and 3 drops rosemary. Then put one drop of the blend into ¼ tsp of water, and rub on bald area and on entire scalp. A gentle night treatment.

Personal Care—**Lavender Volume Shampoo** and **Lavender Volume Conditioner** (with clary sage—*see Recipe #2 above*).

Supplements—ComforTone, Essentialzyme, Essentialzymes-4, MultiGreens, Super B (stress), Thyromin.

—FRAGILE HAIR

Oils—[T]Clary sage, [T]lavender, [T]thyme, [T]Roman chamomile, [T]sandalwood, [T]wintergreen.

Personal Care—KidScents Shampoo, Lavender Volume Shampoo, and **Lavender Volume Conditioner**.

—GREASY

Oils—[T]Petitgrain.

—GROWTH (STIMULATE)

Oils—[T]Thyme[266], [T]rosemary[266], [T]lavender[266], [T]cedarwood[266], [T]ylang ylang (promotes), [T]basil, [T]western red cedar, [T]cypress, [T]geranium, [T]ginger, [T]grapefruit, [T]hyssop, [T]lemon, [T]sage.

H

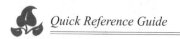
Personal Care—**Lavender Volume Shampoo** and **Lavender Volume Conditioner**.

Supplements—Sulfurzyme. A deficiency in sulfur can result in hair loss or poor hair growth.

—**ITCHING**

Oils—^T_F**Peppermint** (skin), ^Tlavender.

—**LOSS** *See also BALDNESS above*

Oils—^T_F**Rosemary**[266], ^T_F**lavender**[266], ^T_F**cedarwood**[266], ^T**thyme**[266], ^T_F**ylang ylang**, ^T**clary sage**, ^T**cypress**, ^T**laurel** (after infection), ^Tlemon, ^TRoman chamomile, ^Tsage, ^Tsage lavender, ^Twintergreen.

> *In males, hair loss can often be blamed on heredity, hormones (high levels of testosterone), and aging. Other reasons for hair loss may include poor circulation, hypertension, acute illness, surgery, radiation, scarlet fever, syphilis, stress, sudden weight loss, iron deficiency, diabetes, hypothyroidism, drugs, poor diet, and vitamin deficiency.*
>
> *Avoid hair products that are not natural on the hair. Avoid chlorinated swimming pools or polluted seas. Chemical products may also leave a residue buildup which can cause hair loss. Correcting a hormonal imbalance or hypertension (dilate blood vessels and stimulate cell division) may help.*

–**ALOPECIA AREATA (INFLAMMATORY HAIR LOSS DISEASE)**

Oils—^T**Thyme**[266], ^T**rosemary**[266], ^T**lavender**[266], ^T**cedarwood**[266].

T—Add any or all of these oils to jojoba and grapeseed carrier oils, and massage into scalp daily.

Personal Care—Lavender Volume Shampoo and Lavender Volume Conditioner.

Supplements—Sulfurzyme, Super B, Thyromin.

***Comments**—*Refer to the chapter entitled "How to Use—The Personal Usage Reference" in the* <u>Essential Oils Desk Reference</u> *under "Hair Loss" for some excellent blend recipes.*

—**SILKY AND SHINY**

Oils—^T**Tamanu**.

Personal Care—**KidScents Shampoo**.

—**SPLIT ENDS**

Personal Care—**KidScents Shampoo**.

T—Apply 1–2 drops of oil to hands, and massage into hair and scalp before bath or shower; then shampoo and rinse hair as normal. Add 1–2 drops of oil to 2 Tbs. of an unscented shampoo or shower gel, and use to shampoo hair.

Halitosis: *See Oral Conditions: Halitosis.*

Hands: *See also Skin.*

> Oils—^TGeranium, ^Tlemon, ^Tsandalwood, ^Teucalyptus, ^Tlavender, ^Tpatchouli, ^Trosemary.
>
> —**DRY**
>
>> Oils—^TGeranium, ^Tpatchouli, ^Tsandalwood.
>>
>> Personal Care—Genesis Hand & Body Lotion, Rose Ointment.
>
> —**NEGLECTED**
>
>> Oils—^TGeranium, ^Tlemon, ^Tpatchouli.
>
> —**TINGLING IN**
>
>> Recipe #1—Lemongrass in Genesis Hand & Body Lotion.
>
> **T**—Dilute as necessary, and apply 1–2 drops to hands. Dilute 1–2 drops in 1 Tbs. almond or olive oil, and use as massage oil to massage into hands.

Hangovers:

> Oils—^{TA}Lemon, ^{TA}grapefruit, ^{TA}fennel, ^{TA}lavender, ^{TA}rose, ^{TA}rosemary, ^{TA}sandalwood.
>
> **T**—Add 3–4 drops to warm bathwater, and bathe. Dilute as recommended, and apply 1–2 drops to back of neck or over liver. Dilute with V-6 Oil to create massage oil, and massage onto back and neck.
>
> **A**—Inhale directly or applied to hands, tissue, or a cotton wick. Drop 1–2 drops in a bowl of hot water, and inhale vapors. Diffuse into the air.
>
> Supplements—Super C / Super C Chewable.

Happiness:

> Oils—^{AT}Christmas Spirit, ^{AT}Joy.
>
> **A**—Diffuse into the air. Inhale directly or applied to tissue or a cotton wick.
>
> **T**—Apply to auricular emotion points. Dilute with V-6 Oil to create a massage oil, and massage onto the skin.

Harmony in Body Systems:

> Oils—^{AT}Acceptance, ^Aclove, ^{AT}geranium (harmonizing), ^{AT}Harmony, ^{AT}Inspiration, ^{AT}Lady Sclareol (women), ^{AT}Roman chamomile.
>
> Personal Care—Sensation Hand & Body Lotion. Sensation Massage Oil creates an exotic arousal and increases sexual desire. The fragrance creates a peaceful and harmonious feeling that is helpful in easing relationship stress. Relaxation Massage Oil also creates a peaceful and harmonious feeling.

A=Aromatic   **T**=Topical   **I**=Internal

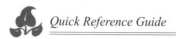

—Of Mind and Body

　　Oils—^{AT}Release.

A—Diffuse into the air. Inhale directly or applied to tissue or a cotton wick.

T—Apply to auricular emotion points or to chakras. Dilute with V-6 Oil to create a massage oil, and massage onto the skin.

Harshness:

　　Oils—^{AT}Jasmine.

A—Diffuse into the air. Inhale directly or applied to tissue or a cotton wick.

T—Apply to auricular emotion points. Dilute with V-6 Oil to create a massage oil, and massage onto the skin.

Hashimoto's Disease: *See also Thyroid: HYPERTHYROIDISM.*

▸▸ *Hashimoto's disease is an autoimmune disorder where the immune system attacks the thyroid, causing it to swell up and become irritated. Possible symptoms include abnormal fatigue, weight gain, muscle pain and stiffness, a hoarse voice, prolonged menstrual bleeding, constipation, a feeling of tightness in the throat, sensitivity to cold, dry skin, and depression.*

　　Oils—^{TA}Lemongrass, ^{TA}EndoFlex, ^{TA}myrrh, ^{TA}blue tansy, ^{TA}spruce.

T—Dilute as necessary, and apply over thyroid area or to Vita Flex points on the feet.

A—Diffuse into the air. Inhale oil applied to hands.

Supplements—Thyromin, ImmuPro, EndoGize, Inner Defense, Mineral Essence, Multi-Greens, Sulfurzyme (helps mitigate effects of autoimmune diseases), Master Formula.

Hate:

　　Oils—^{AT}Acceptance, ^{AT}Forgiveness, ^{AT}Release.

A—Diffuse into the air. Inhale directly or applied to tissue or a cotton wick.

T—Apply to auricular emotion points. Dilute with V-6 Oil to create a massage oil, and massage onto the skin.

Hay Fever: *See Allergies: Hay Fever.*

Headaches:

　　Oils—^{TA}ᵣPeppermint[267], ^{TA}Aroma Siez, ^{TA}M-Grain, ^{TA}ᵣrosemary, ^TDeep Relief (roll-on), ^{TA}basil,

> *Clarity may cause headaches when chemicals or metals are in the brain. To break this blockage, put Aroma Life or helichrysum on arteries in the neck.*

^TA^<u>Aroma Life</u> (massage on arteries in neck), ^TA^calamus, ^TA^cardamom, ^TA^<u>Clarity</u>, ^TA^clove, ^TA^cumin, ^TA^eucalyptus, ^TA^<u>Dragon Time</u>, ^TA^frankincense, ^TA^<u>Gentle Baby</u>, ^TA^lavender[268], ^TA^marjoram, ^TA^<u>Mister</u>, ^TA^<u>Relieve It</u>, ^TA^sage lavender.

***Comments—According to the <u>Essential Oils Desk Reference</u>, "For headaches, put one drop [Thieves] on tongue and push tongue against the roof of the mouth." (<u>EDR</u>-June 2002; Ch. 8; Thieves; Application) Also, refer to the chapter entitled "How to Use—The Personal Usage Reference" in the <u>Essential Oils Desk Reference</u> under "Headaches" for some excellent blend recipes and supplement recommendations for several different types of headaches.

—Cold/Flu Headaches

> **Oils**—^TA^Cumin.

—Emotional Headaches

> **Oils**—^TA^<u>Joy</u>.

—Menstrual Migraines *See also Hormonal Imbalance*

>> *Many women find that their migraine headaches are closely related to their menstrual cycles, occurring when their estrogen and progesterone levels are at their lowest.*

> **Oils**—^TA^Sage lavender.

—Children's Migraines

> **Blend #1**—5 drops Roman chamomile, 10 drops grapefruit, 5 drops peppermint, 3 drops rosemary, and 4 oz. V-6 Oil for children under age seven, or 2 oz. V-6 Oil for children over age seven.

—Migraine Headaches

>> *A migraine is a severe and painful type of headache. Symptoms of migraines include throbbing pain accompanied by nausea, vomiting, and heightened sensitivity to light. Migraines can be triggered by stress, anxiety, sleep or food deprivation, bright lights, loud noises, and hormonal changes.*

> *My husband has been bothered by migraine headaches for much of his adult life. Doctors have treated this condition with various medications—all with their own bag of side effects. So one day I decided to have him try peppermint oil, a drop on each temple. To his amazement, the headache was gone in seconds, and the cooling feel of the peppermint gave him a feeling of energy and revitalization.*
>
> *–Submitted by Kathleen Mueller, Menomonee Falls, WI (July 2004)*

> **Oils**—^TA^<u>M-Grain</u>, ^TA^~F~peppermint[267], ^TA^~F~basil, ^TA^~F~eucalyptus, ^TA^PanAway, ^T^<u>Deep Relief</u> (roll-on), ^TA^<u>Aroma Siez</u>, ^TA^cumin, ^TA^German chamomile, ^TA^grapefruit, ^TA^lavender[268], ^TA^marjoram, ^TA^<u>Peace & Calming</u>, ^TA^<u>Relieve It</u>, ^TA^<u>Release</u>, ^TA^Roman chamomile, ^TA^spearmint, ^TA^valerian, ^TA^wintergreen, ^TA^ylang ylang.

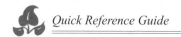
*****Comments**—May be caused by problems in the colon. Cleanse the colon using supplements.

Supplements—AlkaLime (if caused from acidosis), Balance Complete, Cleansing Trio (ComforTone, Essentialzyme, and ICP), Digest + Cleanse. Do not use ComforTone and JuvaTone together (*See ComforTone in the Supplements section of the Reference Guide for Essential Oils*).

Personal Care—Progessence/Progessence Plus.

—Stress (Tension) Headaches

▸▸ *Stress headaches (or tension headaches) are the most common type of headache. Tension headaches are characterized by dull, constant pressure or pain (usually on both sides of the head). Tension headaches can last from thirty minutes to several days and tend to come back when a person is under stress.*

Oils—^{TA}M-Grain, ^TDeep Relief (roll-on), ^{TA}Roman chamomile.

—Sugar Headaches

Oils—^{TA}Thieves (for low blood sugar headaches).

Supplements—Allerzyme (aids the digestion of sugars, starches, fats, and proteins), AlkaLime, Digest + Cleanse, Mineral Essence.

T—Dilute as recommended, and apply to temples, back of neck, and forehead

A—Diffuse into the air.

Healing:

Oils—^TThe Gift, ^Tfrankincense, ^{AT}PanAway, ^{AT}tea tree, ^Aclary sage, ^TAcceptance, ^Tclove, ^Tcypress, ^Aeucalyptus, ^{AT}Humility, ^Alemon, ^{AT}sage.

T—Dilute with V-6 Oil to create a massage oil, and massage on location, on feet, or on back and neck.

A—Diffuse into the air.

Recipe #1—Combinations of sandalwood, frankincense, and lavender or frankincense and balsam fir (add myrrh if dealing with infection) have been used to help heal after surgery or major injuries. Also, combine the following oils (ratio in drops) in a 5 ml bottle: 20 valerian, 5 vetiver, 2 helichrysum, 1 clove, 1 peppermint. Applying several drops of this blend to the brain stem area (cervical vertebrae on back of neck) before surgery has been shown to maintain normal white blood cell counts during surgery, thereby speeding recovery by up to 30%. Any of these combinations may be used both internally and externally.

Health:

Oils—**A**<u>Abundance</u>, **A**lavender, **A**lemon.

A—Diffuse into the air.

Supplements—**Balance Complete,** Cleansing Trio (**ComforTone, Essentialzyme,** and **ICP**), **Digest + Cleanse, Longevity Capsules, NingXia Red, Omega Blue/OmegaGize[3]** (omega-3 essential fatty acids). The following is a recommended daily regimen to help maintain and promote optimal health: NingXia Red and Longevity Capsules (for optimal antioxidant support), Omega Blue (to support cell membranes and optimal brain function), and Balance Complete (to replace the least nutritional meal; for nutritional support, toxin removal, and healthy elimination).

—Promotes

Oils—**A**Eucalyptus, **A**juniper.

A—Diffuse into the air. Inhale directly or applied to hands, tissue, or a cotton wick.

Hearing: *See Ears.*

Heart: *See Cardiovascular System: Heart.*

Heartburn: *See Digestive System: Heartburn.*

H

Hematoma: *See also Bruise.*

>> *A hematoma is a collection of blood outside of the blood vessels. The most common form of a hematoma is a bruise. Hematomas can also form into hard, blood-filled sacs that look like welts and can move to different locations. These often dissolve on their own.*

Oils—**T**F Helichrysum, **T**<u>Aroma Life</u>, **T**German chamomile.

T—Dilute as necessary, and apply on location.

Hemorrhaging: *See also Blood: Hemorrhaging, Female Specific Conditions: Hemorrhaging.*

>> *Hemorrhaging is excessive or uncontrollable blood loss.*

Oils—**T**Helichrysum, **T**rose, **T**ylang ylang.

T—Massage around ankles, lower back, and stomach. Cayenne pepper may also help.

Hemorrhoids:

>> *Hemorrhoids are swollen, twisted veins that occur in the rectum or anus. They are caused by increased pressure within the veins, often due to pregnancy, frequent lifting, or constipation.*

Oils—^T_FCypress, ^T_Fclary sage, ^T_Fpatchouli, ^T_Fpeppermint, ^T_Fsandalwood, ^{T}<u>Aroma Life</u>, ^{T}basil, ^{T}frankincense, ^{T}helichrysum, ^{T}juniper, ^{T}myrrh.

T—Dilute as necessary, and apply 1–2 drops on location. Mix 1–2 drops with 1 tsp. V-6 Oil, and apply using a rectal syringe.

Recipe #1—Put cypress and helichrysum inside and on location.

Hepatitis: *See Liver: Hepatitis.*

Hernia:

>> *A hernia is the protrusion of a tissue or organ through tissue or muscle outside of the body cavity in which it is normally contained. There are several different types of hernias, and the symptoms vary with each type.*

—HIATAL HERNIA

>> *A hiatal (hiatus) hernia is when a portion of the stomach protrudes through the diaphragm into the chest cavity above. This can cause pain, acid reflux, and heartburn. This type of hernia can be caused by a birth defect or may be brought on by heavy lifting, stress, or being overweight.*

Oils—^{T}Basil, ^{T}peppermint, ^{T}cypress, ^{T}fennel, ^{T}geranium, ^{T}ginger, ^{T}hyssop, ^{T}lavender, ^{T}rosemary, ^{T}vitex.

Recipe #1—Drink water. Put the first two fingers of each hand just below the sternum (under center of rib cage), press in firmly, and brush down quickly and firmly. This can also be done after raising up on toes and while dropping down on heels to more firmly emphasize the effect.

Supplements—Essentialzyme/Essentialzymes-4 before meal, ComforTone, ICP (fiber beverage) after meal.

—INCISIONAL HERNIA

>> *An incisional hernia is caused by a protrusion through scar tissue from an abdominal wound or incision that has not healed correctly.*

Oils—^{T}Basil, ^{T}helichrysum, ^{T}lemongrass, ^{T}geranium, ^{T}ginger, ^{T}lavender, ^{T}lemon, ^{T}tea tree.

—INGUINAL HERNIA

>> *An inguinal hernia is when the intestines protrude into the inguinal canal (a small opening that leads from the abdominal cavity into the groin area). This can sometimes be seen as a bulge in the groin area and is usually painless, but it may become painful if the blood supply to the herniated portion of the intestine is restricted (strangulated).*

Oils—[T]Lemongrass, [T]lavender.

T—Dilute as necessary, and apply oil(s) on location, lower back, and Vita Flex points on feet.

Herpes Simplex:

>> *Herpes simplex type 1 and type 2 viruses are the two viruses that cause genital and oral herpes infections. These viruses cause painful outbreaks of blisters and sores to occur in the affected area when the virus is active in the skin or mucus membranes, followed by periods of latency when the virus resides in the nerve cells around the in[fected]*

Oils—[T]Peppermint[269], [T]tea tree[270], [T]helichrysum[271], [T]clove[272], [T][F]lavender, [T][F]ravintsara, [T]melissa[273], [T]manuka[274], [T]__Australian Blue__, [T]blue cypress, [T]bergamot (with Eucalyptus radiata), [T]eucalyptus, [T]geranium, [T]lemon, [T]rose.

> *Jean Valnet, MD, a French physician, recommends a blend of lemon and geranium. Tisserand suggests eucalyptus and bergamot. Dr. Wabner says that a one-time application of either true rose oil or true melissa oil led to complete remission of herpes simplex lesions. Apply the oil directly on the lesions at the first sign of an outbreak. (Alternative Medicine—The Definitive Guide, p. 56).*

H

Hiccoughs/Hiccups:

Oils—[AT][F]Tarragon, [AT]sandalwood.

A—Diffuse into the air. Inhale directly or applied to hands, tissue, or a cotton wick.

T—Dilute as necessary, and apply to the diaphragm area or to Vita Flex points on the feet.

High Blood Pressure: *See Blood.*

Hives: *See Acidosis, pH Balance.*

>> *Hives are itchy patches of inflamed spots on the skin surrounded by redness, typically caused by an allergic reaction or a viral infection.*

Oils—[T]Tea tree[275], [T]peppermint[276], [T]lavender[277], [T]patchouli (may relieve itching), [T]Roman chamomile.

T—Dilute as necessary, and apply on location. Dilute with V-6 Oil to create a massage oil, and massage on location.

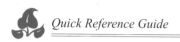
*****Comments**—Hives may be the result of too much acid in the blood or the result of a niacin flush (vitamin B3 taken on empty stomach).

Supplements—AlkaLime (combat yeast and fungus overgrowth and preserve the body's proper pH balance), MultiGreens, Super Cal (may prevent).

*****Comments**—One woman broke out in hives over her entire body. She used peppermint oil diluted with V-6 Oil for a body massage; and almost instantly her body cooled off, and the hives diminished until gone.

Hodgkin's Disease: *See Cancer: LYMPHOMA.*

Hope:

Oils—^{AT}<u>Hope</u> (restores).

A—Diffuse into the air. Inhale directly or applied to tissue or a cotton wick.

T—Apply to auricular emotion points. Dilute with V-6 Oil to create a massage oil, and massage onto the skin.

Hormonal Imbalance:

Oils—^{AT}<u>SclarEssence</u>, ^{AT}ylang ylang, ^{AT}dorado azul, ^{AT}anise.

A—Diffuse into the air. Inhale directly or applied to tissue or a cotton wick.

T—Dilute as necessary, and apply to Vita Flex points on the ankles, to the lower back, thyroid, liver, kidneys, gland areas, center of the body and along both sides of the spine, or to the clavicle area.

Personal Care—Prenolone/Prenolone+, Progessence/Progessence Plus.

Supplements—FemiGen, Mineral Essence, Sulfurzyme (lowered libido).

Hormonal System: *See also Endocrine System..*

Oils—^{TA}_FSpearmint (hormone-like), ^{TA}ylang ylang, ^{TA}clary sage, ^{TA}<u>Acceptance</u>, ^{TA}<u>Aroma Life</u>, ^{TA}<u>Clarity</u>, ^{TA}davana, ^{AT}dorado azul, ^{TA}<u>Dragon Time</u>, ^{TA}<u>EndoFlex</u>, ^{TA}fennel, ^{TA}goldenrod, ^{TA}<u>Gentle Baby</u>, ^{TA}<u>Mister</u>, ^{TA}<u>M-Grain</u>, ^{TA}myrrh, ^{TA}myrtle, ^{TA}peppermint, ^{TA}<u>Relieve It</u>, ^{TA}sage, ^{TA}sage lavender, ^{TA}sandalwood, ^{TA}<u>SclarEssence</u>.

Personal Care—Dragon Time Massage Oil, Prenolone/Prenolone+, Progessence/Progessence Plus.

Supplements—CortiStop (Women's), EndoGize, Estro Tincture, FemiGen (female), Prostate Health (male), Slique Tea, Thyromin, Ultra Young+.

—BALANCE

Oils—$^{TA}_F$Clary sage, ^{TA}ylang ylang, ^{AT}dorado azul, ^{TA}Mister (creates greater balance), ^{TA}Legacy, ^{TA}bergamot, ^{A}clove, ^{TA}EndoFlex, ^{TA}fennel, ^{TA}geranium, ^{TA}nutmeg, ^{TA}sage.

Personal Care—Dragon Time Massage Oil, Prenolone / Prenolone+, Progessence/Progessence Plus.

Supplements—CortiStop (Women's), EndoGize, Estro Tincture, FemiGen (female), Prostate Health (male), MultiGreens, Super B, Super Cal, Thyromin, Ultra Young+.

> *A hormonal imbalance can cause many problems, including PMS, pre- and post-menopausal conditions, depression, endometriosis, fibromyalgia, fibrocysts, infertility, insomnia, irregular menstrual cycles, lowered libido, menstrual migraines, osteoporosis, ovarian cysts, unexplained first-trimester miscarriages, water retention, etc. Carbonated water can cause hormone deficiency. But most often it is a result of estrogen dominance; that is, not enough progesterone to balance out the amount of estrogen. Estrogen is manufactured in several places of the body, even after menopause, and is also found in much of our food, especially in animal and dairy products. Progesterone is secreted by the corpus luteum, by the placenta, and in small amounts by the adrenal glands. If the ovaries are not functioning properly, have been removed, or if they have atrophied because of menopause or hysterectomy, the woman is undoubtedly estrogen dominant. Therefore, she is a candidate for the problems listed above. One successful approach for the above problems is NATURAL PROGESTERONE (obtained from the Wild Yam or SOY). Two good books to read about natural progesterone are What Your Doctor May Not Tell You About Premenopause and What Your Doctor May Not Tell You About Menopause. Both books were written by John R. Lee, MD.*

—DISTURBANCES

Supplements—EndoGize, Prostate Health (male), or FemiGen (female).

—FEMALE

Oils—^{TA}Lady Sclareol, ^{AT}dorado azul (balances estrogen), ^{TA}Mister (for estrogen).

Supplements—CortiStop (Women's), EndoGize, Estro Tincture, FemiGen, Ultra Young+.

—MALE

Oils—^{TA}Mister

Supplements—EndoGize, Prostate Health, Ultra Young+.

—SEXUAL ENERGY

Oils—^{TA}Goldenrod, ^{TA}Lady Sclareol, ^{TA}ylang ylang.

Supplements—EndoGize.

T—The most common places to apply oils for hormonal balance are on the Vita Flex points on the ankles, on the lower back, thyroid, liver, kidneys, gland areas, on the center of the body and along both sides of the spine, and on the clavicle area. Dilute as necessary, and apply on these areas.

A—Diffuse into the air.

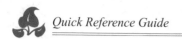

Hot Flashes: *See Female Specific Conditions:* HOT FLASHES.

Housecleaning:

— BATHROOMS/KITCHENS

Oils—^TFir, ^Tlemon, ^Tspruce, or ^Thinoki for cleaning and disinfecting.

— CARPETS

Oils—^T<u>Purification</u>, ^Tlemon (has been used to remove black shoe polish)

— DISHES

Personal Care—Thieves Dish Soap

Recipe #1—A couple of drops of <u>Melrose</u> or lemon in the dishwater make for sparkling dishes and a great smelling kitchen.

— FURNITURE POLISH

Oils—^TFir, ^Tlemon, or ^Tspruce work well for polishing furniture.

— GUM/GREASE

Oils—^TLemon (is terrific for dissolving gum and grease).

— LAUNDRY

Oils—^TLemon, ^T<u>Purification</u>.

Personal Care—Thieves Laundry Soap

***Comments—Adding oils to the washer can increase the antibacterial benefits, provide greater hygiene, and make the clothes come out with a fresh, clean smell. A few drops of oil can also be placed on a washcloth and put in the dryer with laundry or added to a bottle of water, shook well, and sprayed into the dryer before drying the laundry.

— MOLD/FUNGUS *SEE ALSO ANTIFUNGAL*

Oils—^T<u>Purification</u>, ^T<u>Thieves</u>.

T—Put a few drops of oil on your dust cloth; or put 10 drops in a spray bottle of water, and spray as a mist.

Hyperactivity: *See Calming:* HYPERACTIVITY.

Hyperpnea (Abnormal rapid breathing): *See Respiratory System:* HYPERPNEA.

Hypertension (High blood pressure): *See Blood.*

Hypoglycemia: *See also Blood: Low Blood Sugar. See also Protein.*

>> *Hypoglycemia is a condition of low levels of sugar in the blood. It is most common in people with diabetes but can be caused by drugs or by a tumor in the pancreas that causes the pancreas to create too much insulin. Symptoms of hypoglycemia can include hunger, sweating, weakness, palpitations, shaking, dizziness, and confusion.*

> *Protein deficiency causes **hypoglycemia**. Honey enters the blood stream faster than sugar and can cause hypoglycemia. When flu and virus enter the body and mix with problems of hypoglycemia, they can cause candida, Epstein-Barr virus, allergies, etc. There is a progressive deterioration from hypoglycemia. Signs of hypoglycemia include headaches, fatigue, PMS, orneriness, moodiness, weakness, light-headedness, and a lack of hunger in the morning because the body is still digesting its food from the night before.*

Oils—^T_FEucalyptus, ^TThieves, ^Tcinnamon bark, ^Tclove, ^TGentle Baby, ^TGratitude, ^Tthyme.

T—Dilute as necessary, and apply over pancreas and on Vita Flex points on the feet.

Supplements—Allerzyme (aids the digestion of sugars, starches, fats, and proteins), Alka-Lime, Balance Complete, Digest + Cleanse, MultiGreens, Power Meal, Pure Protein Complete, Stevia, Sulfurzyme, Wolfberry Crisp Bars, Yacon Syrup.

Hysteria:

Oils—^{AT}Lavender[278], ^{TA}tea tree, ^{TA}neroli.

T—Dilute as necessary, and apply to heart and to bottoms of feet

A—Diffuse into the air.

Immune System:

>> *The Immune System is the body's defense against disease. The immune system protects the body by identifying and killing bacteria, viruses, parasites, other microorganisms, and tumor cells that would harm the body. The immune system is comprised of several different types of white blood cells (lymphocytes) that recognize, process, or destroy foreign objects; the bone marrow that creates several types of white blood cells; the thymus that creates white blood cells and teaches them to recognize foreign objects and to distinguish them from the body's cells; lymphatic vessels that help transport lymph and white blood cells; and several other organs, such as the lymph nodes, tonsils, spleen, and appendix, that filter out foreign objects and serve as a place for white blood cells to gather, interact, and share information about infections.*

Oils—^{TA}Thieves (enhances; massage on feet and body), ^{TA}ImmuPower, ^{ITA}oregano[279], ^{TA}frankincense[280], ^{TA}lemon[281], ^{TA}Abundance, ^{TA}cistus, ^{TA}clove, ^{TA}cumin, ^{TA}Exodus II, ^{TA}geranium, ^{TA}Idaho tansy, ^{TA}lavender, ^{TA}ledum (supports), ^{TA}tea tree, ^{TA}mountain savory, ^{TA}Raven, ^{TA}ravintsara, ^{TA}rosemary (supports), ^{TA}thyme (immunological functions), ^{TA}white lotus.

H

I

A=Aromatic **T**=Topical **I**=Internal

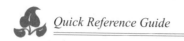

Supplements—**ImmuPro, Inner Defense,** AlkaLime (designed to combat yeast and fungus overgrowth and to preserve the body's proper pH balance), Cleansing Trio (ComforTone, Essentialzyme, and ICP), Digest + Cleanse, Longevity Capsules, Master Formula, Mineral Essence, MultiGreens, NingXia Red, NingXia Wolfberries (dried), Power Meal, Super B, Super C / Super C Chewable, Thyromin, Ultra Young+ (may help raise levels of cytokines, interleukin 1 & 2, and tumor necrosis factor), Wolfberry Crisp Bars (*Refer to the Wolfberry Crisp Bar in the Supplements section of the <u>Reference Guide for Essential Oils</u> for more information on the benefits of the Ningxia Wolfberry*).

—**Stimulates**

Oils—^A<u>Thieves</u> (diffuse with clove), ^{TA}Foregano[279], ^{TA}Ffrankincense[280], ^{TA}<u>ImmuPower</u>, ^{TA}FCinnamon bark, ^{TA}Ftea tree, ^T<u>Breathe Again</u>, ^T<u>The Gift</u>, ^{TA}lavender (for immune system), ^{TA}mountain savory.

—**Boosting Immune Defense**

Oils—^{TA}Cumin, ^{TA}ledum.

T—Dilute as necessary, and apply oil(s) to bottoms of feet, along spine, or under arms. Dilute with V-6 Oil to create massage oil, and massage into the skin.

A—Diffuse into the air for ½ hour at a time.

Impetigo: *See Skin: Impetigo.*

Impotency:

Oils—^TFClary sage, ^{TI}Fclove, ^I<u>SclarEssence</u> (taken internally as a dietary supplement; helps to raise testosterone levels), ^TFsandalwood, ^{TI}<u>Mister</u>, ^{TI}Fginger, ^Tgoldenrod, ^Tjasmine, ^Tnutmeg, ^Trose, ylang ylang.

T—Dilute as necessary, and apply to Vita Flex points on the feet, to groin area, or to abdomen.

I—Add 2–4 drops oil to an empty capsule with 2–4 drops V-6 Oil, and swallow.

Supplements— Prostate Health.

Personal Care—Prenolone+.

Incontinence: *See Bladder.*

Indifference:

Oils—^{AT}Jasmine.

A—Diffuse into the air. Inhale directly or applied to tissue or a cotton wick.

T—Apply to auricular emotion points. Dilute with V-6 Oil to create a massage oil, and massage onto the skin.

Indigestion: *See Digestive System: INDIGESTION.*

Infection: *See also Antibacterial, Antifungal, Antiviral.*

> Oils—^{TA}_FCinnamon bark, ^{TA}<u>Thieves</u>, ^{TA}_Fclary sage, ^{TA}_Fbergamot, ^{TA}_Fpine (severe), ^{TA}<u>Mel-rose</u> (prevents growth of all infections), ^{TA}myrrh (with oregano), ^{TA}cajeput (urethra), ^{TA}clove, ^{TA}cypress, ^{AT}elemi (chest/bronchial infections), ^{TA}Idaho tansy, ^{TA}jasmine (bacterial infection), ^{TA}juniper, ^{TA}fennel, ^{TA}lavender, ^{TA}lemongrass, ^{TA}Tea tree quinquenervia (viral), ^{TA}oregano, ^{TA}peppermint, ^{AT}<u>Raven</u>, ^{TA}ravintsara, ^{TA}rosemary (with myrrh for oral infection), ^{TA}thyme (urinary infection).

Supplements—Inner Defense.

—ANTI-INFECTIOUS

> Oils—^{TA}_FCinnamon bark, ^{AT}_Fspruce, ^{TA}_Fbasil, ^{TA}_Fpine, ^{TA}_Fthyme, ^{TA}_Frosemary, ^{TA}myrrh (with oregano), ^{TA}_Fravintsara, ^{TA}_Fcypress, ^{TA}<u>Purification</u>, ^{TA}_Flavender, ^{TA}_Frosewood, ^{TA}_Fpatchouli, ^{TA}cassia, ^{TA}clove, ^{TA}davana, ^{TA}elemi, ^{TA}eucalyptus, ^{TA}hyssop, ^{TA}Idaho tansy, ^{TA}marjoram, ^{TA}tea tree, ^{TA}Tea tree ericifolia, ^{TA}petitgrain, ^{TA}rose, ^{TA}Roman chamomile, ^{TA}spearmint, ^{TA}spikenard, ^{TA}tarragon.

> ***Comments—See the "Single Oil Property Chart" in the Appendix of this book for additional anti-infectious oils and their strengths.

Supplements—Super C / Super C Chewable.

—INFECTED WOUNDS

> Oils—^TFrankincense, ^Ttea tree, ^Tbasil[282], ^Tpatchouli.

> Blend #1 *(to draw infection out)*—1 drop thyme. Apply hot compress twice daily. Mix together 3 drops lavender, 2 drops tea tree, and 2 drops thyme with 1 tsp. V-6 Oil. After the infection and pus have been expelled, apply a little of the mixture twice daily on the infected area.

Supplements—ImmuPro, Inner Defense, Super C / Super C Chewable.

Infectious Disease:

> Oils—^{TA}Cinnamon bark, ^{TA}<u>ImmuPower</u>, ^{TA}tea tree, ^A<u>Raven</u>, ^ARC, ^{TA}thyme (bacterial infection), ^{TA}bergamot, ^{TA}clove, ^{TA}<u>Exodus II</u>, ^{TA}ginger, ^{TA}hyssop (viral infections), ^{TA}juniper (viral infections), ^{TA}lemon, ^{TA}myrtle.

> **T**—Dilute as necessary, and apply on location and on bottoms of feet.

> **A**—Diffuse into the air.

> ***Comments—Dr. Young uses <u>Raven</u>, <u>RC</u>, and <u>ImmuPower</u> together for infectious diseases.

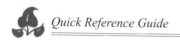
Inferiority (Overcoming):

Oils—[TA]Peppermint, [TA]<u>Transformation</u>.

A—Diffuse into the air. Inhale directly or applied to tissue or a cotton wick.

T—Apply to auricular emotion points. Dilute with V-6 Oil to create a massage oil, and massage onto the skin.

Infertility: *See also Female Specific Conditions, Hormonal Imbalance, Male Specific Conditions.*

Oils—[T]Clary sage, [T]<u>Dragon Time</u> (place on ankles, lower abdomen, and in vagina for women), [T]<u>Mister</u> (for men, place in rectum, across lower back, around and under ankles), [T]**geranium**, [T]anise, [T]bergamot, [T]cypress, [T]fennel, [T]melissa, [T]nutmeg, [T]Roman chamomile, [T]sage, [T]thyme, [T]yarrow, [T]ylang ylang.

T—Dilute as necessary, and apply as indicated, or apply on Vita Flex points, groin area, or lower abdomen.

***Comments—Feed the thyroid.

Supplements— **Prostate Health** (male) or **FemiGen** (female), **Prenolone/Prenolone+ / Progessence/Progessence Plus**, and 1–3 **MultiGreens** three times a day.

Inflammation: *See Anti-inflammatory.*

Influenza: *See also Antiviral, Colds, Respiratory System.*

» *Influenza, commonly referred to as "the flu," is a highly contagious viral infection of the respiratory system. Influenza is marked by a sudden onset of high fever, dry cough, sore throat, muscle aches and pains, headache, fatigue, loss of appetite, nausea, and nasal congestion.*

Oils—[AT]RC, [TA]<u>Raven</u> (apply to thymus area, Vita Flex points on feet, chest, back, and on any place where the flu has settled), [AT]tea tree[283], [AT]peppermint, [AT]<u>Thieves</u>, [AT]rosemary, [TA]<u>ImmuPower</u>, [AT]myrtle, [AT]Eucalyptus radiata, [T]blue cypress (aches and pains), [AT]clove, [AT]copaiba, [AT]<u>Exodus II</u>, [T]fir

> One Sunday after church a friend commented that I looked "exhausted." I thought that strange because I had gotten a good night's sleep. I walked over to a meeting for a mission trip I would be participating in, and an hour later I started getting a headache and felt something happening to my throat. About 30 minutes later, I knew I was coming down with the flu as the headache and sore throat intensified and I started feeling shaky. Fortunately, I had peppermint, oregano and <u>Thieves</u> in my truck; and as soon as I got in, I rubbed several drops of oregano on my feet, rubbed <u>Thieves</u> on my neck and throat, and put several drops of peppermint in my water and started drinking it. By the time I got home, the headache and sore throat had lessened. That evening and for the next several days I took by capsule a combination of lemon, mountain savory, and oregano three times a day. While I could tell my body was fighting an infection (as indicated by my desire to take naps), the oils completely stopped the flu in its tracks, and the headache and sore throat never returned.
>
> *–Submitted by Kevin Dunn*
> *Los Angeles, California (July 2004)*

(aches and pains), ᴬᵀgoldenrod, ᴬᵀginger, ᵀIdaho tansy (on bottoms of feet), ᴬᵀlavender, ᴬᵀledum, ᴬᵀTea tree ericifolia, ᴬᵀonycha (benzoin), ᴬᵀorange, ᴬᵀoregano, ᴬᵀpine, ᴬᵀsage lavender, ᴬᵀthyme, ᴬᵀtsuga.

A—Diffuse into the air

T—Dilute as necessary, and apply to chest, back, neck, sinuses, or Vita Flex points on the feet..

***Comments**—According to the <u>Essential Oils Desk Reference</u>, "[Idaho] tansy should be applied topically on stomach and bottom of feet." (<u>EDR</u>-June 2002; Ch. 28; Flu) It may be best to dilute Idaho tansy first in one teaspoon V-6 Oil before topical application.

Bath Recipe #1—2 Tbs. Evening Peace Bath & Shower Gel with drops of the following oils: 1 wintergreen, 20 eucalyptus, 5 frankincense, 3 helichrysum, 15 ravintsara, and 6 spruce. Mix together, and put mixture under the faucet while running HOT bathwater. SOAK until cool. Also consider using Thieves Cleansing Soap to wash hands with, especially during cold and flu season.

Supplements—Essentialzyme, Essentialzymes-4, Master Formula, ParaFree, Super C / Super C Chewable.

Injuries: *See also Cuts, Pain, Scarring, Tissue, Wounds. See also Blend #2 under Pain for pain reduction.*

Oils—ᵀBalsam fir (with frankincense, sandalwood, myrrh, and helichrysum for pain and inflammation), ᵀcistus (promotes healing of scar tissue), ᵀhelichrysum (reduces scarring and discoloration), ᵀ<u>Melrose</u> (regenerates tissue), ᵀsandalwood (for any DNA repair).

—Sᴘᴏʀᴛ

Oils—ᵀBalsam fir, ᵀhelichrysum, ᵀ<u>Melrose</u>, ᵀ<u>PanAway</u>.

Personal Care—Ortho Ease Massage Oil, Ortho Sport Massage Oil.

T—Dilute as necessary, and apply on location.

Inner Knowing:

Oils—ᴬᵀ<u>Inner Child</u> (reconnects you with your inner child), ᴬᵀ<u>SARA</u>.

A—Diffuse into the air. Inhale directly or applied to tissue or a cotton wick.

T—Apply to auricular emotion points. Dilute with V-6 Oil to create a massage oil, and massage onto the skin.

Insanity:

Oils—ᵀᴬ<u>Hope</u> (ears), ᵀᴬ<u>Release</u> (liver), ᵀᴬ <u>Relieve It</u>.

T—Dilute as necessary, and apply on area indicated or on temples or brain stem area.

A—Inhale directly. Diffuse into the air.

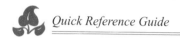
Insect:

—BITES *See also Bites.*

> *Dr. Jean Valnet says that basil, cinnamon, garlic, lavender, lemon, onion, sage, savory, and thyme are effective against insect bites because of their antitoxic and antivenomous properties.*

    Oils—ᵀIdaho tansy, ᵀcajeput, ᵀbergamot.

    Blend #1—Combine 3 drops Roman chamomile, 4 drops eucalyptus, 10 drops lavender, and 1 drop thyme with 1 Tbs. V-6 Oil.

    ***Comments—*Refer to the chapter entitled "How to Use—The Personal Usage Reference" in the Essential Oils Desk Reference under "Insect Bites" for some excellent blend recipes for bites/stings from different types of insects.*

—CHIGGERS

    Oils—ᵀLavender.

—COCKROACHES

    Oils—ᵀCumin[284].

> *My husband was bitten by a spider on his stomach. The bite swelled with a large blister, and it itched terribly. I used lavender oil—about a drop—on the area. In about 4 hours my husband asked for another application of the "magic oil". My husband has an allergy and reacts to any type of a bite. In fact, he usually has to go to the Dr. and get shots and prescriptions.*
> *–Submitted by Mary Rynicki (July 2004)*

    Blend #2—Combine 10 drops peppermint and 5 drops cypress in ½ cup of water; spray.

—POISONS FROM BROWN RECLUSE SPIDER OR WASPS

    Oils—ᵀBasil (known to neutralize poisons), ᵀ<u>Purification</u> (removes poisons from the body).

—INSECTICIDAL

    Oils—ᵀCitronella, ᵀpatchouli[285], ᵀclove[286], ᵀlavender[287], ᵀbasil[288], ᵀtea tree[289], ᵀpink pepper[290], ᵀrosemary[291], ᵀeucalyptus radiata[292], ᵀcaraway[293], ᵀeucalyptus citriodora[294], ᵀdorado azul[295].

—ITCHING

    Oils—ᵀLavender.

    Personal Care—Lavender Hand & Body Lotion (with lavender).

—REPELLENT

    Oils—ᵀᴬCitronella[296], ᵀᴬclove[297], ᵀᴬpatchouli[298], ᵀᴬ<u>Purification</u>, ᵀᴬlavender[299], ᵀᴬlimette[300], ᵀᴬplectranthus oregano,

> *My husband was stung by a wasp last year on the inside of the hand. He removed the stinger and asked me to put something on it. I put <u>Purification</u> on it, and the itching stopped. After his shower that evening, I put <u>Purification</u> on it again. The next morning, you couldn't see or even tell that he'd been stung. I've also put <u>Purification</u> on coworkers who have had mosquito/bug bites that itched. After the <u>Purification</u> went on the bites, the itching stopped.*
> *–Submitted by Christie Krajewski*
> *Batesville, Arkansas (July 2004)*

^{AT}mastrante, ^{TA}micromeria, ^{TA}pink pepper[301], ^{TA}basil, ^{TA}bergamot, ^{TA}cassia[302], ^{TA}cedarwood, ^{TA}geranium[303].

Blend #3—Combine 5 drops lavender, 5 drops lemongrass, 3 drops peppermint, and 1 drop thyme; put on feet, or add to a cup of water and spray on.

Blend #4—Clove, lemon, and orange.

Blend #5—Put 5 drops lemon and 5 drops <u>Purification</u> in a little spray bottle of water, and mist on your skin to protect yourself against insects, flies, and mosquitoes. *1 or 2 oz. glass or plastic spray bottles work very well and are small enough to take with you.*

***Comments—Dr. Friedmann came in contact with a person who had bugs growing on her face and scalp. Somehow she was subjected to a fungus to which the bugs were attracted. The bugs established their nest and laid and hatched their eggs on her skin. She had been using many products and was only able to suppress the problem but not correct it. Dr. Friedmann applied <u>Melrose</u>, helichrysum, lavender, and <u>ImmuPower</u> on her thymus. She stopped using all other chemicals, and several weeks later the bugs were almost gone.

T—Dilute as necessary, and apply on location. Dilute with V-6 Oil to create a massage oil, and apply to skin. Add 3–5 drops to 1 oz. water in a small spray bottle, and mist onto the skin.

A—Diffuse into the air. Apply 1–2 drops on a ribbon or string and hang from windows, branches, or vents.

Insomnia:

Oils—^{AT}_FLavender[304] (best when combined with Roman chamomile and dill), ^{AT}<u>RutaVa-La</u>, ^{AT}valerian[305], ^{AT}_Fbergamot, ^{AT}<u>Citrus Fresh</u>, ^{AT}_Forange, ^{AT}<u>Peace & Calming</u>, ^{AT}_Fylang ylang, ^{AT}_Fcypress, ^{AT}_Fmarjoram, ^{AT}_Fravintsara, ^{AT}_Fmyrtle (for hormone-related insomnia), ^{AT}angelica, ^{AT}basil, ^{AT}clary sage, ^{AT}lemon, ^{AT}Tea tree ericifolia, ^{AT}neroli, ^{AT}nutmeg (small amount), ^{AT}petitgrain, ^{AT}Roman chamomile (small amount), ^{AT}rosemary, ^{AT}sandalwood, ^{AT}<u>Surrender</u> (behind the ears).

Blend #1—Combine 6 drops <u>Citrus Fresh</u> with 6 drops lavender or 6 drops <u>Peace & Calming</u>. Apply blend to big toes, bottoms of feet, 2 drops around navel, and 3 drops on back of neck.

Blend #2—2 drops Roman chamomile, 6 drops geranium, 3 drops lemon, and 4 drops sandalwood. Mix together, and add 6 drops in your bath at bedtime and 5 drops with 2 tsp. V-6 Oil for a massage after bath.

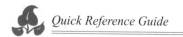

Blend #3—Combine 20 ml valerian, 5 ml vetiver, 2 ml helichrysum, 1 ml clove, and 1 ml peppermint in a 1 oz. dropper bottle. Add several drops (up to 3 droppers full) to 2–3 oz. of water, and drink—followed by ½ tsp. AlkaLime in water.

Supplements—ImmuPro.

*****Comments**—Refer to the chapter entitled "How to Use—The Personal Usage Reference" in the <u>Essential Oils Desk Reference</u> under "Insomnia" for some excellent blend recipes.

—**For Children**

    –**12 months to 5 years**

        Oils—^{AT}Lavender, ^{AT}Roman chamomile

    –**5 to 12 years**

        Oils—^{AT}Lavender, ^{AT}clary sage, ^{AT}geranium, ^{AT}Tea tree ericifolia, ^{AT}ylang ylang (infection).

A—Diffuse into the air. Place 1–2 drops on a pillow or stuffed animal. Add 1–3 drops to 1 oz. distilled water in a spray bottle, and mist into the air.

T—Dilute as necessary, and apply to bottoms of feet or back of neck. Dilute with V-6 Oil to create a massage oil, and massage onto back of legs, feet, and arms. Add 1–2 drops to bathwater, and bathe.

Intestinal Problems: *See Digestive System: Intestinal Problems.*

Invigorating:

Oils—^{TA}Wintergreen.

—**In Summer**

    Oils—^{TA}Eucalyptus, ^{TA}peppermint.

T—Dilute in V-6 Oil to create massage oil, and massage onto the skin. Add 1–2 drops to 1 oz. cool distilled water in a spray bottle, and mist onto the skin.

A—Diffuse into the air.

Ions:

—**Increase Negative Ions**

    Oils—When dispersed into the air through a cool-air nebulizing diffuser, the following oils ionize negatively: Bergamot,

> *Negative ions* are produced naturally by wind and rain. They help stimulate the parasympathetic nervous system, which controls rest, relaxation, digestion, and sleep. However, if you live in an environment with an overabundance of negative ions, such as in the country or by the ocean, you may benefit greatly from diffusing the oils listed under **Positive Ions**. The production of more positive ions can help bring greater balance to the area and provide a more healthy environment.

cedarwood, citronella, *Eucalyptus citriodora*, grapefruit, lavandin, lavender, lemon, lemongrass, mandarin, orange, patchouli, sandalwood.

—INCREASE POSITIVE IONS

Oils—When dispersed into the air through a cool-air nebulizing diffuser, the following oils ionize positively: Cajeput, clove, cypress, eucalyptus, frankincense, helichrysum,

> *Positive ions* are produced by electronic equipment and are typically found in man-made environments. They help stimulate the sympathetic nervous system, necessary for recovering, strengthening, and energizing. However, an overabundance of positive ions can lead to stress and agitation. The diffusion of the oils listed under **Negative Ions** can help balance the ions and help produce a more stress-free environment.

juniper, marjoram, *Tea tree quinquenervia*, palmarosa, pine, ravintsara, rosemary, thyme, ylang ylang.

Iron:

***Comments—Iron is important for learning. **Raisins** are a good natural source.

Supplements— **Master Formula, KidScents MightyVites** (chewable).

Irritability: *See also Calming.*

Oils—ᴬᵀLavender, ᴬᵀForgiveness, ᴬᵀHope, ᴬᵀHumility, ᴬᵀInspiration, ᴬᵀmyrrh, ᴬᵀPresent Time, ᴬᵀSurrender, ᴬᵀValor.

A—Diffuse into the air. Inhale directly or applied to hands, tissue, or a cotton wick.

T—Dilute with V-6 Oil to create massage oil, and massage into the skin.

***Comments—All single oils can help **except** eucalyptus, pepper, peppermint, and rosemary.

Supplements—AlkaLime.

Irritable Bowel Syndrome: *See Digestive System: IRRITABLE BOWEL SYNDROME.*

Itching:

Oils—ᵀPeppermint (ears), ᵀlavender, ᵀPeace & Calming (ears).

T—Dilute as necessary, and apply on location or on ears.

Blend #1—6 drops lavender and 3 drops rosemary with Lavender Hand & Body Lotion.

Personal Care—Rose Ointment, Lavender Hand & Body Lotion.

Jaundice: *See Liver: JAUNDICE*

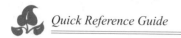
Jealousy:

Oils—^{AT}Bergamot, ^{AT}eucalyptus, ^{AT}<u>Forgiveness</u>, ^{AT}frankincense, ^{AT}<u>Harmony</u>, ^{AT}<u>Humility</u>, ^{AT}<u>Joy</u>,
^{AT}lemon, ^{AT}marjoram, ^{AT}orange, ^{AT}rose, ^{AT}rosemary, ^{AT}<u>Sacred Mountain</u>, ^{AT}sandalwood, ^{AT}thyme, ^{AT}<u>Valor</u>, ^{AT}<u>White Angelica</u>.

A—Diffuse into the air. Inhale directly or applied to hands, tissue, or a cotton wick.

T—Apply to auricular emotion points. Dilute with V-6 Oil to create massage oil, and massage into
the skin.

Jet Lag:

≫ *Jet lag is the disruption of normal sleep patterns experienced while the hypothalamus (the body's internal clock) adjusts to rapid changes in daylight and nighttime hours when flying to different areas of the world. Jet lag can cause tiredness, fatigue, and insomnia during normal sleeping hours. It is recommended to drink lots of fluids and to avoid alcohol or caffeine while flying to help prevent jet lag. Avoiding naps and forcing yourself to stay awake until your normal bedtime the first day can also help the body recover more quickly.*

Oils—^T<u>Valor</u>, ^Tpeppermint, ^T<u>Brain Power</u>, ^Teucalyptus, ^T<u>Clarity</u>, ^T<u>En-R-Gee</u>, ^Tgeranium, ^Tgrapefruit, ^T<u>ImmuPower</u> (for protection), ^Tlavender, ^Tlemongrass, ^T<u>Present Time</u>.

T—Dilute as necessary, and apply to temples, thymus, and bottoms of feet. It is best to not eat heavy foods and to drink as much water as possible.

Supplements—Power Meal, Sulfurzyme, Super C / Super C Chewable.

Joints: *See also Rotator Cuff, Shoulder (Frozen), Tennis Elbow.*

Oils—^TWintergreen (discomfort), ^Tspruce (aching), ^Tcajeput (stiff), ^Tbalsam fir (pain from exercising), ^TDouglas fir (calming to tired and overworked joints), ^Tnutmeg, ^TRoman chamomile (inflamed).

T—Dilute as necessary, and apply on location or on Vita Flex points on the feet. Dilute with V-6 Oil and massage on location.

Supplements— Master Formula.

***Comments**—Refer to the chapter entitled "How to Use—The Personal Usage Reference" in the Essential Oils Desk Reference under "Joint Stiffness and Pain" for some excellent blend recipes.

Joyous:

Oils—**ᴬᵀ**Joy, **ᴬᵀ**Abundance, **ᴬᵀ**bergamot (turns grief to joy), **ᴬᵀ**Christmas Spirit, **ᴬᵀ**Citrus Fresh (brings joy to children), **ᴬ**orange.

A—Diffuse into the air. Inhale directly or applied to hands, tissue, or a cotton wick.

T—Apply to auricular emotion points. Dilute with V-6 Oil to create massage oil, and massage into
the skin.

Kidneys: *See also Diuretic.*

>> *The kidneys are paired organs located just below the rib cage on either side of the spine that function to filter waste and extra water from the blood. The kidneys convert the waste and extra water into urine that is then excreted through urination. The kidneys also play an important role in hormone production.*

Oils—**ᵀ_F**Lemongrass (combine with juniper for greater synergistic effect), **ᴵ**thyme[306], **ᵀ**Aroma Life, **ᴵ**bergamot[307], **ᵀ**calamus (reduces congestion after intoxication), **ᵀ**clary sage, **ᵀ**EndoFlex, **ᵀ**geranium, **ᵀ**grapefruit, **ᵀ**juniper (for better function of kidneys), **ᵀ**JuvaFlex, **ᵀ**ledum (strengthen), **ᵀ**Release.

T—Apply over kidneys as a hot compress. Dilute as necessary, and apply over kidneys or on Vita Flex points on the feet.

I—Add 1–2 drops to an empty capsule, and swallow. Use as flavoring in food.

*****Comments**—Drink plenty of distilled water (3–4 quarts each day). When kidneys start producing ammonia, the ammonia can go to the brain—and people have died from that alone. Do the **MASTER CLEANSER** (*See Cleansing*).

Supplements—**Longevity Capsules** (contains thyme oil to help preserve omega-3 fatty acids in the kidneys), **K&B Tincture**, EndoGize, MultiGreens (turns blood back to alkaline).

*****Comments**—Refer to the chapter entitled "How to Use—The Personal Usage Reference" in the Essential Oils Desk Reference under "Kidney Disorders" for some excellent blend recipes and supplement recommendations.

—**Blockage**

Recipe #1—Massage Release and other oils onto the kidney points on the feet twice a day.

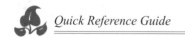

Supplements—Cleansing Trio (ComforTone, Essentialzyme, and ICP), JuvaTone (First week: 2 tablets a day; Second week: 3 tablets a day for 90 days).

—CAPILLARIES BEING ATTACKED IN KIDNEYS

Supplements—Need to support the body and cleanse the blood with **MultiGreens, Cleansing Trio (ComforTone, Essentialzyme, and ICP)**.

—INFECTION IN

Oils—ᵀRosemary.

T—Dilute as necessary, and apply to kidneys and to Vita Flex points.

Blend #1—Cypress, marjoram, and <u>Thieves</u> or <u>JuvaFlex</u>. Apply as a hot compress.

Nutrition—Drink one gallon of distilled water and 2 quarts of cranberry juice in a day.

Supplements—**Inner Defense, NingXia Red** (1–3 oz. followed by 8–10 oz. of water 3 times daily).

—INFLAMMATION (NEPHRITIS)

Oils—ᵀ<u>Aroma Life</u>, ᵀjuniper, ᵀ<u>JuvaFlex</u>.

T—Dilute as necessary, and apply to kidneys and to Vita Flex points.

***Comments—Do a colon cleanse (*see Cleansing*).

Nutrition—Drink one gallon of distilled water and 2 quarts of cranberry juice in a day.

Supplements—**K&B Tincture,** MultiGreens, Power Meal, Rehemogen Tincture, Super C / Super C Chewable.

***Comments—*Refer to the chapter entitled "How to Use—The Personal Usage Reference" in the* <u>Essential Oils Desk Reference</u> *under "Kidney Disorders," subcategory "Inflammation in the Kidneys (Nephritis)," for a very specific regimen of supplements and blends.*

—MUSCLES THAT WON'T WORK IN THE KIDNEYS

Oils—ᵀ<u>Aroma Siez</u>, ᵀ<u>EndoFlex</u>.

Blend #2—8 drops fennel and 10 drops juniper.

T—Dilute as necessary, and apply to kidneys and to Vita Flex points.

—STONES

 ⮞ *A kidney stone is a solid piece of material that forms as chemicals in the urine crystallize and adhere together in the kidney. Small stones may pass through urination without causing pain. Larger stones with sharp edges and corners, however, can cause an extreme amount of pain as they are passed out of the body through the urinary tract.*

Oils—ᵀEucalyptus, ᵀhyssop, ᵀjuniper.

T—Dilute as necessary, and apply to kidneys and to Vita Flex points. Apply as a hot compress over kidney area.

Blend #3—10 drops juniper and 10 drops geranium. Apply as a hot compress over kidneys once a day.

Supplements—After being on the Cleansing Trio (ComforTone, Essentialzyme, and ICP) for 10 days, add Super C / Super C Chewable.

Recipe #2—To pass (without edges), drink 4 oz. distilled water with juice from ½ lemon every 30 minutes for 6 hours straight. Then take 2 Tbs. extra light virgin olive oil with the juice from 1 full lemon. Repeat daily until stone passes.

Knee Cartilage Injury:

Blend #1—8 drops clove, 12 drops ginger, and 10 drops nutmeg with 2 oz. V-6 Oil. Massage three times a day. Apply ice for swelling and inflammation. Wrap knee and elevate when sitting. Use the ice method three times a day, and alternate with a hot compress and the oils.

Personal Care—Ortho Ease Massage Oil, Ortho Sport Massage Oil, Regenolone.

Supplements—BLM

Labor: *See also Pregnancy/Motherhood.*

Oils—ᵀ<u>Gentle Baby</u>, ᵀjasmine (pain).

T—Dilute as necessary, and apply on ankles and abdomen.

Lactation (Secretion of breast milk): *See also Pregnancy/Motherhood: Nursing.*

Oils—ᵀ_FFennel or ᵀbasil (increase flow), ᵀpeppermint (with cold compress—decrease flow).

T—Apply above the breasts on the lymph area, and apply 2–3 drops on the spine, about breast level.

Supplements—PD 80/20, Prenolone/Prenolone+, Progessence/Progessence Plus.

Lactose Intolerance:

►► *Lactose intolerance is the inability of the body to fully digest lactose, a sugar found in milk and in other dairy products. Symptoms of lactose intolerance include abdominal pain and bloating, diarrhea, nausea, and gas.*

K

L

A=Aromatic **T**=Topical **I**=Internal

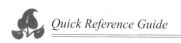

Oils—[IT]Lemongrass (reported to help eliminate lactic acid from fermentation of lactose in milk).

I—Add 1–2 drops to 1 tsp. honey, and swallow; or add 1–2 drops to 4 oz. rice or almond milk, and drink. Place 1–2 drops in an empty capsule, and swallow.

T—Dilute as recommended, and apply 1–2 drops on abdomen or on reflex points on the feet.

Supplements—Allerzyme, Essentialzyme, Essentialzymes-4, Life 5 (probiotic), Power Meal.

Laryngitis:

➤➤ *Laryngitis is an inflammation and swelling of the voice box (called the larynx) that causes the voice to sound hoarse or raspy. Laryngitis is most commonly caused by viruses, allergies, or overuse of the voice and will generally go away by itself within two weeks.*

Oils—[AT]Sandalwood, [A]frankincense, [AI]lavender, [AT]thyme, [ATI]<u>Melrose</u>, [AT]jasmine, [AT]ledum, [AT]onycha (benzoin), [AT]sage.

A—Diffuse into the air.

T—Dilute as necessary, and apply to neck and to Vita Flex points on the feet.

I—Add 1–2 drops to 1 tsp. honey, and swallow

Blend #1—Add one drop each of <u>Melrose</u> and lemon to 1 tsp. honey. Swish around in mouth for a couple of minutes to liquefy; then swallow.

Laundry: *See Housecleaning: LAUNDRY.*

Laxative:

Oils—[T]Hyssop, [T]jasmine, [TI]tangerine.

T—Apply to abdomen with warm compress. Dilute as necessary, and massage on abdomen; or apply to Vita Flex points on the feet.

I—Add 1–2 drops to 8 oz. rice or almond milk, and drink.

Blend #1—Dilute equal parts rosemary, lemon, and peppermint oils[308] in V-6 Oil, and massage on abdomen.

Supplements—Balance Complete, Cleansing Trio (ComforTone, Essentialzyme, and ICP), Digest + Cleanse.

Legs, Restless:

Restless legs are caused by the body dumping acid into the system at night. The following recipe was recommended to counteract this reaction to the over-acidification of the body.

Recipe #1—In the evening before bed, take 1 Tbs of JuvaPower (in almond, rice or soy milk, or water), followed by ½ tsp of AlkaLime in water. Then apply 2–3 drops each of valerian, Roman chamomile, and lavender to the brain stem area (back of neck from shoulders to base of skull), and work them in with the Vita Flex technique.

Leg Ulcers: *See Ulcers: Leg.*

Lethargy:

Oils—^{AT}Jasmine, ^{AT}<u>Transformation</u>.

A—Diffuse into the air. Inhale directly or applied to hands.

T—Dilute with V-6 Oil to create massage oil, and massage into skin. Add 1–2 drops to 1 Tbs. bath or shower gel, and use in bath or shower.

Libido (Low): *See also Frigidity, Sex Stimulant.*

Oils—^{AT}Ylang ylang, ^{AT}<u>Sensation</u>, ^{AT}<u>Dragon Time</u>, ^{AT}<u>Live with Passion</u>, ^{AT}<u>Mister</u>, ^{AT}<u>Joy</u>, ^{AT}nutmeg, ^{AT}rose, ^I<u>SclarEssence</u>.

***Comments—Do the MASTER CLEANSER (*See Cleansing*).

Supplements— **Progessence/Progessence Plus**, PD 80/20, Prenolone/Prenolone+, Sulfurzyme.

—MEN *See also Prostate.*

Oils—^{AT}Cinnamon, ^{AT}black pepper, ^{AT}ginger, ^{AT}myrrh, ^{AT}pine.

Personal Care—Protec (combine with frankincense to decongest the prostate).

—WOMEN

Oils—^{AT}Jasmine, ^{AT}<u>Lady Sclareol</u>, ^{AT}clary sage, ^{AT}geranium.

A—Diffuse into the air. Dissolve 8–10 drops in 2 tsp. pure grain or perfumers alcohol, combine with distilled water in a 1 or 2 oz. spray bottle, and spray into the air or on clothes or bed linens.

T—Dilute as necessary, and apply on temples, neck, or wrists. Dilute with V-6 Oil to create a massage oil, and massage into the skin. Combine 1–2 drops with 1/4 cup Epsom salts, and dissolve in warm bathwater for a romantic bath.

I—Place 2–5 drops in an empty capsule, and swallow.

A=Aromatic **T**=Topical **I**=Internal | 231

Lice:

Oils—^TTea tree[309], ^Tcitronella[310], ^Tpine (repels), ^Teucalyptus[292], ^Tgeranium, ^Tlavender, ^Tlemon, ^Trosemary.

T—Apply oil(s) to scalp and to bottoms of feet three times a day.

Ligaments: *See also Muscles.*

Oils—^TLemongrass (torn or pulled: combine with marjoram to stimulate torn ligaments; combine with basil if torn ligaments produce spasms), ^T<u>Deep Relief</u> (roll-on), ^Tpalo santo.

Supplements—BLM

—Torn

Oils—^TLemongrass, ^T<u>PanAway</u>, ^Twintergreen, ^Tclove, ^hhelichrysum, ^Tmarjoram.

Personal Care—Ortho Sport Massage Oil.

T—Dilute as necessary, and apply on location or on Vita Flex points on the feet.

Lipoma: *See Tumors: Lipoma.*

Lips:

Oils—^TGerman chamomile, ^Tlavender, ^Tlemon, ^Ttea tree.

T—Dilute as necessary, and apply on lips.

—Dry Lips

Blend #1—Combine 2–5 drops geranium with 2–5 drops lavender, and apply 1–2 drops on lips.

Personal Care—Cinnamint or Lavender Lip Balms, LBrianté Lip Gloss

Listlessness: *See also Calming.*

Oils—^{AT}Jasmine.

A—Diffuse into the air. Inhale directly or applied to hands.

T—Dilute with V-6 Oil to create massage oil, and massage into skin. Add 1–2 drops to 1/4 cup Epsom salts, and dissolve in warm bathwater before bathing.

Liver:

≫ *The liver is the largest internal organ of the body. It is located in the upper abdomen and helps with digestion, produces cholesterol used to make several hormones and cellular membranes, re-*

moves waste products and old cells from the blood, and metabolizes harmful substances and toxins into harmless chemicals.

Oils—^{TA}Ledum (powerful detoxifier), ^{TA}dill³¹¹, ^{TA}rosemary³¹², ^{TA}caraway³¹¹, ^{TA}JuvaFlex (detoxification), ^{TA}Juva Cleanse, ^{TA}_Fsage (for liver problems), ^{TA}_Fhelichrysum, ^{TA}_Fgeranium (cleanses and detoxifies the liver), ^{TA}_FGerman chamomile, ^{TA}thyme³¹³, ^{TA}Acceptance, ^{TA}cypress, ^{TA}Di-Gize, ^{TA}fleabane, ^Iginger³¹⁴, ^{TA}GLF, ^{TA}goldenrod (supports liver function), ^{TA}grapefruit (liver disorders), ^{TA}myrrh, ^{TA}Peace & Calming, ^{TA}ravintsara, ^{TA}sage lavender (congestion), ^TRelease (apply to liver and to Vita Flex points), ^{TA}Roman chamomile, ^{TA}3 Wise Men (on crown).

Supplements—JuvaTone, Balance Complete, Digest + Cleanse, Longevity Capsules (contains thyme oil to help preserve omega-3 fatty acids in the liver). Also NingXia Red, Omega Blue, OmegaGize³, and Power Meal.

***Comments—**When the liver is toxic, it makes the mind lethargic and slows the emotions. For those who have liver problems, be careful about the oils used and the amounts. Ease into a liver cleanse!

—CIRRHOSIS OF THE LIVER

>> *Cirrhosis is scarring of the liver that occurs as the liver tries to repair damage done to itself. When extensive liver damage occurs, the massive scar tissue buildup makes it impossible for the liver to function. The most common causes of cirrhosis are fatty liver (resulting from obesity or diabetes) and alcohol abuse; but any damage done to the liver can cause cirrhosis.*

Oils—^{TA}Frankincense, ^{TA}myrrh, ^{TA}geranium, ^{TA}juniper, ^{TA}lavender, ^{TA}Roman chamomile, ^{TA}rosemary³¹⁵, ^{TA}rose.

Supplements—JuvaTone, NingXia Red, Super C / Super C Chewable.

—CLEANSING

Oils—^{TA}Juva Cleanse, ^{TA}clove (increases detoxification), ^{TA}GLF, ^{TA}JuvaFlex, ^{TA}carrot seed, ^{TA}helichrysum, ^{TA}geranium, ^{TA}German chamomile, ^{TA}ledum (with JuvaTone), ^{TA}myrrh, ^{TA}sage lavender.

Supplements—Longevity Capsules, NingXia Red, Sulfurzyme (may help detoxify the liver).

—FUNCTION (IMPROVE)

Recipe #1—GLF, JuvaFlex, goldenrod, and myrrh. Do a compress over the liver, and alternate the oils on the liver Vita Flex points.

Supplements—NingXia Red, Omega Blue, OmegaGize³, Power Meal.

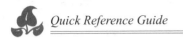

—HEPATITIS *See also Antiviral*

>> *Hepatitis is any swelling or inflammation of the liver. This can interfere with normal liver functioning and can possibly lead to cirrhosis or cancer over time. The most common cause of hepatitis is from one of the five different forms of hepatitis viruses, but it can also be caused by alcohol consumption, other viruses, or medications. Possible symptoms of hepatitis include diarrhea, jaundice, stomach pain, loss of appetite, dark-colored urine, pale bowel movements, nausea, and vomiting.*

Oils—^{TA}GLF, ^{T}JuvaFlex (over the liver), ^{I}myrrh (with ledum internally for hepatitis B & C), ^{TA}cinnamon bark, ^{TA}cypress^{316}, ^{TA}eucalyptus, ^{TA}ImmuPower (on spine and liver), ^{TA}tea tree, ^{TA}oregano, ^{TA}patchouli, ^{TA}ravintsara (viral), ^{T}Release (on feet and liver), ^{TA}Roman chamomile, ^{TA}rosemary, ^{TA}thyme.

Supplements—NingXia Red.

Recipe #2—The following regimen has been useful: Use the Cleansing Trio (ComforTone, Essentialzyme, and ICP) for 1 week, 4 Life 5 (probiotic) a day, Master Formula, 1 MultiGreens a day, 4 Super C / Super C Chewable three times a day. Add JuvaTone on the 3rd day.

***Comments—Refer to the chapter entitled "How to Use—The Personal Usage Reference" in the Essential Oils Desk Reference under "Liver," subcategory "Hepatitis," for a specific daily program using supplements and blends.

–DETOXIFY LIVER

Oils—^{T}Ledum and ^{TA}JuvaTone together.

–VIRAL

Oils—$^{I}_{F}$Myrrh and ^{ITA}JuvaFlex, ^{TA}frankincense^{317}, $^{TA}_{F}$ravintsara, $^{TA}_{F}$rosemary, ^{TA}GLF, ^{TA}ledum.

Supplements—Super C / Super C Chewable.

—JAUNDICE

>> *Jaundice is a condition characterized by a yellow appearance of the skin and the whites of the eyes. Jaundice is a result of excessive levels in the blood of a chemical called bilirubin. Bilirubin is a pigment that is made when hemoglobin from old or dead red blood cells is broken down. Jaundice occurs when the liver is unable to pass bilirubin from the body as fast as it is being produced. Jaundice is often a symptom of other diseases or conditions.*

Oils—$^{TA}_{F}$Geranium, ^{TA}GLF, ^{TA}Juva Cleanse, ^{TA}lemon, ^{TA}rosemary, ^{TA}sage lavender.

—REGENERATION

Supplements—NingXia Red

*****Comments**—*One individual had total liver regeneration using JuvaTone, Rehemogen, and JuvaFlex.*

—SPOTS

>> *Liver spots are gray, black, or brown spots that appear on the skin in areas that have had a lot of sun exposure over the years. Liver spots are not harmful, but many people wish to eliminate them for cosmetic reasons.*

Personal Care—Prenolone/Prenolone+, Progessence/Progessence Plus.

—STIMULANT FOR LIVER CELL FUNCTION

Oils—^{TA}_FHelichrysum, ^{TA}GLF, ^{TA}ledum (combine with JuvaTone).

Supplements—Balance Complete, Cleansing Trio (ComforTone, Essentialzyme, and ICP), JuvaTone (helps increase digestion in the liver), NingXia Red, Omega Blue, OmegaGize³.

T—Dilute as necessary, and apply 1–2 drops over liver area and on Vita Flex points on the feet. Apply along the spine for viral infections, alternating oils. Apply as a hot compress over the liver area.

A—Diffuse into the air. Inhale directly or applied to hands.

I—Add 3–5 drops oil to an empty capsule with 3–5 drops V-6 Oil; swallow.

Longevity:

Oils—^AFennel, ^{IA}Longevity.

A—Diffuse into the air. Inhale directly or applied to hands, tissue, or a cotton wick.

I—Add 3–5 drops to an empty capsule; swallow.

Supplements—NingXia Red (whole wolfberry puree), Longevity Capsules (Longevity blend + frankincense in gel caps for internal consumption), Omega Blue/OmegaGize³ (omega-3s).

Loss of Loved One:

Oils—^{AT}Basil, ^{AT}cedarwood, ^Acypress, ^{AT}fir, ^{AT}Forgiveness, ^{AT}jasmine, ^{AT}Joy, ^{AT}rose, ^{AT}spruce, ^{AT}Transformation, ^{AT}Valor, ^{AT}ylang ylang.

A—Diffuse into the air. Inhale directly or applied to hands, tissue, or a cotton wick.

T—Apply to auricular emotion points. Dilute with V-6 Oil to create massage oil, and massage into skin.

Personal Care—Sensation Hand & Body Lotion, Sensation Bath & Shower Gel, Sensation Massage Oil.

L

A=Aromatic   **T**=Topical   **I**=Internal

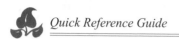
Loss of Smell:

Oils—^ABasil.

A—Inhale directly. Diffuse into the air.

Lou Gehrig's Disease: *See also Alzheimer's Disease, Brain, Multiple Sclerosis, Parkinson's Disease, Pineal Gland, Pituitary Gland.*

» *Lou Gehrig's disease (also known as amyotrophic lateral sclerosis) is a progressive and fatal neurological disease that affects nerve cells in the brain and spinal cord. As the disease progresses, motor neurons die, and the brain loses its ability to control muscle movement. Later stages of the disease can lead to complete paralysis. Eventually, control is lost of the muscles needed to breathe, to speak, and to eat.*

Oils—^{TA}Cypress (circulation), ^{TA}Valor, ^{TA}frankincense, ^{TA}sandalwood, ^{TA}Acceptance (may help to oxygenate the pineal and pituitary glands), ^{TA}Clarity (for brain function), ^{TA}Egyptian Gold, ^{TA}Peace & Calming.

*****Comments**—Use the same oils as you would if you were handling Multiple Sclerosis, Alzheimer's, and Parkinson's Disease. Drink distilled water.

T—Dilute as necessary, and apply 1–2 drops on brain stem area, neck, spine, and Vita Flex points on the feet. Add 1–2 drops to 1 Tbs. V-6 Oil, and massage on back, neck, and feet.

A—Diffuse into the air. Inhale directly or applied to hands.

Supplements—Cleansing Trio (ComforTone, Essentialzyme, and ICP), Digest + Cleanse, JuvaPower/JuvaSpice, JuvaTone, Omega Blue, OmegaGize³, Sulfurzyme.

Love:

Oils—^{AT}Forgiveness, ^{AT}Joy, ^{AT}juniper, ^{AT}Lady Sclareol, ^{AT}lavender, ^{AT}Oola Family, ^{AT}Sensation, ^{AT}ylang ylang.

Personal Care—Sensation Massage Oil, Sensation Hand & Body Lotion, Sensation Bath & Shower Gel (contains oils used by Cleopatra to enhance love and to increase the desire to be close to that someone special).

—ATTRACTS

Oils—^{AT}Joy.

—SELF LOVE

Oils—^{AT}Joy.

A—Diffuse into the air. Inhale directly or applied to hands, tissue, or a cotton wick.

T—Apply to auricular emotion points. Dilute with V-6 Oil to create massage oil, and massage into skin.

Lumbago: *See Back:* LOWER BACK PAIN.

Lungs: *See Respiratory System:* LUNGS.

Lupus: *See also Adrenal Glands, Digestive System, Endocrine System, Immune System, Thyroid.*

>> *Lupus is an autoimmune disease that occurs when the immune system begins attacking its own tissues and organs. Lupus can cause pain, damage, and inflammation in the joints, blood vessels, skin, and organs. Common symptoms include joint pain or swelling, fever, muscle pain, and red rashes (often on the face).*

> *Lupus is a collagen breakdown that may effect the skin, joints, and other systems of the body. It occurs because of thyroid and adrenal malfunction. The immune system cells malfunction and some of the good immune cells turn and destroy other good immune cells. This attack leads to an allergic reaction. The immune cells go crazy and attack whatever is convenient for them. The endocrine systems are usually affected and may shut down. In order to heal Lupus, it is necessary to cleanse the body, reduce the toxins, increase blood circulation, and nutritionally support the endocrine functions. When this happens, the adrenal glands can secrete the cortisone that is necessary for connective tissue repair and maintenance.*
>
> *To determine whether or not the thyroid needs help, you must monitor your basal cell temperature. Place a mercury thermometer under your arm pit, and leave it there for 10 minutes. If your temperature is below 97.6°, you need to work on the thyroid (See Recipe #2 below).*

Oils—^{TA}Clove, ^{TA}Joy, ^{TA}Thieves (every 2 hours on the feet), ^{TA}Present Time (key oil for lupus), ^{TA}Valor (always use first on the feet for courage to overcome fear and build self esteem), ^{TA}Acceptance, ^{TA}EndoFlex, ^{TA}ImmuPower (alone has cleared up Lupus).

Bath—Put 30 drops EndoFlex in softened bath gel.

Massage—Thieves (every 2 hours on feet).

Personal Care—A·R·T Skin Care System, Regenolone (may help reverse symptoms).

Supplements—Balance Complete, ComforTone, Digest + Cleanse, EndoGize, ICP, and Essentialzyme (cleanses the body of toxins and supports the digestive function), Thyromin (is a main stay for lupus as it feeds and regulates the thyroid), ImmuPro, Inner Defense, MultiGreens (high in chlorophyll; contains melissa, which supports the connective tissue and the immune function), NingXia Red (contains mannose, an essential sugar that helps to prevent infection—lupus patients are all deficient in this), Power Meal (predigested protein that contains wolfberry), Master Formula. Carrot juice is also very supportive.

L

A=Aromatic   **T**=Topical   **I**=Internal | 237

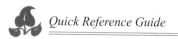
***Comments**—Refer to the chapter entitled "How to Use—The Personal Usage Reference" in the <u>Essential Oils Desk Reference</u> under "Lupus" for a specific daily regimen using supplements and blends.

—**Adrenal Glands** *See also Adrenal Glands*

> **Recipe #1**—Nutmeg has adrenal cortex properties and is contained in EndoFlex. EndoFlex or Blend #1 can be applied over the adrenal gland area using a hot compress. Also, apply on and massage the Vita Flex points.

> **Blend #1**—3 drops clove (rub in), 5 drops nutmeg (rub in), 7 drops rosemary (rub in), and 20 drops V-6 Oil. Apply a hot compress.

> **Blend #2**—30 drops cypress, 30 drops lemongrass, and 30 drops <u>EndoFlex</u> in 4 oz. V-6 Oil. Massage whole body every day.

—**Fluid Retention** (caused by steroids)

> **Oils**—ᵀᴬ<u>EndoFlex</u>.

—**Endocrine System Support** *See Endocrine System.*

> **Oils**—ᵀᴬ<u>EndoFlex</u>.

> The following is a recipe that has been used for individuals with Lupus:

> **Recipe #2**—If your basal cell temperature is below 97.6° F (36.5° C), you need to work on the thyroid. Take 2 Thyromin at bedtime. If your temperature does not come up in three days, you will need to increase the amount of Thyromin you are taking. Take 1 upon arising along with the 2 at bedtime. When your temperature gets back up to 97.6° F, stop taking the one in the morning. Gradually go off the 2 at night. Check regularly to see that your temperature continues to stay at 97.6° F. In addition, choose one of the following oils to work as a tissue generator: <u>Acceptance</u>, <u>Joy</u>, <u>Present Time</u>, or <u>Valor</u>; apply to Vita Flex points and to thyroid. To support the adrenal glands, use Blend #1. To determine the adrenal area, lay a yard stick across the back from elbow to elbow, and go up 2". Apply <u>ImmuPower</u> on the spine and Vita Flex points. Finally, supplement with Super C / Super C Chewable and 2 Thyromin, or more if needed.

> **Case History #1**—After taking Thyromin in the following manner for two months, one individual was totally free from Lupus: 2 capsules in the morning and 2 in the evening until temperature stayed down for three days; then increased to 3 capsules in the morning and 3 in the evening. Also, oils used included <u>ImmuPower</u> and <u>Valor</u>, among others.

> **Case History #2**—A nurse in a hospital in the East gave <u>ImmuPower</u> to a patient who was leaving the hospital after another serious bout with Lupus. The patient had suffered from Lupus for 22 years, but she felt better very soon after she started

using <u>ImmuPower</u>. And no symptoms of Lupus were found in her at all after eight days.

Case History #3—After suffering from systemic lupus for some time, one lady decided there was nothing left to try from the doctors. She turned to the oils and started applying <u>ImmuPower</u>, <u>EndoFlex</u>, and <u>Joy</u> over her thymus and on her feet over the Vita Flex points for the pineal and pituitary glands. She also began taking Thyromin supplements. After only a day and a half of applying <u>EndoFlex</u> to her toes, she began to have some feeling return. After a while (specific time unknown), the "butterfly" on her face disappeared, and blood tests returned "just fine".

Thought Patterns and Emotions—Some feelings you experience may be subconscious or may be patterns that you inherited from your ancestors in the DNA. A feeling of giving up. Feeling that it is better to die than to stand up for one's self. Anger and a need to be punished. Feelings of deep grief. Laughing on the outside, but crying on the inside. Self destructive programming; an internal cannibalism; a loss of self worth. (Remember it may not have begun with you; we carry in our cells the programming of our ancestors for 4 generations back). You may feel one or more of the above. Reprogram your cells by claiming your power, loving and approving of yourself (no judgment). You are free and safe; speak up for yourself freely and easily. Visualize your body healed or healing. Learn the reason you chose this lesson, and learn from it so you can get past it and be healed. Put as little energy as possible into your affliction.

Lyme Disease: *See also Antibacterial, Insect: REPELLENT.*

▸▸ *Lyme Disease is an inflammatory illness caused by the bite of a tick carrying the bacterium Borrelia burgdorferi. Signs of Lyme disease include flu-like symptoms, joint pain, neurological problems, and a rash.*

Oils—ᵀ<u>Clarity</u> (back of ears), ᵀ<u>Joy</u> (over heart), ᵀᴬ<u>RC</u> (on chest), ᵀ<u>Sacred Mountain</u> (on back of neck), ᵀ<u>Thieves</u> (on feet and thymus), ᵀ<u>White Angelica</u> (on forehead).

T—Dilute as necessary, and apply on location indicated.

A—Inhale directly.

Supplements—Cleansing Trio (ComforTone, Essentialzyme, and ICP), Inner Defense.

Lymphatic System: *See also Immune System.*

▸▸ *The lymphatic system is made up of the tissues and organs (bone marrow, thymus, spleen, lymph glands, etc.) that produce and store the cells used to fight infection and disease. The lymphatic system transports immune cells through a fluid called lymph.*

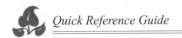

Oils—^A_FCypress, ^{TA}_Fsage, ^{TA}sandalwood (supports), ^{TA}<u>Di-Gize</u>, ^{TA}<u>JuvaFlex</u> (detoxifying), ^{TA}ledum (inflamed lymph nodes), ^{TA}tangerine.

—**BALANCE AND LONGEVITY**

   Oils—^{TA}<u>Aroma Life</u>, ^{TA}<u>Mister</u>.

   Blend #1—5 drops Roman chamomile, 5 drops lavender, and 5 drops orange in 2 Tbs. V-6 Oil. Apply a few drops of blend, and massage.

—**CLEANSING**

   Oils—^{TA}Lemon, ^{TA}lime.

—**DECONGESTANT FOR**

   Oils—^A_FCypress, ^{TA}_Fgrapefruit, ^{TA}<u>Aroma Life</u>, ^{TA}<u>Citrus Fresh</u>, ^{TA}cumin, ^{TA}helichrysum, ^{TA}lemongrass, ^{TA}myrtle, ^{TA}orange, ^{TA}rosemary, ^{TA}tangerine, ^{TA}thyme.

   Personal Care—Cel-Lite Magic.

—**DRAINAGE OF**

   Oils—^{TA}_FHelichrysum, ^{TA}_Flemongrass.

—**ELIMINATES WASTE THROUGH**

   Oils—^{TA}_FLavender.

—**INCREASE FUNCTION OF**

   Oils—^{TA}Lemon.

   Personal Care——Cel-Lite Magic (stimulates lymph), **Relaxation Massage Oil**.

   Supplements— **Master Formula, MultiGreens,** Power Meal.

T—Dilute as necessary, and apply on neck, arms, thyroid area, and Vita Flex points on the feet. Add 1–2 drops to warm bathwater, and bathe.

A—Diffuse into the air. Inhale directly or applied to the hands.

Lymphoma: *See Cancer: LYMPHOMA, HODGKIN'S DISEASE.*

Malaria:

   Recipe #1—Lemon with honey in water to prevent.

Male Specific Conditions: *See also Aftershave, Impotence, Skin, Sterility.*

   Oils—^{AT}<u>Shutran</u>, ^{AT}<u>Awaken</u>.

   Personal Care—PD 80/20, Prenolone/Prenolone+, Lavender Hand & Body Lotion (moisturizes skin leaving it soft, silky, and smooth), Sensation Hand & Body Lotion (moisturizes and protects skin with an alluring fragrance). KidScents Lotion makes a great aftershave as it soothes and rehydrates the skin.

—GENITAL AREA

–INFECTION

Oils—ᵀTea tree, ᵀoregano, ᵀeucalyptus, ᵀlavender, ᵀpatchouli.

–INFLAMMATION

Oils—ᵀLavender, ᵀRoman chamomile, ᵀhyssop.

–SWELLING

Oils—ᵀEucalyptus, ᵀlavender, ᵀrosemary, ᵀcypress, ᵀhyssop, ᵀjuniper.

—HORMONAL SYSTEM (MALE)

Oils—ᵀMister (balances), ᵀSclarEssence (increases testosterone levels).

—INFERTILITY (MALE)

Oils—ᵀBasil, ᵀclary sage, ᵀSclarEssence, ᵀcedarwood, ᵀᴵcinnamon[318], ᵀᴵgeranium[319], ᵀsage, ᵀthyme.

Supplements— Master Formula, MultiGreens.

—JOCK ITCH

Recipe #1—Put 2 drops of either cypress, lavender, tea tree, or patchouli in 1 tsp. V-6 Oil, and apply to area morning and night; or put 2 drops of any one of these oils in a small bowl of water, and wash and dry area well.

Supplements— Prostate Health, Master Formula, MultiGreens.

T—Dilute as necessary, and apply on location or on Vita Flex points on the feet. Dilute with V-6 Oil to create massage oil, and massage on location. Add 1–2 drops to warm bathwater, and bathe.

A—Diffuse into the air. Inhale directly or applied to hands, tissue, or a cotton wick.

Massage:

Personal Care—Any of the different Massage Oils; Ortho Ease and Ortho Sport are excellent.

Blend #1—5 drops Roman chamomile, 5 drops lavender, and 5 drops orange with 2 Tbs. V-6 Oil. Apply as a relaxing massage.

***Comments—A simple massage oil can be made by mixing 2–10 drops essential oil with 1 Tbs. of any carrier oil, such as V-6 Oil, jojoba, sweet almond, olive, or sesame.

L

M

Measles: *See Childhood Diseases: Measles.*

Medication:

Supplements—Super C / Super C Chewable.

Meditation:

Oils—**AT**Sacred frankincense, **AT**western red cedar, **AT**<u>Dream Catcher</u> (also for sweat lodges), **A**elemi, **AT**<u>Gratitude</u>, **AT**<u>Humility</u>, **AT**<u>Inspiration</u>, **A**myrrh, **AT**Roman chamomile, **AT**sandalwood, **AT**<u>Sacred Mountain</u>, **AT**tsuga (uplifting and grounding).

A—Diffuse into the air. Inhale directly or applied to hands, tissue, or a cotton wick.

T—Dilute with V-6 Oil to create massage oil, and massage into skin. Add 1–3 drops to 1/4 cup Epsom salts, and dissolve in warm bathwater for bathing.

Melanoma: *See Cancer: MELANOMA.*

Memory:

Oils—**TA**Rosemary[320], **TA**sage lavender[321], **TA**peppermint[322], **TA**<u>Clarity</u>, **TA**<u>Aroma Life</u>, **TA**basil (for poor memory)[323], **TA**bergamot, **TA**calamus, **TA**clove (memory deficiency)[324], **TA**<u>Dragon Time</u>, **TA**<u>En-R-Gee</u>, **TA**<u>Gentle Baby</u>, **TA**ginger, **TA**grapefruit, **TA**<u>Joy</u> (of love), **TA**lavender, **TA**lemon (improves), **TA**lemongrass, **TA**<u>Mister</u>, **TA**mountain savory (may bring back good memories), **TA**<u>M-Grain</u>, **TA**<u>Relieve It</u>, **TA**rose[325], **IA**dill[326].

Blend #1—Add a drop of lemongrass to 1–3 drops of <u>Clarity</u>. May be best to dilute with a few drops of V-6 Oil. Apply to forehead, temples, behind ears, and on back of neck. Cup hands over nose and mouth, and breathe deeply.

Blend #2—Add a drop of rosemary to 1–3 drops of <u>M-Grain</u>. Apply as described in Blend #1.

Supplements— MindWise, Omega Blue, OmegaGize³, Master Formula.

—**AMNESIA**

   » *Amnesia is a condition where a person experiences either complete or partial loss of memory. Most commonly, Amnesia is caused by a head injury. But amnesia can also be caused by traumatic experiences, strokes, brain tumors, exposure to toxic substances, seizures, etc.*

   Oils—**TA**Rosemary, **TA**basil, **TA**clove.

—**FORGETFULNESS**

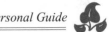
Oils—^{TA}Sage lavender, ^{TA}rosemary, ^T<u>Brain Power</u> (1 drop under tongue), ^{TA}<u>Accep-</u>
<u>tance</u> (over heart and liver), ^{TA}cedarwood, <u>Clarity</u>, ^{TA}cypress, ^{TA}<u>Dream Catcher</u>, ^{TA-}
<u>Highest Potential</u>, ^{TA}<u>Hope</u>, ^{TA}fir, ^{TA}<u>Gathering</u>, ^{TA}geranium, ^{TA}juniper, ^{TA}marjoram,
^{TA}myrrh, ^{TA}orange, ^{TA}<u>Present Time</u>, ^{TA}Roman chamomile, ^{TA}rose, ^{TA}sandalwood,
^{TA}<u>3 Wise Men</u>, ^{TA}rose, ^{TA}<u>Valor</u>, ^{TA}<u>White Angelica</u>, ^{TA}ylang ylang.

Supplements—Omega Blue, OmegaGize³, Ultra Young+, MultiGreens.

—IMPROVE

Oils—^{TA}_FClove, ^{TA}sage lavender, ^Aclary sage, ^{TA}lime.

Blend #3—5 drops basil, 2 drops peppermint, 10 drops rosemary, and 1 oz. V-6 Oil.

—RELEASES NEGATIVE

Oils—^{TA}<u>Forgiveness</u> (has high frequencies), ^Ageranium, ^{TA}palo santo, ^{TA}<u>3 Wise Men</u>.

—RETENTION

Oils—^{TA}<u>Clarity</u>.

—STIMULATE

Oils—^{TA}Calamus, ^Arosemary.

Blend #4—2 drops blue tansy, 2 drops Roman chamomile, 3 drops geranium, 4 drops
lavender, 3 drops rosemary, 3 drops rosewood, 1 drop spearmint, 2 drops tangerine,
and 1 oz. V-6 Oil. Apply a few drops of blend to back of neck, wrist, and heart.

T—Wear as a perfume or cologne. Dilute as necessary, and apply to temples.

A—Diffuse into the air. Inhale directly or applied to hands, tissue, or a cotton wick. *See*
COMMENTS under Asthma for a discussion on using **plastic nasal inhalers**. *These work well*
if used while studying material that needs to be remembered (i.e. school exams) and then used
again during testing to help recall studied material[327].

Menopause: *See Female Specific Conditions: Menopause.*

Menstruation: *See Female Specific Conditions: Menstruation.*

Mental: *See also Alertness, Energy, Memory, Brain, Stress.*

Oils—^{AT}<u>Brain Power</u> (increases capacity and clarity by dissolving petrochemicals),
^{AT}_Foregano (mental diseases), ^A<u>Common Sense</u> (clarity and focus), ^Asage (strain), ^{AT}vitex
(unrest). **M**

Supplements— MindWise, Omega Blue (a powerful blend of EPA and DHA from fish
oil, plus essential oils to preserve and support delivery to the brain; critical nutrients for
proper brain function), OmegaGize³, Master Formula.

—ACCURACY

>   Oils—^{AT}Clarity, ^{AT}peppermint. Diffuse or inhale.

—ALERTNESS

>   Oils—^{AT}Clarity, ^{AT}En-R-Gee, ^{AT}sacred frankincense, ^Ahong kuai.
>
>   ***Comments—*These oils are good for night driving.*

—FATIGUE

>   Oils—^{AT}_FBasil, ^{AT}_Frosemary, ^{AT}_Fylang ylang, ^{AT}sacred frankincense, ^{AT}Awaken, ^{AT}Aroma Life, ^{AT}cardamom, ^{AT}Clarity, ^{AT}Dragon Time, ^{AT}Gentle Baby, ^{AT}lemongrass, ^{AT}Mister, ^{AT}M-Grain, ^{AT}Relieve It, ^Asage.
>
>   Blend #1—Basil and lemongrass together are a good combination.

—IMPAIRMENT

>   Supplements—Sulfurzyme.

—RETARDATION

>   Supplements—Can be due to a mineral deficiency. **KidScents MightyVites, Mineral Essence.**

—STRESS

>   Oils—^{AT}Clary sage,^{AT}Evergreen Essence, ^Apine, ^ACommon Sense, ^{AT}Surrender, ^TTranquil (roll-on).
>
>   Supplements—ImmuPro.

A—Diffuse into the air. Inhale directly or applied to hands, tissue, or a cotton wick. *See COMMENTS under Asthma for a discussion on using* **plastic nasal inhalers**.

T—Wear as a perfume or cologne. Dilute as necessary, and apply to temples.

Metabolism:

—BALANCE

>   Oils—^AClove, ^{AT}Valor, ^{AT}EndoFlex (increases), ^{AT}spearmint, ^{AT}oregano.

—INCREASE (OVER ALL)

>   Oils—^ISpearmint (add to water, and freeze to emulsify throughout), ^{AT}eucalyptus blue, ^{AT}spikenard.

—LIPID

>   Oils—^THyssop (regulates).

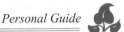

—STRENGTHEN (VITAL CENTERS)

    Oils—^{AT}Sage.

    Supplements—Thyromin (regulates metabolism), **Power Meal**.

A—Diffuse into the air. Inhale oil applied to tissue or a cotton wick.

T—Dilute as recommended, and apply 1–2 drops on neck or on bottoms of the feet.

Metals: *See Detoxification: METALS. See also Chelation.*

Mice (Repel):

Oils—^A<u>Purification</u>.

A—Diffuse into the air. Apply to cotton balls, and place in small openings where mice may enter.

Migraine Headaches: *See Headaches: MIGRAINE.*

Mildew: *See also Antifungal.*

  ›› *Mildew is a whitish fungus that forms a flat growth on plants and organic material. Mildew attacks clothing, leather, paper, ceilings, walls, floors, shower walls, windowsills, and other places with high moisture levels. Mildew can produce a strong musty odor, especially in places with poor air circulation.*

    Recipe #1—Place a few drops of <u>Purification</u> in a spray bottle, and spray into the air or directly onto a wall to neutralize mildew.

Mind: *See also Alertness, Brain, Energy, Memory, Mental.*

Oils—^{AT}Basil (absentminded), ^{AT}<u>Believe</u> (stimulates), ^{AT}<u>Surrender</u> (clearing), ^A<u>Common Sense</u> (soothes and focuses), ^{AT}western red cedar (powerful effects on subconscious and unconscious mind), ^{AT}sacred frankincense.

A—Diffuse into the air. Inhale directly or applied to hands, tissue, or a cotton wick. *See COMMENTS under Asthma for a discussion on using* **plastic nasal inhalers**.

T—Wear as a perfume or cologne. Dilute as necessary, and apply to temples.

Minerals (deficiency):

Supplements—Cleansing Trio (ComforTone, Essentialzyme, and ICP), Mineral Essence.

Miscarriage: *See Pregnancy/Motherhood.*

M

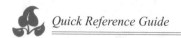

Mold: *See Antifungal: M*OLD*.*

Moles:

   Oils—ᵀFrankincense, ᵀ<u>Melrose</u>,
     ᵀgeranium,
     ᵀlavender.

   T—Dilute as necessary, and apply on
     location.

> *I used a combination of lavender and frankincense on a new mole that grew in with a very crusty surface. By the time I was able to have an appointment with my doctor, it had totally disappeared.*
>   *-Submitted by Judi Arndt*
>   *Colorado Springs, Colorado (July 2004)*

Moment:

   —B*EING* I*N*

     Oils—ᴬ<u>Present Time</u>.

     A—Inhale directly or applied to hands. Diffuse into the air.

Mono (Mononucleosis): *See also Antiviral, Chronic Fatigue, Epstein-Barr.*

>> *Mononucleosis is viral disease caused by the Epstein-Barr virus and usually spread through contact with infected saliva, tears, and mucous. Symptoms of this disease include fatigue, weakness, severe sore throat, fever, swollen lymph nodes, swollen tonsils, headache, loss of appetite, and a soft or swollen spleen. Once individuals are exposed to the Epstein-Barr virus, they carry the virus for the rest of their lives.*

   Oils—ᵀᴬ<u>ImmuPower</u>, ᵀᴬ<u>RC</u>, ᵀᴬ<u>Thieves</u>.

   Blend #1—3 drops oregano, 3 drops <u>Thieves</u>, and 3 drops thyme. Rub on feet.

   —I*NFECTIOUS*

     Oils—ᵀᴬ_F_Ravintsara.

     Supplements—Build immune system. **Inner Defense,** Cleansing Trio (ComforTone,
     Essentialzyme, and ICP), ImmuPro, Power Meal, Super C / Super C Chewable,
     Master Formula.

   T—Dilute as necessary, and apply on throat and on feet.

   A—Diffuse into the air. Inhale directly or applied to the hands.

Mood Swings: *See also Hormonal Imbalance.*

   Oils—ᴬClary sage, ᴬ<u>Peace & Calming</u>, ᴬlavender, ᴬ<u>Valor</u>, ᴬylang ylang, ᴬ<u>Acceptance</u>,
   ᴬbergamot, ᴬ<u>Dragon Time</u> or ᴬ<u>Mister</u>, ᴬfennel, ᴬ<u>Gathering</u>, ᴬgeranium, ᴬ<u>Harmony</u>,
   ᴬjasmine, ᴬ<u>Joy</u>, ᴬjuniper, ᴬlemon, ᴬpeppermint, ᴬ<u>Present Time</u>, ᴬrose, ᴬrosemary, ᴬsage,
   ᴬsage lavender, ᴬsandalwood, ᴬspruce, ᴬ<u>Trauma Life</u>, ᴬyarrow.

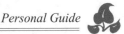

A—Diffuse into the air. Inhale directly or applied to hands, tissue, or a cotton wick.

*****Comments**—Can be due to a vitamin B deficiency.

Supplements—AlkaLime (if due to over-acidification), Super B.

Morning Sickness: *See Pregnancy/Motherhood.*

Mosquitoes: *See also Insect.*

   *****Comments**—Frequent mosquito bites could be due to a vitamin B deficiency.

   Supplements—Super B.

Mother (Problems with):

Oils—^{TA}Acceptance, ^{TA}geranium, ^{TA}Valor.

T—Apply to mother auricular emotion point. Dilute with V-6 Oil to create massage oil, and massage into skin. Add 1–3 drops to 1/4 cup Epsom salts, and dissolve in warm bathwater for bathing.

A—Diffuse into the air. Inhale directly or applied to hands, tissue, or a cotton wick.

Motion Sickness: *See also Nausea.*

▸▸ *Motion sickness is a feeling of illness that occurs as a result of repeated movement, such as that experienced in a car, on a boat, or on a plane. These motions interfere with the body's sense of balance and equilibrium. The most common symptoms of motion sickness include dizziness, fatigue, and nausea.*

Oils—^{TA}_FPeppermint, ^{TA}ginger, ^{TA}Di-Gize, ^{AT}AromaEase, ^{TA}M-Grain, ^{TA}nutmeg, ^{TA}spearmint.

T—Apply to feet, temples, and wrists.

A—Inhale directly or applied to hands, tissue, or a cotton wick. Diffuse into the air. *See COMMENTS under Asthma for a discussion on using plastic nasal inhalers.*

Recipe #1—Apply a drop or two of Di-Gize to the hands; stir in a clockwise motion, apply behind both ears, rub hands together, cup over nose and mouth, and breathe deeply.

*****Comments**—According to the Essential Oils Desk Reference, "Mix 4 drops peppermint and 4 drops ginger in 1 ounce V-6 Oil. Rub on chest and stomach before traveling." (EDR–June 2002; Ch. 28; Digestion Problems; Travel Sickness)

M

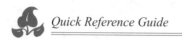

Motivation:

—To Move Forward

Oils—**AT**<u>Envision</u> (emotional support), **AT**<u>Magnify Your Purpose</u> (empowering and uplifting), **AT**<u>Motivation</u>, **AT**myrrh, **AT**<u>Live with Passion</u>.

A—Diffuse into the air. Inhale directly or applied to hands, tissue, or a cotton wick.

T—Dilute with V-6 Oil to create massage oil, and massage into skin.

Supplements—Sulfurzyme.

MRSA (Methicillin Resistant Staphylococcus Aureus): *See Antibacterial: MRSA.*

Mucus: *See Congestion: Mucus. See also Anticatarrhal.*

Multiple Sclerosis (M.S.): *See also Myelin Sheath.*

>> *Multiple sclerosis (MS) is an autoimmune disease in which the immune system attacks and gradually destroys the myelin sheath (which covers and insulates the*

> *According to D. Gary Young, progesterone is absolutely necessary in manufacturing, building, repairing, and rejuvenating the myelin sheath. Progesterone is naturally produced from pregnenolone.*

nerves) and the underlying nerve fibers of the central nervous system. This destruction of the myelin sheath interferes with communication between the brain and the rest of the body. Symptoms of MS include partial or complete loss of vision, tingling, burning, pain in parts of the body, tremors, loss of coordination, unsteady gait, dizziness, and memory problems.

Oils—**TA**Frankincense, **TA**sandalwood, **TA**peppermint, **TA**<u>Aroma Siez</u>, **TA**<u>Clarity</u>, **TA**copaiba[328], **TA**cypress, **TA**elemi, **TA**geranium, **TA**helichrysum, **TA**Idaho tansy, **TA**juniper, **TA**oregano, **TA**<u>Peace & Calming</u>, **TA**rosemary, **TA**sage, **TA**thyme, **TA**wintergreen.

T—Dilute as necessary, and apply on spine, back of neck, and feet. Dilute with V-6 Oil to create a massage oil, and massage on back and neck.

A—Diffuse into the air. Inhale directly or applied to hands.

***Comments**—Do the Raindrop Technique.

Personal Care—PD 80/20, Prenolone/Prenolone+, Progessence/Progessence Plus.

Supplements—Cleansing Trio (ComforTone, Essentialzyme, and ICP), ImmuPro, Inner Defense, JuvaPower/JuvaSpice, JuvaTone, Mineral Essence, MultiGreens, Omega Blue/OmegaGize[3] (a powerful blend of EPA and DHA from fish oil plus essential oils to preserve and support delivery to the brain; critical nutrients for proper brain function), Power Meal, Sulfurzyme, Super B, Super C / Super C Chewable, Master Formula.

The following are recipes that have been used successfully:

Recipe #1—Supplement with MultiGreens, Cleansing Trio (ComforTone, Essentialzyme, and ICP), and Super C / Super C Chewable. Blend 10 drops cardamom, 10 drops peppermint, and 10 drops rosemary with 1 oz. V-6 Oil for a full body massage. Finally, diffuse <u>Acceptance</u> and <u>Awaken</u>.

Recipe #2—Supplement with 8 Super Cal, 2 Super B (after breakfast), 6 Super C / Super C Chewable, 6 MultiGreens four times a day, and Master Formula. Apply juniper and peppermint, one at a time, on the spine. If the M.S. is in the neck, work up the spine. If it is in the legs, work down the spine. Do a cold compress, and wait for 30 minutes. Remove the compress and repeat again.

Recipe #3—Take 2 droppers full of Mineral Essence morning and evening to conduct the current to reconnect the nerve tissues. Take ½ Super B in the morning and evening with meals for the first week. Then increase the dosage. Use juniper, geranium, and peppermint on the bottoms of the feet and up the legs and spine. Apply juniper and cypress on the base of the neck; then add <u>Aroma Siez</u>. Next do the Raindrop Technique on the spine using oregano and thyme. Use <u>Peace & Calming</u> and <u>Clarity</u> for brain function and cypress for circulation. Use the Cleansing Trio (ComforTone, Essentialzyme, and ICP) and JuvaTone. Also use Super C / Super C Chewable for six days. Then start on Super B morning and evening with a meal, 6 MultiGreens four times a day.

Blend #1—6 drops juniper, 4 drops sandalwood, 2 drops peppermint, and 12 drops geranium. Mix, and massage into neck, spine, and bottoms of feet.

***Comments—Avoid hot baths, etc. Heat is the worst thing you can do. If anything, insulate the body with ice packs. Lowering the body temperature with cold packs helps to regenerate the myelin sheath. The person can be kept in the cold packs either for as long as they can stand it or until their body temperature drops 3 degrees. The body temperature must be monitored closely to avoid lowering it too far. This process can be repeated until the person can only stand being in the cold packs for 20 minutes. It is also best to avoid diet foods, especially those that contain aspartame, as it is known to cause MS, brain damage, and other problems.

Mumps: *See Childhood Diseases: Mumps.*

Muscles:

Oils—ᵀMarjoram, ᵀ<u>Aroma Siez</u>, ᵀpeppermint[329], ᵀ<u>Cool Azul</u>, ᵀwintergreen, ᵀ<u>Deep Relief</u> (roll-on), ᵀbasil, ᵀcypress, ᵀbalsam fir, ᵀlavender, ᵀlemongrass, ᵀpalo santo, ᵀ<u>Valor</u>, ᵀwhite fir.

Personal Care—Ortho Ease Massage Oil, Ortho Sport Massage Oil, Relaxation Massage Oil (these oils are great for all problems associated with muscles). ᵀ<u>Cool Azul Sports Gel.</u>

M

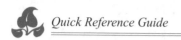

Supplements—**BLM,** Mineral Essence, NingXia Red, Power Meal, Pure Protein Complete (the ideal blend of 5 ultraclean, ultrabioactive whey proteins; provides prolonged assimilation for better protein synthesis), Sulfurzyme, Super Cal, Super C Chewable, Wolfberry Crisp Bars (*Refer to the Wolfberry Crisp Bar in the Supplements section of the <u>Reference Guide for Essential Oils</u> for more information on the benefits of the Ningxia Wolfberry*).

*****Comments**—*One professional trainer for body builders used Be-Fit, Power Meal, and Wolfberry Bars to increase muscle mass and strength beyond anything he had previously achieved!*

—ACHES AND PAINS

Oils—ᵀ<u>PanAway</u>, ᵀ<u>Deep Relief</u> (roll-on), ᵀ<u>Cool Azul</u>, ᵀwintergreen, ᵀ_Fclove, ᵀ<u>Aroma Siez</u>, ᵀwhite fir (with inflammation), ᵀcopaiba, ᵀblue cypress, ᵀbalsam fir, ᵀDouglas fir, ᵀginger, ᵀhelichrysum, ᵀlavender, ᵀlemongrass (especially good for ligaments), ᵀmarjoram, ᵀnutmeg, ᵀoregano, ᵀpalo santo, ᵀpeppermint, ᵀ<u>Relieve It</u>, ᵀRoman chamomile, ᵀrosemary, ᵀspearmint, ᵀthyme, ᵀvetiver.

Supplements—ᵀSulfurzyme.

Personal Care—ᵀ<u>Cool Azul Sports Gel</u>.

*****Comments**—*Refer to the chapter entitled "How to Use—The Personal Usage Reference" in the <u>Essential Oils Desk Reference</u> under "Muscles" for some excellent blends to help sore and tight muscles.*

—ANTI-INFLAMMATORY *See also Anti-inflammatory*

Oils—ᵀFrankincense, ᵀpeppermint, ᵀ<u>Deep Relief</u> (roll-on), ᵀ<u>Cool Azul</u>, ᵀbasil, ᵀbalsam fir, ᵀwhite fir.

*****Comments**—*Refer to the chapter entitled "How to Use—The Personal Usage Reference" in the <u>Essential Oils Desk Reference</u> under "Muscles" for an excellent blend to help reduce inflammation.*

—CARDIAC MUSCLE *See also Cardiovascular System: HEART*

Oils—ᵀᴬMarjoram, ᵀᴬlavender, ᵀᴬrosemary verbenon (helps regulate), ᵀᴬgoldenrod, ᵀᴬneroli, ᵀᴬpeppermint, ᵀᴬrose.

—CRAMPS/CHARLEY HORSES

>> *A muscle cramp or charley horse is the sudden, involuntary contraction of a muscle. Muscle cramps can occur in any muscle in the body, but they usually occur in the thigh, calf, or arch of the foot. Cramps can be caused by excessive strain to the muscle, injury, overuse, dehydration, a lack of neces-*

Every fall when the weather is hot, then cold here in Florida, I get chest pains that my doctor has characterized as charley horses in the deep muscles of my chest. Unlike a leg or foot muscle, you can't massage these or walk to stretch them, so there was nothing to do but "endure" these annoying episodes, which sometimes lasted for two hours. One night I woke up with this chest pain, and as I lay there thinking about what I could do for it, I remembered the instant results I had had with Aroma Siez on other people's leg cramps. So I got up and rubbed a few drops of Aroma Siez on my chest, and the pain went away in about 10 minutes!
—Submitted by Jan Early
Tallahassee, Florida (July 2004)

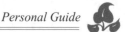

sary salts or minerals, or a lack of blood flow to the muscle. Muscle cramps can happen during or after a physical activity and while lying in bed.

Oils—[T]Aroma Siez, [T]marjoram, [T]Cool Azul, [T]Deep Relief (roll-on), [T]rosemary, [T]basil, [T]clary sage, [T]coriander, [T]cypress, [T]grapefruit, [T]jasmine, [A]lavender, [T]pine, [T]Roman chamomile, [T]thyme, [T]vetiver.

Personal Care—[T]Cool Azul Sports Gel.

Supplements—BLM, Mineral Essence, Sulfurzyme, Super Cal.

Blend #1—Equal parts rosemary and Aroma Siez. Apply neat; or mix with V-6 Oil, and massage.

—DEVELOPMENT

▸▸ *When muscles are stretched or used during exercise, they produce a substance that activates stem cells already present in the tissue. Once these cells are activated, they begin to divide—creating new muscle fiber, and thereby increasing the size and strength of the muscles.*

Oils—[T]Wintergreen (with spruce), [T]PanAway.

Supplements— MultiGreens (stimulates and strengthens), Power Meal, Pure Protein Complete, Super Cal.

—FATIGUE

Oils—[T]Marjoram, [T]balsam fir, [T]cypress, [T]Douglas fir, [T]peppermint, [T]Aroma Siez, [T]eucalyptus, [T]grapefruit, [T]ravintsara, [T]rosemary, [T]thyme.

Supplements—Mineral Essence, Super Cal.

—INFLAMMATION: *SEE ANTI-INFLAMMATORY*

—OVER-EXERCISED

Oils—[T]Balsam fir, [T]white fir (with inflammation), [T]eucalyptus, [T]Deep Relief (roll-on), [T]mastrante, [T]Douglas fir, [T]ginger, [T]lavender, [T]thyme.

Personal Care—[T]Cool Azul Sports Gel.

Bath—3 drops marjoram and 2 drops lemon in a tub of water. Soak.

Blend #1—Equal parts of eucalyptus, peppermint, and ginger. Mix with V-6 Oil, and massage.

—RHEUMATISM (MUSCULAR) *SEE ALSO FIBROMYALGIA*

Oils—[T]Palo santo, [T]rosemary, [T]thyme.

—SMOOTH MUSCLE

Oils—[T]Marjoram, [T]rosemary[330], [T]peppermint, [T]bergamot, [T]black pepper, [T]clary sage, [T]cypress, [T]fennel, [T]juniper, [T]lavender, [T]melissa, [T]neroli, [T]Roman chamomile, [T]sandalwood.

***Comments—*Essential oils with high proportions of ester compounds are especially effective.*

M

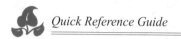

—SPASMS

    Oils—ᵀBasil, ᵀ<u>Cool Azul</u>, ᵀmarjoram, ᵀ<u>PanAway</u>, ᵀRoman chamomile, ᵀmastrante, ᵀ<u>Aroma Siez</u>, ᵀclary sage, ᵀcypress, ᵀlavender, ᵀjasmine, ᵀpeppermint.

    Personal Care—Cel-Lite Magic, Ortho Ease Massage Oil ᵀ<u>Cool Azul Sports Gel</u>.

    Supplements—Super Cal.

—SPRAINS

    >> *A sprain is an injury to a ligament caused by excessive stretching. The ligament can have little tears in it, or it can be completely torn apart and still be considered a sprain. The most common areas to receive a sprain are the ankle, knee, and wrist. After a person receives a sprain, the area will swell rapidly and be quite painful.*

    Oils—ᵀ_FMarjoram, ᵀlemongrass, ᵀ<u>PanAway</u>, ᵀwhite fir, ᵀ<u>Aroma Siez</u>, ᵀ<u>Cool Azul</u>, ᵀmastrante, ᵀblack pepper, ᵀclove, ᵀeucalyptus, ᵀginger, ᵀhelichrysum, ᵀIdaho tansy, ᵀjasmine, ᵀlavender, ᵀ<u>Peace & Calming</u>, ᵀnutmeg, ᵀpine, ᵀRoman chamomile, ᵀrose, ᵀrosemary, ᵀthyme, ᵀvetiver.

—STIFFNESS

    Oils—ᵀ<u>Aroma Siez</u>, ᵀ<u>PanAway</u>, ᵀ<u>Deep Relief</u> (roll-on).

—TENSION (ESPECIALLY IN SHOULDERS AND NECK)

    Oils—ᵀ<u>Cool Azul</u>, ᵀMarjoram, ᵀ<u>Aroma Siez</u>, ᵀ<u>Relieve It</u>, ᵀpeppermint[329], ᵀ<u>Deep Relief</u> (roll-on), ᵀmastrante, ᵀDouglas fir, ᵀhelichrysum, ᵀjuniper, ᵀlavender, ᵀRoman chamomile, ᵀspruce.

    Personal Care—Ortho Ease and Ortho Sport Massage Oils, Evening Peace Bath & Shower Gel (relaxes tired, fatigued muscles and helps alleviate tension). ᵀ<u>Cool Azul Sports Gel.</u>

—TISSUE

    Supplements—Pure Protein Complete and Power Meal (contain a complete amino acid and vitamin profile and have a high level of predigested protein to maintain a good food supply for muscle tissue), BLM, Ultra Young+ (increase production of growth hormone, which increases formation of lean muscle tissue).

    *****Comments**—*Refer to the chapter entitled "How to Use—The Personal Usage Reference" in the <u>Essential Oils Desk Reference</u> under "Muscles" for some excellent blends to help improve circulation in the muscles and to aid in the regeneration of muscle tissue.*

—TONE

    Oils—Apply these oils before exercise. ᵀCypress, ᵀwintergreen, ᵀmarjoram, ᵀbasil, ᵀblack pepper, ᵀginger, ᵀgrapefruit, ᵀjuniper, ᵀlavender, ᵀlime, ᵀorange, ᵀpeppermint, ᵀpetitgrain, ᵀpine, ᵀrosemary, ᵀthyme.

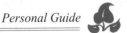
Supplements— Pure Protein Complete, Sulfurzyme.

***Comments—*Poor muscle tone may indicate a sulfur deficiency.*

—Torn Muscles

Oils—^THelichrysum and ^Tspruce (take pain away—use hot packs), ^T<u>Cool Azul</u>, ^Tlemongrass, ^Tginger (circulation), ^Tlemon myrtle.

Personal Care—Ortho Sport Massage Oil.

T—Dilute as necessary, and apply on location. Dilute with V-6 Oil to create a massage oil, and massage into desired muscles. Add 1–2 drops to warm bathwater, and bathe. Apply as hot (or cold for strains or sprains) compress.

A—Diffuse into the air.

Muscular Dystrophy:

≫ *Muscular dystrophy is any of several genetic diseases that cause gradual weakening of the skeletal muscles. The most common forms, Duchenne and Becker muscular dystrophies, are caused by a gene defect that inhibits or alters the production of dystrophin, a protein necessary for proper muscle cell structure.*

Oils—^TLemongrass, ^Tmarjoram (combine with equal parts lemongrass), ^Tbasil, ^Trosemary, ^T<u>Aroma Siez</u>, ^Teucalyptus, ^Tgeranium, ^Tginger, ^Tlavender, ^Tlemon, ^Torange, ^Tpine, ^T<u>Relieve It</u>.

Personal Care—Ortho Ease Massage Oil, Ortho Sport Massage Oil.

Supplements—Essentialzyme, Essentialzymes-4, Mineral Essence, MultiGreens, Power Meal, Sulfurzyme, Thyromin, Ultra Young+.

T—Dilute as necessary, and apply on location. Dilute with V-6 Oil to create a massage oil, and massage on location. Add 1–2 drops to warm bathwater, and bathe. Apply as cold compress.

Myelin Sheath:

≫ *The myelin sheath is an insulating layer of protein and fatty substances that forms around nerves (including those in the brain), increasing the speed of nerve impulses. Damage to the myelin sheath interrupts these nerve impulses and can cause diseases such as multiple sclerosis, peripheral neuropathy, central pontine myelinolysis, and other neurological diseases.*

Oils—^T<u>ImmuPower</u>, ^Tpeppermint, ^Tjuniper, ^Tgeranium

T—Apply with **cold** compress *(remember, **no heat!**)*.

Supplements—Omega Blue/OmegaGize³ (contains DHA, which helps support the myelin sheath), ImmuPro.

M

A=Aromatic **T**=Topical **I**=Internal

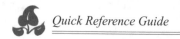

Nails:

Oils—ᵀ<u>Citrus Fresh</u>, ᵀlemon (repeated use may help harden), ᵀtea tree³³¹ (infection), ᵀfrankincense, ᵀmyrrh, ᵀeucalyptus, ᵀgrapefruit, ᵀlavender, ᵀlime, ᵀtea tree, ᵀoregano, ᵀpatchouli, ᵀpeppermint, ᵀravintsara, ᵀrosemary, ᵀthyme.

T—Dilute as necessary, and apply on nails.

Blend #1—Equal parts frankincense, lemon, and myrrh. Mix with a couple drops of wheat germ oil, and apply 2–3 times per week.

Supplements—**Sulfurzyme** (helps with growth and removal of ridges and cracks), **Mineral Essence, Super Cal**.

***Comments**—*A deficiency in sulfur can cause poor nail growth.*

Narcolepsy:

⯈ *Narcolepsy is a disorder that is characterized by sudden and uncontrollable drowsiness and attacks of sleep at unexpected and irregular intervals. It is frequently misdiagnosed as hypothyroidism (insufficient thyroid hormone), hypoglycemia (insufficient blood sugar), epilepsy, or multiple sclerosis. Proper diagnosis requires overnight monitoring with a device used to detect brain waves called an electroencephalograph.*

Oils—ᴬᵀ<u>Brain Power</u>

A—Diffuse into the air. Inhale directly or applied to hands.

T—Apply to the brain stem, neck, and Vita Flex points on the feet.

Supplements—Mineral Essence, MultiGreens, Thyromin, Ultra Young+.

***Comments**—*Establishing a routine of strict bedtimes and daytime naps may also help reduce the number of unexpected sleep attacks.*

Nasal: *See Nose.*

Nausea: *See also Motion Sickness, Pregnancy/Motherhood:* MORNING SICKNESS, *Vomiting.*

Oils—ᴵᴬᵀGinger³³², ᴬ_Fpeppermint³³³, ᴬᵀAromaEase, ᴬᵀ_Flavender, ᴬᵀcalamus, ᴬᵀcardamom, ᴬᵀclove, ᵀ<u>Di-Gize</u> (over stomach and colon), ᴬᵀjuniper, ᴬᵀ<u>M-Grain</u>, ᴬᵀnutmeg, ᴬᵀrosewood, ᴬᵀspearmint, ᴬᵀtarragon.

A—Diffuse. Inhale directly. *See COMMENTS under Asthma for a discussion on using plastic nasal inhalers.*

I—Place 2–5 drops in an empty capsule, and swallow.

T—Apply behind ears and on Vita Flex points.

> Blend #1—2 drops lavender, 2 drops spearmint, and 2 drops of another oil for your type of nausea. Mix together, and put a little on a cotton ball; inhale three times a day, or diffuse.

Neck:

Oils—ᵀGeranium, ᵀclary sage, ᵀlemongrass, ᵀbasil, ᵀlemon, ᵀorange, ᵀhelichrysum.

T—Dilute with V-6 Oil to create a massage oil, and massage on neck.

Supplements—BLM.

—CHRONIC PAIN

Oils—ᵀ<u>PanAway</u>.

T—Apply to base of big toe.

Negative Ions: *See Ions: Negative.*

Negativity:

Oils—ᴬᵀSandalwood (removes negative programming from the cells), ᴬᵀ<u>Transformation</u>.

—BREAKS UP

Oils—ᴬᵀ<u>Dream Catcher</u>, ᴬᵀ<u>Forgiveness</u>, ᴬᵀpalo santo.

—DROWNING IN OWN

Oils—ᴬGrapefruit.

A—Diffuse into the air. Inhale directly or applied to tissue or a cotton wick.

T—Apply to auricular emotion points. Dilute with V-6 Oil to create a massage oil, and massage onto the skin.

Nervous System: *See also Lou Gehrig's Disease, Carpal Tunnel Syndrome, Multiple Sclerosis, Paralysis, Parkinson's Disease*

>> *The nervous system is a network of nerve cells that regulates the body's reaction to external and internal stimuli. The nervous system sends and receives nerve impulses to and from organs and muscles throughout the body. The body relies on these impulses to function. The nervous system is comprised of the **central nervous system** (the brain and spinal cord) and the **peripheral nervous system** (all other nerves). The peripheral nervous system is comprised of the **somatic nervous system** (nerves that connect to the skeletal muscles and sensory nerve receptors in the skin) and the **autonomic nervous system** (nerves that connect to the cardiac and smooth muscles and other organs, tissues, and systems that don't require conscious effort to control). The autonomic system is divided further into two main parts as well: the sympathetic and parasympathetic nervous systems. The **sympathetic nervous system** functions to accelerate heart rate, increase blood pressure,*

A=Aromatic **T**=Topical **I**=Internal 255

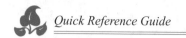
*slow digestion, and constrict blood vessels. It activates the "fight or flight" response in order to deal with threatening or stressful situations. The **parasympathetic nervous system** functions to slow heart rate, store energy, stimulate digestive activity, and relax specific muscles. It allows the body to return to a normal and calm state after experiencing pain or stress.*

Oils—[TA]Peppermint[334] (soothes and strengthens; place on wrists or location of nerve damage),
[TA]Fbasil (stimulant and for nervous breakdown), [TA]lavender[335], [AT]lemon[336], [AT]grapefruit[337], [AT]pepper[337] (stimulant), [TA]frankincense[338], [TA]Fsage, [TA]copaiba[339], [TA]lemongrass (for nerve damage; activates), [AT]<u>RutaVaLa</u>, [TA]juniper[340] (better nerve function), [TA]rosemary[341], [TA]balsam fir, [AT]bergamot, [AT]<u>Brain Power</u>, [TA]calamus, [TA]cedarwood (nervous tension), [TA]cinnamon bark, [TA]cumin (stimulant), [TA]<u>Di-Gize</u>, [TA]geranium (regenerates nerves), [TA]ginger, [A]jasmine (nervous exhaustion), [TA]marjoram (soothing), [TA]Tea tree ericifolia (nervous tension), [TA]nutmeg (supports), [TA]orange, [TA]palmarosa (supports), [AT]<u>Peace & Calming</u>, [TA]petitgrain (reestablishes nerve equilibrium), [TA]pine (stimulant), [TA]ravintsara, [TA]Roman chamomile, [TA]sage lavender, [TA]sandalwood, [TA]spearmint, [TA]spruce (fatigue), [TA]valerian (central nervous system depressant), [TA]vetiver.

Personal Care—Regenolone (helps nerve regeneration).

Supplements—Mineral Essence, Omega Blue, OmegaGize³, Sulfurzyme, Super B.

—NERVOUSNESS *See also Calming*

    Oils—[AT]Orange[342], [AT]cypress, [AT]goldenrod, [AT]<u>Surrender</u>, [AT]tangerine.

—NEURALGIA

    » *Neuralgia is intense pain felt along the path of a nerve. Neuralgia results from damage or irritation to a nerve. Causes can include certain drugs, diabetes, infections, inflammation, trauma, and chemical irritation.*

    Oils—[TA]FMarjoram, [TA]eucalyptus[341], [TA]FRoman chamomile, [TA]cajeput, [TA]cedarwood, [TA]helichrysum, [TA]juniper, [TA]lavender, [TA]nutmeg, [TA]pine, [TA]sage lavender.

—NEURITIS

    » *Neuritis is the inflammation of a nerve or of a group of nerves. Neuritis causes pain, poor reflexes, and muscle atrophy.*

    Oils—[TA]FRoman chamomile, [TA]eucalyptus[341], [TA]lavender, [TA]cedarwood, [TA]clove, [TA]juniper, [TA]yarrow.

—NEUROLOGICAL PROBLEMS

    Oils—Limit the use of oils with high *ketone* content.

    ***Comments**—A 4 year old child was in a car accident where she suffered severe brain damage. The surgeon removed part of her brain, which sent her into a coma.

After being in a coma for two months, Dr. Friedmann was asked to help her. He used oils that are commonly used for neurological problems. He put <u>Valor</u> on the back of her neck, skull, and feet. He also used <u>Present Time</u> and <u>Awaken</u>. She came out of the coma and started doing physical therapy.

—Neuropathy

>> *Neuropathy is the broad term for any of a series of diseases that adversely affect the nerves or nerve cells. Some forms of neuropathy include peripheral neuropathy (the most common), cranial neuropathy, auditory neuropathy, and optic neuropathy.*

Oils—^{TA}Lemongrass, ^{TA}peppermint, ^{TA}eucalyptus, ^{TA}lavender, ^{TA}Roman chamomile, ^{TA}<u>Brain Power</u>, ^{TA}cedarwood, ^{TA}cypress, ^{TA}geranium, ^{TA}helichrysum, ^{TA}juniper, ^{TA}<u>JuvaFlex</u>, ^{TA}<u>Valor</u>.

Personal Care—PD 80/20, Prenolone/Prenolone+, Progessence/Progessence Plus, Regenolone.

Supplements—Mineral Essence, Sulfurzyme, Super B.

*****Comments**—Refer to the chapter entitled "How to Use—The Personal Usage Reference" in the <u>Essential Oils Desk Reference</u> under "Nerve Disorders," subcategory "Neuropathy," for some excellent blends.

–Pain

Recipe #1—Apply <u>Relieve It</u>, helichrysum, and/or <u>PanAway</u> with a cold compress. Massage with peppermint, juniper, and geranium, and reapply cold compresses.

—Neurotonic

Oils—^{AT}Tea tree, ^{AT}_Fravintsara, ^{AT}thyme.

—Parasympathetic Nervous System

Oils—^{AT}Lavender[335], ^{AT}_Flemongrass (regulates), ^{AT}_Fmarjoram (increases tone of), ^{AT}<u>Peace & Calming</u>, ^T<u>Tranquil</u> (roll-on), ^{AT}<u>Valor</u>.

Diffusion—*See Ions: Negative for a list of oils that ionize negatively when diffused to help stimulate the parasympathetic nervous system.*

*****Comments**—See the Autonomic Nervous System chart in the Science and Application section of the <u>Reference Guide for Essential Oils</u>.

—Sympathetic Nervous System

Oils—^{AT}Grapefruit[337], ^{AT}black pepper[337], ^{AT}fennel[337], ^{AT}<u>Brain Power</u>, ^{AT}<u>Clarity</u>, ^{AT}Eucalyptus radiata, ^{AT}ginger, ^{AT}peppermint.

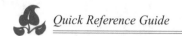

***Comments**—Stimulation of certain areas of the Sympathetic Nervous System can be achieved by application of any of the above oils at the appropriate places along the spinal column (*refer to the Autonomic Nervous System chart in the Science and Application section of the* <u>*Reference Guide for Essential Oils*</u>).

Supplements—Mineral Essence, Power Meal, Sulfurzyme, Super Cal, Ultra Young+.

***Comments**—*Stress can create a condition that has been termed as "Sympathetic System Override," where the production of cortisol, adrenalin, and 5HT (serotonin) skyrockets and heavily overloads the lymphatic and cardiovascular systems. Essential oils can help suppress "Sympathetic System Override"; and the following recipe has been used to do just that— and to bring the body back into a parasympathetic state.*

Recipe #2—Apply frankincense to the top of the spine (at the base of the skull), and work it in. This is the "gatekeeper," and it helps prepare the body to more effectively transmit and utilize the oils that follow. Then apply 3–5 drops of each of the following oils, one at a time, up the back of the neck, and work each one in individually: valerian, vetiver, and balsam fir. Other oils can be added, such as Roman chamomile, helichrysum, clove, and peppermint.

—**Virus of Nerves**

Blend #1—Clove and frankincense.

T—Dilute as necessary, and apply on location, spine, back of neck, or Vita Flex points on the feet. Dilute with V-6 Oil to create a massage oil, and massage on location. Add 1–2 drops to warm bathwater, and bathe.

A—Diffuse into the air. Inhale directly or applied to the hands.

Neuralgia: *See Nervous System:* Neuralgia.

Neuritis: *See Nervous System:* Neuritis.

Neurological Problems: *See Nervous System:* Neurological Problems.

Neuromuscular:

Oils—^TRoman chamomile, ^Ttarragon.

T—Dilute as necessary, and apply on location, spine, back of neck, or Vita Flex points on the feet. Dilute with V-6 Oil to create a massage oil, and massage on location. Add 1–2 drops to warm bathwater, and bathe.

Neuropathy: *See Nervous System:* Neuropathy.

Neurotonic: *See Nervous System: NEUROTONIC.*

Night Sweats: *See also Hot Flashes and Hormonal Imbalance.*

Oils—^{TA}ᴴSage, ^{TA}EndoFlex.

T—Dilute as necessary, and apply on temples, forehead, or bottoms of feet. Dilute with V-6 Oil to create a massage oil, and massage on back of neck or spine. Add 1–2 drops to warm bathwater, and bathe.

A—Diffuse into the air. Inhale directly or applied to the hands.

Nose:

Oils—^{TA}Tea tree, ^{TA}rosemary.

—BLEEDING

Oils—^THelichrysum, ^Tcypress, ^Tfrankincense, ^Tlavender, ^Tlemon.

Blend #1—2 drops cypress, 1 drop helichrysum, and 2 drops lemon in 8 oz. ice water. Soak cloth, and apply to nose and to back of neck.

—NASAL MUCUS MEMBRANE

Oils—Both ^{AT}eucalyptus and ^{AT}peppermint may help reduce inflammation. ^{AT}Lemon[343].

—NASAL NASOPHARYNX

Oils—^{AT}Eucalyptus.

—POLYPS *See also Polyps.*

  ⯈⯈ *A nasal polyp is an abnormal tissue growth inside the nose. Since nasal polyps are not cancerous, very small polyps generally do not cause any problems. But larger polyps can obstruct the nasal passage and make it difficult to breath or smell and can cause frequent sinus infections. Possible symptoms of polyps include runny nose, decreased sense of smell, decreased sense of taste, snoring, facial pain or headache, itching around the eyes, and persistent congestion.*

Oils—^{TA}Frankincense, ^{TA}RC (can be applied to inside of nose with cotton swab), ^{TA}oregano, ^{TA}basil, ^Tcitronella, ^{TA}peppermint, ^{TA}Purification.

***Comments**—A colon and liver cleanse may be helpful. Wintergreen or Valor may also be applied to bridge of nose for possible structural realignment.

***Comments**—Nasal polyps are caused by an overproduction of fluid in the mucous membranes. They are seen with asthma, hay fever, chronic sinus infections, and cystic fibrosis. In fact, one source stated that one out of four people with cystic

---

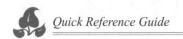

fibrosis have nasal polyps. They may also be a result of blockages in the brain or of some trauma to the nose in which structural integrity has been compromised. Diet may also be a factor.

T—Dilute as necessary, and apply to exterior of nose (use caution because of close proximity to eyes)

A—Diffuse into the air, and breathe in diffused mist.

Nursing: *See Pregnancy/Motherhood:* Nursing.

Obesity: *See also Diet, Weight.*

Oils—[AI]Grapefruit[344], [A]fennel[337], [AI]orange, [AI]oregano[345], [IA]<u>Slique Essence</u>, [AI]thyme[345], [A]rosemary, [A]<u>GLF</u>, [A]juniper, [A]<u>Juva Cleanse</u>, [AI]tangerine.

Supplements—Balance Complete, Digest + Cleanse, JuvaPower/JuvaSpice, NingXia Red, Power Meal (eat for breakfast as a meal replacement), Slique Tea, Slique Bar, Slique Gum, Slique Slim Caps, Wolfberry Crisp Bars.

—Reduce

Oils—[A]<u>Juva Cleanse</u>, [AI]orange, [AI]tangerine.

A—Diffuse into the air. Inhale directly or applied to hands, tissue, or a cotton wick.

I—Add 1 drop to 8–12 oz. of water, and drink.

Obsessiveness:

Oils—[AT]<u>Acceptance</u>, [AT]<u>Awaken</u>, [AT]clary sage, [AT]cypress, [AT]<u>Forgiveness</u>, [AT]geranium, [AT]helichrysum, [AT]<u>Humility</u>, [AT]<u>Inner Child</u>, [AT]<u>Joy</u>, [AT]lavender, [AT]marjoram, [AT]<u>Motivation</u>, [AT]<u>Present Time</u>, [AT]rose, [AT]<u>Sacred Mountain</u>, [AT]sandalwood, [AT]<u>Valor</u>, [AT]ylang ylang.

A—Diffuse into the air. Inhale directly or applied to tissue or a cotton wick.

T—Apply to auricular emotion points. Dilute with V-6 Oil to create a massage oil, and massage onto the skin.

Odors: *See also Deodorant.*

Oils—[AT]<u>Purification</u> (neutralizes and eliminates), [AT]bergamot, [AT]lavender.

Personal Care—AromaGuard Deodorants.

—Body

Oils—[T]<u>Purification</u> (obnoxious odors).

—Controlling

Oils—**AT**Cedarwood.

A—Diffuse into the air. Dissolve 8–10 drops in 1 tsp. perfumers or pure grain alcohol, and combine with distilled water in a 1 oz. spray bottle. Spray into the air or on affected surface.

T—Dilute as necessary, and apply on skin or under arms. Add 2–3 drops to 1 Tbs. baking soda, and apply under the arms, on the feet, or on other areas of the body.

Opening (to receive):

Oils—**A**Fir, **AT**<u>Transformation</u>.

A—Diffuse into the air. Inhale directly or applied to tissue or a cotton wick.

T—Apply to chakras. Dilute with V-6 Oil to create a massage oil, and massage onto the skin.

Opposition:

Oils—**AT**<u>Valor</u>.

A—Diffuse into the air. Inhale directly or applied to tissue or a cotton wick.

T—Apply to auricular emotion points. Dilute with V-6 Oil to create a massage oil, and massage onto the skin.

Oral Conditions: *See also Gums, Teeth.*

Oils—**T**$_F$Rosewood.

T—Dilute as necessary, and swab on location in mouth. Mix 1–2 drops with 4 oz. of water, and use as mouth-rinse. Place 5–6 drops with 1 oz. distilled water in a small spray bottle, and mist into the mouth.

—Abscess

Recipe #1—Apply helichrysum, <u>Purification</u>, or Roman chamomile using a hot compress on face. It may also help to apply one drop of oil to a cotton ball and apply it directly to the abscess. Put <u>Thieves</u> on a rolled-up gauze, and place over abscess to pull out the infection.

Blend #1—Use clove, wintergreen, myrrh, and helichrysum to help with infection.

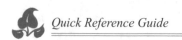

—**GINGIVITIS**

>> *Gingivitis is an inflammation of the gums because of bacteria associated with plaque buildup. When infected with gingivitis, the gums become red and swollen and often bleed during teeth brushing.*

Oils—ᵀThieves, ᵀ_F_sage[346], ᵀtea tree[347], ᵀMelrose, ᵀForgiveness, ᵀHarmony, ᵀhelichrysum, ᵀmyrrh, ᵀPresent Time, ᵀrose, ᵀrosemary.

T—Dilute as necessary, and apply on throat and gums.

Personal Care—Thieves AromaBright or Dentarome/Dentarome Plus Toothpaste, Thieves Fresh Essence Plus Mouthwash, KidScents Toothpaste (for children).

—**GUM DISEASE**

>> *Gum disease is an infection of the tissue and bones surrounding the teeth and is caused by a buildup of plaque. Gum disease consists of two parts: first gingivitis and then periodontal disease.*

Oils—ᵀThieves, ᵀ_F_tea tree[347], ᵀMelrose (fights infection), ᵀForgiveness, ᵀHarmony, ᵀmyrrh, ᵀPresent Time, ᵀtsuga.

T—Dilute as necessary, and apply on throat and gums.

Personal Care—Thieves AromaBright or Dentarome/Dentarome Plus Toothpaste, Thieves Fresh Essence Plus Mouthwash.

—**HALITOSIS (BAD BREATH)**

Oils—ᵀ_F_Peppermint[348], ᵀThieves, ᵀ_F_nutmeg, ᵀcardamom, ᵀlavender.

T—Mix 1–2 drops with 4 oz. of water, and use as mouth-rinse. Combine 5–6 drops with 1 oz. distilled water in a small spray bottle, and mist into the mouth.

> *Don't you just love the feel of clean teeth and fresh breath! Try putting a drop of **Thieves** on your toothbrush instead of toothpaste. At first it is a little warm, but it sure feels refreshing. If this doesn't work for you, try putting a drop on your toothpaste; or put 10 drops of Thieves in a small spray bottle full of distilled water, and mist it in your mouth before brushing your teeth.*

Supplements—AlkaLime.

Personal Care—Thieves AromaBright or Dentarome/Dentarome Plus Toothpaste, Thieves Fresh Essence Plus Mouthwash, KidScents Toothpaste (for children).

—**INFECTION**

Oils—ᵀTea tree, ᵀThieves, ᵀclove and ᵀfrankincense, ᵀhelichrysum, ᵀmyrrh.

T—Dilute as necessary, and apply to jaws and gums.

Personal Care—Thieves AromaBright or Dentarome/Dentarome Plus Toothpaste, Thieves Fresh Essence Plus Mouthwash, KidScents Toothpaste (for children).

Osteomyelitis: *See Bones: OSTEOMYELITIS.*

O

Osteoporosis: *See Bones: Osteoporosis.*

Ovaries: *See also Female Specific Conditions, Hormonal Imbalance.*

Oils—^{TA}_FRosemary (regulates), ^{TA}_Fmyrtle, ^{TA}Di-Gize, ^{TA}geranium,^{TA} Gratitude.

—OVARIAN CYSTS

Oils—^{TA}Basil.

Blend #1—5 drops frankincense and 5 drops Melrose. Mix, and apply to lower back and abdomen. May also consider adding this blend to 2 tsp. of olive oil and, before going to bed, while lying down, inserting blend into vagina and retaining with a tampon throughout the night.

Personal Care—PD 80/20, Prenolone/Prenolone+, Progessence/Progessence Plus, Protec.

Supplements—FemiGen (helps feed the body), Master Formula.

T—Dilute as necessary, and apply on abdomen and on Vita Flex points on the feet. Dilute with V-6 Oil to create a massage oil, and massage onto abdomen and lower back. Add 1–2 drops to 2 tsp. olive oil, insert into vagina, and retain overnight with a tampon.

A—Diffuse into the air. Inhale directly or applied to hands, tissue, or a cotton wick.

Overcome and Release Unpleasant, Difficult Issues in Life:

Oils—^{AT}Acceptance, ^{AT}Release, ^{AT}Roman chamomile, ^{AT}SARA, ^{AT}Transformation, ^{AT}Trauma Life.

A—Diffuse into the air. Inhale directly or applied to tissue or a cotton wick.

T—Apply to auricular emotion points. Dilute with V-6 Oil to create a massage oil, and massage onto the skin.

Overeating: *See Eating Disorders.*

Overweight: *See Obesity and Weight.*

Overwhelmed:

Oils—^{AT}Acceptance, ^{AT}Hope, ^{AT}Release, ^{AT}Valor.

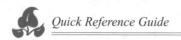

A—Diffuse into the air. Inhale directly or applied to tissue or a cotton wick.

T—Apply to auricular emotion points. Dilute with V-6 Oil to create a massage oil, and massage onto the skin.

Oxygen:

—OXYGENATING

Oils—**AT**Sandalwood (increases oxygen around pineal and pituitary glands), **AT**frankincense, **AT**fennel, **AT**fir, **AT**oregano.

> *All essential oils increase the ability of the body to take oxygen to the cells and to push toxins out. The oils pick up more oxygen and take it to the site of discomfort.*

Personal Care—**Satin Facial Scrub - Mint** (deep cleansing that dispenses nutrients and oxygen).

—OXYGEN EXCHANGE

Oils—**AT**Tsuga (increases by opening and dilating respiratory tract).

A—Diffuse into the air. Inhale directly or applied to tissue or a cotton wick.

T—Dilute as recommended, and apply 1–2 drops to forehead, chest, and sinuses.

Pain:

Oils—**T**PanAway, **T**Relieve It, **T**Deep Relief (roll-on), **T**Cool Azul, **TA**lavender[349], **T**eucalyptus[350], **A**lemon[351], **T**rosemary[352], **T**clove[353], **T**copaiba[354], **T**laurel[355], **T**mastrante, **T**blue cypress, **T**balsam fir, **T**sage lavender.

Blend #1—Vetiver & valerian together make a powerful pain killer as do palo santo and frankincense.

Personal Care—**Ortho Ease** or **Ortho Sport** (stronger) Massage Oils. These massage oils help seal in and enhance the effectiveness of the single oils or oil blends. **T**Cool Azul Sports Gel

Supplements—Sulfurzyme contains MSM, which has been shown to be very effective in controlling pain, especially in the joints and tissues.

Blend #2—20 drops valerian, 5 drops vetiver, 2 drops helichrysum, 1 drop clove, and 1 drop peppermint. Combine this ratio (in drops) in a 5 ml bottle, and then apply 3–6 drops of this blend on the back of the neck (up the cervical vertebrae—top of shoulders to base of skull), and work oils in with Vita Flex. *Working this into the brain stem helps stop pain and reduces the production of noradrenaline and cortisol.*

—ANALGESIC

>> *An analgesic is a substance that acts as a pain reliever.*

Oils—[T]PanAway, [TA]lavender[349], [T]eucalyptus[350], [A]lemon[351], [T]rosemary[352], [T]clove[353], [T]copaiba[354], [T]laurel[355], [T]bergamot, [T]geranium, [T]helichrysum, [T]lemongrass, [T]marjoram, [T]tea tree, [T]oregano, [T]peppermint, [T]Roman chamomile, [T]wintergreen.

***Comments—See the "Single Oil Property Chart" in the Appendix of this book for additional analgesic oils and their strengths.

—ANESTHESIA

>> *Anesthesia is an artificially induced insensitivity to pain or other sensation. Anesthesia is commonly used before surgeries and other procedures so that the patient does not feel pain.*

Oils—[T]PanAway, [T]clove[353], [T]helichrysum.

***Comments—One individual applied helichrysum every 15 minutes during gum surgery, and there was no bleeding and no pain. No other anesthetic was used.

—BONE

Oils—[T]PanAway, [T]wintergreen, [T]spruce, [T]cedarwood, [T]cypress, [T]fir, [T]helichrysum, [T]juniper, [T]peppermint, [T]sandalwood; [T]all the tree oils.

Supplements—Super Cal, Master Formula.

—CHRONIC

Oils—[T]PanAway (add 1–2 drops wintergreen for extra strength), [T]wintergreen, [T]cypress, [T]fir, [T]Relieve It, [T]helichrysum, [T]basil, [T]clove, [T]cedarwood, [T]elemi, [T]Idaho tansy, [T]ginger[356], [T]juniper, [T]peppermint, [T]rosemary cineol, [T]sandalwood, [T]spruce, [T]valerian.

Blend #2—Equal parts of wintergreen, elemi, and Idaho tansy.

Personal Care—Ortho Ease or Ortho Sport (stronger) Massage Oils.

Supplements—Super Cal.

—GENERAL

Oils—[T]PanAway, [T]Relieve It, [T]Deep Relief (roll-on), [TA]lavender[349], [T]eucalyptus[350], [T]rosemary[352], [T]wintergreen, [TA]Aroma Siez, [T]blue cypress, [T]balsam fir, [T]frankincense, [T]ginger, [T]helichrysum, [T]marjoram, [T]Roman chamomile, [T]sage lavender, [T]white fir (pain from inflammation).

—GROWING

Recipe #1—Massage with wintergreen, cypress, and peppermint. Wait 5 minutes, and then apply PanAway or Deep Relief (roll-on). Seal with Ortho Ease.

Personal Care—Ortho Ease Massage Oil.

Supplements—Sulfurzyme, Super Cal.

—JOINTS

    Oils—^T<u>PanAway</u>, ^Twintergreen, ^T<u>Deep Relief</u> (roll-on), ^Tspruce, ^Tbalsam fir, ^Tnutmeg, ^TRoman chamomile (inflamed).

—MUSCLE

    Oils—^T<u>Aroma Siez</u>, ^T<u>PanAway</u>, ^T<u>Cool Azul</u>, ^T<u>Deep Relief</u> (roll-on), ^T_Fclove[353], ^Twintergreen, ^Twhite fir (pain from inflammation), ^Tmastrante, ^Tbasil, ^Tbalsam fir, ^Tginger, ^Thelichrysum, ^Tlavender, ^Tlemongrass (especially good for ligaments), ^Tmarjoram, ^Tnutmeg, ^Toregano, ^Tpalo santo, ^Tpeppermint, ^T<u>Relieve It</u>, ^TRoman chamomile, ^Trosemary verbenon, ^Tsage lavender, ^Tspearmint, ^Tspruce (torn muscles), ^Tthyme, ^Tvetiver.

—SURGICAL

    Recipe #2—Valerian, vetiver, helichrysum, clove, and peppermint. Balsam fir and frankincense (equal parts); up to 3 droppers full in water 4 times daily. Also <u>GLF</u>, topically and internally, 3–4 times daily.

    Blend #3—20 ml valerian, 5 ml vetiver, 2 ml helichrysum, 1 ml clove, 1 ml peppermint. Combine oils in a 1 oz. dropper bottle. In postsurgical experiments, 3 droppers full of this blend have been taken in water (internally) up to 6 times daily for effective pain control.

—TISSUE

    Oils—^T<u>PanAway</u>, ^T<u>Cool Azul</u>, ^Tbalsam fir (good for deep tissue pain), ^T<u>Deep Relief</u> (roll-on), ^T<u>Relieve It</u>, ^Thelichrysum.

T—Dilute as necessary, and apply on location. Dilute with V-6 Oil to create a massage oil, and massage on location. Apply as a warm compress on affected area. Add 3–5 drops to 1/4 cup Epsom salts, and dissolve in warm bathwater before bathing.

A—Diffuse into the air. Inhale directly or applied to hands.

Painting:

    Recipe #1—Add one 15 ml bottle of your favorite essential oil (or oil blend) to any five gallon bucket of paint. Stir vigorously, mixing well, and then either spray paint or paint by hand. This should eliminate the paint fumes and after-smell.

Palpitations: *See Cardiovascular System:Heart.*

Pancreas:

    ›› *The pancreas is a gland organ located behind the stomach. The pancreas is responsible for producing insulin and other hormones and for producing "pancreatic juices" that aid in digestion.*

Oils—^T_FCypress (for insufficiencies), ^Trosemary, ^{TA}RC, ^Tcoriander, ^Tdill, ^Tfleabane, ^{TA}lemon, ^TRaven, ^{TA}Thieves.

—Pancreatitis

>> *Pancreatitis is the term used to describe pancreas inflammation. Pancreatitis occurs when the pancreatic juices that are designed to aid in digestion in the small intestine become active while still inside the pancreas. When this occurs, the pancreas literally begins to digest itself. Acute pancreatitis lasts for only a short time and then resolves itself. Chronic pancreatitis does not resolve itself but instead gradually destroys the pancreas.*

Oils—^{TA}Lemon, ^{TA}marjoram.

—Stimulant For

Oils—^{TA}_FHelichrysum, ^{TA}fleabane.

—Support

Oils—^{TA}Cinnamon bark, ^{TA}EndoFlex, ^{TA}geranium, ^{TA}fennel, ^{TA}coriander.

Supplements—EndoGize, Essentialzyme, Essentialzymes-4, MultiGreens, Stevia, Thyromin, Yacon Syrup.

T—Dilute as necessary, and apply over pancreas area or on Vita Flex points on the feet.

A—Diffuse into the air. Inhale directly or applied to the hands.

Pancreatitis: *See Pancreas: Pancreatitis.*

Panic: *See Anxiety: Panic. See also Calming.*

Paralysis: *See also Nervous System.*

Oils—^{TA}Peppermint, ^{TA}lemongrass, ^{TA}geranium, ^{TA}Valor, ^{TA}Awaken, ^{TA}cypress, ^{TA}ginger, ^{TA}helichrysum, ^{TA}juniper, ^{TA}nutmeg, ^{TA}Purification.

Blend #1—Combine 6 drops cypress, 15 drops geranium, 10 drops helichrysum, 5 drops juniper, 2 drops peppermint, and V-6 Oil. May rejuvenate nerve damage up to 60%. Put on location and on feet.

Supplements—Support the body with MultiGreens, Super B, Master Formula, Mineral Essence. When the paralysis starts to reverse, there will be pain; apply PanAway on location and on feet.

T—Dilute as necessary, and apply on location and on feet. Dilute with V-6 Oil to create a massage oil, and massage on location.

A—Diffuse into the air. Inhale directly or applied to the hands.

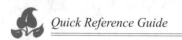

Parasites: *See also Digestive System, Intestinal Problems.*

>> *A parasite is an organism that grows on or in another organism at the host organism's expense. A parasite cannot live independently and is fed and sheltered by the host organism without making any helpful contribution itself.*

> *ParaFree was specifically designed to help the body rid itself of parasites. The essential oils contained in this supplement are black cumin, anise, fennel, laurel, vetiver, nutmeg, Melaleuca alternifolia, Idaho tansy, clove, and thyme.*
>
> *Since this product is to be used orally, and contraindications do exist, one would be well-advised to review the book, <u>Essential Oil Safety—A Guide for Health Care Professionals</u> by Robert Tisserand and Tony Balacs or <u>Aromatherapy for Health Professionals</u> by Shirley and Len Price.*

Oils—$^{IT}_F$Oregano[357], ^T_Fthyme, $^{TI}_F$fennel, ^{IT}<u>Di-Gize</u>, ^T_Ftarragon, ^{IT}lavender[358], ^T_Fcinnamon bark, ^{T}copaiba[359] (skin), ^T_FRoman chamomile, ^T_Fnutmeg, ^{IT}lemon, ^{T}anise, ^{T}clove, ^{T}eucalyptus citriodora[360], ^{IT}ginger, ^{T}hyssop, ^{T}lemongrass, ^{T}tea tree[361], ^{T}mountain savory, ^{T}mugwort (blend with thyme), ^{T}rosemary, ^{T}rosewood, ^{T}spearmint, ^{T}spikenard, ^{T}tangerine, ^{T}tarragon.

*****Comments**—See the "Single Oil Property Chart" in the Appendix of this book for additional antiparasitic oils and their strengths.

    Supplements—Cleansing Trio (ComforTone, Essentialzyme, and ICP), Digest + Cleanse (contains oils that create an unfriendly environment for parasites), ParaFree.

—Intestinal

    Oils—$^{IT}_F$Lemon, ^{IT}oregano[357], $^{IT}_F$Roman chamomile, ^{T}ravintsara.

    Supplements—Cleansing Trio (ComforTone, Essentialzyme, and ICP), Digest + Cleanse, ParaFree.

    *****Comments**—*Individuals have passed parasites within 12 hours using <u>Di-Gize</u> on stomach.*

I—Add 2–4 drops oil to an empty capsule with 2–4 drops V-6 Oil, and swallow.

T—Dilute as necessary, and apply oil on stomach, liver, intestines, and Vita Flex points on the feet to help pass parasites. Dilute as necessary, and apply on location

Parasympathetic Nervous System: *See Nervous System: Parasympathetic.*

Parathyroid:

>> *The parathyroid gland is responsible for secreting a hormone necessary for the metabolism of calcium and phosphorus. It is located near or within the posterior surface of the thyroid gland.*

Oils—^{T}<u>EndoFlex</u>.

T—Apply over the thyroid gland at the bottom of the throat or on the parathyroid Vita Flex point on the feet.

Supplements—EndoGize.

Parkinson's Disease: *See Brain, Pineal Gland, Pituitary Gland, and Alzheimer's Disease.*

▸▸ *Parkinson's disease is a progressive neurodegenerative disease marked by impairment of muscle movement and speech. Symptoms of Parkinson's disease include slowed motion, muscle stiffness, difficulty maintaining balance, impaired speech, loss of automatic movements (such as blinking, smiling, and swinging the arms while walking), and hand tremors.*

> *Cedarwood, vetiver, sandalwood, black pepper, myrrh, patchouli, ginger, German chamomile, spikenard, galbanum, and frankincense all contain sesquiterpenes which have the ability to go beyond the blood-brain barrier. See* Pineal Gland *and* Pituitary Gland.

Oils—[T][I]Cinnamon[362], [T][A]Clarity (brain function), [T]marjoram, [A][T]frankincense, [T][A]lavender, [T][A]Valor, [A][T]Acceptance, [A][T]basil, [A][T]bergamot, [A][T]cypress (circulation), [A][T]Gathering (high in sesquiterpenes and in frequency), [A][T]geranium, [A][T]helichrysum, [A][T]juniper, [A][T]Juva Cleanse, [A][T]lemon, [A][T]nutmeg, [A][T]orange, [A][T]Peace & Calming, [A][T]peppermint, [A][T]rosemary, [A][T]sandalwood, [A][T]thyme, [T]Tranquil (roll-on), [A][T]vitex.

T—Dilute 5–10 drops oil in 1 Tbs. V-6 Oil, and massage on affected muscles, back, legs, and neck. Dilute as necessary, and apply on base of neck or on Vita Flex points on the feet. Add 3–5 drops to warm bathwater before bathing.

A—Diffuse into the air. Inhale directly or applied to hands, tissue, or a cotton wick.

Supplements—BLM, Cleansing Trio (ComforTone, Essentialzyme, and ICP), JuvaPower/JuvaSpice, JuvaTone, Omega Blue, OmegaGize[3], Power Meal (contains choline, which is beneficial for Parkinson's disease), Sulfurzyme.

The following recipe has been used by Dr. Terry Friedmann of Paradise Valley, Arizona:

Recipe #1—Use the Cleansing Trio (ComforTone, Essentialzyme, and ICP) for one week; then add JuvaTone and 10 MultiGreens along with it. Drink 10 glasses of distilled water daily. Diffuse the oil of helichrysum and frankincense together for one hour at night.

Recipe #2—Apply frankincense to the top of the spine (at the base of the skull), and work it in. Then apply 3–5 drops of each of the following oils, one at a time, up the back of the neck, and work each one in individually: valerian, vetiver, balsam fir, Roman chamomile, and western red cedar. This will help to suppress the override of the sympathetic system and bring about a change in attitude and ability.

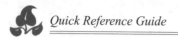

—To Prevent

> **Recipe #1**—Keep liver and blood clean with Juva Cleanse, JuvaTone, and the Cleansing Trio (ComforTone, Essentialzyme, and ICP). Massage with helichrysum and sandalwood to help chelate metallics out of the body.

Past:

Oils—**ᴬᵀ**<u>Present Time</u> (helps to bring you into the present so you can go forward), **ᴬᵀ**<u>Transformation</u>.

A—Diffuse into the air. Inhale directly or applied to tissue or a cotton wick.

T—Apply to auricular emotion points. Dilute with V-6 Oil to create a massage oil, and massage onto the skin.

Peace: *See also Calming.*

Oils—**ᴬᵀ**<u>Peace & Calming</u>, **ᴬ**lavender, **ᴬᵀ**ylang ylang, **ᵀ**<u>Tranquil</u> (roll-on), **ᴬ**juniper, **ᴬᵀ**marjoram, **ᴬᵀ**<u>Release</u>, **ᴬᵀ**<u>Trauma Life</u>, **ᵀᴬ**<u>Oola Balance</u>.

—Finding

> **Oils**—**ᴬ**Tangerine.

—Promote

> **Oils**—**ᴬᵀ**Roman chamomile.

> **Supplements**—Cleansing Trio (ComforTone, Essentialzyme, and ICP) and JuvaTone.

A—Diffuse into the air. Inhale directly or applied to hands, tissue, or a cotton wick.

T—Dilute with V-6 Oil to create a massage oil, and massage onto the skin. Add 3–5 drops to Epsom or bath salts, and dissolve in warm bathwater before bathing.

Pelvic Pain Syndrome:

>> *Pelvic pain syndrome is characterized by pain in the pelvis area that continues for several months. Symptoms include severe and steady pain, dull aching, a feeling of pressure deep in the pelvis, painful bowel movements, pain during intercourse, and pain when sitting down.*

Oils—**ᵀ**Ginger, **ᵀ**geranium, **ᵀ**bergamot, **ᵀ**clove, **ᵀ**nutmeg, **ᵀ**thyme.

T—Place 2–3 drops in warm bathwater, and soak for 10 minutes. Dilute with V-6 Oil to create a massage oil, and massage on location.

Periodontal Disease: *See Oral Conditions:Gum Disease.*

Personal Growth:

Oils—**AT**Transformation.

—ELIMINATING BLOCKED

Oils—**AT**Helichrysum, **AT**frankincense.

A—Diffuse into the air. Inhale directly or applied to tissue or a cotton wick.

T—Dilute with V-6 Oil to create a massage oil, and massage onto the skin.

Personality (Multiple):

Oils—**AT**Inner Child, **AT**SARA, **AT**Sensation.

A—Diffuse into the air. Inhale directly or applied to tissue or a cotton wick.

T—Apply to auricular emotion points. Dilute with V-6 Oil to create a massage oil, and massage onto the skin.

Perspiration:

Oils—**T**Purification, **T**Petitgrain.

T—Dilute as necessary, and apply on location. Combine 3–4 drops oil with 4 oz. unscented talcum powder and 2 oz. baking soda, and apply under the arms, on the feet, or on other areas prone to perspire.

Supplements—Cleansing Trio (ComforTone, Essentialzyme, and ICP).

Pest Troubles: *See also Insect, Mice.*

Oils—**A**Ravintsara.

A—Diffuse into the air. Apply to cotton balls or strips of fabric, and place in areas where pests may enter.

pH Balance: *See also Acidosis and Alkalosis.*

Supplements—AlkaLime (combats yeast and fungus overgrowth and preserves the body's proper pH balance), Balance Complete, ComforTone (to help clean out the colon), Digest + Cleanse, Essentialzyme, Essentialzymes-4, JuvaTone

> *According to Dr. Robert O. Young in his book, <u>One Sickness, One Disease, One Treatment</u>, "disease is an expression of pH." Dr. Robert Young believes that there is only one disease, which is "the constant over-acidification of the blood and tissues which disturbs the central regulation of the human body, all of which is mainly the result of an inverted way of living and eating." All sickness and disease that leads to death begins with an over-acidification of the blood and tissues and culminates with yeast and fungus. A normal healthy body should have a pH of about 7.2. (The use of saliva and urine test strips will show a much lower pH level due to the protein present in the solution. Saliva and urine tests from a healthy body should be about 6.6 to 6.8.) To maintain this pH, our diet should consist of 80% alkaline foods and 20% acid foods. "In the healing of disease, when the individual is acidic, the higher the ratio of alkaline elements in the diet, the faster will be the recovery."*

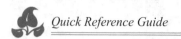

(to clean the liver) and Mineral Essence (if body is too alkaline), MultiGreens (brings blood back to an alkaline pH).

Personal Care—Genesis Hand & Body Lotion (balances pH on skin).

Pharyngitis: *See also Rhinopharyngitis.*

›› *Pharyngitis is an inflammation of the back of the throat (the pharynx). Symptoms of pharyngitis include sore throat, fever, skin rashes, muscle aches, headache, joint pain, and swollen lymph nodes.*

Oils—^{AT}Goldenrod.

A—Diffuse into the air, and inhale the vapors.

T—Dilute as necessary, and apply to sinuses, neck, and Vita Flex points on the feet.

Phlebitis: *See Cardiovascular System: Phlebitis.*

Pimples: *See Acne.*

Pineal Gland:

›› *The pineal gland is a tiny endocrine gland located close to the center of the brain. It is responsible for producing the hormone melatonin that regulates the sleep/wake cycle. The pineal gland also serves to regulate blood pressure, sexual development, growth, body temperature, and motor function. The pineal gland is also involved*

> *Oils containing sesquiterpenes are especially effective in oxygenating the pineal and pituitary glands. These include cedarwood, vetiver, sandalwood, black pepper, myrrh, patchouli, ginger, German chamomile, spikenard, galbanum, and frankincense (in order of sesquiterpene content). Blends include 3 Wise Men, Acceptance, Brain Power, Forgiveness, Gathering, Harmony, Inspiration, Into the Future, and Trauma Life.*

in the process of creativity and planning things to do. If the pineal gland is not open, negative emotions will be attracted back to the aura.

—Opens and Increases Oxygen

Oils—^AFrankincense, ^Asandalwood (increases oxygen), ^A3 Wise Men (same frequency as pineal), ^AAcceptance, ^ABrain Power, ^Acedarwood, ^AForgiveness, ^AGathering, ^AHarmony, ^AInspiration, ^AInto the Future, ^ARelease, ^Aspruce, ^ATransformation, ^ATrauma Life.

A—Inhale directly or applied to hands, tissue, or a cotton wick. Diffuse into the air.

***Comments—*Just smelling the essential oils will increase the oxygen production, particularly around the pineal and pituitary glands, and will help increase the secretion of antibodies, endorphins, and neurotransmitters.*

Pink Eye: *See Eyes: Conjunctivitis.*

Pituitary Gland: *See also Endocrine System.*

▸▸ *The pituitary gland is located at the base of the brain and is considered to be the master gland because its secretions stimulate the other endocrine glands. The pituitary has an anterior and a posterior lobe. The anterior lobe secretes the human growth hormone (stimulates overall body growth), adrenocorticotropic hormone (controls steroid hormone secretion by the adrenal cortex), thyrotropic hormone (stimulates the activity of the thyroid gland), and three gonadotropic hormones (control growth and reproductive activity of the ovaries and testes). The posterior lobe secretes the antidiuretic hormone and oxytocin. The antidiuretic hormone causes water retention by the kidneys. Oxytocin stimulates the mammary glands to release milk and also causes uterine contractions. An overactive pituitary during childhood can cause a child to be extremely tall, while an underactive pituitary can result in the opposite.*

Supplements—Ultra Young+ (a new spray nutraceutical, which contains ingredients that are necessary for stimulating the pituitary gland into producing the human growth hormone (hGH) and allowing the body to utilize it).

—BALANCES

    Oils—ᴬᵀGeranium, ᴬᵀylang ylang.

—INCREASES OXYGEN

    Oils—ᴬᵀ<u>3 Wise Men</u>, ᴬᵀfrankincense, ᴬᵀsandalwood, ᴬᵀ<u>Acceptance</u>, ᴬᵀ<u>Brain Power</u>, ᴬᵀ<u>Egyptian Gold</u>, ᴬᵀ<u>Forgiveness</u>, ᴬᵀ<u>Gathering</u>, ᴬᵀ<u>Harmony</u>, ᴬᵀ<u>Inspiration</u>, ᴬᵀ<u>Into the Future</u>, ᴬᵀ<u>Trauma Life</u>.

A—Inhale directly or applied to hands, tissue, or a cotton wick. Diffuse into the air. Can also rub a couple drops of oil between hands, cup hands over nose and mouth, and breathe deeply *(see Comments under Pineal above)*.

T—Apply to the forehead, back of neck, and Vita Flex points on big toes.

Plague: *See also Antibacterial.*

▸▸ *Plague is a potentially deadly bacterial disease that is caused by the Yersinia pestis bacteria, which is transmitted to humans and animals through close contact or through bites from fleas that have previously bitten infected animals. Symptoms include fever, headaches, and extremely swollen and hot lymph nodes. If left untreated, plague can quickly invade the lungs, causing severe pneumonia, high fever, bloody coughing, and death.*

Oils—ᵀᴬ_FClove, ᵀᴬ<u>Thieves</u> (annihilates bacteria), ᵀᴬ<u>Abundance</u>.

T—Dilute as necessary, and apply to neck, chest, and Vita Flex points on the feet.

A—Diffuse into the air.

Supplements—**Inner Defense.**

A=Aromatic **T**=Topical **I**=Internal |

Pleurisy: *See also Antibacterial, Antiviral, Respiratory System.*

»» *Pleurisy is an inflammation of the moist membrane (pleura) that surrounds the lungs and lines the rib cage. Pleurisy is characterized by a dry cough, chest pain, and difficulty breathing. Viral infection is the most common cause of pleurisy; but bacterial lung infections, chest injuries, and drug reactions are also possible causes.*

Oils—^{AT}_FCypress, ^{AT}_Fthyme.

A—Diffuse into the air.

T—Dilute as necessary, and apply to chest or to Vita Flex points on the feet. Apply to chest with a warm compress.

PMS: *See Female Specific Conditions: PMS.*

Pneumonia: *See also Antibacterial, Respiratory System.*

»» *Pneumonia is an illness characterized by lung inflammation. The lungs are infected by a bacteria, fungus, or virus. The result is a cough, chest pain, difficulty breathing, fever, shaking chills, headache, muscle pain, and fatigue. Pneumonia is a special concern for young children and for individuals over the age of sixty-five. Pneumonia ranges in seriousness from mild to life threatening.*

> *Recently I got **Poison Ivy/Oak** for the first time. I looked in my <u>Reference Guide for Essential Oils</u> and decided to use <u>Melrose</u> on my poison ivy. The itching would stop for about 5 minutes and then start up again. I decided to put <u>Purification</u> on, which stopped the itching for maybe an hour or two before it would start up again. Getting desperate, I used <u>Joy</u> and sometimes <u>Harmony</u> (since I had more <u>Harmony</u>) on the poison ivy. The itching would stop for most of the day, and I would forget about having poison ivy. I didn't start the <u>Harmony</u> and <u>Joy</u> until about 3 or 4 days into the poison ivy flare up; but it's now the 6th day, and I'm not itching unless I take a shower or sweat profusely. From this experience with poison ivy, I'm convinced that the presence of rose, rosewood, and palmarosa in <u>Joy</u> and <u>Harmony</u> have all helped in the healing of our "skin conditions." I plan to stock up on <u>Harmony</u> and <u>Joy</u> for future needs.*
> *-Submitted by Christie Krajewski*
> *Batesville, Arkansas (July 2004)*

Oils—^{AT}<u>RC</u>, ^{AT}<u>Thieves</u> (on feet), ^{AT}thyme[363], ^{AT}cinnamon[363], ^{AT}oregano[364], ^{AT}<u>Raven</u> (on back and on feet), ^{AT}ravintsara, ^{AT}eucalyptus, ^{AT}Eucalyptus radiata, ^{AT}tea tree, ^T<u>Tranquil</u> (roll-on), ^{AT}cajeput, ^{AT}<u>Exodus II</u>, ^{AT}frankincense, ^{AT}<u>ImmuPower</u> (on spine), ^{AT}lavender, ^{AT}lemon, ^{AI}tangerine[365], ^{AT}Tea tree ericifolia, ^{AT}myrrh.

A—Diffuse into the air. Place 4 drops in 1/2 cup hot water, and inhale steam vapors deeply.

T—Dilute as necessary, and apply to indicated area or to chest, back, and Vita Flex points on the feet. Apply as a warm compress to the chest. Add 2–3 drops to 1 tsp. V-6 or olive oil; then place in rectum, and retain overnight.

Supplements—Inner Defense, Master Formula, Ultra Young+.

Recipe #1—One or more of the following can be used with great effect:

    1. <u>RC</u> on chest.

2. Put 15 drops of <u>RC</u> in 2 cups of hot water in a bowl; wet towel in the bowl, ring out, and put on chest with a dry towel on top.

3. Put 4 drops of <u>RC</u> or eucalyptus in ½ cup hot water, and inhale steam deeply.

4. <u>Raven</u> in rectum; <u>RC</u> on chest and back (reverse each night).

*****Comments**—Refer to the chapter entitled "How to Use—The Personal Usage Reference" in the <u>Essential Oils Desk Reference</u> under "Lung Infections - Pneumonia" for some excellent blend recipes and supplement recommendations.

P

Poison Oak/Ivy:

>> *Poison oak and poison ivy are plants with an oily sap called urushiol that causes an itchy rash when it comes into contact with the skin. Infection by poison oak or poison ivy is recognized by redness and itching of the skin, a rash, red bumps, and later oozing blisters. A rash caused by poison oak or by poison ivy usually lasts from 5–12 days.*

Oils—^TRose, ^Tlavender, ^T<u>Joy</u>, ^T<u>Harmony</u>, ^T<u>Melrose</u>, ^TRoman chamomile, ^Trosewood, ^Tpalmarosa.

T—Dilute as necessary, and apply on location. Dilute with V-6 Oil to make a massage oil, and apply on location.

Personal Care—Rose Ointment.

Pollution: *See also Purification.*

Oils—^{AT}<u>Purification</u>.

—Air

    Oils—^ALemon, ^Apeppermint, ^{AT}<u>Purification</u>.

—Cigarette Smoke

    Oils—^A<u>Purification</u>.

—Water

    Oils—^ILemon, ^Ipeppermint, ^I<u>Purification</u>.

A—Diffuse into the air.

I—Add 1–2 drops oil to 8–16 oz. of water; allow to sit for 5 minutes, and then drink.

T—Add 3–5 drops to 1 oz. water in a spray bottle, and mist on location.

Polyps: *See also Colon, Nose: Polyps.*

Oils—^{AT}<u>Di-Gize</u>, ^{AT}<u>Exodus II</u>, ^{AT}peppermint, ^{AT}spikenard, and others with strong anti-bacterial properties (*See Antibacterial*).

A=Aromatic   **T**=Topical   **I**=Internal |

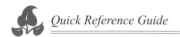

Supplements—ComforTone, Essentialzyme, Essentialzymes-4, Master Formula, Super Cal.

***Comments**—In two separate articles published in 1998, bacterial infection was found to exist when polyps were present. In the case of colorectal (intestinal) polyps, *E. coli* and similar bacteria were found to be adhering to the walls of the large intestine, and even partially penetrating the intestinal mucosa (Gastroenterology 1998; 115: 281-286). In the case of gastric polyps (small growths in the stomach lining), the *Helicobacter pylori* bacteria was found; and when eradicated, the polyps disappeared in 71% of the patients within a 12 to 15 month period (Annals of Internal Medicine 1998; 129: 712-715).

A—Diffuse into the air. Inhale directly or applied to hands, tissue, or a cotton wick.

T—Dilute as necessary, and apply on location.

Positive Feelings:

Oils—^AT^Acceptance, ^AT^Abundance, ^AT^Envision, ^AT^Forgiveness, ^AT^Idaho tansy, ^AT^Joy, ^AT^Motivation, ^AT^Live with Passion, ^AT^3 Wise Men (releases negative memory/trauma and reinforces positive feelings, which creates greater spiritual awareness).

A—Diffuse into the air. Inhale directly or applied to hands, tissue, or a cotton wick.

T—Apply to auricular emotion points. Dilute with V-6 Oil to create a massage oil, and massage onto the skin. Add 3–5 drops to Epsom or bath salts, and dissolve in warm bathwater before bathing.

Positive Ions: *See Ions: Positive Ions.*

Post Traumatic Stress Disorder (PTSD):

Oils— ^AT^Freedom, ^AT^AromaSleep, ^AT^Inner Harmony, ^AT^Divine Release, ^AT^T.R. Care, ^AT^Valor, ^AT^Transformation, Joy, (All of these blends can help release negative memory/ trauma and allowing one the freedom to move forward with achieving their dreams).

A—Diffuse into the air. Inhale directly or applied to hands, tissue, or a cotton wick.

T—Apply to auricular emotion points. Dilute with V-6 Oil to create a massage oil, and massage onto the skin. Add 3–5 drops to Epsom or bath salts, and dissolve in warm bathwater before bathing.

Potassium Deficiency:

≫ *Potassium is important for a healthy nervous system and a regular heart rhythm.*

> *Potassium* is important for a healthy nervous system and a regular heart rhythm. It works with sodium to control the body's water balance and regulates the transfer of nutrients to the cells.

It works with sodium to control the body's water balance and regulates the transfer of nutrients to the cells.

Supplements— Master Formula, Mineral Essence, Thyromin.

Potential:

Oils—**AT**<u>Acceptance</u>, **AT**<u>Awaken</u> (realize our highest potential), **AT**<u>Believe</u> (release our unlimited potential), **AT**<u>Gathering</u>, **AT**<u>Transformation</u>, **AT**<u>White Angelica</u> (greater awareness of one's potential).

A—Diffuse into the air. Inhale directly or applied to hands, tissue, or a cotton wick.

T—Apply to auricular emotion points. Dilute with V-6 Oil to create a massage oil, and massage onto the skin.

Power:

Oils—**A**<u>Sacred Mountain</u>, **A**<u>Surrender</u> (calming and relaxing to dominant personalities), **A**<u>Valor</u>.

A—Diffuse into the air. Inhale directly or applied to hands, tissue, or a cotton wick.

Power Surges: *See Hot Flashes.*

Prayer:

Oils—**AT**Frankincense, **AT**<u>Inspiration</u>, **AT**<u>Sacred Mountain</u>.

A—Inhale directly or applied to hands, tissue, or a cotton wick. Diffuse into the air.

T—Apply to crown chakra. Dilute with V-6 Oil to create a massage oil, and massage onto the skin.

Pregnancy/Motherhood:

Oils—**AT**<u>Gentle Baby</u> (relieves stress during pregnancy; can also be used by fathers to relieve stress during delivery), **AT**geranium, **AT**ylang ylang, **AT**lavender[366], **AT**Roman chamomile, **AT**jasmine, **AT**grapefruit, **AT**tangerine, **AT**elemi.

A—Diffuse into the air. Inhale directly or applied to hands, tissue, or a cotton wick.

T—Dilute with V-6 Oil, and massage gently on abdomen, chest, arms, legs, feet, back, or area of concern. Add 1–2 drops to 1/4 cup Epsom salt, and dissolve in warm bathwater before bathing.

Supplements—PD 80/20, Prenolone/Prenolone+, Progessence/Progessence Plus, Thyromin (use before, during, and after).

A=Aromatic   **T**=Topical   **I**=Internal | 277

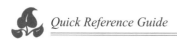

Personal Care—ClaraDerm (essential oil spray—apply topically to stressed skin before and after childbirth).

—ANXIETY/TENSION *SEE ALSO CALMING*

> **Oils—**^A<u>Into the Future</u> (help let go of fear and trauma), ^T<u>Tranquil</u> (roll-on), ^A<u>Present Time</u> (help mother focus on giving birth).
>
> **A—**Diffuse into the air. Inhale directly or applied to hands, tissue, or a cotton wick.
>
> **Blend #1—**Add 10 drops lavender, 10 drops orange, 2 drops marjoram, 2 drops cedarwood, and 1 drop Roman chamomile to 4 oz. sweet almond oil or to V-6 Oil. Use as a massage oil or in bathwater.
>
> **Supplements—**PD 80/20, Prenolone/Prenolone+, Progessence/Progessence Plus.

—BABY (NEWBORN)

> **Recipe #1—**Frankincense (1 drop on the crown for protection), myrrh (on remaining umbilical cord and around navel to protect from infection), <u>Valor</u> (1 drop divided between both feet and 1–2 drops rubbed up spine to help ensure proper alignment).

—BREASTS *SEE ALSO BREASTS*

> **Oils—**^TFennel (tone), ^TRoman chamomile (sore nipples).
>
> **T—**Dilute 3–5 drops in 1 Tbs. V-6 Oil, and massage on location.

—CONCEPTION

> **Recipe #2—**Do a proper cleansing for one year before. You may want to start with the Master Cleanser (See Cleansing for more information).

> *PREGNANCY SAFETY DATA*
>
> <u>*Avoid During Pregnancy*</u>
>
> *Single Oils: Basil, birch, calamus, cassia, cinnamon bark, hyssop, Idaho tansy, lavandin, rosemary, sage, tarragon.*
> *Blends: <u>Di-Gize</u>, <u>Dragon Time</u>, <u>Exodus II</u>, <u>Grounding</u>, <u>Mister</u>.*
> *Other: Estro, FemiGen, ParaFree, Protec,*
>
> <u>*Use Cautiously During Pregnancy*</u>
>
> *Single Oils: Angelica, cedarwood, chamomile (German/blue), cistus, citronella, clary sage, clove bud, cumin (black), cypress, davana, fennel, laurel, marjoram, mountain savory, myrrh, nutmeg, peppermint, rose, spearmint, vetiver, yarrow.*
> *Blends: <u>Aroma Siez</u>, <u>Clarity</u>, <u>Harmony</u>, <u>ImmuPower</u>, <u>Relieve It</u>, <u>Thieves</u>.*
> *Other: Prenolone/Prenolone+, ComforTone, Essentialzyme, Dragon Time Massage Oil.*
>
> *It was very difficult to compile a list of oils and products to be avoided during pregnancy. Each aromatologist has a different opinion. We feel that an oil that is unsafe is an oil that has been adulterated or one that is used improperly. Oils that are diluted, applied externally, and used in moderation should not create a problem. This list is a compilation of the safety data contained in aromatherapy books written by the following authors: Ann Berwick, Julia Lawless, Shirley & Len Price, Jeanne Rose, Robert Tisserand, and Tony Balacs.*

Supplements—Balance Complete (*refer to the 5-Day Nutritive Cleanse program listed under Balance Complete in the Supplements section of the <u>Reference Guide for Essential Oils</u>. This program also uses Digest + Cleanse and NingXia Red to help enhance detoxi-*

fication while maintaining energy levels), Cleansing Trio (especially ComforTone for the colon and ICP for the intestines), Digest + Cleanse, JuvaTone (cleanses liver).

—CONSTIPATION *SEE ALSO DIGESTIVE SYSTEM: Constipation*

Supplements—**ComforTone** can be taken during pregnancy as long as you do not get diarrhea. Diarrhea can cause cramping which could bring on labor. Essentialzyme, Essentialzymes-4, JuvaTone (helps change genetics in the colon and purge the liver).

—DELIVERY

Oils—**ᵀᴬLavender** (circulation stimulating, calming, antibiotic, anti-inflammatory, antiseptic),
ᴬᵀnutmeg (balances hormones, calms the central nervous system, alleviates anxiety, increases circulation, and does good to the blood supply), **ᵀValor** (Align mother's hips: apply along inside and bottom of each foot; then have someone hold feet—right palm to right foot and left palm to left foot—to balance energy flows. Rub a couple drops along newborn's spine for alignment.), **ᵀclary sage, ᴬForgiveness, ᴬGentle Baby, ᴬHarmony.**

T—Dilute as necessary, and apply as indicated or on hips, bottoms of feet, or abdomen. Dilute with V-6 Oil to create massage oil, and massage on hips, bottoms of feet, or abdomen.

A—Diffuse into the air. Inhale directly or applied to hands, tissue, or a cotton wick.

***CAUTION—*Nutmeg is generally nontoxic, nonirritant, and nonsensitizing. However, large doses may cause nausea, stupor, and tachycardia. Use in moderation and with great care during pregnancy. See the safety data about nutmeg in the Appendix of this book.*

–AVOID EPISIOTOMY

Recipe #2—ClaraDerm Spray (spray onto and massage into perineum three times daily), Gentle Baby or geranium (neat or added to olive oil; massage perineum).

Blend #2—8 drops geranium, 5 drops lavender, 1 oz. V-6 Oil. Prepare three weeks before delivery, and rub on perineum three times a day. One week before delivery, prepare the same blend and add 5 drops fennel. Continue applying three times daily.

Diffuse—Hope, Joy, Motivation, Live with Passion, Peace & Calming.

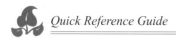

–Uᴛᴇᴘᴜᴍ

–Uterus

    Recipe #2—Tone uterus with 1–3 drops of clary sage around ankles (one
        woman dilated and had her baby in 1 ½ hours), <u>Dragon Time</u>, fennel, <u>Gathering</u>, sage.

–Transition

    Oils—ᵀBasil.

    T—Dilute as necessary, and apply 1–2 drops to temples, abdomen, or Vita Flex
        points on feet.

—Early Labor

    Oils—ᵀLavender

    T—Rub on tummy to stop early labor.

—Energy

    Blend #3—Equal portions of Roman chamomile, geranium, and lavender in V-6 Oil.

—Hemorrhaging

    »» *Postpartum Hemorrhaging is excessive bleeding following childbirth. It is commonly defined
        as losing 500 ml of blood after vaginal birth and 1000 ml of blood after a cesarean birth.
        Postpartum hemorrhaging generally occurs within 24 hours following the birth and can be
        life threatening if not stopped.*

    Blend #4—Helichrysum and <u>Gentle Baby</u> together on lower back (prevent).

—High Blood Pressure

    »» *High blood pressure can potentially be dangerous in pregnancy. High blood pressure can
        cause a decreased flow of blood to the placenta, slowing down the baby's growth; premature
        placenta separation from the uterus, taking away the baby's oxygen and nutrients and caus-
        ing heavy bleeding in the mother; premature birth; and the risk of future disease.*

    Oils—ᵀ<u>Aroma Life</u> (over heart), ᴬᵀylang ylang[367].

    ***Comments—Avoid using hyssop, rosemary, sage, thyme, and possibly peppermint.

    T—Dilute as necessary, and apply on area indicated or over heart area and on Vita
        Flex points.

    A—Diffuse into the air or applied to hands, tissue, or a cotton wick.

—Keep Baby In Birth Canal

    Oils—ᵀ<u>Gentle Baby</u>.

    T—Dilute as necessary, and apply to Vita Flex points on hands and feet.

***Comments—*One mother would rub <u>Gentle Baby</u> on her little fingers and little toes when contracting. Then she would squeeze the sides of her little fingers while someone else squeezed her little toes. This was repeated during contractions until the baby decided to stay in the birth canal.*

—LABOR (DURING)

Oils—^{TA}Clary sage (kick labor into gear; some have combined with fennel), ^T<u>Gentle Baby</u> (apply to ankles and hands when labor starts), ^A<u>Into the Future</u> (to help move past fear and trauma), ^{TA}jasmine (speed up contractions), ^A<u>Present Time</u> (to help focus).

T—Dilute as necessary, and apply on indicated area or on ankles, lower abdomen, or hands.

A—Inhale directly or applied to hands. Diffuse into the air.

Blend #5—**(Use only when ready to deliver.)** 2 oz. V-6 Oil, 8 drops clary sage, 8 drops lavender, 8 drops jasmine. May be useful when trying to induce labor or augment a slow, lazy labor.

–PAIN

Oils—^T<u>PanAway</u>

T—Apply to lower back and tummy area.

***Comments—*Refer to the chapter entitled "How to Use—The Personal Usage Reference" in the <u>Essential Oils Desk Reference</u> under "Pregnancy" for a wonderful blend to use during labor.*

—LABOR (POST)

Oils—^TGeranium, ^Tlavender.

T—Dilute as necessary, and apply on abdomen, ankles, or bottoms of feet.

***Comments—*Lavender is calming and has a slight analgesic effect. It also stimulates circulation, which is great for both mother and baby, and has anti-inflammatory and antiseptic properties. Geranium is one of the best oils to stimulate circulation, which in turn facilitates easy breathing. It has a contractive effect and helps pull together dilated tissues, so it is healing for the uterus and endometrium after the birth. Geranium is also an antidepressant and is known for its uplifting effect (<u>Alternative Medicine—A Definitive Guide</u>, pp. 806-7).*

—LACTATION *See* NURSING/LACTATION *below*

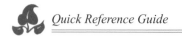

—**MASTITIS (BREAST INFECTION)** *SEE ALSO ANTIBACTERIAL*

» *Mastitis is a breast infection occurring in women who are breast-feeding. Mastitis causes the breast to become red, swollen, and very painful. Symptoms of mastitis include breast tenderness, fever, general lack of well-being, skin redness, and a breast that feels warm to the touch. Mastitis generally occurs in just one breast, not in both.*

Oils—ᵀLavender, ᵀ<u>Citrus Fresh</u> (with lavender), ᵀ<u>Exodus II</u>, ᵀtangerine, ᵀpatchouli[368].

T—Dilute as necessary, and apply on location.

Blend #6—Equal amounts of lavender and tangerine. Dilute with some V-6 Oil, and apply to breasts and under arms twice a day.

Supplements—MultiGreens, Power Meal.

—**MISCARRIAGE (AFTER)**

Oils—ᵀᴬFrankincense, ᵀᴬgrapefruit, ᵀᴬgeranium, ᵀᴬlavender (may help prevent), ᵀᴬRoman chamomile, ᵀspruce (2 drops on solar plexus).

T—Dilute with V-6 Oil to create a massage oil, and massage on back, legs, and arms. Add 3–4 drops to warm bathwater before bathing. Apply as indicated.

A—Inhale directly or applied to hands. Diffuse into the air.

Supplements—JuvaTone, Cleansing Trio (ComforTone, Essentialzyme, and ICP).

—**MORNING SICKNESS** *SEE ALSO NAUSEA.*

» *Morning sickness is the nauseated feeling accompanying the first trimester of pregnancy for many women. Morning sickness can often include vomiting. For most women, morning sickness begins around the sixth week of pregnancy and ends around the twelfth week. Although it is called "morning" sickness, the symptoms can occur at any time during the day.*

Oils—ᴵᵀᴬGinger[369], ᴵᵀ<u>Di-Gize</u> (Sip 1–2 drops in water or apply 1–2 drops around the navel), ᴬᵀpeppermint, ᴵlemon[370], ᴬᵀcalamus, ᴬᵀ<u>M-Grain</u>.

> *Caution: Although <u>Di-Gize</u> is recommended for morning sickness, it contains some oils which some aromatologists strongly discourage using. It may have a lot to do with purity. Use at your own risk. I did, and it worked for me!*

T—Dilute as necessary, and apply on or behind ears, down jaw bone, over stomach as a compress, and on Vita Flex points on feet.

I—Take as indicated; or place 1–3 drops in an empty capsule, and swallow.

A—Inhale directly or applied on hands (rub together and smell); or put a drop on your pillow.

Recipe #3—Can also put 4–6 drops of spearmint in a bowl of boiled and cooled water and place the bowl on floor beside the bed overnight to keep the stomach calm.

Supplements—ComforTone, Essentialzyme, Essentialzymes-4.

—NURSING/LACTATION

Oils—^T**Clary sage** (brings in milk production), ^T_F**fennel** or ^T**basil** (increases milk production),
^T**geranium**.

T—Apply above breasts on lymph area and on spine at breast level.

Caution: Fennel should not be used for more than 10 days, as it will excessively increase flow through the urinary tract.

–INCREASE MILK PRODUCTION

Blend #7—7–15 drops fennel and either 7–15 drops geranium or 5–10 drops clary sage. Dilute 1–2 drops of blend in 2 Tbs. V-6 Oil.

Supplements— Master Formula, MultiGreens.

–DECREASE MILK PRODUCTION

Oils—^T**Peppermint**, ^T**jasmine**[371].

T—Apply with cold compress over breasts. Refer to Methods of Application under the Science and Application section of the <u>Reference Guide for Essential Oils</u> for instructions on using cold compresses.

—ON CHAKRAS

Oils—^T<u>Awaken</u> (after pregnancy).

T—Dilute as necessary, and apply on chakras.

—PLACENTA

›› *The placenta is the organ responsible for sustaining life in an unborn baby. The placenta attaches to the uterus wall and connects to the mother's blood supply to provide nutrients and oxygen for the fetus. The placenta plays other essential roles as well: It removes waste created by the fetus, triggers labor and delivery, and protects the fetus against infection.*

Oils—^T**Basil** (has been used to help retain), ^T**jasmine** (helps expulsion).

T—Dilute as necessary, and apply on lower abdomen and on Vita Flex points on the feet.

—POSTPARTUM DEPRESSION (BABY BLUES)

›› *Postpartum depression is depression sometimes experienced by mothers shortly after giving birth. New mothers may experience symptoms such as irritableness, sadness, uncontrollable*

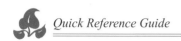

emotions, fatigue, anxiety, difficulty sleeping, thoughts of suicide, hopelessness, and guilt. Postpartum depression is typically thought to result from a hormonal imbalance caused by the pregnancy and childbirth.

Oils—[AT]Joy, [AT]lavender[372], [AT]lemon[373], [AT]grapefruit, [AT]Peace & Calming, [AT]Hope, [AT]Valor, [AT]basil, [AT]bergamot, [AT]clary sage, [AT]fennel, [AT]frankincense, [AT]geranium, [AT]Gentle Baby, [AT]Harmony, [AT]jasmine, [AT]myrrh, [AT]nutmeg (use in moderation), [AT]orange, [AT]patchouli, [AT]vetiver, [AT]White Angelica.

> *Natural Progesterone or Pregnenolone may help prevent postpartum depression. Just before a woman has a baby her body produces about 400 mg of progesterone each day to help hold the placenta in place. When the baby is born, the production of progesterone falls dramatically. The body's inability to produce high doses of progesterone can help induce postpartum depression.*

A—Diffuse into the air. Inhale directly or applied to hands, tissue, or a cotton wick.

T—Apply to auricular emotion points. Dilute as necessary, and apply to temple or forehead. Dilute with V-6 Oil to create a massage oil, and massage into skin. Add 1–3 drops to warm bathwater before bathing.

Personal Care—Prenolone/Prenolone+, Progessence/Progessence Plus.

Supplements—ImmuPro, Omega Blue, OmegaGize[3].

Some women have had wonderful results with the following recipe:

Recipe #1—Valor first (2–5 drops on each foot; hold to balance energies), Harmony (use finger to dab a small amount onto each energy center [chakra]), Joy (apply a drop between and just above the breasts), and White Angelica (on the crown of the head and over the top of the shoulders).

—SELF LOVE

Oils—[TA]Joy.

T—Apply to auricular emotion points. Dilute with V-6 Oil to create a massage oil, and massage into skin.

A—Diffuse into the air. Inhale directly.

—SKIN ELASTICITY

Oils—[T]Aroma Life, [T]Clarity, [T]Dragon Time, [T]Gentle Baby, [T]Mister, [T]M-Grain, [T]Relieve It.

Caution: Many of these blends contain oils that many aromatologists feel should be avoided or used with caution during pregnancy (which may have to do with purity). Use at your own risk and with caution.

T—Dilute with V-6 Oil to create a massage oil, and apply on location.

Personal Care—A·R·T Skin Care System, ClaraDerm (essential oil spray—apply topically to stressed skin before and after childbirth).

—**STRETCH MARKS** *SEE ALSO SKIN*

>> *Stretch marks are thin purple or red lines on the skin that appear as the skin is rapidly stretched over a short period of time. Many women notice the appearance of stretch marks in the last few months of pregnancy. These marks most often appear on the breasts, stomach, buttocks, thighs and hips. Stretch marks tend to fade over time, but it is difficult to eliminate them completely. The best way to avoid serious stretch marks in pregnancy is to keep the skin well moisturized and as elastic as possible.*

Oils—**T**Gentle Baby

T—Dilute as necessary, and apply every day on tummy.

Personal Care—ClaraDerm (essential oil spray—apply topically to stressed skin before and after childbirth).

—**TOXEMIA/PREECLAMPSIA**

>> *Preeclampsia, also known as toxemia, is pregnancy-induced high blood pressure. Symptoms include protein in the urine, elevated blood pressure levels, sudden weight gain, blurred vision, abdominal pains in the upper-right side, and swelling in the hands and face.*

Oils—**TA**Aroma Life.

T—Dilute with V-6 Oil, and apply on bottoms of feet and on abdomen.

A—Diffuse into the air. Inhale directly or applied to hands, tissue, or a cotton wick.

Pride:

Oils—**AT**Peppermint (dispels).

A—Inhale directly or applied to hands. Diffuse into the air.

T—Apply to auricular emotion points. Apply to crown chakra.

Procrastination:

Oils—**AT**Motivation (easier to take action; gets you out of the mood of procrastination), **AT**Magnify Your Purpose (empowering and uplifting), **AT**Acceptance, **AT**Envision (emotional support).

A—Inhale directly or applied to hands. Diffuse into the air.

T—Apply to auricular emotion points. Dilute with V-6 Oil to create a massage oil, and massage into skin. Apply to crown chakra.

A=Aromatic **T**=Topical **I**=Internal

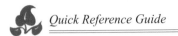

Progesterone:

Oils—**ᴬᵀ**<u>EndoFlex</u>, **ᴬᵀ**<u>Grounding</u>.

A—Inhale directly. Diffuse into the air.

T—Dilute as necessary, and apply to lower abdomen, lower back, or to Vita Flex points on the feet.

***Comments—Progesterone is made from cholesterol and helps to protect against cancer.

Personal Care—PD 80/20, Prenolone/Prenolone+, Progessence/Progessence Plus.

Prosperity:

Oils—**ᴬᵀ**<u>Abundance</u>, **ᴬᵀ**bergamot, **ᴬ**cinnamon bark, **ᴬᵀ**cypress.

A—Inhale directly or applied to hands. Diffuse into the air. Wear as perfume or cologne.

T—Apply to auricular emotion points. Apply to crown and heart chakra. Add 1–3 drops to 1/4 cup Epsom salts, and dissolve in warm bathwater before bathing.

Prostate:

▸▸ *The prostate gland is a small organ just beneath that bladder that is part of the male reproductive system. Its primary function is to create and store fluid that helps nourish and protect the sperm.*

Oils—**ᵀ**Frankincense, **ᵀ**<u>Mister</u>, **ᵀ**<u>Australian Blue</u>, **ᵀ**<u>EndoFlex</u>, **ᵀ**blue cypress, **ᵀ**<u>Gratitude</u>, **ᵀ**helichrysum, **ᵀ**juniper, **ᵀ**<u>Juva Cleanse</u>, **ᵀ**yarrow.

T—Dilute as necessary, and apply to the posterior, scrotum, ankles, lower back, or bottoms of feet. Add 5 drops to 1 Tbs. V-6 Oil or olive oil; insert into rectum, and retain throughout the night.

Personal Care—Progessence/Progessence Plus, PD 80/20, Prenolone/Prenolone+, Protec (designed to accompany the night long retention enema, it helps buffer the prostate from inflammation, enlargement, and tumor activity).

Supplements—Prostate Health (an herbal support for the male glandular system; it may prevent prostate atrophy and malfunction and protect men from prostate cancer), Master Formula.

—DECONGESTANT

Oils—ᵀMister (decongests prostate and balances hormones), ᵀ_Fcypress, ᵀ_Fspruce, ᵀ_Fmyrtle, ᵀImmuPower, ᵀDi-Gize, ᵀDragon Time, ᵀmyrrh, ᵀsage, ᵀyarrow.

T—Apply oils to inside ankle and heel. ImmuPower on lower spine and in rectum.

Blend #1—Combine 15 drops frankincense and 5 drops Mister with 2 tsp. V-6 Oil. Insert blend into rectum with bulb syringe or pipet, and retain throughout night.

P

Blend #2—Combine 10 drops frankincense and 10 drops lavender with 2 tsp. V-6 Oil. Insert blend into rectum with bulb syringe, and retain throughout night.

Blend #3—Combine 10 drops frankincense, 5 drops myrrh, and 3 drops sage with 2 tsp. V-6 Oil. Insert blend into rectum with bulb syringe or pipet, and retain through night.

***Comments—*Abundant Health offers dispensing syringes with rectal insertion tips.*

—ENLARGEMENT (BENIGN PROSTATIC HYPERPLASIA)

▸▸ *The size of the prostate begins at about the same size as a walnut, but the size increases as a male ages. If the prostate grows too large, it can block passage of urine from the bladder through the urethra. This blockage can lead to an increased risk for developing urinary tract stones, infections, or damaged kidneys.*

Recipe #1—Mix 10 drops of Mister with 1 Tbs. of V-6 Oil; insert in rectum, and retain overnight. May also apply either sage, fennel, or yarrow to posterior, scrotum, ankles, lower back, and bottoms of feet.

—INFLAMED/PROSTATITIS

▸▸ *Prostatitis is an inflamed prostate, typically due to infection. This can cause pain in the lower back and groin area, painful urination, and the need to urinate frequently.*

Oils—ᵀCypress, ᵀlavender, ᵀthyme (Alternative Medicine—A Definitive Guide, p. 742).

T—Dilute as necessary, and apply to the posterior, scrotum, ankles, lower back, or bottoms of feet. Add 5 drops to 1 Tbs. V-6 Oil or olive oil; insert into rectum, and retain throughout the night.

—STRENGTHEN

Supplements—PD 80/20, Prenolone/Prenolone+, Prostate Health, Protec.

—THOUGHT PATTERNS AND EMOTIONS

***Comments—The prostate represents the masculine principle. Men's **prostate problems** have a lot to do with low self-worth and with an incorrect belief that as they get older they become less of a man. Ideas may be in conflict about sex, refus-

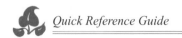

ing to let go of the past, fearing aging, and feeling like throwing in the towel. They may be feeling inadequate in their sexual role, may be holding onto unpleasant memories of previous relationships, or may be feeling unfulfilled in love.

Prostate Cancer: *See Cancer: PROSTATE.*

Protection: (from negative influence)

Oils—^AClove, ^{AT}cypress, ^{AT}fennel (protection from psychic attack), ^Afir, ^{AT}frankincense, ^{AT}<u>Harmony</u>, ^{AT}<u>Joy</u>, ^{AT}palo santo,^{AT}<u>Sacred Mountain</u>, ^{AT}<u>Valor</u>, ^{AT}<u>White Angelica</u>.

A—Diffuse into the air. Inhale directly or applied to hands.

T—Dilute as necessary, and apply to temples, forehead, heart, or crown of the head.

Protein:

*****Comments**—Carbonated water prevents the absorption of protein. Protein deficiency causes hypoglycemia.

> *A **protein deficiency**, either from the lack of protein intake or from the inability to digest it, creates an acidic pH in the blood. A high acidity level in the blood creates an environment for cell mutation and disease. See Acidosis.*

Supplements—**Digest + Cleanse, Essentialzyme, Essentialzymes-4, MultiGreens, Power Meal** (pre-digested protein), **Pure Protein Complete, Sulfurzyme** (helps digest protein).

Psoriasis: *See also Skin.*

≫ *Psoriasis is a skin condition characterized by patches of red, scaly skin. The most commonly affected areas are the elbows, knees, scalp, back, face, palms, and feet. But other areas can be affected as well. Psoriasis does not have a known cure, but there are medications and creams to lessen the symptoms. Psoriasis tends to be less severe in the warmer months.*

Oils—^T_F**Helichrysum,** ^T_F**thyme,** ^Tbergamot, ^Tcajeput, ^Tcedarwood, ^Tlavender, ^Ttea tree, ^Tpatchouli, ^TRoman chamomile.

T—Dilute as necessary, and apply on location.

Blend #1—Combine 2–3 drops each of Roman chamomile and lavender for use as an ointment for pH Balance.

Personal Care—**A·R·T Skin Care System, Rose Ointment** (helps soften cracking skin), **Essential Beauty Serum - Dry Skin Blend, Lavender Volume Shampoo** and **Lavender Volume Conditioner** for psoriasis of the scalp.

Supplements—AlkaLime, Balance Complete, Cleansing Trio (ComforTone, Essentialzyme, and ICP), Digest + Cleanse, JuvaPower/JuvaSpice, JuvaTone, Sulfurzyme.

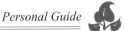

Psychic:

Oils—**^ACinnamon bark** (awareness), **^Afennel** (protect from attack), **^Alemongrass**.

—Centers

Oils—**^AElemi** (balances, strengthens, fortifies).

A—Diffuse into the air.

Puberty:

Oils—**^{TA}Fleabane** (stimulates retarded puberty).

T—Dilute as necessary, and apply to lower abdomen, lower back, and bottoms of feet.

A—Diffuse into the air. Inhale directly.

Pulmonary: *See Respiratory System:* Lungs.

Purge: *See Cleansing.*

Purification:

Oils—**^{AT}Purification,** **^{AT}lemon,** **^{AT}**<u>Abundance</u>, **^{AT}**<u>Acceptance</u>, **^{AT}cedarwood,** **^{AT}**<u>En-R-Gee</u>, **^Aeucalyptus,** **^Afennel,** **^Alemongrass,** **^{TA}tea tree,** **^Aorange,** **^{AT}sage**.

—Air

Oils—**^ALemon,** **^{TA}Hong Kuai** (diffuse, or add to a spray bottle of water to deodorize and sterilize the air).

—Cigarette Smoke

Oils—**^A**<u>Purification</u>.

—Dishes

Recipe #1—2 drops of <u>Melrose</u> or lemon in the dishwater for sparkling dishes and a great-smelling kitchen.

—Water

Oils—**^I_FLemon,** **^Ipeppermint**.

—Clothing

Recipe #2—Adding oils to the washer or dryer decreases bacteria, improves hygiene, and gives clothes a fresh, clean smell.

—Furniture

Recipe #3—A few drops of fir, lemon, or spruce oil on a dust cloth, or 10 drops in a 1 oz. glass or plastic spray bottle filled with distilled water, works well for polish-

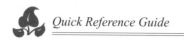

ing, cleaning, and disinfecting furniture, kitchens, and bathrooms. You may also consider adding <u>Abundance</u> to increase your abundance. Lemon oil works for dissolving gum and grease. Use <u>Purification</u> for mold and fungus. If you don't have a diffuser, you may want to add 10–12 drops of <u>Purification</u> to 8 oz. of distilled water in a spray bottle, and spray into the air.

A—Diffuse into the air. Add 10–15 drops to 1–2 oz. distilled water in a spray bottle; shake, and mist into the air.

T—Add 3–5 drops to 1 oz. water; soak rag in water, and apply on location. Add 1–2 drops to warm bathwater before bathing. Add 1–2 drops to a bowl of water, and use to soak fruits and vegetables.

I—Add 1–2 drops to 8–16 oz. water; wait 5 minutes, and drink.

Pus: *See also Antibacterial, Infection, and Anti-infectious.*

Oils—Tea tree is useful in healing pus-filled wounds.

Radiation: *See Cancer.*

>> *Radiation is energy emitted from a source and sent through space or matter. Different forms of radiation can include light, heat, sound, radio, microwaves, gamma rays, or X-rays, among others. While many forms of radiation are around us every day and are perfectly safe (such as light, sound, and heat), frequent or prolonged exposure to high-energy forms of radiation can be detrimental to the body, possibly causing DNA mutation, damaged cellular structures, burns, cancer, or other damage.*

Oils—ᴵᵀPeppermint[374] (gamma), ᵀsandalwood[375] (UV), ᵀtamanu[376] (UV), ᵀᴬTea tree quinquenervia, ᵀᴬ<u>Melrose</u>, ᵀᴬpatchouli.

—Cᴏᴍᴘᴜᴛᴇʀ, TV, Mɪᴄʀᴏᴡᴀᴠᴇ

    Recipe #3—Fill a wooden bowl half full of peat moss and half full of hazelnuts. Add 30 drops of <u>Melrose</u>, and then set the bowl on top of the appliance. Using an equipment diode may also help (available from Abundant Health).

    Comments— *<u>Melrose</u> may help protect the body during radiation treatments if used 10 days before, during, and 10 days after.* **Do not use on the day** *of* **radiation treatment***. According to Dr. Pénoël, massage with Tea tree quinquenervia helps to prevent radiation side effects. Remember to keep all massage light and away from trauma area.*

—RADIATION BURNS

>> *A radiation burn is skin damage due to radiation exposure. Radiation burns include anything from sunburns to burns caused by medical radiation treatments. Radiation burns are generally recognized by their red appearance and can be quite painful.*

Recipe #1.

—SIDE-EFFECTS

>> *The possible side effects of radiation therapy are numerous and depend, in part, on which area of the body is being treated. Some common side effects include nausea, hair loss (if the head is exposed to radiation), fatigue, low blood count, skin damage, scarring, diarrhea, swelling, and difficulty swallowing. The majority of these side effects will only last for a couple of months after the treatment has been completed. Other side effects, although more rare, can potentially appear six or more months after the treatment has been completed. These later side effects may include infertility, secondary cancer, lymphedema (swelling in the arm or leg), joint problems, and mouth problems.*

Recipe #2.

—TREATMENTS

> *Valerie Worwood suggests Recipe #1 below to be used at least two to three weeks before the radiation treatments begin. Don't use it during the treatment, but use it between treatments and for at least a month after your last treatment.*

> ***RECIPE #1***—*10 drops lavender, 5 drops German chamomile, 5 drops Roman chamomile, 5 drops tagetes, 5 drops yarrow, and 2 tsp. of vinca infused oil. Massage the entire torso, including the back and abdomen and the trauma area. This treatment will not conflict with the doctor's treatment. Note: Vinca is made from periwinkle, which is known to contain alkaloids that in some cases can suppress the cancerous cells. (The Complete Book of Essential Oils & Aromatherapy, pp. 249–50).*

> *The following Dr. Westlake formula utilizes Bach Flower Remedies to counteract the side effects of cancer patients who have received radiation therapy.*

> ***RECIPE #2***—*"Mix 3.5 grams of sea salt with 100 ml of distilled water. In a 10 ml dropper bottle, combine 2 drops of each of the following Bach Flower Remedies: Cherry Plum, Gentian, Rock Rose, Star of Bethlehem, Vine, Walnut and Wild Oat. Top off the bottle with the sea salt solution. Take 2 drops 3 to 4 times a day, or add 10 to 15 drops to a bath. People who have been exposed to radiation sources, such as X-rays, cobalt therapy or other medical radiation therapies, or who have been contaminated in an escape from a nuclear power station, or who regularly use office or domestic equipment that gives out low-level radiation, such as color television sets, microwaves, and visual display units, would do well to use this formula in a bath once or twice a week." (Aromatherapy—An A to Z by Patricia Davis, p. 269)*

*****Comments**—Radiation treatments can produce tremendous toxicity within the liver. Cut down on the use of oils with high phenol content to prevent increasing the liver toxicity.

–CHEMOTHERAPY

>> *Chemotherapy is the use of chemical drugs to treat cancer. Chemotherapy attacks rapidly dividing cells, so it can often negatively affect normal cells as well, such as those related to bone marrow, hair, skin, mouth, stomach, and intestines.*

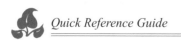

          *****Comments**—Because of the greater amounts of toxicity produced, even greater care should be taken to limit the use of oils with high *phenol* content.

—WEEPING WOUNDS FROM

    Oils—ᵀTea tree, ᵀoregano, ᵀthyme.

    Supplements—The apple pectin that is contained in **ICP** helps remove unwanted metals and toxins. It is also valuable in radiation therapy.

T—Dilute as necessary, and apply on location, bottoms of feet, kidneys, or thyroid.

I—Place 2–3 drops in an empty capsule, and swallow.

A—Diffuse into the air.

Rashes: *See Skin:* RASHES.

Raynaud's Disease:

>> *Raynaud's disease is a condition that causes the arteries supplying blood to the skin to suddenly narrow and inhibit blood circulation. As a result, specific areas of the body feel numb and cool. The most commonly affected areas are the toes, fingers, nose, and ears. During an attack, the skin turns white and then blue. As circulation returns and warms the affected areas, a prickling, throbbing, stinging, or swelling sensation often accompanies it. These attacks are often triggered by cold temperatures and by stress.*

    Oils—ᵀᴬCypress, ᵀᴬ<u>Aroma Life</u>, ᵀᴬclove, ᵀᴬfennel, ᵀᴬgeranium, ᵀᴬhelichrysum, ᵀᴬlavender, ᵀᴬnutmeg, ᵀᴬrosemary.

T—Dilute as necessary, and apply on the affected area, carotid arteries, and on Vita Flex points on the feet.

A—Diffuse into the air. Inhale oil directly or applied to hands, tissue, or a cotton wick.

Regenerating:

    Oils—ᵀHelichrysum, ᵀlavender, ᵀ<u>Melrose</u>.

T—Dilute as necessary, and apply on location. Dilute with V-6 Oil to create a massage oil, and massage into skin.

Blend #1—Blend equal parts of <u>Thieves</u> and V-6 Oil, and apply on location.

Supplements—Power Meal, Master Formula.

Rejection:

    Oils—ᵀᴬ<u>Acceptance</u>, ᵀᴬ<u>Joy</u>, ᴬᵀOola Family.

T—Apply to rejection auricular emotion point. Dilute with V-6 Oil to create a massage oil, and massage into skin.

A—Inhale directly or applied to hands. Diffuse into the air.

Relationships:

Oils—^{AT}Oola Family,

Personal Care—**Sensation Bath & Shower Gel** contains oils used by Cleopatra to enhance love and to increase the desire to be close to that someone special. **Sensation Massage Oil** creates an exotic arousal and increases sexual desire. The fragrance creates a peaceful and harmonious feeling that is helpful in easing relationship stress. **Sensation Hand & Body Lotion.**

—ENHANCING

Oils—^{TA}<u>Lady Sclareol</u> (especially for the woman—best if applied by male partner), ^{TA}ylang ylang.

—ENDING RELATIONSHIPS

Oils—^ABasil.

T—Dilute with V-6 Oil, and massage onto skin.

A—Diffuse into the air. Inhale directly or applied to hands.

Relaxation:

Oils—^{AT}Lavender[377], ^T<u>Tranquil</u> (roll-on), ^{TA}ylang ylang[378], ^Alemon[379], ^T<u>Stress Away</u>, ^{AT}<u>Peace & Calming</u>, ^A<u>Citrus Fresh</u>, ^Trose[380], ^{AT}mastrante, ^{AT}clary sage, ^{AT}frankincense, ^{AT}<u>Gentle Baby</u>, ^{AT}geranium, ^{AT}jasmine, ^{AT}Roman chamomile, ^{AT}sandalwood, ^{AT}<u>Trauma Life</u> (calming).

Supplements—SleepEssence (short-term only).

Personal Care—Relaxation Massage Oil, Evening Peace Bath & Shower Gel.

—DIFFUSION *See Negative Ions for oils that produce negative ions when diffused to help promote relaxation.*

Oils—^ALavender, ^A<u>Peace & Calming</u>.

—SENSE OF

Oils—^{AT}Ylang ylang.

Blend #1—1 drop bergamot, 2 drops lavender, 2 drops marjoram, and 4 drops rosewood.

A—Diffuse into the air. Inhale directly or applied to hands, tissue, or a cotton wick.

T—Dilute with V-6 Oil to create a massage oil, and massage into skin. Place 3–5 drops in 1/4 cup Epsom salts or other bath salts, and dissolve in warm bathwater before bathing.

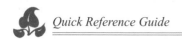

Release Negative Trauma:

Oils—**AT**Inspiration, **AT**Release, **AT**Transformation.

A—Diffuse into the air. Inhale directly or applied to hands.

T—Dilute as necessary, and apply to temples, forehead, heart, or crown of the head.

Resentment:

Oils—**AT**Forgiveness, **AT**Harmony, **AT**Humility, **AT**Idaho tansy, **AT**jasmine, **AT**Release, **AT**rose, **AT**White Angelica.

A—Diffuse into the air. Inhale directly or applied to tissue or a cotton wick.

T—Apply to auricular emotion points. Dilute with V-6 Oil to create a massage oil, and massage onto the skin.

Respiratory System: *see also Bronchitis, Pleurisy, Pneumonia.*

▸▸ *The Respiratory System's primary purposes are to supply the blood with oxygen, which is then delivered to all parts of the body, and to remove waste carbon dioxide from the blood and eliminate it from the body. The Respiratory system consists of the mouth, nose, and pharynx (through which air is first taken in), larynx (voice box),*

> *Vita Flex points for the bronchial tubes are located between the bones on the tops of the feet. The sinus points are located at the base of the middle three toes on the bottoms of the feet. One of the most effective ways to handle a respiratory problem is by doing rectal implants. There is a nerve that goes from the rectum to the lungs. The oils will travel in this manner in 3 seconds. The next best method is through inhalation.*

trachea (airway leading from the larynx to the lungs), bronchi (which branch off from the trachea and go into the lungs), bronchiole (smaller tubes that branch off from the bronchi), alveoli (tiny sacs filled with capillaries that allow inhaled oxygen to be transferred into the blood and carbon dioxide to be expelled from the blood into the air in the lungs), pleura (which covers the outside of the lungs and the inside of the chest wall), and diaphragm (a large muscle at the bottom of the chest cavity that moves to pull air into the lungs (inhale), and to push air out of the lungs (exhale).

Oils—**AT**RC, **AT**Raven (all respiratory problems), **AT**_Feucalyptus[381] (general stimulant and strengthener), **AT**Eucalyptus radiata, **AT**_Fpeppermint[382] (aid), **AT**eucalyptus blue (infection), **AT**_Ffir (opens respiratory tract, increases oxygenation, decongests, and balances), **AT**_Fmyrtle, **AT**_Fspearmint, **T**Breathe Again, **AT**dorado azul, **AT**cinnamon[383], **AT**Thieves (diffuse with *Eucalyptus radiata*; add spruce to help push the oils deeper into the lungs), **AT**Abundance, **AT**anise, **AT**basil (restorative), **AT**bergamot (infections), **AT**cajeput (infections), **AT**clary sage (strengthens), **AT**clove, **AT**Di-Gize, **AT**EndoFlex, **AT**fennel (stimulant), **AT**frankincense, **AT**goldenrod (discharges mucus), **AT**GLF, **AT**helichrysum (relieves), **AT**hyssop (opens respiratory system and discharges toxins and mucus),

^{AT}JuvaFlex, ^{AT}ledum (supports), ^{AT}lemon, ^{AT}marjoram (calming), ^{AT}tea tree, ^{AT}Tea tree ericifolia, ^{AT}Melrose, ^{AT}oregano (antiseptic), ^{AT}pine (dilates and opens bronchial tract), ^{AT}ravintsara, ^{AT}rosemary verbenon, ^{AT}Sacred Mountain (soothing), ^{AT}sage lavender, ^{AT}spruce (combine with any eucalyptus oils, especially *Eucalyptus polybractea*), ^{AT}tsuga (dilates and opens tract).

Supplements—Inner Defense, Super C / Super C Chewable.

Recipe #1—Dr. Young alternates the oils of <u>Raven</u> and <u>RC</u> in rectal implants. He uses 20 drops of the oil in 1 Tbs. of V-6 Oil and implants it rectally using a pipet (glass dropper) or a syringe with a rectal insertion tip (*available at Abundant Health*).

Blend #1—3 drops wintergreen, 8 drops eucalyptus, 6 drops fir, 6 drops frankincense, 1 drop peppermint, 10 drops ravintsara, and 1 oz. V-6 Oil.

Blend #2—3 drops German chamomile, 10 drops fir, and 5 drops lemon.

R

—ACUTE

Oils—^{AT}RC and ^{AT}Raven, ^{AT-}Thieves.

Blend #3—5 drops eucalyptus, 8 drops frankincense, and 6 drops lemon. Add to 1 oz. V-6 Oil for a hot compress on chest, and rub neat (without V-6) on bottoms of feet under toes.

Blend #4—3 tsp. *Eucalyptus radiata* (or any oil from the Myrtaceae botanical family)

> *My 18-year-old daughter has had **respiratory problems** for years, and finally the doctors put her on inhalers. These helped, but she did not like the way they made her feel. Soon after I started using therapeutic grade essential oils, we began using them on her. After a few weeks, she was off her inhalers and has never needed them since. She has, however, had the occasional upper-respiratory infection, which in the past has always led to a bout with bronchitis and several months of coughing. Now, we apply oils and the infection goes away without bronchitis ever showing up. This has saved vacations and more! We apply the oils to her chest, back, and feet twice a day. The oils we use are hyssop, myrrh, and two Young Living blends—<u>RC</u> and <u>Raven</u>.*
> *-Submitted by Lauren Martin (July 2004)*

and 1 tsp. balsam fir (or any conifer oil). Apply to Vita Flex points on the feet; add to V-6 Oil, and apply to chest area; or diffuse.

Blend #5—10 drops each of *Eucalyptus radiata* and myrrh. Add to 1 Tbs. of V-6 Oil, and insert rectally with a syringe for an overnight retention enema. Works well for all lung conditions, including emphysema, pneumonia, and tuberculosis.

—BREATHING

Oils—^{AT}Raven, ^{AT}RC (may work instead of an inhaler), ^{AT}frankincense, ^{AT}cinnamon bark, ^{AT}Exodus II, ^{AT}ginger, ^{AT}hyssop, ^{AT}juniper, ^{AT}marjoram, ^{AT}nutmeg, ^{AT}Roman chamomile, ^{AT}rosemary, ^{AT}thyme.

—HYPERPNEA (ABNORMAL RAPID BREATHING)

Oils—^{TA}_FYlang ylang (lung area and Vita Flex points).

A=Aromatic   **T**=Topical   **I**=Internal

—LUNGS

    Oils—^{AT}<u>Raven</u> (stronger than <u>RC</u>), ^{AT}_Feucalyptus, ^{AT}<u>RC</u> (diffuse to open lungs and to send oxygen to red blood cells),^{AT}<u>Aroma Life</u>, ^{AT}<u>Believe</u>, ^{AT}copaiba (stimulates), ^{AT}<u>Forgiveness</u>, ^{AT}frankincense (stimulates), ^{AT}hyssop (diffuse to clear lungs of mucus), ^{AT}<u>Joy</u>, ^{AT}ravintsara, ^{AT}<u>Thieves</u>.

    Blend #5—Equal parts *Tea tree ericifolia* and either <u>RC</u> or <u>Raven</u> (depending on strength desired). Add to 1 oz. V-6 Oil, and insert into rectum for retention (at least 15 min., if not overnight). Rectal implant is one of the quickest ways to affect the lungs.

    –PULMONARY ARTERY/VEIN

        Oils—^{TA}<u>Aroma Life</u>, ^{TA}_Fsage, ^{TA}_Fsandalwood, ^{TA}cypress, ^{TA}eucalyptus, ^{TA}pine (antiseptic).

> *The pulmonary is the designated artery conveying blood from the right ventricle of the heart to the lungs or any of the veins conveying oxygenated blood from the lungs to the left atrium of the heart.*

—OXYGEN

    Oils—^{AT}Cedarwood, ^{AT}frankincense, ^{AT}sandalwood, ^{AT}all essential oils.

    Personal Care—Satin Facial Scrub - Mint (deep cleansing that dispenses nutrients and oxygen). Mix with Orange Blossom Facial Wash for a milder cleanse.

—SHORTNESS OF BREATH

    Oils—^{AT}<u>Aroma Life</u>.

    Blend #1—For shortness of breath due to overexertion (lots of work, no sleep, etc.), add 10 drops each of eucalyptus and peppermint to a basin of lukewarm water. Soak some cloths in this water, and wring them out—leaving them fairly moist. Then wrap the joints (ankles, knees, wrists, elbows, and neck) with the cloths. While relaxing and allowing the compresses to cool the joints, have another person do Vita Flex on the Pineal Gland and Adrenal Gland points on the feet.

A—Diffuse into the air. Inhale directly; or apply to hands, tissue, or a cotton wick, and inhale. Add 3–4 drops to a small bowl of steaming-hot water, and inhale the vapors.

T—Dilute as necessary, and apply to chest, sinuses, neck, or Vita Flex points on the feet. Add 2–3 drops to water, and gargle. Apply to chest as a warm compress.

Restlessness: *See also Calming.*

    Oils—^{AT}<u>RutaVaLa</u>, ^{AT}lavender, ^{AT}<u>Peace & Calming</u>, ^T<u>Tranquil</u> (roll-on), ^{AT}orange, ^{AT}valerian, ^{AT}<u>Acceptance</u>, ^{AT}angelica, ^{AT}basil, ^{AT}bergamot, ^{AT}cedarwood, ^{AT}frankincense, ^{AT}<u>Gathering</u>, ^{AT}geranium, ^{AT}<u>Harmony</u>, ^{AT}<u>Inspiration</u>, ^{AT}<u>Joy</u>, ^{AT}rose, ^{AT}rosewood, ^{AT}<u>Sacred Mountain</u>, ^{AT}spruce, ^{AT}<u>Trauma Life</u>, ^{AT}<u>Valor</u>, ^{AT}ylang ylang.

A—Diffuse into the air. Inhale directly or applied to hands.

T—Dilute with V-6 Oil to create a massage oil, and massage onto the skin. Add 3–5 drops to 1/4 cup bath salts, and dissolve salts in warm bathwater before bathing. Dilute as necessary, and apply to wrists.

Rheumatic Fever:

▸▸ *Rheumatic fever is a complication of strep throat or scarlet fever. It is an inflammatory disease that can cause permanent damage to the heart. Symptoms of rheumatic fever include painful and swollen joints, chest pain, fever, fatigue, the sensation of a pounding heartbeat, shortness of breath, rash, sudden jerky body movements, and unusual displays of emotion. Rheumatic fever is most common in children between ages 5 and age 15.*

Oils—^T_FTarragon, ^Tginger. Both help with pain.

T—Dilute as necessary, and apply on location or on Vita Flex points on the feet.

R

Rheumatism: *See Muscles, Arthritis.*

Rhinitis:

▸▸ *Rhinitis is inflammation of the nasal mucus membrane. Rhinitis is commonly caused by viral infections and allergies and can be acute (short-term) or chronic (long-term). Symptoms of Rhinitis may include runny nose, sneezing, congestions, and ear problems.*

Oils—^{AT}Basil, ^{AT}sage lavender.

A—Diffuse into the air and inhale mist through nose.

T—Dilute as necessary, and apply to sinuses, sides of nose, or to Vita Flex points on the feet.

Rhinopharyngitis:

▸▸ *Rhinopharyngitis is an inflammation of the mucus membrane and the pharynx. Symptoms include high fever, reduced sense of smell, runny nose, sneezing, and a red, swollen throat. Rhinopharyngitis is the precursor of the common cold.*

Oils—^A_FRavintsara.

A—Diffuse into the air, and inhale mist through nose.

Ringworm: *See Antifungal: Ringworm.*

Romantic Touches:

Oils—^TJasmine, ^T<u>Lady Sclareol</u>, ^Tpatchouli, ^T<u>Sensation</u>, ^Tylang ylang.

A=Aromatic   **T**=Topical   **I**=Internal |

T—Dilute with V-6 Oil, and apply a small amount on location.

Personal Care—Sensation Massage Oil, Sensation Bath & Shower Gel, Sensation Hand & Body Lotion.

Rosacea (Acne Rosacea): *See Acne: ROSACEA*

Sacredness:

Oils—^{AT}Sacred Mountain (sacred place of protection within self).

A—Inhale directly or applied to hands, tissue, or a cotton wick. Diffuse into the air.

T—Apply to crown chakra. Dilute with V-6 Oil to create a massage oil, and massage onto the skin.

Sadness:

Oils—^{AT}Joy (over heart), ^{AT}Acceptance, ^{AT}helichrysum, ^{AT}Inspiration, ^Tonycha (combine with rose in V-6 Oil for calming/uplifting massage), ^{AT}orange (overcome), ^{AT}3 Wise Men, ^{AT}Transformation, ^{AT}Valor.

A—Diffuse into the air. Inhale directly or applied to tissue or a cotton wick. Wear as a perfume or cologne.

T—Apply to auricular emotion points. Dilute with V-6 Oil to create a massage oil, and massage onto the skin.

Saint Vitus' Dance (Chorea):

▸▸ *Chorea is a neurological disorder that is characterized by rapid, irregular, involuntary movements of the body. These movements can affect the hands, feet, neck, trunk, and face. They are irregular and seem to move randomly from one body part to another. The quick movements of the feet and hands are similar to dancing and piano playing.*

Blend #1—5 drops Aroma Siez, 3 drops basil, 6 drops juniper, and 8 drops peppermint.

Sanitation: *See also Antibacterial, Antifungal, Antiviral.*

Oils—^TPurification, ^Tcitronella, ^Tlemongrass.

T—Add 5–10 drops to a small bowl of water, and use water to clean counters and other surfaces.

Scabies: *See Skin: SCABIES.*

Scarring:

>> *Scars are fibrous connective tissue that is used to quickly repair a wound or injury and replace the damaged skin or tissue Scar tissue is often not as strong or as functional as the regular tissue.*

Oils—^T_F**Lavender** (burns), ^T**helichrysum** (reduces), ^T__Gentle Baby__, ^T**rose** (prevents), ^T**frankincense** (prevents), ^T**geranium**, ^T**hyssop** (prevents), ^T__Melrose__, ^T**rosehip** (reduces).

Personal Care—**A·R·T Skin Care System, Lavender Hand & Body Lotion** (moisturizes skin and promotes healing).

Blend #1—Equal parts helichrysum and lavender mixed with liquid lecithin.

Blend #2—3 drops rosemary, 15 drops rosewood, and 1¾ oz. hazelnut oil.

Blend #3—6 drops lavender, 3 drops patchouli, 4 drops rosewood, and vitamin E oil.

—PREVENT FORMATION

Oils—^T**Frankincense**, ^T**helichrysum**, ^T**rose**, ^T**hyssop**, ^T**myrrh**, ^T**rosehip seed**.

Blend #4—5 drops helichrysum, 2 drops patchouli, 4 drops lemongrass, and 3 drops lavender in ¼–½ oz. V-6 Oil.

Blend #5—Equal parts lavender, lemongrass, and geranium.

T—Dilute as necessary, and apply on location.

Schmidt's Syndrome: *See Adrenal Glands: ADDISON'S DISEASE.*

Sciatica:

>> *The sciatic nerve (the longest nerve in the body) runs from the spinal cord through the buttock and hip area and down the back of each leg. When this nerve is pinched or irritated due to something such as a herniated disc, it can cause pain in the area, numbness and weakness, tingling sensations, or a loss of bladder or bowel control.*

Oils—^T**Cistus** (followed by peppermint), ^T_F**thyme**, ^T_F**helichrysum**, ^T_F**tarragon** (with Idaho tansy—can promote sciatic regeneration), ^T**peppermint**, ^T__Aroma Life__, ^T**cardamom**, ^T**fir**, ^T__Gentle Baby__, ^T**hyssop**, ^T__M-Grain__, ^T__PanAway__, ^T__Relieve It__, ^T**sandalwood**, ^T**spruce** (alleviates pain), ^T__Valor__.

T—Apply over area with a cold compress. Dilute as necessary, and apply on lower back, buttocks, or legs. Dilute with V-6 Oil to create a massage oil, and massage on location.

Recipe #1 Apply one (or more) of the above oils with a cold compress, and lightly massage with Roman chamomile or lavender and wintergreen. Relief can also be obtained by applying Joy and lavender to the bottoms of the feet.

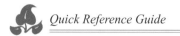

Blend #1—Tarragon, balsam fir, and spearmint (small amount) or tarragon, basil, and peppermint.

Personal Care—Ortho Ease Massage Oil.

Recipe #2—Apply frankincense to the top of the spine (at the base of the skull), and work the oil in. Then apply 3–5 drops of each of the following oils, one at a time, up the back of the neck, and work each one in individually: valerian, vetiver, balsam fir, and tarragon. While working each one into the spine, a glass probe or glass dropper can be used to gently stimulate the tops of each of the vertebrae.

Scoliosis: *See Back: Scoliosis.*

Scrapes: *See also Cuts, Wounds.*

Oils—^TLavender, ^Travintsara.

T—Dilute as necessary, and apply on location.

Scurvy:

» *Scurvy is a disease caused by a deficiency of ascorbic acid (vitamin C). Some results of scurvy are general weakness, anemia, gum disease (gingivitis), skin hemorrhages, spots on the skin (usually the thighs and legs), and bleeding from the mucus membranes.*

Oils—^T_FGinger.

T—Dilute as necessary, and apply over kidneys, liver, and on corresponding Vita Flex points on the feet.

Supplements—Super C / Super C Chewable.

Security:

Oils—^{AT}<u>Christmas Spirit</u>, ^{AT}<u>Sacred Mountain</u>.

—Creating

    Oils—^{AT}Acceptance, ^{AT}Roman chamomile.

—Feeling Of

    Oils—^ACypress.

—In the Home

    Oils—^{AT}Bergamot.

—Self Secure

    Oils—^{AT}Oregano.

A—Diffuse into the air. Inhale directly or applied to hands, tissue, or a cotton wick.

T—Dilute with V-6 Oil to create a massage oil, and massage into skin. Apply to auricular emotion points. Add 3–5 drops to 1/4 cup Epsom salts, and dissolve in warm bathwater before bathing.

Sedative: *See Calming:* SEDATIVE.

Seizure:

>> *A seizure is an uncontrolled, abnormal electrical discharge in the brain that may produce physical convulsions, minor physical signs, thought disturbances, or a combination of symptoms. The symptoms depend on what parts of the brain are involved.*

—CONVULSIONS

>> *A convulsion is the repeated, rapid contracting and relaxing of muscles resulting in the uncontrollable shaking of the body. Convulsions usually last about 30 seconds to 2 minutes and are often associated with seizures.*

Oils—[TA]Clary sage, [TA]lavender[384], [TA]Valor, [TA]Brain Power, [TA]neroli, [TA]Roman chamomile.

Supplements—KidScents MightyVites, Mineral Essence, Ultra Young+.

—EPILEPSY

>> *Epilepsy is a neurological condition where the person has recurring, unpredictable seizures. Epilepsy has many possible causes, although in many cases the cause is unknown. Possible causes may include illness, injury to the brain, or abnormal brain development.*

> **OILS TO AVOID IF EPILEPTIC**
>
> *There are several oils that should not be used if prone to epilepsy. Please see the Appendix for safety data on the oils and products mentioned in this book. For further contraindication information, please consult the following books:*
>
> *Essential Oil Safety—A Guide for Health Care Professionals by Robert Tisserand and Tony Balacs and Aromatherapy for Health Professionals by Shirley and Len Price.*

Oils—[TA]Brain Power, [TA]clary sage.

Supplements—Cleansing Trio (ComforTone, Essentialzyme, ICP), JuvaPower/ JuvaSpice.

—GRAND MAL

>> *The grand mal seizure, also known as the tonic-clonic seizure, is the most common seizure. The tonic phase last about 10–20 seconds. During this stage, the person looses consciousness and the muscles contract, causing the person to fall down. During the clonic phase, the person experiences violent convulsions. This phase usually lasts less than two minutes.*

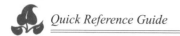
    Recipe #1—Need to support the body. <u>Aroma Siez</u> (apply using the Raindrop Technique up the spine), <u>Brain Power</u> and <u>Peace & Calming</u> (diffuse, and apply around naval), <u>Joy</u> (over the heart), <u>Sacred Mountain</u> (back of neck and crown), and <u>Valor</u> (on feet).

    Supplements—Cleansing Trio (ComforTone, Essentialzyme, and ICP), JuvaPower, Omega Blue, OmegaGize³.

    *****Comments**—Grand Mal seizures can sometimes be caused by zinc and copper imbalance. Mineral Essence provides zinc and copper in both ionic and colloidal form for optimal assimilation.

T—Dilute as necessary, and apply to back of neck and to brain Vita Flex points on bottoms of feet.

A—Inhale directly or applied to hands. Diffuse into the air.

Self Adjustment:

Oils—^{TA}<u>Awaken</u>.

    T—Dilute with V-6 Oil to create a massage oil, and massage into skin. Apply to auricular emotion points. Add 3–5 drops to 1/4 cup Epsom salts, and dissolve in warm bathwater before bathing.

    A—Diffuse into the air. Inhale directly or applied to hands, tissue, or a cotton wick.

Self Esteem:

Oils—^{AT}<u>Acceptance</u>, ^{AT}<u>Forgiveness</u>, ^{AT}<u>Joy</u>, ^{AT}Oola Field, ^{AT}<u>Valor</u>.

—Build

    Oils—^{AT}<u>Joy</u>, ^{AT}<u>Transformation</u>, ^{AT}Oola Field, ^{AT}<u>Valor</u>.

—Self Love

    Oils—^{TA}<u>Joy</u>, ^{TA}<u>Valor</u>.

A—Diffuse into the air. Inhale directly or applied to hands, tissue, or a cotton wick.

T—Apply to auricular emotion points. Dilute with V-6 Oil to create a massage oil, and massage into skin. Add 3–5 drops to 1/4 cup Epsom salts, and dissolve in warm bathwater before bathing.

Self Hypnosis:

Oils—^AClary sage, ^Ageranium, ^Apatchouli.

    A—Inhale directly or applied to hands. Diffuse into the air.

Self Pity:

Oils—**AT**<u>Acceptance</u>, **AT**<u>Motivation</u>, **AT**<u>Transformation</u>, **AT**<u>Valor</u>.

A—Diffuse into the air. Inhale directly or applied to hands, tissue, or a cotton wick.

T—Apply to auricular emotion points. Dilute with V-6 Oil to create a massage oil, and massage into skin.

Sensory System (Senses): *See also Awareness.*

Oils—**AT**Wintergreen.

A—Inhale directly or applied to hands, tissue, or a cotton wick. Diffuse into the air.

T—Dilute with V-6 Oil to create a massage oil, and massage into skin.

Sexual Abuse:

Oils—**AT**<u>SARA</u> (its fragrance, when inhaled, may enable a person to relax into a mental state such that he or she may be able to let go of the memory trauma of sexual and/or ritual abuse).

A—Inhale directly. Diffuse into the air, and inhale.

T—Apply on auricular emotion points.

Sexually Transmitted Diseases (STD): *See AIDS, Herpes Simplex*

Sexual Stimulant:

Oils—**AT**<u>Sensation</u>, **AT**Fcinnamon bark (general), **AT**Fylang ylang (sex drive problems), **AT**ginger, **AT**goldenrod, **AT**rose, **AT**<u>SclarEssence</u>.

Personal Care—**Sensation Bath & Shower Gel** (contains oils used by Cleopatra to enhance love and to increase the desire to be close to that someone special), **Sensation Massage Oil** (creates an exotic arousal and increases sexual desire. The fragrance creates a peaceful and harmonious feeling that helps to ease relationship stress.), **PD 80/20**, **Prenolone/Prenolone+** (for both males and females), **Progessence/Progessence Plus** (for females only), **Sensation Hand & Body Lotion**.

Supplements—EndoGize, Master Formula, Mineral Essence, MultiGreens.

—Arousing Desire

Oils—**AT**Clary sage, **AT**<u>Lady Sclareol</u>.

—Frigidity *See Frigidity.*

Oils—**AT**<u>Lady Sclareol</u>, **AT**nutmeg (overcome).

A=Aromatic   **T**=Topical   **I**=Internal

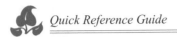
—Impotence

    Oils—^{AT}Goldenrod, ^I<u>SclarEssence</u> (use capsules to take internally).

—Influences

    Oils—^{AT}<u>Lady Sclareol</u>, ^Apatchouli.

A—Wear as perfume or cologne. Diffuse into the air.

T—Dilute with V-6 Oil to create a massage oil, and massage into the skin. Add 3–5 drops to 1/4 cup Epsom or bath salts, and dissolve in warm water before bathing. Dilute as necessary, and apply on skin.

I—Add 2–3 drops to an empty capsule, and swallow.

Shingles: *See also Antiviral, Childhood Diseases:* Chicken Pox.

>> *Shingles is an acute viral infection with inflammation of certain spinal or cranial nerves and the eruption of vesicles along the affected nerve path. It usually strikes only one side of the body and is often accompanied by severe neuralgia. Also called herpes zoster. Some say it is necessary to cleanse the liver to eliminate/avoid shingles.*

> *Dr. Schnaubelt says that his greatest success in helping individuals with shingles came from applying a blend of 50 percent Ravintsara aromatica and 50 percent Calophyllum inophyllum (Tamanu). "Drastic improvements and complete remission occur within seven days." (Alternative Medicine—The Definitive Guide, p. 56).*

Oils—^T<u>Australian Blue</u>, ^Travintsara, ^Ttea tree, ^Teucalyptus, ^Tblue cypress, ^Tbergamot, ^Tgeranium, ^Tlavender, ^Tlemon, ^Ttamanu, ^TRoman chamomile.

Blend #1—10 drops lavender, 10 drops tea tree (tea tree), and 10 drops thyme mixed in Genesis Hand & Body Lotion. Rub on feet.

Personal Care—Ortho Sport Massage Oil, PD 80/20, Prenolone/ Prenolone+, Progessence/Progessence Plus.

Supplements—Cleansing Trio (ComforTone, Essentialzyme, and ICP).

—Herpes Zoster

    Oils—^T<u>Australian Blue</u>, ^Ttea tree (*See Alternative Medicine—The Definitive Guide, p. 972*), ^Tblue cypress, ^TEucalyptus radiata, ^Tbergamot, ^Tgeranium, ^Tlavender, ^TRoman chamomile.

T—Dilute as necessary, and apply on location. Dilute with V-6 Oil to create a massage oil, and massage on location and on bottoms of feet.

Shock: *See also Fainting.*

>> *Shock is a potentially life-threatening condition where the body suffers from severely low blood pressure. This can be caused by low blood volume due to bleeding or dehydration, inadequate*

pumping of the heart, or dilation of the blood vessels due to head injury, medications, or poisons from bacterial infections. Shock can cause pale or bluish skin that feels cold or clammy to the touch, confusion, rapid breathing, and a rapid heartbeat. Without the needed oxygen being sent to the body's tissues and cells, the organs can shut down and, in severe cases, can lead to death. Shock often accompanies severe injuries or other traumatic situations. A person suffering from shock should be made to lie down with the feet elevated above the head, kept warm, and have the head turned to the side in case of vomiting. Check breathing often, and ensure that any visible bleeding is stopped. Get emergency medical help as soon as possible.

Oils—^{TA}_FPeppermint, ^{TA}_FRoman chamomile, ^{TA}helichrysum, ^{TA}<u>Aroma Life</u>, ^{TA}<u>Joy</u>, ^{TA}<u>Australian Blue</u>, ^{TA}basil, ^{TA}<u>Clarity</u> (to keep from going into shock), ^{TA}<u>Gathering</u>, ^{TA}<u>Grounding</u>, ^{TA}<u>Highest Potential</u>, ^{TA}<u>Inspiration</u>, ^{TA}tea tree, ^{TA}melissa, ^{TA}myrrh, ^{TA}neroli, ^{TA}rosemary, ^{TA}<u>Valor</u>, ^{TA}ylang ylang.

T—Dilute as necessary, and apply on back of neck, feet, over heart, or on front of neck.

A—Inhale directly or applied to hands. Diffuse into the air.

S

Shoulder (Frozen):

Oils—^TBasil, ^Twintergreen, ^Tlemongrass, ^Toregano, ^Tpeppermint, ^Twhite fir, ^T<u>Deep Relief</u> (roll-on).

Recipe #1—Begin by applying white fir to shoulder Vita Flex point on foot (same side of body as frozen shoulder) to deal with any inflammation. Work it in with Vita Flex technique. Then check for improvement in pain reduction and/or range of motion (check after each oil to help determine what the problem really was). In a similar manner, apply lemongrass (for torn or pulled ligaments), basil (for muscle spasms), and wintergreen (for bone problems) on the same Vita Flex point on the foot. After applying the oils to the foot and determining which oil(s) get the best results, apply the same oil(s) on the shoulder, and work the oil into the area with Vita Flex. Then apply peppermint (for nerves) and oregano (create thermal reaction to enhance elasticity of muscle and help it to stretch) on the shoulder, and work each one into the area with Vita Flex. Finally, apply white fir to the other shoulder to create balance as the opposite shoulder will compensate for the sore one. Drink lots of water.

T—See Recipe #1 above. Dilute as necessary, and apply on shoulder and on Vita Flex points on the feet.

Personal Care—Regenolone.

Supplements—Sulfurzyme.

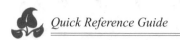

Sinuses:

>> *Sinuses are several hollow cavities within the skull that allow it to be more lightweight, while still maintaining strength. These cavities are connected to the nasal cavity through small channels. When the mucous membrane lining these channels becomes swollen or inflamed due to colds or allergies, these channels can become blocked, making it difficult for the sinuses to drain correctly. This can lead to infection and inflammation of the mucous membrane within the sinuses (sinusitis). There are sinus cavities behind the cheek bone and forehead, and near the eyes and nasal cavity.*

Oils—^{AT}_FHelichrysum, ^{AT}_Fmyrtle, ^T<u>Breathe Again</u>, ^{AT}eucalyptus, ^{AT}peppermint, ^{AT}<u>RC</u>, ^{AT}cedarwood, ^{AT}<u>PanAway</u>, ^T<u>Thieves</u> (on feet).

A—Inhale directly or applied to hands. Diffuse into the air. Place 1–2 drops in a bowl of hot water, and inhale vapors.

T—Dilute as necessary, and apply on sides of nose or on forehead.

***Comments**—Eucalyptus and other sinus oils work really well when rubbed on each side of the nose. It seems to clear the sinuses almost immediately.

Sinusitis: *See also Respiratory System.*

Oils—^{AT}_FEucalyptus, ^{AT}_Frosemary, ^{AT}_Fpine, ^T<u>Breathe Again</u>, ^{AT}<u>RC</u>, ^{AT}cajeput, ^{AT}elemi, ^{AT}Eucalyptus radiata, ^{AT}fir, ^{AT}ginger, ^{AT}Tea tree ericifolia, ^{AT}myrtle, ^{AT}peppermint, ^{AT}ravintsara, ^{AT}sage lavender.

A—Inhale directly or applied to hands. Diffuse into the air. Place 1–2 drops in a bowl of hot water, and inhale vapors.

T—Dilute as necessary, and apply on sides of nose or on forehead.

Skeletal System: *See Bones. See also Scoliosis.*

Skin: *See also Acne, Allergies, Boils, Bruises, Burns, Cancer: SKIN, Cuts, Dermatitis, Eczema, Facial Oils, Feet: CORNS, MOLES, Psoriasis, Wounds, Wrinkles.*

>> *The skin is the organ that covers the body, offering the first layer of protection to the internal organs and tissues from exposure to the environment and fungal, bacterial, and other infections. It helps regulate body heat and helps prevent evaporation of water from the body. The skin also carries nerve endings that allow the body to sense touch, heat, and pain. The skin is comprised of three layers. The upper layer is the epidermis, the middle layer is the dermis, and the deeper layer is the hypodermis, or subcutis layer.*

Oils—^T_FPeppermint (itching skin), ^T_Ftea tree (healing), ^T_Fmyrtle (antiseptic), ^Tsandalwood (regenerates), ^Tfrankincense, ^Tlavender, ^Tmyrrh (chapped and cracked), ^TRoman and German chamomile (inflamed skin), ^T<u>Acceptance</u>, ^T<u>Aroma Life</u>, ^Tcajeput, ^Tcedarwood,

^TClarity, ^Tcypress, ^TDragon Time, ^TGentle Baby (youthful skin), ^Tgeranium, ^Thelichrysum, ^TInner Child, ^Tjasmine (irritated skin), ^Tjuniper, ^Tledum (all types of problems), ^Tlemon, ^Tmarjoram, ^TMelrose, ^TMister, ^TM-Grain, ^Tonycha (chapped and cracked), ^Torange, ^Tpalmarosa (rashes, scaly, and flaky skin), ^Tpatchouli (chapped; tightens loose skin and prevents wrinkles), ^TRelieve It, ^Trosehip, ^Trosemary, ^Trosewood (elasticity and candida), ^Tsage, ^Tsage lavender, ^TSensation, ^TValor, ^Tvetiver, ^Twestern red cedar (nourishing), ^{TA}Build Your Dream (vibrant) ^Tylang ylang.

T—Dilute as necessary, and apply on location. Dilute with V-6 Oil to create massage oil, and massage on location. Add 1–2 drops to 1 tsp. unscented lotion, and apply on location. Add 1–2 drops to bath or shower gel, and apply to the skin.

> *Contact-sensitization* is a type of allergic reaction which can occur when a substance comes into contact with the body. A few essential oils applied to the skin may cause sensitization, perhaps only after repeated application (the amount used is not significant). The skin reaction appears as redness, irritation, or vesiculation. A rule of thumb when applying oils to someone is that people with darker hair usually have less sensitive skin while those with blond or red hair are generally more sensitive.
>
> *Single oils:* Bergamot, cassia, cinnamon bark, citronella, clove, fennel, Laurus nobilis, ylang ylang.
>
> *(For a list of possible skin irritants, please see the Appendix of this book.)*

S

Personal Care—A·R·T Skin Care System, AromaGuard Deodorants, Boswellia Wrinkle Cream, Clara-Derm, Essential Beauty Serums (Dry, & Acne-Prone Skin Blends), **Genesis Hand & Body Lotion** (hydrates, heals, and nurtures the skin), **Satin Facial Scrub - Mint** (eliminates layers of dead skin cells and slows down premature aging of the skin), **Orange Blossom Facial Wash combined with Sandalwood Moisture Cream** (cleans and moisturizes dry or prematurely aging skin), **Prenolone , Progessence/Progessence Plus, Regenolone** (helps moisturize and regenerate tissues), **Rose Ointment** (for skin conditions and chapped skin), **Lavender Hand & Body Lotion** (moisturizes skin, leaving it feeling soft, silky, and smooth), Sensation Hand & Body Lotion (moisturizes, softens, and protects the skin from weather, chemicals, and household cleaners).

Bar Soaps—Lavender Rosewood Moisturizing Soap, Lemon Sandalwood Cleansing Soap, Peppermint Cedarwood Moisturizing Soap, Sacred Mountain Moisturizing Soap for Oily Skin, Thieves Cleansing Soap.

Bath & Shower Gels—**Dragon Time** (for women who have lower back pain, stress and sleeping problems due to menstruation), **Evening Peace** (relaxes tired, fatigued muscles and helps to alleviate tension), **Morning Start** (dissolves oil and grease), and **Sensation** (aphrodisiac).

Supplements for Skin—JuvaTone, Sulfurzyme, Ultra Young+ (helps firm and tighten skin by activating the production of skin proteins, collagen, and elastin).

A=Aromatic   **T**=Topical   **I**=Internal

—AFTERSHAVE

Recipe #1—<u>Awaken</u> can be used instead of aftershave lotion. Try adding <u>Awaken</u> to Sandalwood Moisture Cream, Lavender Hand & Body Lotion, Sensation Hand & Body Lotion, or Genesis Hand & Body Lotion as an aftershave. KidScents Lotion makes a great aftershave, as it soothes and rehydrates the skin (and smells good too).

—AGING *See also* WRINKLES *below*

Oils—^TFrankincense, ^Tpatchouli (prevents wrinkles), ^Trosehip (retards), ^Trosewood (slows), ^Tcarrot, ^Trose.

T—Dilute as necessary, and apply on location. Dilute with V-6 Oil or other carrier oil, such as jojoba, apricot, hazelnut, or sweet almond, to create massage oil, and apply to areas of concern. Add 3–4 drops to 1/4 cup Epsom salts, and dissolve in warm bathwater before bathing.

> *For years, I had been troubled with an **actinic keratosis** on the back of my hand. It had been caused by excessive sun exposure when I was younger. Farmers often get them on their foreheads. My dermatologist said there was no way to get rid of it—unless I wanted to freeze it off with liquid nitrogen. He didn't want to do that because it was over 1/2 inch in diameter, and freezing it would have made a hole in my hand. The growth continued to bother me. It was red, scaly, and itchy. One day, in desperation, I put some "Thieves" blend on it. The Thieves seemed to make it feel better, so I continued to apply it once a day. It is now several months later, and the growth has almost disappeared. I intend to continue using Thieves on it until it is gone. It doesn't bother me anymore, and the redness and itching have disappeared.*
>
> *-Submitted by Judy Brown*
> *Geneva, New York (July 2004)*

Personal Care— A·R·T Beauty Masque, Boswellia Wrinkle Cream, A·R·T Sheerlumé, Genesis Hand & Body Lotion, Satin Facial Scrub - Mint, PD 80/20, Prenolone/Prenolone+, Progessence/Progessence Plus, Rose Ointment, Sandalwood Moisture Cream.

Supplements—Ultra Young+ (helps firm and tighten skin by activating the production of skin proteins, collagen, and elastin).

—CALLUSES

>> *A callus is a flat, thick growth of skin that develops on areas of the skin where there is constant friction or rubbing. Calluses typically form on the bottoms of the feet, but they can also form on the hands or on other areas of the bodies that are exposed to constant friction.*

Oils—^TMelrose and ^Toregano (calluses on feet), ^Tcarrot, ^Tpeppermint, ^TRoman chamomile.

T—Dilute as necessary, and apply on location.

—Chapped/Cracked

>> *Chapped or cracked skin is the result of the depletion of natural oils (sebum) in the skin, leading to dehydration of the skin beneath it. Some common causes for chapped skin include exposure to the cold or wind, repeated contact with soap or chemicals that break down oils, or a lack of essential fatty acids in the body.*

Oils—^TMyrrh, ^Telemi, ^Tdavana,^T onycha (benzoin), ^Tpatchouli.

T—Dilute as necessary, and apply on location. Dilute with V-6 Oil to create a massage oil, and apply on location.

Blend #1—1 drop geranium, 1 drop patchouli, and 1 drop rosemary in Genesis Hand & Body Lotion or Lavender Hand & Body Lotion.

Blend #2—1–3 drops of both onycha (benzoin) and rose in Genesis Hand & Body Lotion, Lavender Hand & Body Lotion (makes a wonderful hand cream), or Rose Ointment. May also add lemon and/or lavender for their additional healing properties.

Personal Care—Cinnamint or Lavender Lip Balms

—Complexion

Personal Care—A·R·T Skin Care System

–Dull

Oils—^TJasmine,^T orange.

–Oily (Greasy)

Oils—^TBergamot, ^Torange, ^Tcajeput, ^Tclary sage, ^Tcypress, ^Tjasmine, ^Tlavender, ^Tlemon, ^Tnutmeg, ^Tylang ylang.

T—Dilute as necessary, and apply oils to face, neck, and intestines.

—Dermatitis *See Eczema/Dermatitis below*

—Diaper Rash: *See Children/Infants: Diaper Rash*

—Disease

Oils—^TRose, ^TMelrose.

T—Dilute as necessary, and apply on location.

—Dry

Oils—^T_FRosewood, ^Tgeranium, ^Tlavender, ^TGentle Baby, ^TRoman chamomile, ^Tmastrante, ^Tdavana, ^Tjasmine, ^Tlemon, ^Tneroli, ^Tpatchouli, ^Tsandalwood.

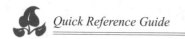
T—Dilute as necessary, and apply on location. Dilute with V-6 Oil to create massage oil, and massage on location. Add 1–2 drops to 1 tsp. unscented lotion, and apply on location.

Personal Care— A·R·T Renewal Serum, **Genesis Hand & Body Lotion** (hydrates, heals, and nurtures), **Orange Blossom Facial Wash** (gently cleanses the skin), **PD 80/20, Prenolone/Prenolone+, Progessence, Sandalwood Moisture Cream** (hydrates), **Lavender Hand & Body Lotion** (nourishes and moisturizes), **A·R·T Sheerlumé, Sensation Massage Oil** (silky and youthful skin)

—ECZEMA/DERMATITIS

>> *Dermatitis is any inflammation of the upper layers of the skin that results in redness, itching, pain, or possibly blistering. It can be caused by contact with an allergen or irritating substance, fungal infection, dehydration, or possibly another medical condition.*

Oils—^T_F**Helichrysum,** ^T_F**German chamomile,** ^T_F**rosewood,** ^T_F**thyme,** ^T_F**patchouli,** ^T_F**juniper,** ^{T}**bergamot,** ^{T}**eucalyptus,** ^{T}**geranium,** ^{T}**hyssop,** ^{T}**lavender,** ^{T}**Tea tree ericifolia,** ^{T}**melissa,** ^{T}**onycha (benzoin),** ^{T}**pine,** ^{T}**sage,** ^{T}**sage lavender.**

Supplements—Essentialzyme, Essentialzymes-4, JuvaPower/JuvaSpice, Sulfurzyme.

***Comments—Eczema or dermatitis may indicate a sulfur deficiency.

–DRY

Oils—^T_F**German chamomile,** ^{T}**bergamot,** ^{T}**geranium,** ^{T}**hyssop,** ^{T}**rosemary.**

–WET

Oils—^T_F**German chamomile,** ^{T}**hyssop,** ^{T}**juniper,** ^{T}**lavender,** ^{T}**myrrh.**

T—Dilute with V-6 Oil to create a massage oil, and apply on location. Dilute as necessary, and apply oil on location.

—FACIAL MASK

Oils—^{T}**Myrrh,** ^{T}**patchouli,** ^{T}**sandalwood,** ^{T}**vetiver.**

T—Add 2–3 drops to a facial mask. Can use individually or together. Frankincense is too drying to the skin alone, but it can be combined with any or all of these others.

Personal Care— A·R·T Creme Masque, A·R·T Beauty Masque, **Orange Blossom Facial Wash, Satin Facial Scrub - Mint.**

—FEEDS SKIN AND SUPPLIES NUTRIENTS

Personal Care—Boswellia Wrinkle Cream, Rose Ointment.

—Impetigo

>> *Impetigo is a bacterial skin infection that causes sores and blisters filled with a yellowish fluid. These sores can be itchy and painful and can easily be spread to other areas of the skin or to another person.*

Recipe #2—Lavender, myrrh. Boil 4 ounces water; let water cool. Add 5–10 drops lavender, and wash infected skin. You may also use myrrh (cover for an hour). Do hot compress on site.

—Itching

Oils—^T**Peppermint,** ^Tlavender, ^T<u>Peace & Calming</u>.

T—Dilute as necessary, and apply on ears and on location.

Personal Care—ClaraDerm (essential oil spray), **Lavender Hand & Body Lotion**.

—Rashes

>> *A rash is an area of irritated skin, redness, or red bumps on the body. Rashes may be localized or may cover large patches of the body. A rash may be caused by a chemical or allergen irritating the skin, or as a symptom of another medical condition or infection.*

> *If the rash occurs from application of oils to the skin, it may be due to the oils reacting with accumulated synthetic chemicals (toxins) that are trapped in the fatty layers of the skin. Take the following steps: 1) Try diluting the oils first (1–3 drops of oil to ½ tsp. V-6 Oil), 2) reduce the number of oils used with each application (use oils one at a time), 3) reduce the amount of oils (number of drops) used, and 4) reduce the frequency of application (more time between applications). Drinking pure (steam-distilled) water helps promote the elimination of accumulated toxins from the body. Initiating programs to cleanse the bowels and blood will also help remove accumulated toxins and reduce the possible recurrences of the rash. If the rashes persist, discontinue use of the oils and consult your health care professional.*

Oils—^T_FTea tree, ^T<u>Melrose</u>, ^T**elemi** (allergic), ^T**hinoki,** ^Tlavender, ^Tpalmarosa, ^T<u>Release</u> (on Vita Flex points of feet), ^TRoman chamomile.

T—Dilute as necessary, and apply on location.

*****Comments**—Red spots on body may indicate a biotin deficiency; take Super C or Super C Chewable.

Personal Care—KidScents Tender Tush, Rose Ointment.

*****Comments**—Dr. Friedmann had a patient who had a rash for three years on the side of the face and arms, and the eyes were weeping. The patient had gone to five physicians for treatments and had no success. Dr. Friedmann did the following: 1) Did a culture of the eye and face and determined that the patient had staphylococcus. 2) Had the patient apply <u>Melrose</u> and lavender alternately morning and night. 3) Had the patient take Mineral Essence and Colloidal Essence (a colloidal silver

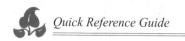

product). After a short period of time, the patient's face and eyes totally cleared up and the arms were healing.

—RINGWORM: *See Antifungal: RINGWORM*

—SAGGY SKIN

> **Blend #1**—Combine 8 drops each of sage, pine, and lemongrass with 1 oz. V-6 Oil. Rub on areas.

—SCABIES

> ▸▸ *Scabies is an infestation of the skin by mites (Sarcoptes scabei) that burrow into the upper layers of the skin, causing small, extremely itchy bumps.*
>
> **Oils**—ᵀ<u>Thieves</u> (needs to be diluted), ᵀ**tea tree,** ᵀ**lavender** and ᵀ**peppermint,** ᵀbergamot, ᵀlaurel, ᵀpine.
>
> **T**—Add 5–10 drops to 1 Tbs. V-6 Oil, and apply a small amount on location morning and night.

—SCARRING *SEE SCARRING*

—SENSITIVE

> **Oils**—ᵀ**Geranium,** ᵀ**German chamomile,** ᵀ**jasmine,** ᵀ**lavender,** ᵀ**neroli.**
>
> **Personal Care**—Lavender Hand & Body Lotion.

—STRETCH MARKS *See Stretch Marks*

—SUNBURN *See Sunburn*

—TONES

> **Oils**—ᵀ**Patchouli.**
>
> **T**—Dilute with V-6 Oil to create a massage oil, and massage into the skin.
>
> **Personal Care**—Cel-Lite Magic, Satin Facial Scrub - Mint, Sandalwood Moisture Cream, A·R·T Sheerlumé.
>
> **Supplements**—Ultra Young+ (helps firm and tighten skin by activating the production of skin proteins, collagen, and elastin).

—VITILIGO

> ▸▸ *Vitiligo is white patches of the skin caused by the death or dysfunction of pigment-producing cells in the area. While the exact cause is unknown,*

> *Vitiligo may be due to a malfunction of the pineal gland and possibly the pituitary gland as well. See Pineal and Pituitary for oils and products that can help oxygenate these glands. Another possible remedy includes daily exposure of the eyes to full-spectrum light without contacts or eyeglasses.*

it may be caused by an immune or genetic disorder, or may have a relationship to thyroid problems.

Oils—^TSandalwood, ^Tvetiver, ^Tfrankincense, ^TMelrose, ^Tmyrrh, ^TPurification, ^Tsage.

T—Apply behind ears and to back of neck. Then rub hands together, cup hands over nose and mouth, and breathe deeply. Can also be applied to Vita Flex points relating to the pineal and pituitary glands on the feet and hands.

—WRINKLES

Oils—^TFrankincense, ^Tpatchouli, ^Tlavender, ^Tmyrrh[385], ^Tcarrot, ^Tfennel, ^Tdill[386], ^Tgeranium, ^Thelichrysum, ^Tlemon, ^Trosewood, ^Tsandalwood, ^Tcistus, ^Tclary sage, ^Tcypress, ^Telemi, ^Tgalbanum, ^Tmyrrh, ^Tneroli, ^Torange, ^Toregano, ^Trose, ^Trosemary, ^Tspikenard, ^Tthyme, ^Tylang ylang.

> *Wrinkles occur as we mature and as we lose oxygen to the tissues. Essential oils oxygenate the tissues and thereby slow down the premature aging of the skin.*

Blend #1—3 drops lavender, 4 drops geranium, 2 drops patchouli, 6 drops rosewood, and 1 oz. V-6 Oil. Rub on wrinkles in an upward, lifting motion.

Blend #2—1 drop frankincense, 1 drop lavender, and 1 drop lemon. It's like magic for wrinkles. Rub on morning and night around the eyes.

Blend #3—5–10 drops frankincense added to Sandalwood Moisture Cream.

Blend #4—Equal amounts of sandalwood, helichrysum, geranium, lavender, and frankincense. Combine with either Genesis Hand & Body Lotion or Lavender Hand & Body Lotion, and apply to skin.

Personal Care— A·R·T Creme Masque, A·R·T Skin Care System (repairs DNA damage, builds collagen), Boswellia Wrinkle Cream (collagen builder), Essential Beauty Serums (Dry, & Acne-Prone Skin Blends), Rose Ointment, Sandalwood Moisture Cream, Lavender Hand & Body Lotion, Satin Facial Scrub - Mint, Wolfberry Eye Cream. The following three items can be used together to help tone the skin and prevent wrinkles: Orange Blossom Facial Wash, Rose Ointment, Sandalwood Moisture Cream, Lavender Hand & Body Lotion.

Supplements—Essentialzyme, Essentialzymes-4, PD 80/20, Prenolone/Prenolone+, Progessence/Progessence Plus, Thyromin (thyroid function affects the skin), Ultra Young+.

–PREVENT

Oils—^TGentle Baby and ^Tpatchouli (prevents and retards).

Personal Care—A·R·T Skin Care System, Boswellia Wrinkle Cream (collagen builder), Essential Beauty Serums (Dry, & Acne-Prone Skin Blends), Satin

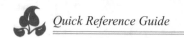

Facial Scrub - Mint, Wolfberry Eye Cream. The following three items can be used together to help tone the skin and to prevent wrinkles: **Orange Blossom Facial Wash, Sandalwood Moisture Cream.**

–SMOOTH

Recipe #3—Add 2 drops frankincense to a little Genesis Hand & Body Lotion or Lavender Hand & Body Lotion, and apply.

Personal Care—**A·R·T Skin Care System, Boswellia Wrinkle Cream** (collagen builder), **Essential Beauty Serums** (Dry, & Acne-Prone Skin Blends).

T—Dilute as necessary, and apply on location. Dilute with V-6 Oil or other carrier oil, such as jojoba, apricot, hazelnut, or sweet almond, to create massage oil, and apply to areas of concern. Add 3–4 drops to 1/4 cup bath salts, and dissolve in warm bathwater before bathing.

Sleep:

Oils—^(AT)Lavender[387] (on spine), ^(AT)RutaVaLa, ^(AT)Peace & Calming, ^(TA)valerian[388] (disturbances), ^(T)Tranquil (roll-on), ^(AT)mastrante, ^(A)marjoram, ^(A)Roman chamomile[389], ^(T)Stress Away.

A—Diffuse into the air. Apply 1–2 drops to pillow or stuffed animal. Add 2–5 drops to 1 oz. distilled water in a small spray bottle, and mist into the air or on linens before sleeping. *See also Negative Ions for oils that produce negative ions when diffused to help promote sleep.*

T—Dilute as necessary, and apply on area indicated or on back, bottoms of feet, or back of neck. Add 3–4 drops to 1/4 cup Epsom or bath salts, and dissolve in warm bathwater before bathing. Dilute with V-6 Oil to create massage oil, and massage into the skin.

Supplements—SleepEssence, Ultra Young+ (restores deep sleep).

—ANIMALS

Oils—^(T)Peace & Calming, ^(T)Trauma Life.

T—Oils can be used on the paws of animals to help them relax and sleep when in pain.

—GOOD NIGHTS SLEEP

Recipe #1—*See also Insomnia for additional blends.* 1/4 cup bath salts and 10 drops geranium or lavender in bath; soak in tub. Bathe with Evening Peace Bath Gel.

—RESTLESS *See also Legs, Restless for recipe*

Oils—^(AT)Lavender, ^(AT)Gathering.

A—Diffuse into the air. Apply 1–2 drops to pillow or stuffed animal.

T—Dilute as necessary, and apply on area indicated or on legs, back, bottoms of feet, or back of neck. Dilute with V-6 Oil to create massage oil, and massage into the skin.

—Sleeping Sickness

>> *Sleeping sickness is swelling of the brain caused by an infection carried by tsetse flies. Symptoms include fever, anxiety, drowsiness, insomnia at night, sweating, mood changes, swollen lymph nodes, and an uncontrollable urge to sleep. Without treatment, this disorder can be fatal.*

Oils—ᵀJuniper, ᵀpeppermint, ᵀ<u>Peace & Calming</u> (on big toes, back of neck, and navel), ᵀgeranium, ᵀ<u>Valor</u> (on feet).

T—Dilute as necessary, and apply on area indicated or on back of neck, lymph nodes, and Vita Flex points on the feet.

Slimming and Toning Oils: *See also Weight.*

Oils—ᴬᴵGrapefruit[390], ᴵsage[391], ᴬlemongrass, ᴬᴵorange, ᴬbasil, ᴬlavender, ᴬrosemary, ᴬthyme.

A—Inhale directly. Diffuse into the air.

I—Add 1 drop to 12–16 oz. of water, and drink. Add 1–2 drops to empty capsule, and swallow.

Slivers (Splinters):

Recipe #1—Mix 10 drops <u>Thieves</u> with 4 Tbs. V-6 Oil, and massage bottoms of feet, armpits, throat, and lower stomach. Put 30 drops of <u>Thieves</u> in bath gel, and use the gel in the shower each day (this helps pull the slivers to gently massage them out).

Smell, Loss of:

Oils—ᴬBasil (helps when loss of smell is due to chronic nasal catarrh), ᴬpeppermint.

A—Inhale directly or applied to hands. Diffuse into the air.

—Stimulate Sensory Cortex

Oils—ᵀ<u>Brain Power</u>.

> *Just smelling the oils helps stimulate the sense of smell. To smell the oils, first close the eyes; then hold the left nostril closed, breathe in the smell of the oil through the right nostril, and then breathe out through the mouth. Breathing in the fragrance of the oils in this manner stimulates every endocrine gland in the brain. Next hold the right nostril closed and repeat the process.*

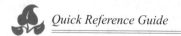
T—Place under the tongue, behind the ears, and on the forehead. Can also place a couple drops of oil in the hands, rub hands together in a clockwise motion, cup hands over the nose and mouth, and breathe deeply.

***Comments**—*According to the <u>Essential Oils Desk Reference</u>, "Massage 1 or 2 drops [of Brain Power] with a finger on the insides of cheeks in the mouth. Doing this 1 or 2 times a day will immediately improve the smell sensory cortex." (<u>EDR</u>-June 2002; Ch. 8; Brain Power; Application)*

Smoking: *See also Addictions: Smoking, Air Pollution, Purification.*

Oils—^ABlack pepper³⁹², ^A<u>Purification</u>.

—Cigarette

Oils—^ABlack pepper³⁹², ^A<u>Purification</u>.

—Purify Air

Oils—^A<u>Purification</u>, ^Alemon.

—Stop Smoking *See also Addictions.*

Oils—^ABlack pepper³⁹², ^Aclove (removes desire), ^T<u>Thieves</u> (on tongue before lighting up helps remove desire), ^A<u>GLF</u>, ^A<u>Peace & Calming</u>, ^A<u>Present Time</u> (helps with insecurity), ^A<u>Purification</u>.

Supplements—JuvaPower/JuvaSpice, JuvaTone, Super C / Super C Chewable.

***Comments**—One individual used JuvaTone to break a habit of smoking 2½ packs of cigarettes a day for 20 years. Another individual who used JuvaTone went from smoking a pack a day to 1 cigarette in 1½ weeks.*

A—Inhale directly or applied to hands. Diffuse into the air.

T—Apply as indicated.

Snoring:

Oils—^T<u>RC</u>.

T—Rub on throat before sleeping to help keep the airway open.

Soothing:

Oils—^{TA}<u>Gentle Baby</u>, ^{TA}Roman chamomile, ^{TA}myrrh, ^{TA}onycha (benzoin), ^{AT}<u>Release</u>.

T—Dilute with V-6 Oil, and apply on area of concern or on back, legs, feet, and arms.

A—Diffuse into the air. Inhale directly or applied to hands, tissue, or a cotton wick.

Sores: *See also Antibacterial, Antifungal, Antiviral, Cuts, Wounds.*

Oils—^TTea tree, ^Tbasil[393], ^T<u>Thieves</u>, ^Tpine.

T—Dilute as necessary, and apply on location.

Sore Throat: *See Throat.*

Spacing Out:

Oils—^A<u>Grounding</u>, ^A<u>Acceptance</u>, ^A<u>Present Time</u>, ^A<u>Sacred Mountain</u>.

A—Inhale directly or applied to hands, tissue, or a cotton wick. Diffuse into the air.

Spasms: *See also Digestive System, Muscles, Antispasmodic.*

Oils—^TBasil, ^T_Fcypress, ^T<u>Aroma Siez</u>, ^Tcalamus, ^T<u>Deep Relief</u> (roll-on), ^Tjasmine (muscle), ^Tlavender (antispasmodic), ^Tmarjoram (relieves), ^Toregano, ^T<u>Peace & Calming</u>, ^Tpeppermint, ^TRoman chamomile, ^Tspikenard, ^Ttarragon, ^Tthyme.

—SPASTICITY

Oils—^TCypress, ^Tginger, ^Tjuniper, ^Tlavender, ^Tlemon, ^Trosemary, ^Tsandalwood.

T—Dilute as necessary, and apply on location of spasm or on Vita Flex points on the feet. Apply as a warm compress over area of concern.

Spina Bifida:

≫ *Spina bifida is a birth defect in which the vertebrae of the lower spine do not form correctly, leaving a gap or opening between them. In the most severe cases, this can cause the meninges (the tissue surrounding the spinal cord), or even the spinal cord itself, to protrude through the gap. If the spinal cord protrudes through the gap, it can prevent the nerves from developing normally, causing numbness, paralysis, back pain, and loss of bladder and bowel control and function. This later type often also develops along with a defect in which the back part of the brain develops in the upper neck rather than within the skull, often causing a mental handicap.*

Oils—^{TA}Eucalyptus, ^{TA}lavender, ^{TA}Roman chamomile, ^{TA}lemon, ^{TA}nutmeg, ^{TA}orange, ^{TA}rosemary, ^{TA}<u>3 Wise Men</u>.

T—Apply oil(s) to bottoms of feet, forehead, back of neck, along spine.

A—Diffuse into the air.

***Comments**—Do the Raindrop Technique.

Spine: *See Back.*

Spiritual:

Oils—^{AT}Awaken, ^{AT}Believe, ^{AT}Dream Catcher, ^{AT}Gathering, ^{AT} Gratitude, ^{AT}Humility, ^{AT}Inspiration, ^{AT}Oola Faith.

—AWARENESS

Oils—^{AT}Acceptance, ^{AT}western red cedar, ^{AT}cedarwood, ^{AT}juniper, ^{AT}hinoki, ^{AT}m-yrrh, ^{AT}Sacred Mountain, ^{AT}spruce, ^{AT}Transformation, ^AWhite Angelica, ^{AT}white lotus.

—BALANCING

Oils—^{AT}Joy, ^{AT}Into the Future, ^{AT}Oola Faith, ^{AT}spruce.

—INCREASE

Oils—^{AT}Believe, ^{AT}cedarwood (enhances), ^Afrankincense (opening and enhancing spiritual receptivity), ^{AT}Oola Faith, ^{AT}Gratitude, ^{AT}Transformation.

—INNER AWARENESS

Oils—^{AT}Believe, ^{AT}Gratitude, ^{AT}Inner Child, ^{AT}Inspiration.

—MEDITATION

Oils—^{AT}Believe, ^{AT}Oola Faith, ^{AT}western red cedar, ^{AT}frankincense, ^{AT}Inspiration, ^{AT}tsuga, ^{AT}White Angelica.

—PRAYER

Oils—^{AT}Gratitude, ^{AT}Oola Faith, ^{AT}Inspiration, ^{AT}White Angelica.

—PROTECTION

Oils—^T3 Wise Men (on crown and shoulders).

—PURITY OF SPIRIT

Oils—^{AT}Myrrh.

—SPIRITUALLY UPLIFTING

Oils—^{AT}Believe, ^{AT}Gratitude, ^{AT}Sacred Mountain, ^{AT}Oola Faith, ^{AT}Transformation.

A—Inhale directly or applied to hands, tissue, or a cotton wick. Diffuse into the air.

T—Dilute as necessary, and apply on indicated areas or on crown, forehead, or heart.

Spleen:

›› *The spleen is a fist-sized spongy tissue that is part of the lymphatic system. Its purpose is to filter bacteria, viruses, fungi, and other unwanted substances out of the blood and to create lymphocytes (white blood cells that create antibodies).*

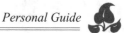
Oils—ᵀLaurel, ᵀmarjoram.

T—Dilute as necessary, and apply over spleen or on Vita Flex points on the feet. Apply as a warm compress over upper abdomen.

Sports: *See Aches/Pains, Bones, Injuries, Muscles, Tissue.*

—Excel In

Oils—ᵀ<u>Clarity</u> (on forehead), ᵀ<u>Peace & Calming</u> (back of neck), ᵀ<u>PanAway</u> (injuries), ᵀ<u>Valor</u> (on feet for courage and confidence), ᵀ<u>Tranquil</u> (roll-on).

—Injuries

Oils—ᵀHelichrysum, ᵀ<u>PanAway</u>, ᵀ<u>Deep Relief</u> (roll-on), ᵀlemongrass, ᵀ<u>Melrose</u>, ᵀ<u>Peace & Calming</u>.

Supplements—BLM

—Track Competition

Oils—ᴵBalsam fir

I—Take 2–3 drops in a capsule before the competition to help reduce muscle soreness afterward.

Blend #1—5 drops basil, 5 drops bergamot, and 2 tsp. V-6 Oil.

Personal Care—Ortho Ease Massage Oil, Ortho Sport Massage Oil. Massage into the muscles to increase oxygen and elasticity in the tissues to prevent the muscles and ligaments from tearing during strenuous exercise. It may also be used after to prevent the muscle from cramping.

Supplements—MultiGreens.

T—Dilute as necessary, and apply on area indicated or on area of concern.

Sprains: *See Muscles: Sprain.*

Spurs, Bone: *See also Bones.*

Oils—ᵀLavender, ᵀ<u>RC</u> (dissolves).

T—Apply directly on location.

Stains: *See also Housecleaning.*

Oils—ᵀLemon (removes).

T—Apply 1–2 drops on location.

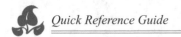

Staph Infection: *See Antibacterial:*STAPH INFECTION, MRSA.

Sterility:

    Oils—^TClary sage, ^T_Fgeranium, ^Trose (wonderful for both men and women), ^Tjasmine, ^Tneroli, ^Tsage lavender, ^Tsandalwood, ^T<u>SclarEssence</u> (taken internally, helps increase estradiol and testosterone levels), ^Trosewood, ^Tvetiver.

    T—Apply several together (or alternate individually) by massage or aromatic bath.

    I—Add 1–3 drops to an empty capsule, and swallow.

    Personal Care—**Prenolone/Prenolone+, Progessence/Progessence Plus** (for women only).

    Supplements—Power Meal.

Stimulating:

    Oils—^T_FPeppermint, ^T<u>En-R-Gee</u>, ^T_Fsage, ^Teucalyptus[394], ^Trosemary[394], ^Tbasil, ^Tblack pepper, ^Tfir, ^Tginger, ^Tgrapefruit, ^Torange, ^Tpatchouli, ^Trose, ^T<u>Transformation</u>.

    T—Dilute with V-6 Oil to create a massage oil for a stimulating massage. Can also add a few drops of an oil (or of a couple oils) to bath gel, and then add the gel to the bathwater as the tub is filling.

    ***Comments—Adding a little black pepper to an oil like rosemary can give it a little more power.

Stings: *See Bites/Stings.*

Stomach: *See also Digestive System.*

    Oils—^T_FBasil, ^Tginger, ^Tpeppermint, ^Tcalamus (supports).

    T—Apply to stomach Vita Flex points on feet, or apply as a hot compress over the stomach area.

    —ACHE

        Oils—^T<u>Di-Gize</u> (behind ears and down jaw bone), ^{TI}peppermint, ^Teucalyptus, ^Tgeranium, ^{TI}lavender, ^Trosemary.

        T—Dilute as necessary, and apply as indicated; or apply over stomach area and on Vita Flex points on the feet.

        I—Add 1–2 drops to an empty capsule, and swallow.

    —ACID

        Oils—^IPeppermint

        I—Put drop on finger, and place on tongue.

Recipe #1—Put several drops of fresh lemon juice in warm water, and sip slowly.

Supplements—AlkaLime (acid-neutralizing mineral formula).

—BACTERIA OR GERMS

Oils—^IPeppermint

I—Add 1–2 drops to an empty capsule, and swallow.

—BLOATING

Oils—^IFennel

I—Add 1–2 drops to almond or rice milk, water, or other liquid; drink.

—CRAMPS

Oils—^T_FHelichrysum, ^T_Fthyme (general tonic for), ^Tblue cypress, ^Tginger, ^Tlavender, ^Tonycha (benzoin), ^Trosemary cineol.

T—Apply as a warm compress over stomach area. Dilute as necessary, and apply over stomach area or on Vita Flex points on the feet.

Recipe #2—Flavor water with 5 drops of Di-Gize, and drink for stomach pains **or** add 3 drops basil in a capsule with Di-Gize.

—TONIC

Oils—^ITangerine.

I—Add 1–2 drops to 12–16 oz. of water; drink.

—UPSET

Oils—^{TIA}<u>Di-Gize</u>, ^Iginger[395].

T—Apply over stomach and colon, behind the ears, on Vita Flex points on the feet

I—Add 1 drop to 8 oz. rice or almond milk, and drink. Place 1–2 drops in an empty capsule, and swallow.

A—Place a couple of drops on the palms of the hands, rub the hands together clockwise, cup hands over nose and mouth, and breathe deeply.

Strength:

Oils—^{TA}_FPeppermint, ^Acypress, ^{TA}<u>Hope</u>, ^{TA}oregano, ^{TA}patchouli, ^{TA}<u>Raven</u>, ^{TA}Roman chamomile (strengthens positive imprinting in DNA), ^{TA}<u>Sacred Mountain</u>, ^{TA}<u>White Angelica</u>.

T—Add 1–2 drops to warm bathwater, and bathe. Dilute with V-6 Oil to create a massage oil, and massage onto the skin.

A—Diffuse into the air.

A=Aromatic **T**=Topical **I**=Internal 321

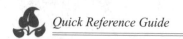

Supplements— NingXia Red, Power Meal, Pure Protein Complete, Wolfberry Crisp Bars.

Strep Throat: *See Throat: Strep.*

Stress: *See also Calming.*

Oils—[AT]Lavender[396], [AT]ylang ylang[397], [T]Stress Away, [T]Tranquil (roll-on), [AT]Peace & Calming, [AT]₍ᵣ₎bergamot, [AT]lemon[398] [AT]Common Sense, [AT]Aroma Life, [AT]basil, [AT]Believe, [AT]Clarity, [AT]clary sage, [AT]cypress, [AT]elemi, [AT]Evergreen Essence, [AT]frankincense, [AT]geranium, [AT]grapefruit, [AT]Harmony, [AT]Inspiration, [AT]Joy, [AT]marjoram, [AT]neroli, [AT]onycha (benzoin), [AT]pine, [AT]Roman chamomile (relieves stress), [AT]rosewood, [AT]Sacred Mountain, [AT]spruce, [AT]Surrender, [AT]tangerine, [AT]3 Wise Men, [AT]Valor, [AT]White Angelica.

Personal Care—Evening Peace or Sensation Shower Gel, Relaxation or Sensation Massage Oil, Sensation Hand & Body Lotion.

Supplements—ImmuPro, Inner Defense, Master Formula, Thyromin, Super B, and Super Cal.

***Comments—You can't change the stressful situations that come, but you can change your response to those situations. Focus on resolution not on recrimination! *(See Forgive)*

—CHEMICAL

Oils—[AT]Lavender, [AT]rosemary, [AT]clary sage, [AT]geranium, [AT]grapefruit, [AT]lemon, [AT]patchouli.

—EMOTIONAL STRESS

Oils—[AT]Joy, [AT]clary sage, [AT]bergamot, [T]Tranquil (roll-on), [AT]Evergreen Essence, [AT]Forgiveness, [AT]Gathering, [AT]geranium, [AT]AromaEase, [AT]ravintsara, [AT]sandalwood (layer on navel and chest), [AT]Surrender, [AT]Transformation, [AT]Trauma Life.

—ENVIRONMENTAL STRESS

Oils—[AT]Bergamot, [AT]geranium, [AT]Roman chamomile, [AT]cypress, [AT]basil, [AT]cedarwood.

—MENTAL STRESS

Oils—[AT]Lavender[396], [AT]bergamot, [AT]grapefruit, [T]Tranquil (roll-on), [AT]basil, [AT]Evergreen Essence, [AT]geranium, [AT]patchouli, [AT]pine, [AT]sandalwood, [AT]Surrender.

—PERFORMANCE STRESS

Oils—[AT]Grapefruit, [AT]bergamot, [T]Tranquil (roll-on), [AT]ginger, [AT]rosemary.

—PHYSICAL STRESS

Oils—^{AT}Peace & Calming, ^{AT}lavender, ^{AT}marjoram, ^{AT}bergamot, ^{AT}geranium, ^{AT-}Believe, ^{AT}fennel, ^{AT}Gentle Baby, ^{AT}Harmony, ^{AT}Roman chamomile, ^{AT}rosemary, ^{AT}thyme, ^TTranquil (roll-on), ^{AT}Trauma Life (calming).

Supplements—ImmuPro.

—RELATIONSHIP STRESS *See also Sex Stimulant.*

Personal Care—Sensation (Hand & Body Lotion, Massage Oil, Bath & Shower Gel) creates an exotic arousal, increasing sexual desire. The fragrance creates a peaceful and harmonious feeling that helps ease relationship stress. **Relaxation Massage Oil** also creates a peaceful and harmonious feeling. You may want to add jasmine and ylang ylang.

—STRESS THAT STARTS WITH TIREDNESS, IRRITABILITY, OR INSOMNIA

Blend #1—15 drops clary sage, 10 drops lemon, 5 drops lavender, and 1 oz. V-6 Oil.

Supplements—ImmuPro, Inner Defense, Super B.

Stretch Marks: *See also Pregnancy/Motherhood: STRETCH MARKS.*

Oils—^TGentle Baby, ^T_Flavender, ^T_Fmyrrh, ^Tmandarin, ^Tneroli.

T—Dilute as necessary, and apply on location.

Blend #1—3 drops rosemary, 15 drops rosewood, and 1¾ oz. hazelnut oil.

Blend #2—6 drops lavender, 4 drops rosewood, 3 drops patchouli, and vitamin E Oil.

***Comments—Patricia Davis recommends adding mandarin and neroli to either rosehip seed oil or almond oil to massage over tummy and hips.

Stroke: *See also Blood: CLOTS, Blood: BROKEN BLOOD VESSELS, Brain.*

➤➤ *A stroke occurs when the blood supply to the brain is interrupted. Within a few minutes, brain cells begin to die. The affected area of the brain is unable to function, and one or more limbs on one side of the body become weak and unable to move. Strokes can cause serious disabilities, including paralysis and speech problems.*

Oils—^{AT}Aroma Life, ^{AT}cypress, ^{AT}helichrysum, ^Ifennel[399], ^Ibasil[400], ^{AT}black pepper[401], ^{AT}calamus.

A—Inhale oil deeply either directly from bottle or applied to hands, tissue, or a cotton wick. *See Comments under Asthma for a discussion on using* **plastic nasal inhalers**.

T—Apply to neck and forehead.

I—Add 1–3 drops to an empty capsule, and swallow.

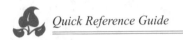

Supplements— Master Formula, NingXia Red, Power Meal, Sulfurzyme, Ultra Young+, Wolfberry Crisp Bars.

—HEAT

Oils—ᵀPeppermint, ᵀlavender

T—Rub on neck and on forehead.

—MUSCULAR PARALYSIS

Oils—ᵀLavender.

T—Apply on affected muscles, spine, and back of neck.

Blend #1—Mix together equal parts of basil, lavender, and rosemary. Rub spinal column and paralyzed area (*Alternative Medicine—The Definitive Guide*, p. 978).

Structural Alignment:

Oils—ᵀ<u>Valor</u>, ᵀwintergreen (apply on feet to reduce time and effort neces-

> *Valor is considered a "chiropractor in a bottle." It may help to realign the spine and keep the body in balance.*

sary for alignments and to increase the amount of time the alignment remains effective), ᵀ<u>Aroma Siez</u>, ᵀbasil, ᵀcypress, ᵀpeppermint.

T—Dilute as necessary, and apply to spine and to bottoms of feet.

***Comments—Do the Raindrop Technique.

Personal Care—Ortho Ease Massage Oil.

Subconscious:

Oils—ᴬᵀBelieve, ᴬᵀbalsam fir, ᴬᵀ<u>Gratitude</u>, ᴬᵀhelichrysum (uplifts when diffused), ᴬᵀ<u>Transformation</u>, ᴬᵀwestern red cedar.

A—Inhale directly or applied to hands, tissue, or a cotton wick. Diffuse into the air.

T—Dilute with V-6 Oil to create a massage oil, and massage into the skin. Add 1–2 drops to warm bathwater before bathing.

Sudorific:

Oils—ᵀThyme, ᵀhyssop, ᵀjuniper, ᵀlavender, ᵀRoman chamomile, ᵀrosemary.

> *A sudorific is an agent that causes sweating. It may be helpful in times of fever or when toxins need to be released through the skin.*

T—Dilute with V-6 Oil to create a massage oil, and apply to the skin.

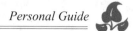
Sugar:

*****Comments**—White sugar creates acid in the body.

Honey goes into the blood stream faster than sugar and can be harder on the system than sugar. Maple syrup is one of the most perfect sugars because it has equal proportions of positive and negative ions. It also has the same pH as the blood, and it doesn't go into the blood as fast as honey or sugar. Diabetics and pre-diabetics should use blackstrap molasses instead of maple syrup.

Supplements—Allerzyme (aids the digestion of sugars, starches, fats, and proteins). **NingXia Red** (contains 4 of the 8 essential sugars that heal the body and are necessary for cell-to-cell communication).

Substitute—Stevia (liquid), **Yacon Syrup**.

—**REMOVE ADDICTIONS TO SUGAR**

Oils—^{T}Dill

T—Apply on wrists.

—**STOP EATING**

Oils—^{A}Peace & Calming, ^{A}Purification.

A—Inhale directly or applied to tissue or a cotton wick.

Supplements—JuvaTone.

Suicide: *See Depression and Emotions.*

Sunburn: *See also Burns.*

Oils—^T_FTea tree, ^{T}lavender ^{T}Australian Blue, ^{T}peppermint, ^{T}tamanu (mix with helichrysum).

My niece came to me in a panic. She had been at the beach all day and had acquired a nasty sunburn on her face, chest, and arms. She was planning to go to a fancy party the next day and decided that she absolutely could not go to the party unless the sunburn was gone. I immediately applied a layer of lavender oil, followed a few minutes later by a layer of peppermint oil. The next day to her amazement the sunburn had vanished and she was able to enjoy her party.

–Submitted by J. S., Florida (July 2004)

T—Dilute as necessary, and apply on location.

Recipe #1—Spray or rub with Roman chamomile and lavender. Add 5–6 drops of Roman chamomile to lukewarm bathwater to help reduce the burning sensation.

Recipe #2—Add a little lavender or tamanu oil to some Lavender Hand & Body Lotion.

Blend #1—Put 10 drops of lavender in a 4 oz. glass or plastic spray bottle full of distilled water. Shake well; then spray on location. This is effective for pain and healing.

Supplements—Mineral Essence (can apply directly on affected area).

Personal Care—LavaDerm Cooling Mist (use as often as needed to keep skin cool and moist), A·R·T Skin Care System, Lavender Hand & Body Lotion (later to help maintain moisture).

A=Aromatic **T**=Topical **I**=Internal

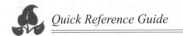

–P<small>REVENT</small> B<small>LISTERING</small>

Recipe #3—Apply 2–3 drops of lavender with Lavender Hand & Body Lotion.

Sun Screen:

Oils—^T_FHelichrysum, ^Ttamanu[402] (used by Polynesians as a natural sunscreen for centuries).

T—Dilute with V-6 Oil, and apply to the skin.

Personal Care—A·R·T Skin Care System.

Supportive:

Oils—^{TA}Myrrh.

T—Dilute with V-6 Oil to create a massage oil, and massage into the skin. Apply to Vita Flex points on the feet.

A—Diffuse into the air. Inhale directly or applied to hands.

Swelling: *See also Edema (for swelling from water retention), Inflammation.*

» *Swelling is the enlargement of organs, skin, or other body parts. It is caused by an excess of fluids in the tissues. Swelling can be throughout the body (generalized) or only in a specific part of the body (localized). Swelling can occur due to an injury, infection, or disease.*

Oils—^{TI}Tangerine, ^Thelichrysum, ^Tlemongrass, ^Tocotea.

T—Dilute as necessary, and apply on location.

I—Add 1 drop to 8 oz. of water, and drink.

Blend #1—Layer myrrh, frankincense, balsam fir, and helichrysum directly on location.

Sympathetic Nervous System: *See Nervous System: S<small>YMPATHETIC</small>.*

Sympathy:

Oils—^{AT}<u>Acceptance</u>, ^{AT}<u>Awaken</u>, ^{AT}<u>Present Time</u>.

A—Inhale directly or applied to hands. Diffuse into the air.

T—Apply to auricular emotion points. Add 1–2 drops to warm bathwater, and bathe.

Tachycardia (Rapid Heartbeat): *See Cardiovascular System: T<small>ACHYCARDIA</small>.*

Talkative:

Oils—^ACypress (for over-talkative).

A—Inhale directly or applied to hands.

Taste:

Oils—^THelichrysum, ^Tpeppermint (for impaired taste).

T—Apply 1 drop on tongue, or on Vita Flex points on the feet.

Supplements—Mineral Essence, Super B, Super C / Super C Chewable (enhances flavor).

Teeth: *See also Oral Conditions.*

—CAVITIES

Recipe #1—Brush teeth with <u>Thieves</u>. Put a drop on your toothpaste if you can't handle it straight.

Personal Care—Thieves Dentarome/Dentarome Plus Toothpaste, Thieves Fresh Essence Plus Mouthwash, KidScents Toothpaste (for children).

***Comments—*People have had regeneration of their teeth in as little as four months by brushing their teeth with <u>Thieves</u>.*

> *My husband has very cavity prone teeth that have needed much dental work in the past 5 years. He has been going in for cleanings every 3 months. His dentist had once prescribed a special mouth wash that was supposed to help his decaying teeth. He didn't use the mouthwash regularly enough to see any improvement. About a year ago, he started using Dentarome Plus toothpaste instead of the brand he had been using from the local grocer. That was the only change he made to his dental hygiene routine. At his cleaning in March, his dentist wanted to know what he was doing differently, because his x-rays showed no dental work needed to be done and they didn't have to work as hard to polish his teeth. He told them that all he changed was the toothpaste he was using. They wanted to know if it had fluoride in it, because to be any good (in their eyes) it must have fluoride in it; he brushed them off not wanting to get into the dangers of fluoride with them that day. Then at his cleaning just last week, the dentist had to look at his x-rays twice as well as call on two other colleagues to look at his x-rays to be sure that nothing was being missed because they could not find anything that needed to be fixed. They also told him to come back in six months (instead of 3) for his next cleaning. Now, if I could only get him to use the Fresh Essence Plus mouthwash...*
> *-Submitted by A. Corn*
> *Machesney Park, Illinois (July 2004)*

—FILLINGS

Recipe #2—To help eliminate toxins from mercury in the system, place 22 drops of balsam fir in a capsule, and take once in the morning and once at night. Can also combine balsam fir with helichrysum and/or frankincense.

Supplements—Super C / Super C Chewable, Cleansing Trio (ComforTone, Essentialzyme, and ICP), Detoxzyme (5 in morning and 5 at night until body says stop! Then back off to 1 or 2 per day).

—GUM SURGERY

Recipe #3—Helichrysum every 15 minutes for the pain.

—TEETHING PAIN

Oils—^TGerman chamomile, ^T<u>Thieves</u>.

A=Aromatic   **T**=Topical   **I**=Internal

—TOOTHACHE

Oils—$^\text{T}_\text{F}$Clove, $^\text{T}$cajeput, $^\text{T}$tea tree, $^\text{T}$Purification (antibacterial), $^\text{T}$Roman chamomile.

Personal Care—Thieves Dentarome / Dentarome Plus Toothpaste, Thieves Fresh Essence Plus Mouthwash.

—TOOTHPASTE

Oils—$^\text{T}$Thieves.

***Comments—*You may want to put 10-12 drops of Thieves in a 2 oz. spray bottle filled with distilled water. Shake well, then mist in mouth or on toothbrush and brush.*

Personal Care—Thieves Dentarome / Dentarome Plus Toothpaste, Thieves Fresh Essence Plus Mouthwash, KidScents Toothpaste (for children).

Recipe #4—Combine 4 tsp. green or white clay with 1 tsp. salt, 1–2 drops peppermint, and 1–2 drops lemon; mix clockwise.

—NERVE PAIN

Recipe #5—Put 1 drop tea tree in a small amount of water, and hold in mouth for 1–2 minutes to help calm nerves.

T—Dilute as necessary, and apply on location (on gums) and along jawbone. Mix 1–2 drops with 4 oz. water, and use as mouth rinse.

Temperature: *See also Cooling Oils, Fever, Thyroid, Warming Oils.*

Supplements—Thyromin (balances the temperature in the body).

—LOWER

Oils—$^\text{T}$Peppermint, $^\text{T}$bergamot, $^\text{T}$eucalyptus, $^\text{T}$lavender, $^\text{T}$melissa. $^\text{T}$Cypress and $^\text{T}$rosemary induce sweating to lower temperature indirectly.

T—Use oils in baths; or mix oils with cool water, and sponge over body or area.

—RAISE

Oils—$^\text{T}$Marjoram, $^\text{T}$thyme, $^\text{T}$onycha (benzoin).

T—Add to V-6 Oil for brisk massage.

***Comments—*Locally warming (rubefacient) oils like black pepper, juniper, and rosemary help raise temperature in cold extremities.

Tendinitis:

Oils—^TWintergreen, ^Tmarjoram,
^TPanAway, ^TRelieve It, ^Tbasil,
^Tcypress, ^Tbalsam fir, ^Tginger, ^Tlavender, ^Tpeppermint, ^Trosemary.

Supplements—BLM

—PAIN RELIEF

Oils—^TWintergreen, ^TPanAway,
^Tbalsam fir, ^Tfrankincense,
^Tpeppermint.

> **Tendinitis Blend**
>
> *This has worked for my tendinitis and for several other people I have given it to. In a 15 ml amber glass bottle, I mix the following essential oils: 3 drops each of helichrysum, pepper, bergamot, and geranium, 5 drops each of Idaho balsam fir and lemongrass, then 3 drops each of hyssop, blue tansy, pine, and myrtle. Then I fill the rest of the bottle with V-6 Mixing Oil. This is applied to the area where the pain is and followed with a layer of peppermint oil. This can be done several times per day. If a sensitivity develops, stop using it for a few weeks.*
>
> **-Submitted by J. S.**
> **West Saint Paul, Minnesota (July 2004)**

*****Comments**—If pain and inflammation are results of torn or infected ligaments or tendons, then lemongrass and helichrysum can be helpful when added to any of the above oils.

T—Apply oils in Raindrop fashion on location and apply an ice pack. Can also try alternating cold and hot packs.

Tennis Elbow:

>> *Tennis Elbow is the painful inflammation of the tendon on the outer side of the elbow that usually results from excessive strain on and twisting of the forearm.*

Oils—^TPanAway, ^Teucalyptus, ^Tpeppermint, ^Thelichrysum, ^Trosemary, ^Twintergreen.

T—Dilute as necessary, and apply on location. Apply as cold compress.

Blend #1—10 drops eucalyptus, 10 drops peppermint, 10 drops rosemary, and 1 Tbs. V-6 Oil. Mix and apply; then apply ice pack. Can also try alternating cold and hot packs.

Blend #2—Equal parts lemongrass, helichrysum, marjoram, and peppermint. Mix and apply; then apply ice pack.

Tension:

Oils—^{AT}Peace & Calming, ^{AT}_rcedarwood, ^TStress Away, ^{AT}lavender, ^{AT}ylang ylang, ^TTranquil (roll-on), ^{AT}basil (nervous), ^{AT}bergamot (nervous), ^{AT}frankincense, ^{AT}Harmony, ^{AT}Tea tree ericifolia (nervous), ^{AT}Trauma Life (balances and calms), ^{AT}valerian.

Supplements—SleepEssence (short-term only).

—RELIEVE

Oils—^TTranquil (roll on), ^{AT}Grapefruit, ^{AT}Roman chamomile, ^{AT}Transformation.

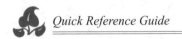

Personal Care—**Ortho Ease Massage Oil, Relaxation Massage Oil,** Prenolone/Prenolone+, Progessence/Progessence Plus.

A—Apply on hands, cup hands over nose and mouth, and breathe deeply; or diffuse. *See COMMENTS under Asthma for a discussion on using plastic nasal inhalers.*

T—Mix a few drops of oil, or oils of choice, in ½ cup Epsom salts, and dissolve in warm bathwater before bathing. Dilute with V-6 Oil to create a massage oil, and massage into skin.

Testicle/Testes:

>> *The testes are the male reproductive organs. The testes are responsible for producing and storing sperm and male hormones such as testosterone. Hormones produced in the testes are responsible for the development of male characteristics: facial hair, wide shoulders, low voice, and reproductive organs.*

Oils—^{TA}_FRosemary.

—REGULATION

Oils—^{TA}<u>Aroma Siez</u> (combine with <u>Mister</u>), ^{TA}clary sage, ^{TA}sandalwood, ^{TA}geranium, ^{TA}yarrow.

Personal Care—Prenolone+.

Supplements—Mineral Essence, Prostate Health, Ultra Young+.

T—Dilute as necessary, and apply on location or on Vita Flex points on the feet.

A—Diffuse into the air. Inhale directly or applied to hands, tissue, or a cotton wick.

Thoughts:

Oils—^A<u>Inspiration</u> (relieves negative), ^Aravintsara (lifts emotions).

A—Diffuse into the air. Inhale directly or applied to hands, tissue, or a cotton wick. Wear as perfume or cologne.

Throat: *See also Antibacterial, Antiviral, Colds.*

Oils—^{TA}_FCypress, ^{TA}calamus (helps remove phlegm), ^{TA}oregano.

***Comments—Myrrh and peppermint are also very effective for removing phlegm and mucus from the throat area.

—Dry

Oils—^{IT}Grapefruit, ^{IT}lemon.

—INFECTION IN

   Oils—^{AI}_FLemon, ^{TAI}_Fpeppermint, ^{TA}clary sage, ^{TA}oregano.

—LARYNGITIS *See Laryngitis.*

—SORE

   Oils—^{TAI}Thieves, ^T_Ftea tree, ^Toregano, ^Aeucalyptus, ^Tbergamot, ^Tcajeput, ^Aclary
   sage, ^Tgeranium, ^Tginger, ^TImmuPower, ^Alavender, ^Tmyrrh, ^TRC, ^{TA}sandalwood,
   ^Athyme.

   Recipe #1—Put 1 drop of Thieves in 32 oz. water, and drink.

   Personal Care—Gargle with **Fresh Essence Plus Mouthwash**.

   Supplements—Inner Defense, Thieves Lozenges.

—STREP *See also Antibacterial*

   ≫ *Strep throat is a throat infection caused by streptococci bacteria. This infection causes the throat and tonsils to become inflamed and swollen, resulting in a severe sore throat. Symptoms of strep throat include a sudden severe sore throat, pain when swallowing, high fever, swollen tonsils and lymph nodes, white spots on the back of the throat, skin rash, and sometimes vomiting.*

   Oils—^{TAI}Thieves (rub on throat every time it feels sore; dilute well!), ^{TA}geranium,
   ^{TA}ginger, ^{TA}hyssop, ^{TA}laurel, ^{TA}tea tree (combine with Thieves, and dilute),
   ^{TA}oregano, ^{TA}ravintsara (combine with Melrose).

   Personal Care—Gargle with **Fresh Essence Plus Mouthwash** (every hour).

   Supplements—Inner Defense, Thieves Lozenges, ImmuPro, Super C / Super C Chewable.

—TONSILLITIS

   ≫ *Tonsillitis is inflammation of the tonsils, typically due to infection. Tonsillitis causes the tonsils to become swollen and painful. Symptoms of Tonsillitis include sore throat, red and swollen tonsils, painful swallowing, loss of voice, fever, chills, headache, and white patches on the tonsils.*

   Oils—^{TA}_FTea tree, ^{TA}Thieves, ^{TA}_Fginger, ^{TA}bergamot, ^{TA}clove, ^{TA}geranium, ^{TA}goldenrod, ^{TA}lavender, ^Tlemon (gargle), ^{TA}onycha (benzoin), ^{TA}Roman chamomile, ^{TA}thyme.

   Personal Care—Fresh Essence Plus Mouthwash.

   Supplements—Thieves Lozenges.

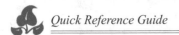

    *****Comments**—Use caution when considering surgery (tonsillectomy) for recurring tonsillitis, as doctors have discovered that the only area of the body that can synthesize the antibody to poliomyelitis (polio) is the tonsils.

T—Dilute as necessary, and apply 1–2 drops on throat, Vita Flex points on the feet, or lungs. Add 1–2 drops to 4 oz. water, and gargle.

A—Diffuse into the air, and inhale vapors deeply. Inhale directly or applied to hands.

I—Add 1 drop to 8 oz. water (32 oz. for <u>Thieves</u>), and drink.

Thrush: *See Antifungal: Candida.*

Thymus:

  » *The thymus is an organ responsible for the development of T cells needed for immune system functioning. The thymus is located just behind the sternum in the upper part of the chest.*

    Oils—ᵀ<u>Thieves</u>, ᵀ<u>ImmuPower</u> (throat and chest), ᵀelemi, ᵀravintsara.

    —**Stimulates**

        Oils—ᵀ_F_Spruce, ᵀ<u>ImmuPower</u>.

        Supplements—Ultra Young+ (reverses aging of the thymus gland).

    T—Dilute as necessary, and apply as indicated or over thymus and on bottoms of feet.

Thyroid:

  » *The thyroid is a gland located in the front of the neck that plays a key role in regulating metabolism. The thyroid produces and secretes the hormones needed to regulate blood pressure, heart rate, body temperature, and energy production.*

    —**Dysfunction**

        Oils—ᵀᴬClove.

    —**Normalizes Hormonal Imbalance Of**

        Oils—ᵀᴬMyrtle.

    —**Hyperthyroidism**

      » *Hyperthyroidism is when the thyroid gland produces too much of its hormones, typically due to the thyroid becoming enlarged. This can result in a noticeably enlarged thyroid gland (goiter), sudden weight loss, sweating, a rapid or irregular heartbeat, shortness of breath, muscle weakness, nervousness, and irritability.*

        Oils—ᵀᴬ_F_Myrrh, ᵀᴬ_F_spruce, ᵀᴬ<u>EndoFlex</u>, ᵀᴬmyrtle.

        Supplements—Sulfurzyme.

Blend #1—Equal parts lemongrass and myrrh. Apply undiluted on thyroid and parathyroid Vita Flex points under big toes; or dilute with a small amount of V-6 Oil, and apply on throat just under the Adam's apple.

Blend #2—Equal parts myrrh and spruce. Apply as directed in **Blend #1** above.

—**HYPOTHYROIDISM**

Oils—$^{TA}_{F}$Myrtle, ^{TA}EndoFlex (on tops of big toes), ^{TA}clove, ^{TA}peppermint, ^{TA}spearmint.

***Comments—Combine lemongrass with any or all of these oils, and apply as directed in Blend #1 above.

> *The **thyroid gland** is situated in the neck and regulates the body's metabolic rate.*
>
> *To determine whether or not the thyroid needs help, you must monitor your basal cell temperature. Place a thermometer under your armpit before getting out of bed in the morning, and rest quietly for 10 minutes. A temperature below 97.6° F (36.5° C) may indicate hypothyroidism (low thyroid function), and a temperature above 98° F (36.7° C) may indicate hyperthyroidism.*

Supplements—Thyromin (regulates metabolism, balances body temperature, prevents fatigue; *follow directions for use as specified in the Supplements section of the* Reference Guide for Essential Oils *under Thyromin*).

***Comments—*One of the signs of thyroid deficiency is rough, dry skin on the bottoms of the feet.*

—**REGULATION**

Oils—^{TA}Ledum.

—**SUPPORTS**

Oils—^{TA}EndoFlex, ^{TA}myrrh (rub on hands and feet), ^{TA}myrtle.

Supplements—Thyromin (regulates metabolism, balances body temperature, prevents fatigue; *follow directions for use as specified in the Supplements section of the* Reference Guide for Essential Oils *under Thyromin*), Cleansing Trio (ComforTone, Essential-zyme, and ICP), EndoGize, MultiGreens (enhances effect of Thyromin), Power Meal.

T—Dilute as necessary, and apply 1–2 drops on base of throat, hands, or Vita Flex points on the feet.

A—Diffuse into the air. Inhale oils applied to hands.

Tinnitus: *See Ears: Tinnitus.*

Tired: *See Energy, Exhaustion, and Fatigue.*

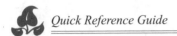

Tissue:

▸▸ *Tissue refers to any group of similar cells that work together to perform a specific function in an organ or in the body. Some types of tissue include muscle tissue, connective tissue, nervous tissue, or epithelial tissue (tissue that lines or covers a surface, such as the skin, or the lining of the blood vessels).*

Oils—ᵀLemongrass, ᵀhelichrysum, ᵀbasil, ᵀelemi (rejuvenates), ᵀlavender, ᵀlime (tightens connective tissue), ᵀmarjoram, ᵀ<u>Melrose</u>, ᵀRoman chamomile, ᵀsandalwood.

Personal Care—Essential Beauty Serums (Dry, & Acne-Prone Skin Blends)

Supplements— Power Meal (predigested protein), **Pure Protein Complete,** Master Formula.

—Aɴᴛɪ-ɪɴꜰʟᴀᴍᴍᴀᴛᴏʀʏ *See Inflammation*

—Bᴏɴᴇ ᴀɴᴅ Jᴏɪɴᴛ Rᴇɢᴇɴᴇʀᴀᴛɪᴏɴ

Blend #1—5 drops wintergreen, 2 drops German chamomile, 1 drop blue tansy, 7 drops fir, 5 drops hyssop, 5 drops helichrysum, 4 drops lemongrass, 8 drops sandalwood, 8 drops spruce, and 1 oz. V-6 Oil.

—Cʟᴇᴀɴsᴇs Tᴏxɪɴs Fʀᴏᴍ

Oils—ᵀFennel.

—Cᴏɴɴᴇᴄᴛɪᴠᴇ Tɪssᴜᴇ, Wᴇᴀᴋ

Oils—ᵀLemongrass, ᵀ<u>Aroma Siez</u>, ᵀhelichrysum, ᵀlavender, ᵀpatchouli.

Personal Care—Ortho Ease Massage Oil.

—Dᴇᴇᴘ Tɪssᴜᴇ Pᴀɪɴ

Oils—ᵀ<u>Deep Relief</u> (roll-on), ᵀ<u>PanAway</u>, ᵀ<u>Relieve It</u>, ᵀhelichrysum, ᵀpalo santo.

Personal Care—Ortho Ease and **Ortho Sport Massage Oils.**

—Rᴇᴘᴀɪʀ

Oils—ᵀLemongrass (repairs connective tissue), ᵀelemi (builds), ᵀhelichrysum (scar tissue; reduces tissue pain), ᵀhyssop (scars), ᵀorange, ᵀrosewood, ᵀsage (firms tissue), ᵀ<u>Relieve It</u> (deep tissue damage).

Personal Care—A·R·T Skin Care System (unique enzymes that work to repair DNA damage), **Rose Ointment** (to help maintain, protect, and keep the scab soft), Lavender Hand & Body Lotion (to moisturize and promote healing).

—Rᴇɢᴇɴᴇʀᴀᴛᴇ

Oils—ᵀ_F_Patchouli, ᵀhelichrysum, ᵀlemongrass, ᵀgeranium, ᵀ<u>Melrose</u>, ᵀrosehip.

***Comments**—*Use helichrysum and <u>Melrose</u> together for traumatized tissue (cuts, wounds, and abrasions).*

—SCARRING: *See Scarring*

T—Dilute as necessary, and apply on location or on Vita Flex points on the feet. Apply as warm compress. Dilute with V-6 Oil to create a massage oil, and massage on location.

TMJ (Temporomandibular Joint Disorder or TMD):

≫ *TMD is a disorder of the temporomandibular joint—the joint connecting the lower jaw to the skull. TMD signs and symptoms include jaw pain or tenderness, difficulty chewing, ear pain, facial pain, difficulty opening and closing the mouth, jaw lock, headache, swelling of the side of the face, and popping or grating sounds when opening or closing the mouth. Some possible causes of TMD are teeth clenching or grinding, osteoarthritis or rheumatoid arthritis, stress, and injury.*

Recipe #1—<u>3 Wise Men</u>. Apply on temple and on side of face, in front of ear and down to the jaw. Cover with ice packs for 10 minutes at a time, 3–4 times a day. May be best to seek advice from a health care professional, especially a dentist.

Tonic:

T

—DIGESTIVE

Oils—$^{TA}_F$German chamomile, ^{TA}Tea tree quinquenervia.

Supplements—**Digest + Cleanse** (very soothing to the digestive system)

—GENERAL

Oils—^{TA}Lemongrass, ^{TA}cinnamon bark, ^{TA}sandalwood, ^{TA}angelica, ^{TA}basil, ^{TA}cajeput, ^{TA}cardamom, ^{TA}cistus, ^{TA}clary sage, ^{TA}cumin, ^{TA}galbanum, ^{TA}geranium, ^{TA}ginger, ^{TA}grapefruit, ^{TA}juniper, ^{TA}lemon, ^{TA}lime, ^{TA}mandarin, ^{TA}marjoram, ^{TA}melissa, ^{TA}Roman chamomile, ^{TA}mountain savory, ^{TA}myrrh, ^{TA}neroli, ^{TA}nutmeg, ^{TA}orange, ^{TA}palmarosa, ^{TA}patchouli, ^{TA}spruce, ^{TA}ylang ylang.

—HEART

Oils—^{TA}Thyme, ^{TA}lavender.

—NERVE

Oils—$^{TA}_F$Ravintsara, ^{TA}tea tree, ^{TA}clary sage, ^{TA}carrot, ^{TA}thyme.

—SKIN

Oils—^{T}Spearmint, ^{T}lemon, ^{T}lime, ^{T}spikenard.

Personal Care—Essential Beauty Serums (Dry, & Acne-Prone Skin Blends)

A=Aromatic **T**=Topical **I**=Internal

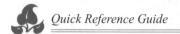
—S<small>TOMACH</small>

>   Oils—^{TA}Tangerine.

—U<small>TERINE</small>

>   Oils—^{TA}Jasmine, ^{TA}thyme.

T—Dilute with V-6 Oil to create a massage oil, and massage into skin and over area of concern. Add 1–2 drops to warm bathwater before bathing. Dilute as necessary, and apply 1–2 drops to area of concern or to Vita Flex points on the feet or hands.

***Comments—The best way to restore tone in a body that is run-down is to apply oils by massage. Baths are next in effectiveness to massage if massage is not possible or in between massages.

Tonsillitis: *See Throat: T<small>ONSILLITIS</small>.*

Toothache: *See Teeth.*

Toxemia: *See also Antibacterial, Pregnancy/Motherhood: T<small>OXEMIA</small>/P<small>REECLAMPSIA</small>.*

>> *Toxemia is the general term for toxic substances in the bloodstream. This is typically caused by a bacterial infection in which bacteria release toxins into the blood.*

>   Oils—^{TA}<u>Aroma Life</u>, ^{TA}cypress.

>   Supplements—Rehemogen tincture.

T—Dilute as necessary, and apply 1–2 drops over neck, over heart, or over bottoms of feet. Dilute with V-6 Oil to create a massage oil, and massage on location.

A—Diffuse into the air. Inhale directly or applied to hands.

Toxins: *See Detoxification: T<small>OXINS</small>.*

Transition in Life:

>   Oils—^{TA}<u>Transformation</u>, ^{TA}<u>Acceptance</u>, ^{TA}<u>Awaken</u> (into achieving success),^{TA} basil, ^{TA}cypress. May also want to concentrate on the emotional blends of ^{TA}<u>Valor</u>, ^{TA}<u>Motivation</u>, ^{TA}<u>Grounding</u>, ^{TA}<u>Release</u>,
>   ^{TA}<u>Hope</u>, and ^{TA}<u>Joy</u> *(refer to the pages on "Auricular Emotional Therapy" and "Emotional Release" in the Science and Application section of the <u>Reference Guide for Essential Oils</u>).*

T—Apply to auricular emotion points. Dilute with V-6 Oil to create a massage oil, and massage into skin.

A—Inhale directly or applied to hands. Diffuse into the air.

Trauma: *See also Shock.*

> **Recipe #1**—Release (feet and liver), Joy (heart), 3 Wise Men (crown); use all three blends in succession. May also diffuse. Australian Blue, Envision, Forgiveness, Hope, and Release can also aid in releasing emotional trauma (*Refer to each blend separately in the Blends section of the Reference Guide for Essential Oils for possible applications*). Trauma Life is an excellent blend for helping to cope with shock or emotional trauma. Apply on forehead and on palms; then rub palms together, cup over nose and mouth, and inhale deeply. Others that may help are Valor (on the feet), SARA (on temples), Peace & Calming (on palms; place hands together over heart in prayer position), or Tranquil (roll-on), .
>
> *****Comments**—Concentrate on relaxing to help release the trauma. Also, if after an emotional or physical trauma you find you don't like the smell of a particular oil, it may be the one you need most to help unlock the trauma. Try exposing yourself to it a little at a time until the healing is finished.
>
> **Supplements**—ImmuPro, Mineral Essence, Super C / Super C Chewable.

Travel Sickness: *See Motion Sickness, Nausea.*

Tuberculosis (T. B.): *See also Antibacterial, Respiratory System: Blend #5.*

> ›› *Tuberculosis is a bacterial disease spread through the air (via coughing, spitting, sneezing, etc.). Tuberculosis most commonly infects the lungs, but it can infect other bodily systems as well. Symptoms of Tuberculosis include a chronic cough (often with blood), fever, chills, weakness and fatigue, weight loss, and night sweats. Tuberculosis is contagious and sometimes deadly.*
>
> **Oils**—[AT][F]Eucalyptus radiata, [AT][F]cedarwood, [AT]melissa, [AT][F]cypress, [AT][F]thyme linalol, [AT][F]myrtle, [AT]cajeput, [AT]lemon, [AT]vetiver[403], [AT]eucalyptus citriodora[404], [AT]peppermint, [AT]rosemary verbenon, [AT]sandalwood.
>
> **Recipe #1**—Exodus II (on spine and Raven on back with a hot compress), ImmuPower (on spine daily), Raven (1–2 drops in V-6 Oil as a rectal implant), RC (on chest and back—reverse each night with Raven), rose, rosemary, Thieves (on feet). A hot compress can be used when applying oils to the chest or back. **Do the Raindrop Technique**.
>
> **Supplements**—ImmuPro, Inner Defense, MultiGreens, Rehemogen Tincture, Super C / Super C Chewable. Do a colon and liver cleanse with Balance Complete or the Cleansing Trio (ComforTone, Essentialzyme, and ICP), and JuvaTone.
>
> **Blend #1**—1–2 drops each of *Eucalyptus radiata*, myrtle, mountain savory, and ravintsara in 1 Tbs. V-6 Oil. Apply as a rectal implant.

A=Aromatic   **T**=Topical   **I**=Internal

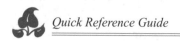
*****Comments**—*Refer to the chapter entitled "How to Use—The Personal Usage Reference" in the* <u>Essential Oils Desk Reference</u> *under "Tuberculosis" for a specific regimen using the blends and supplements.*

—**AIRBORNE BACTERIA**

> Oils—^A<u>Thieves</u>, ^A<u>Purification</u>, ^A<u>RC</u>, ^Alemongrass[405], ^Ageranium[405], ^A<u>Raven</u>, ^A<u>Sacred Mountain</u>.

> *****Comments**—Alternate diffusing different oils to help control the spread of bacteria like *Mycobacterium tuberculosis*.

> **Blend #2**—Equal amounts of cypress and <u>Sacred Mountain</u>. Diffuse.

—**PULMONARY**

> Oils—^{AT}_FOregano, ^{AT}cypress, ^{AT}eucalyptus, ^{AT}<u>Inspiration</u>, ^{AT}ravintsara.

> **Blend #3**—Equal amounts of frankincense and <u>ImmuPower</u>. Diffuse; or dilute with V-6 Oil, and massage on chest or back. Can also apply to Vita Flex lung points on hands and feet.

A—Diffuse into the air. Add 2–3 drops to a bowl of hot water, and inhale vapors. Inhale directly or applied to hands.

T—Dilute as necessary, and apply on chest, back, or Vita Flex points on the feet. Add 1–2 drops to 1 tsp. V-6 Oil or olive oil, and apply as a rectal implant. Dilute with V-6 Oil to create a massage oil, and massage on chest, back, and feet.

Tumors: *See also Cancer.*

—**ANTITUMORAL**

> ➤➤ *An antitumor is a substance used to prevent the development of malignant tumors. A tumor is an abnormal growth of cells in a lump or mass. Some tumors are malignant (cancerous) and some are benign (noncancerous). Benign tumors in most parts of the body do not create health problems. However, both malignant and benign tumors in the brain can cause serious health issues because they press on sensitive areas of the brain.*

> Oils—^T_FFrankincense (can combine with balsam fir), ^Tledum (may be more powerful than frankincense), ^Tclove (inhibits tumor growth).

> **T**—Apply directly on tumor location.

> **Supplements**—**Longevity Capsules** (contains clove, orange-high limonene, and frankincense essential oils)

—Lipoma

>> *A lipoma is a fatty tumor that normally grows between the skin and the muscle. Lipomas are not cancerous and are generally harmless.*

Oils—^TFrankincense and ^Tclove, ^Tledum, ^Tgrapefruit, ^Tginger.

T—Dilute as necessary, and apply on location and on Vita Flex points on the feet.

Personal Care—Prenolone/Prenolone+, Progessence/Progessence Plus.

Typhoid: *See Antibacterial.*

>> *Typhoid fever is a bacterial infection caused by the bacteria Salmonella typhi. Typhoid is spread through food and water infected with the feces of typhoid carriers. Possible symptoms of typhoid include abdominal pain, severe diarrhea, bloody stools, chills, severe fatigue, weakness, chills, delirium, hallucinations, confusion, agitation, and fluctuating mood.*

Oils—^{AT}_FCinnamon bark, ^{AT}peppermint, ^{AT}lemon, ^{AT}<u>Melrose</u>, ^{AT}mountain savory, ^{AT}<u>Purification</u>, ^{AT}<u>Raven</u>, ^{AT}ravintsara, ^{AT}<u>RC</u>.

A—Diffuse into the air.

T—Dilute with V-6 Oil, and apply over intestines and on Vita Flex points on the feet.

Ulcers:

>> *An ulcer is an open sore either on the skin or on an internal mucous membrane (such as that lining the stomach).*

> *While some sources claim that sixty percent of all **ulcers** are caused by bacteria, F. Batmanghelidj, MD, maintains that the majority of ulcers are only dehydration of the stomach lining. In his book, <u>Your Body's Many Cries for Water</u>, Dr. Batmanghelidj shows that rehydration is the simplest cure for this and many other adverse health conditions.*

Oils—^{IT}_FFrankincense, ^{IT}_FGerman chamomile, ^{IT}_Fmyrrh, ^{IT}marjoram[406], ^{IT}lemon[407], ^{IT}dill[408], ^{IT}bergamot, ^{IT}cinnamon bark, ^{IT}clove, ^{IT}elemi, ^{IT}geranium, ^{IT}lemon, ^{IT}oregano, ^{IT}rose, ^{IT}thyme, ^{IT}vetiver.

I—Add one drop of oil to rice or almond milk, and take as a dietary supplement.

T—Apply over stomach with a hot compress.

Supplements—Use **ComforTone** to help destroy the bacteria; then use Essentialzyme, Essentialzymes-4, Master Formula.

—Duodenal

>> *A duodenal ulcer is an ulcer in the upper part of the small intestine.*

Oils—^{IT}_FFrankincense, ^{IT}_FGerman chamomile, ^{IT}_Fmyrrh, ^{IT}bergamot, ^{IT}cinnamon bark, ^{IT}clove, ^{IT}elemi, ^{IT}geranium, ^{IT}lemon, ^{IT}oregano, ^{IT}rose, ^{IT}thyme, ^{IT}vetiver.

I—Add one drop of oil to rice or almond milk, and take as a dietary supplement.

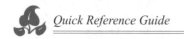

T—Apply over stomach with a hot compress.

Supplements—AlkaLime.

—GASTRIC *See also Gastritis.*

>> *A gastric ulcer is an ulcer in the stomach.*

Oils—**IT**_FGeranium, **IT**bergamot, **IT**marjoram[406], **IT**lemon[407], **IT**dill[408], **IT**frankincense, **IT**geranium, **IT**manuka, **IT**orange, **IT**peppermint.

I—Add one drop of oil to rice or almond milk, and take as a dietary supplement. Add 1 drop as flavoring in food.

T—Applied over stomach with a hot compress. Dilute as necessary, and apply to stomach and Vita Flex points.

Supplements—AlkaLime, Cleansing Trio (ComforTone, Essentialzyme, and ICP), Master Formula.

***Comments—*Manuka Honey is said to naturally kill Helicobacter pylori.*

—LEG

>> *An ulcer on the leg may be due to a lack of circulation in the lower extremities or possibly due to a bacterial, fungal, or viral infection.*

Oils—**T**Purification, **T**Gentle Baby, **T**Melrose, **T**lavender, **T**geranium, **T**German chamomile, **T**patchouli, **T**Roman chamomile, **T**rosewood, **T**Sensation.

T—Dilute as necessary, and apply on location.

***Comments—*Dilute oils with V-6 Oil, and massage lower extremities to stimulate circulation. Thyromin may be needed to help with overall circulation.*

Personal Care—Rose Ointment, Sensation Massage Oil.

Blend #1—Equal drops of lavender and either Melrose or Purification applied on location. Can cover with Rose Ointment.

—MOUTH *See also Cankers.*

>> *Mouth ulcers are open, often painful sores that occur in the mouth. Common mouth ulcers include cancer sores and cold sores. Stress, anxiety, fatigue, injury, illness, hormonal changes, and food allergies can often trigger mouth ulcers.*

Oils—**T**Basil (mouthwash), **T**myrrh, **T**orange.

T—Dilute as necessary, and apply on location. Add 1–3 drops to 4 oz. water, and use as mouthwash.

Blend #1—1 drop each of sage and clove and 1–3 drops lavender. Apply directly on location.

—Peptic

>> *A peptic ulcer is an ulcer that forms in an area of the digestive system where acid is present, such as in the stomach (gastric), esophagus, or upper part of the small intestine (duodenal).*

Recipe #1—Flavor a quart of water with 1 drop of cinnamon bark oil, and sip all day.

Supplements—AlkaLime.

—Stomach *See Gastric above*

—Ulcerations

>> *Ulceration is the process of an ulcer being formed or eroding away at the skin or mucous membrane.*

Oils—ᵀLavender, ᵀMelrose, ᵀrose.

T—Dilute as necessary, and apply on location.

***Comments—Cleanse liver and colon (*See Cleansing*).

Personal Care—Rose Ointment.

—Varicose Ulcers.

Oils—ᵀTea tree, ᵀgeranium, ᵀlavender, ᵀeucalyptus, ᵀthyme, ᵀyarrow.

T—Dilute as necessary, and apply on location.

Unwind: *See also Calming, Massage.*

Oils—ᴬᵀLavender, ᴬᵀPeace & Calming, ᵀTranquil (roll-on).

A—Diffuse into the air. Rub between hands, and inhale deeply,

T—Combine with V-6 Oil or massage oil for a massage. Add 3–5 drops to 1/4 cup Epsom or bath salts, and dissolve in warm bathwater before bathing.

Personal Care—Relaxation Massage Oil, Evening Peace Bath & Shower Gel.

Uplifting:

Oils—ᴬLemon[409], ᴬJoy, ᴬLive with Passion, ᴬorange, ᴬᵀOola Fitness, ᴬjade lemon, ᴬᵀLight the Fire, ᴬᵀOola Fun, ᴬBelieve, ᴬbergamot, ᴬBrain Power, ᴬfir (emotionally uplifting), ᴬbalsam fir, ᴬgrapefruit, ᴬhelichrysum, ᴬIdaho tansy, ᴬjasmine, ᴬlavender, ᴬmyrrh, ᴬravintsara, ᴬSacred Mountain, ᴬSensation, ᴬspruce, 3 Wise Men, ᴬTransformation, ᴬtsuga, ᴬwintergreen.

A—Diffuse or wear as perfume or cologne. *See Comments under Asthma for a discussion on using plastic nasal inhalers.*

Blend #1—3 drops wintergreen, 3 drops lavender, 3 drops orange, 3 drops spruce, and 1 oz. V-6 Oil. Wear a few drops of this blend as a perfume or cologne, or apply it over the heart,

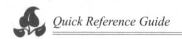
on the chest, neck, and/or shoulders, and behind the ears. Can also apply a few drops on both hands, rub hands together, cup hands over nose and mouth, and breathe deeply.

Personal Care—Morning Start Bath & Shower Gel, Sensation Bath & Shower Gel.

Ureter: *See Urinary Tract: Ureter.*

Urinary Tract: *See also Bladder, Kidneys.*

»» *The urinary tract is the collection of organs and tubes responsible for producing and excreting urine. The urinary tract is comprised of the kidneys, ureters, bladder, and urethra.*

Oils—^{TA}_FSandalwood, ^{TA}_Fthyme (infection), ^{TA}_Fsage, ^{TA}bergamot, ^{TA}copaiba, ^{TA}Immu-Power, ^{TA}lavender, ^{TA}ledum, ^{TA}tea tree, ^{TA}pine (antiseptic), ^{TA}rosemary, ^{TA}tarragon.

T—Dilute as necessary, and apply over lower abdomen, lower back, or pubic area. Dilute with V-6 Oil to create a massage oil, and massage on abdomen, lower back, or pubic area. Apply as a warm compress.

A—Diffuse into the air.

—GENERAL STIMULANT

> **Oils**—^{TA}_FEucalyptus, ^{TA}bergamot.
>
> **T**—Dilute as necessary, and apply over lower abdomen, lower back, or pubic area. Dilute with V-6 Oil to create a massage oil, and massage on location. Apply as a warm compress.
>
> **A**—Diffuse into the air.

—INFECTION *See also Bladder: INFECTION.*

> **Oils**—^T_FCedarwood, ^TPurification (effective by itself), ^TImmuPower, ^TInspiration (effective by itself), ^Tbergamot, ^Tcajeput, ^TDi-Gize, ^TEndoFlex, ^Tgeranium, ^Thyssop, ^Tjuniper, ^Tlemongrass, ^TMelrose, ^Tonycha, ^Ttarragon.
>
> **T**—Apply 2–3 drops of oil directly over bladder. May also apply as a hot compress.
>
> **Blend #1**—Equal parts sage and Purification.
>
> **Blend #2**—Equal parts thyme and Melrose.
>
> **Blend #3**—Equal parts oregano and Thieves.
>
> **Blend #4**—Equal parts juniper and EndoFlex.

With any of these blends, dilute with V-6 Oil, and massage over lower back and pubic area, or apply with a hot compress.

Supplements—AlkaLime, Inner Defense, K&B Tincture.

Recipe #1—Add 1 drop of mountain savory to 3 droppers of K&B tincture in distilled water, and drink every few hours.

***Comments—*Refer to the chapter entitled "How to Use—The Personal Usage Reference" in the <u>Essential Oils Desk Reference</u> under "Urinary Tract/Bladder Infection" for a unique blend of 14 different oils to specifically help with infection.*

—STONES IN

>> *Stones are solid masses that form as minerals and other chemicals crystallize and adhere together. They can form in the bladder or kidneys. While small stones generally cause no problems, larger stones may block the ureters or urethra, causing intense pain and possibly injury.*

Oils—^T_FFennel, ^T_Fgeranium.

T—Apply oils over pubic area and lower back with a hot compress. *See MASTER CLEANSER under Cleansing.*

—SUPPORT

Oils—^{TA}Cypress, ^{TA}geranium, ^{TA}juniper, ^{TA}goldenrod, ^{TA}juniper, ^{TA}laurel, ^{TA}tea tree.

T—Dilute as necessary, and apply over lower abdomen, lower back, or pubic area. Dilute with V-6 Oil to create a massage oil, and massage on location. Apply as a warm compress.

A—Diffuse into the air.

Supplements—K&B Tincture.

—URETER (INFECTIONS IN)

>> *Ureters are the two paired tubes by which urine passes from the kidneys to the bladder.*

Oils—^T_FLemon, ^T_Fmyrtle.

T—Apply 2–3 drops of oil directly over bladder. May also apply a hot compress.

Uterus:

>> *The uterus is the female reproductive organ in which a fetus is formed and develops until birth.*

Oils—^{T}Frankincense, ^{T}lemon, ^{T}cedarwood, ^{T}geranium, ^{T}jasmine, ^{T}myrrh.

—INFLAMMATION

Oils—^{T}Elemi.

—REGENERATION OF TISSUE

Recipe #1—Frankincense, sage, tarragon. Add 1–3 drops of each to 1 tsp. V-6 Oil; insert into vagina, and retain overnight.

U

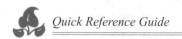

Personal Care—PD 80/20, Prenolone/Prenolone +, Progessence/Progessence Plus.

Supplements—FemiGen.

—**U**UTEROTONIC

Oils—^TThyme.

—**U**TERINE **C**ANCER *See also Cancer.*

Oils—^TFrankincense, ^Tgeranium, ^Tcedarwood, ^T<u>Gratitude</u>, ^T<u>ImmuPower</u>, ^Tlemon, ^Tmyrrh.

T—Oils can be applied to the reproductive Vita Flex points on the feet—mostly around the front of the ankle, on either side of the ankle under the ankle bone, and up the Achilles tendon. The most effective application of oils is by vaginal retention implant. Add 2–5 drops of any of these single oils or a combination of any of them to 1 tsp. V-6 Oil; insert into vagina, and retain overnight. A tampon may be used if necessary to help retain the oil.

—**U**TERINE **C**YSTS *See Ovaries: Ovarian Cysts.*

T—Dilute as necessary, and apply on lower abdomen or on Vita Flex points on the feet and ankles. Add 2–5 drops oil to 1 tsp. V-6 Oil, and insert into vagina for overnight retention (a tampon may be used if necessary to help retain the oil).

Vaginal:

—**C**ANDIDA (**THRUSH**) *See Antifungal: Candida*

—**I**NFECTION

    »» *Vaginal infections occur when there is a disruption in the normal balance of vaginal organisms, such as the sudden presence of yeast, bacteria, or viruses. Common signs of vaginal infection include redness, swelling, itching, pain, odor, change in discharge color or amount, burning sensation when urinating, and pain or bleeding during intercourse. The most common vaginal infections are yeast infection, trichomoniasis, and bacterial vaginosis.*

Oils—^T_FRosemary, ^Ttea tree, ^T_Frosewood, ^T_Fcinnamon bark (be extremely careful; dilute well), ^Tclary sage, ^Tcypress, ^Teucalyptus, ^Thyssop, ^T<u>Inspiration</u>, ^Tjuniper, ^Tlavender, ^Tlaurel, ^T<u>Melrose</u>, ^Tmyrrh, ^Tmountain savory, ^Toregano, ^Tsage, ^T<u>3 Wise Men</u>, ^Tthyme.

Recipe #1—Apply oregano and thyme along the spine using the Raindrop Technique.

Blend #1—Equal parts oregano, thyme, and <u>Melrose</u>. Dilute with V-6 Oil, and apply as described under **T** (Topical application instructions) below.

Blend #2—3 drops rosemary, 2 drops *Tea tree quinquenervia*, 2 drops oregano, and 1 drop thyme. Dilute with V-6 Oil, and apply as described under **T** (Topical application instructions) below. Can also apply as a hot compress over lower abdominal area.

Blend #3—5 drops <u>Melrose</u>, 2 drops oregano, and 1 drop thyme in 1 Tbs. V-6 Oil. Use as douche or vaginal retention implant as described under **T** (Topical application instructions) below.

—INFLAMMATION OF VAGINA *See also Anti-inflammatory*

Oils—**T**Eucalyptus, **T**lavender, **T**tea tree, **T**yarrow.

—RETENTION IMPLANT

*****Comments**—Used to cleanse and nourish the female reproductive system or as a support when taking products like the FemiGen supplement. Best when done after a colon and liver cleanse using the Cleansing Trio (ComforTone, Essentialzyme, ICP). The following blends can be inserted directly into the vagina with a vaginal syringe (available from Abundant Health). A tampon may be necessary to help retain.

Blend #4—Dilute 2 drops *Tea tree quinquenervia*, 1 drop lavender, and 1 drop bergamot in 1 Tbs. V-6 Oil. Insert, and retain overnight.

Blend #5—Dilute 2 drops frankincense and 7 drops <u>Purification</u> in 1 Tbs. V-6 Oil. Insert, and retain overnight.

—VAGINITIS

>> *Vaginitis is vaginal inflammation, typically due to infection, characterized by redness, swelling, itching, irritation, discharge, and pain of the vaginal area.*

Oils—**T**_FRosemary, **T**tea tree, **T**_Frosewood, **T**_Fcinnamon bark (be extremely careful; dilute well), **T**Eucalyptus radiata.

Valerie Worwood suggests the following douche recipe that should be used daily for three days a week only.

Recipe #1—1 drop lavender, 1 drop tea tree (tea tree), 1 tsp. of vinegar, ½ tsp. lemon juice, and 2½ cups of warm water. Mix thoroughly.

T—Mix desired oil(s) with water, and either use in a douche or in a sitz bath. Desired oil(s) may also be mixed with V-6 Oil and either applied directly, inserted with a vaginal syringe (available from Abundant Health) and retained with a tampon, or by soaking a tampon in mixture, inserting and leaving in all day or night.

U

V

A=Aromatic **T**=Topical **I**=Internal | 345

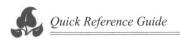

Varicose Ulcers: *See Ulcers:* VARICOSE.

Varicose Veins:

>> *Varicose veins are abnormal swelling of the veins in the legs. They are most often a symptom of poor circulation and of a loss of elasticity of the vascular walls and particularly their valves. If the valves do not work properly, blood accumulates in the veins instead of flowing back to the heart. This accumulation of blood causes*

> *Cleanse the colon.*
>
> *Helichrysum dissolves the coagulated blood inside and outside of the veins. Cypress strengthens the veins. Massage* **above** *the affected vein toward the heart with helichrysum and cypress every morning and night; wear support hose until healed. It may take from three months to a year to heal completely. It is important to vary the essential oils being used. Try using lavender, juniper or rosemary instead of cypress and helichrysum. See Diet, Circulatory System.*
>
> **Caution**: *Do not rub below the affected area, as rubbing may increase the pressure on the vein*

the veins to become swollen and twisted. Hemorrhoids are varicose veins of the anus or rectum usually resulting from constipation.

Oils—^T_FCypress (as bath oil), ^T_Flemongrass, ^T_Flemon (tonic for circulatory system), ^T_Fpeppermint, ^TAroma Life, ^TAroma Siez, ^Tbasil, ^Tbergamot, ^TCitrus Fresh, ^Tgeranium, ^Thelichrysum (especially during pregnancy), ^TIdaho tansy (helps weak veins), ^Tjuniper, ^Tlavender, ^Torange, ^Trosemary, ^Tspikenard, ^Ttangerine, ^Tyarrow.

Personal Care—Cel-Lite Magic (strengthens vascular walls).

Supplements—MultiGreens, Rehemogen Tincture, Super B, Thyromin.

Blend #1—1–3 drops each of lemongrass and Aroma Life with Cel-Lite Magic.

Blend #2—1–3 drops each of basil and Aroma Siez. Massage above the affected vein toward the heart.

***Comments—Refer to the chapter entitled "How to Use—The Personal Usage Reference" in the Essential Oils Desk Reference under "Varicose Veins" for more specific blend recipes and instructions regarding treatment.

T—Dilute as recommended, and apply oils gently from ankles up the legs. Consistent application of oils for an extended period of time is the key. Wearing support hose and elevating the feet can also help keep blood from pooling in the legs.

Vascular System: *See also Cardiovascular System, Lymphatic System, Arteries, Capillaries, Veins.*

>> *The vascular system refers to the vessels or veins that carry and circulate fluids (blood and lymph) throughout the body.*

Oils—^T_FLemongrass (strengthens vascular walls), ^TAroma Life, ^Tcypress, ^Tfrankincense, ^Thelichrysum.

Personal Care—Cel-Lite Magic (strengthens vascular walls).

—CLEANSING *See also Chelation, Metals.*

> Oils—ᵀJuva Cleanse.
>
> Supplements—**JuvaTone**, and **MultiGreens** work very well together. Essential-zyme, Essentialzymes-4, K&B Tincture, Rehemogen Tincture, Super C, Master Formula.
>
> Blend #1—1–3 drops each of helichrysum and Aroma Life with Cel-Lite Magic Massage Oil. Massage on the body to help dilate the blood vessels and to enhance the chelation of metallics.
>
> **T**—Dilute with V-6 Oil to create a massage oil, and apply as a full body massage, over heart, and on bottoms of the feet.

Vasodilator: *See Blood: VASODILATOR.*

Veins: *See also Cardiovascular System, Vascular System.*

>> *A vein is a blood vessel that carries blood from the capillaries back to the heart. Veins may also have one-way valves on the inside that help keep blood from flowing backwards and pooling in the lower extremities due to gravity.*

—CIRCULATION IN VASCULAR WALLS OF VEINS

> Oils—ᵀAroma Life, ᵀcypress, ᵀlemon.
>
> **T**—Dilute as necessary, and apply on location. Dilute with V-6 Oil to create a massage oil, and massage on location.

—BLOOD CLOT IN VEINS

> Blend #1—Cypress and helichrysum (rub neat on location to dissolve).

Vertigo: *See also Ears, Equilibrium, and Dizziness.*

>> *Vertigo refers to the sensation that the environment and objects around an individual are moving or spinning, usually causing a loss of balance or a feelings of nausea. Vertigo may be caused by ear infections, ear disorders, or motion sickness.*

> Oils—ᵀᴬGinger.
>
> **T**—Dilute as necessary, and apply around ears and on Vita Flex points on the feet.
>
> **A**—Inhale directly or applied to hands.

Viral Disease: *See Antiviral: VIRAL DISEASE.*

Viruses: *See Antiviral: VIRUSES.*

V

A=Aromatic   **T**=Topical   **I**=Internal

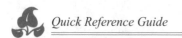

Visualization:

Oils—**ᴬ**<u>Awaken</u>, **ᴬ**<u>Dream Catcher</u>, **ᴬ**helichrysum, **ᴬ**palo santo, **ᴬ**<u>PanAway</u>.

A—Diffuse or wear as perfume or cologne.

Vital Centers:

Recipe #1—Oregano and sage may strengthen the vital centers of the body.

Vitamins: *See the Supplements section of the <u>Reference Guide for Essential Oils</u>.*

Supplements—**Power Meal, Sulfurzyme** (sulfur necessary for proper assimilation of vitamin C), **Super B, Super C / Super C Chewable, Super Cal.**

Children's Supplements—**KidScents MightyVites** (chewable vitamin tablets).

Vitiligo: *See Skin: Vitiligo.*

Voice (Hoarse): *See also Laryngitis.*

Oils—**ᵀ**Bergamot, **ᵀ**jasmine.

T—Add 1 drop to 1 oz. (2 Tbs.) water, and gargle.

Blend #1—Add one drop each of <u>Melrose</u> and lemon to 1 tsp. honey. Swish around in mouth for a couple of minutes to liquefy; then swallow.

Void:

Oils—**ᵀ**<u>3 Wise Men</u> (replaces the void).

T—Apply on crown of head.

Vomiting: *See Nausea.*

Oils—**ᴵᴬ**Ginger⁴¹⁰, **ᴬᵀ**_F_peppermint, **ᵀᴵ**_F_fennel, **ᵀ**nutmeg, **ᵀ**black pepper, **ᵀ**lavender, **ᵀ**Roman chamomile, **ᵀ**rose.

T—Apply as warm compress over stomach. Dilute with V-6 Oil to create a massage oil, and massage on stomach.

I—Place 1–2 drops in an empty capsule, and swallow.

A—Inhale directly or applied to hands. Diffuse into the air.

Warming Oils: *See also Cooling Oils, Temperature.*

Oils—**ᵀ**Cinnamon bark, **ᵀ**oregano, **ᵀ**thyme, **ᵀ**onycha (benzoin), **ᵀ**yuzu.

T—Dilute with V-6 Oil to create a massage oil, and massage briskly into skin.

Warts: *See also Antiviral.*

➤➤ *A wart is a small, firm, hard growth on the skin, usually located on the hands and feet, that is typically caused by a virus.*

> *My son had a really big **wart** on his hand. I started using lavender and Melrose, and they seemed to help. Then I decided to try something new. I used Melrose, Purification, Thieves, and clove—one drop of each—and rubbed them in one by one, and within a few days the wart was gone. I was so impressed and happy!*
>
> *-Submitted by Caroline Rood*
> *Toledo, Ohio (July 2004)*

Oils—ᵀFrankincense (excellent for more stubborn warts), ᵀMelrose, ᵀThieves, ᵀoregano, ᵀcinnamon bark, ᵀclove, ᵀcypress, ᵀjasmine, ᵀlavender, ᵀlemon (may dilute in 2 tsp. apple cider vinegar).

Other—Colloidal silver.

Recipe #1—5 drops cypress, 10 drops lemon, and 2 Tbs. apple cider vinegar. Apply twice daily, and bandage. Keep a bandage on it until the wart is gone.

—GENITAL

➤➤ *A genital wart is a small, painful wart or cluster of warts located in the genital area or in the mouth or throat. This type of wart is typically spread by contact with the skin through sexual conduct.*

Oils—ᵀFrankincense (excellent for more stubborn warts), ᵀtea tree, ᵀoregano, ᵀThieves, ᵀhyssop, ᵀthyme.

—PLANTAR

➤➤ *Plantar warts are painful warts that grow on the bottoms of the feet. They are usually flattened and embedded into the skin due to the pressure caused by walking on them.*

Oils—ᵀOregano.

T—Dilute 1–2 drops of oil in a few drops of V-6 Oil, and apply on location.

> *In late October of last year, Cathy brought her 15-year-old daughter to see me for massage therapy. Amanda was dealing with a huge **plantar's wart** grown deep into the ball of her foot. She suffered a great deal of pain with every step, and Cathy was planning to make an appointment for her to see a medical doctor. Cathy also suffered from these warts and had undergone months of treatment at her doctor's office having them repeatedly cut and burned with liquid nitrogen. She was also told you could never get rid of them. I suggested that Amanda rub essential oil of oregano on the infected area, which Amanda did diligently each day, covering it with a bandage. They were amazed that the wart had completely disappeared in 6 weeks and has had no recurrence of the virus. Amanda's only complaint was that she got tired of going to school every day smelling like a pizza.*
>
> *-Submitted by Ellie Ayers (July 2004)*

Waste: *Refer to the chapter entitled, "Cleansing and Diets" in the Essential Oils Desk Reference for lots of information on cleansing.*

—ELIMINATING

Oils—ᵀ_F Lavender (through lymphatic system).

T—Dilute with V-6 Oil to create a massage oil, and massage into the skin.

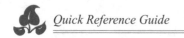

Supplements—**Balance Complete, Cleansing Trio** (ComforTone, Essentialzyme, and ICP), **Digest + Cleanse**. These cleansing products help eliminate toxic waste from the body.

Water Distillation:

Recipe #1—Add 3–5 drops of your favorite oil to the post-filter on your distiller. The oils will help increase the oxygen and frequency of the water. Try lemon or peppermint.

Water Purification:

Oils—^{IT}_FLemon, ^{IT}orange, ^{IT}jade lemon.

—REMOVE NITRATES

>> *Nitrate is a molecule composed of nitrogen and oxygen that shows up in water as a harmful contaminate.*

Oils—^{IT}Peppermint.

I—Add 1 drop to 12–16 oz. of drinking water.

T—Add 1–2 drops to dishwater. Add 1–2 drops to warm bathwater, and bathe. Add 1–2 drops to bowl of water, and use to clean the outside of fruits and vegetables.

Water Retention: *See Edema, Diuretic, and Hormonal Imbalance.*

Weakness: *See also Energy.*

—AFTER ILLNESS

Oils—^{TA}Thyme (physical).

T—Dilute with V-6 Oil to create a massage oil, and massage into the skin.

A—Inhale directly or applied to hands. Diffuse into the air.

Wealth:

Oils—^A<u>Abundance</u>, ^Abergamot.

—ATTRACTS

Oils—^ACinnamon bark.

—MONEY

Oils—^AGinger, ^Apatchouli.

A—Wear as perfume or cologne. Diffuse into the air.

Weight: *See also Hormonal Imbalance, Obesity, pH Balance.*

▸▸ *Proper exercise and nutrition are the most critical factors for maintaining a healthy weight. Other factors that may influence weight include an individual's metabolism, level of stress, hormonal imbalances, low or high thyroid function, or the level of insulin being produced by the body.*

***Comments—**Proper exercise** is absolutely important!

Oils—ᴵᴬSlique Essence.

Supplements—Enzyme products: **Allerzyme** (aids the digestion of sugars, starches, fats, and proteins), **Detoxzyme** (helps maintain and support a healthy intestinal environment), **Digest + Cleanse. Balance Complete** (an excellent meal replacer, nutritive cleanser providing 11 grams of fiber per serving), **Master Formula, MultiGreens, Cleansing Trio (ComforTone, Essentialzyme, and ICP), JuvaPower/JuvaSpice, NingXia Red, Pure Protein Complete, Slique Tea, Slique Bar, Slique Gum, Slique Slim Caps.**

—CONTROL

Recipe #1—EndoFlex (while taking Thyromin, a drop of EndoFlex under the tongue two or three times a day can help).

Supplements—Balance Complete, Digest + Cleanse, EndoGize, Pure Protein Complete, Thyromin, Wolfberry Crisp Bars.

—EMOTIONS

Oils—Excessive weight may be due to unresolved childhood emotions. Any or all of the following may help: Acceptance, Forgiveness, Inner Child, SARA (*Refer to the "Emotional Release" part of the Science and Application section or to the Blend section of the* Reference Guide for Essential Oils *for more information on each of these blends*).

—WEIGHT LOSS

Oils—ᴵᴬSlique Essence, ᵀᴬEndoFlex (on throat, under big toes), ᵀᴬJoy, ᵀᴬMotivation.

T—Apply as indicated or to auricular emotion points.

A—Inhale directly. Diffuse into the air.

Blend #1—Put 5 drops lemon[411] and 5 drops grapefruit[303] in 1 gallon of water, and drink during the day. Add more grapefruit to dissolve fat faster.

Blend #2—4 drops lavender, 4 drops basil, 3 drops juniper, 8 drops grapefruit, 5 drops cypress. Mix, and apply to feet, on location, as a body massage, or use in bath. This blend is used to emulsify fat.

W

A=Aromatic **T**=Topical **I**=Internal

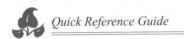
      Personal Care—Massage whole body with **Cel-Lite Magic** after showering. If the weight problem is related to a hormonal imbalance, Prenolone/Prenolone+ / Progessence/Progessence Plus combined with Thyromin and <u>EndoFlex</u> may help.

      Supplements—Use **Balance Complete** (to replace 2 meals and to promote proper elimination) to replace breakfast and dinner, **ComforTone, Digest + Cleanse, ICP,** and **Essentialzyme/ Essentialzymes-4** to promote proper elimination of waste material from the bowels, and **Thyromin** to ensure proper thyroid function. Eat a normal meal at lunch, but watch fat intake. Other products that may help are **AlkaLime** (improves digestion), **JuvaPower/ JuvaSpice, Power Meal, Slique Tea** (helps control cravings), **Slique Bar, Slique Gum, Slique Slim Caps, Sulfurzyme, Ultra Young+** (may help improve fat-to-lean ratios), **Wolfberry Crisp Bars**. Master Formula is also important to use.

—UNDERWEIGHT

      Supplements—Pure Protein Complete. Feed cells with **Mineral Essence**.

Well Being:

      Oils—^A<u>Citrus Fresh</u>, ^AIdaho tansy, ^A<u>Release</u> (emotional), ^Arose, ^A<u>Transformation</u>.

—FEELING OF

      Oils—^A<u>Harmony</u>, ^Aspearmint.

—PROMOTES

      Oils—^AEucalyptus, ^Ageranium, ^Alavender, ^Alemon, ^Alime.

      Supplements—Cleansing Trio (ComforTone, Essentialzyme, and ICP).

    A—Diffuse into the air. Inhale directly or applied to tissue or a cotton wick.

Whiplash: *See also Trauma or Shock.*

  ▸▸ *Whiplash is the over-stretching or tearing of the muscles, ligaments, and/or tendons in the neck and head. This is typically caused by a sudden collision or force pushing the body in one direction, while the head's tendency to remain in the same place causes the head to quickly rock in the opposite direction the body is going.*

      Oils—^TAroma Siez, ^T<u>Deep Relief</u> (roll-on), ^T<u>PanAway</u>, ^Tlemongrass (strained ligaments), ^Tmarjoram (muscles), ^Twintergreen (bones), ^T<u>Relieve It</u>, ^Tbasil, ^Thelichrysum (bruising), ^Thyssop (inflammation), ^Tjuniper, ^TRoman chamomile, ^Tspruce.

    T—Dilute as necessary, and apply on location. Dilute with V-6 Oil to create a massage oil, and gently massage on back of neck, shoulders, and upper back.

Recipe #1—Can also apply valerian, vetiver, helichrysum, clove, and peppermint to the back of the neck (up to the base of the skull) to help calm the sympathetic nervous system and to reduce pain and swelling.

Supplements—Sulfurzyme, Super C / Super C Chewable.

*****Comments**—Remember to think through every physical aspect of the injury (i.e. muscle damage, nerve damage, inflammation, ligament strain, bone injury, fever, and emotions). Select oils for each area of concern.

Wholeness:

Recipe #1—For one's own spirituality and oneness with the Creator. Apply each of the following blends, one right after the other: <u>Awaken</u> over the heart and on the forehead, <u>Sacred Mountain</u> on the crown of the head and over the thymus, and <u>White Angelica</u> on the shoulders. Then rub hands together, cup hands over nose and mouth, and breathe deeply to inhale the aroma of all three blends together.

Whooping Cough: *See Childhood Diseases: WHOOPING COUGH.*

Withdrawal: *See Addictions.*

Workaholic:

Oils—^ABasil, ^Ageranium, ^Alavender, ^Amarjoram.

A—Rub a couple drops between hands, cup hands over nose and mouth, and breathe deeply. Can also be diffused.

Worms: *See also Antifungal: RINGWORM, Parasites.*

Oils—^T<u>Di-Gize</u> (helps expel intestinal worms), ^Tlavender, ^Trosemary verbenon, ^Tbergamot, ^Ttea tree, ^Tpeppermint, ^TRoman chamomile, ^Tthyme.

T—For intestinal worms, apply a few drops over abdomen with a hot compress, or add to V-6 Oil (½–1 oz.) and use as a retention enema for 15 minutes or more. Can also apply on intestine and colon Vita Flex points on the feet.

Blend #1—Mix 6 drops Roman chamomile, 6 drops eucalyptus, 6 drops lavender, and 6 drops lemon with 2 Tbs. V-6 Oil. Apply 10–15 drops of blend over abdomen with a hot compress, and apply on intestine and colon Vita Flex points on the feet.

Supplements—Cleansing Trio (ComforTone, Essentialzyme, and ICP), Digest + Cleanse, ParaFree.

W

Worry:

> Oils—^ABergamot.
>
> **A**—Diffuse into the air.

Wounds: *See also Cuts, Scarring.*

⟫ *A wound is a general term for an injury that involves tissue (typically the skin or underlying skeletal muscles) being torn, cut, punctured, scraped, or crushed.*

Oils—^T_FClove (infected wounds), ^Ttea tree, ^Tlavender (combine with any of these other oils), ^TRoman chamomile (add to Rose Ointment for an excellent first aid salve), ^Tbasil[304], ^TThe Gift, ^Tbergamot, ^Tcajeput, ^Tcistus (to help reduce scarring), ^Tcypress, ^Telemi (infected), ^Teucalyptus, ^Tfrankincense, ^Tgalbanum, ^Tgeranium, ^Tjuniper, ^Tmyrrh (infected), ^Tonycha (benzoin), ^Tpeppermint (when wound has closed; will soothe, cool, and reduce inflammation), ^Trose, ^Trosemary, ^Trosewood, ^Tsandalwood (for DNA repair), ^Tthyme, ^Ttsuga.

Blend #1—Lavender with <u>Purification</u> or <u>Melrose</u>.

Recipe #1—First, 1–3 drops of helichrysum on the fresh wound will help stop the bleeding, and a drop of clove will help with pain. Once bleeding is stopped, a drop of lavender (to help start the healing), a drop of <u>Melrose</u> (to help fight infection), and a drop of lemongrass (for possible ligament damage) can be applied. Other oils such as wintergreen, thyme, or sage may also be applied, depending on the extent of the injury. Rose Ointment can then be applied to help seal the wound and to extend the effectiveness of the applied oils; cover it all with a bandage. When changing the bandage, cistus, myrrh, onycha, sandalwood (for DNA repair), or patchouli can be applied to help promote further healing. <u>Thieves</u>, myrrh, or <u>Purification</u> may be necessary to help fight any occurrence of infection.

> One Sunday morning I tripped and rammed my foot into a dirty pair of grass clippers, cutting my 4th toe at the base where it joins my foot. I washed it out as best I could with hydrogen peroxide, and then I applied lavender oil and a bandage and went on to church. When I came home, I kept my foot elevated and applied more lavender oil throughout the day. My friend looked at my wound and commented that it wasn't just a gash, it was punctured. That evening I also applied clove oil, along with the lavender oil. I slept with it unbandaged, and then I bandaged it during the day while I was at work. I applied the oils morning and night. I had no infection, and by the following Sunday evening, it was almost totally healed. My friend who looked at it again was amazed, and she's an EMT!
>
> *–Submitted by C. Ness*
> *Rapid City, South Dakota (July 2004)*

Personal Care—Rose Ointment (seals and protects).

Supplements—Stevia extract (apply on closed wound to help reduce scarring).

—Children (and Infants)

Oils—ᵀ**Lavender** and/or ᵀ**Roman chamomile**. ᵀHelichrysum and ᵀpeppermint may also be used but are best diluted with lavender or Rose Ointment first to help minimize stinging effect on open wounds.

> *My husband, Tom, was taking apart a rabbit cage, and the roof with the nails poking through fell on his hand and punctured it. Blood was dripping everywhere, and he was becoming sick with pain and weakness. He applied pressure to the wounds, but it still bled until I applied lavender and __PanAway__. Before our very eyes it immediately stopped bleeding. It did swell up, but he kept applying lavender and __PanAway__, and it would take away the pain and bring the swelling down. It was healed in a matter of three days without a trip to the doctor. We feel so blessed to have oils on hand to treat emergencies like this one.*
>
> *–Submitted by Diana Wolford*
> *Olive Branch, Mississippi (July 2004)*

Blend #2—(for Bruises or Wounds) 1–3 drops each of helichrysum and lavender diluted in 1/8 oz. V-6 Oil.

—Bleeding

Oils—ᵀ**Helichrysum**, ᵀrose, ᵀlemon, ᵀlavender.

Blend #3—Equal amounts of Roman chamomile, geranium, and lemon. Can alternate with cypress, hyssop, palmarosa, and rose. Apply directly with a compress 2–3 times a day for 3–4 days, and then reduce to once a day until healed.

—Disinfect

Oils—ᵀ**Tea tree**, ᵀhyssop, ᵀIdaho tansy, ᵀlavender, ᵀmountain savory, ᵀthyme (thymol and linalol).

—Healing *See also Scarring.*

Oils—ᵀ**Basil**[412], ᵀ**helichrysum**, ᵀ**The Gift**, ᵀmyrrh, ᵀIdaho tansy, ᵀlavender, ᵀtea tree (pus-filled wounds), ᵀneroli, ᵀonycha (benzoin), ᵀpatchouli, ᵀravintsara, ᵀsandalwood, ᵀtsuga, ᵀyarrow.

T—Apply directly on wound followed by **Rose Ointment**.

> *Dr. Marcy Foley maintains that "Each person will have a unique picture which created their healing challenges, and will require that each of these areas be addressed for a complete healing to take place." This is especially true for surface **wounds** where each aspect of the trauma must be considered. For example, there may also be damage to muscles, nerves, ligaments, or bones; there may be infection or inflammation; and there may be an emotion or even fever to deal with. Oils should be considered for each of these different areas as well.*

—Inflammation *See also Anti-Inflammatory*

Oils—ᵀ**German chamomile** (helps reduce).

—Surgical

Oils—ᵀ**Peppermint** (cooling and soothing), ᵀ**Melrose**, ᵀ**The Gift**, ᵀPurification, ᵀThieves.

Blend #4—3 drops helichrysum, 3 drops frankincense, and 4 drops lavender in 2 tsp. V-6 Oil. Reapply a few drops of blend when changing bandages.

W

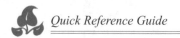

—Weeping

    Oils—ᵀMyrrh, ᵀ<u>The Gift</u>, ᵀjuniper, ᵀpatchouli, ᵀtarragon.

    Blend #5—5 drops Roman chamomile,
       10 drops lavender, 3 drops tarragon, and 2 oz. V-6 Oil. Apply as a hot compress.

T—Dilute as necessary, and apply on location. Apply on location with a warm compress.

Wrinkles: *See Skin:* Wrinkles.

Yeast: *See Antifungal: Candida.*

Yin and Yang:

  ▸▸ *In Chinese philosophy Yin and Yang are two opposing forces in the universe that, when in harmony, create balance.*

    Oils—ᴬYlang ylang (balances)

  A—Inhale directly or applied to hands. Diffuse into the air.

Yoga:

    Oils—ᴬCedarwood, ᴬsandalwood, ᴬspruce, ᴬtsuga.

  A—Diffuse into the air.

Zest (For Life):

    Oils—ᴬ<u>En-R-Gee</u>, ᴬ<u>Motivation</u>, ᴬnutmeg, ᴬ<u>Legacy</u>, ᴬ<u>Live with Passion</u>.

  A—Diffuse into the air.

Endnotes

Note: *This list contains summaries of research articles referenced in this section. For the full article reference, please see Research References in the appendix of this book. Please note that much of this research is still preliminary, and is meant as an educational reference to guide further research and study. It should not be used to attempt to diagnose or prescribe any medical condition. Consult with a certified medical professional with regard to any medical condition.*

1. Rosemary aroma also was found to enhance quality of memory, compared to control (Moss et al., 2003).

2. In human trials, the aroma of peppermint was found to enhance memory and to increase alertness (Moss et al., 2008).

3. In a small human trial, oral administration of sage lavender oil was found to improve speed of memory as well as alertness and calmness in healthy volunteers, compared to a placebo (Tildesley et al., 2005).

4. A gel with 5% tea tree oil was found to be as effective as a 5% benzoyl peroxide (a common chemical used to treat acne) lotion, with fewer side effects (Bassett et al., 1990).

   A topical gel containing 5% tea tree oil was found to be more effective than a placebo at preventing acne vulgaris lesions and at decreasing severity in patients suffering from acne vulgaris (Enshaieh et al., 2007).

   Tea tree oil and several of its main components were found to be active against Propionibacterium acnes, a bacteria involved in the formation of acne. This oil was also found to be active against 2 types of Staphylococcus bacteria (Raman et al., 1995).

5. Mice who inhaled lavender were found to have a decreased motility (natural movement) dependent on exposure time. Additionally, mice injected with caffeine (causing a hyperactivity) were found to reduce their movement to near normal levels after inhaling lavender (Buchbauer et al., 1991).

6. Rats with morphine-induced conditioned place preference that received injections of cumin essential oil demonstrated a decreased morphine-induced conditioning, while rats that received a control substance (Tween-80) did not (Khatibi et al., 2008).

   In mice, repeated administration of cumin fruit essential oil before morphine injection produced a significant decrease in morphine tolerance and dependence, when compared to the control group (Haghparast et al., 2008).

7. Grapefruit and orange: Injection of limonene, a common terpene found in many citrus essential oils, inhibited behavioral manifestations of drug use on rats administered methamphetamine (METH). Examination of the nucleus accumbens of the rats revealed that limonene may produce its effects by regulating dopamine levels and serotonin receptor function (Yun, 2014).

8. Inhaled vapor of black pepper oil was found to reduce craving for cigarettes and symptoms of anxiety in smokers deprived from smoking, compared to a control (Rose et al., 1994).

9. Aging rats fed thyme oil or the constituent thymol were found to have higher levels of the antioxidant enzymes superoxide dismutase and glutathione peroxidase in the brain than aging rats not fed the oil or constituent (Youdim et al., 2000).

   Older rats whose diets were supplemented with thyme oil were found to have a higher level of the antioxidant enzymes superoxide dismutase and glutathione peroxidase in the heart, liver, and kidneys than older rats without this supplementation (Youdim et al., 1999).

10. Based on lemon essential oil's acetylcholinesterase inhibitory activity, butyrylcholinesterase inhibitiory activity, and antioxidant power, this essential oil could be used in the management and/or prevention of neurodegenerative conditions like Alzheimer's disease (Oboh et al., 2014).

    A study using mice demonstrated that pretreatment with lemon essential oil causes an increase in antioxidant enzymatic activities and decreased lipid degradation in the hippocampus (Campelo et al., 2011). Antioxidant and bioprotective activities, like that of lemon essential oil, can reduce damage to neurons produced by neurodegenerative disease (Campelo et al., 2011).

11. Arzanol, extracted from helichrysum, inhibited HIV-1 replication in T cells and also inhibited the release of proinflammatory cytokines (chemical messengers) in monocytes (Appendino et al., 2007).

W

X

Y

Z

A=Aromatic   **T**=Topical   **I**=Internal

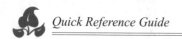

12.   Bergamot extract was found to have potent antiretroviral activity towards HTLV-1 (a human retrovirus that causes T-cell leukemia and lymphoma) and HIV-1 expression in infected cells (Balestrieri et al., 2011).

13.   A formulation of lemongrass and geranium oil was found to reduce airborne bacteria by 89% in an office environment after diffusion for 15 hours (Doran et al., 2009).

14.   In human trials, the aroma of peppermint was found to enhance memory and to increase alertness, while ylang ylang aroma was found to increase calmness (Moss et al., 2008).

15.   In a small human trial, oral administration of sage lavender oil was found to improve speed of memory as well as alertness and calmness in healthy volunteers, compared to a placebo (Tildesley et al., 2005).

16.   Tea tree oil applied to histamine-induced weal and flare in human volunteers was found to decrease the mean weal volume when compared to a control (Koh et al., 2002).

      Tea tree oil was found to reduce swelling during a contact hypersensitivity response in the skin of mice sensitized to the chemical hapten (Brand et al., May 2002).

      Tea tree oil applied to histamine-induced edema (swelling) in mice ears was found to significantly reduce swelling (Brand et al., Jun. 2002).

      Tea tree oil was found to reduce inflammation in the skin of nickel-sensitive human skin exposed to nickel (Pearce et al., 2005).

17.   Lavender oil was found to inhibit immediate-type allergic reactions in mice and rats by inhibiting mast cell degranulation (Kim et al., 1999).

18.   L-menthol was found to inhibit production of inflammation mediators in human monocytes (a type of white blood cell involved in the immune response) (Juergens et al., 1998).

19.   Inhalation of coriander volatile oil was found to possess antianxiety, antidepressant, and antioxidant properties in Alzheimer's disease conditions in a rat model of beta-amyloid Alzheimer's disease (Cioanca et al., 2014).

      Repeated inhalation of coriander oil was found to prevent memory impairment and oxidative damage in a rat model of beta-amyloid Alzheimer's disease, when compared to control (Cioanca et al., 2013).

20.   Based on lemon essential oil's acetylcholinesterase inhibitory activity, butyrylcholinesterase inhibitory activity, and antioxidant power, this essential oil could be used in the management and/or prevention of neurodegenerative conditions like Alzheimer's disease (Oboh et al., 2014).

21.   A blend of ethanol extracts from 8 herbs, including sandalwood, orally administered to a mice model of Alzheimer's disease was shown to improve amyloid beta protein-induced memory impairment, suppress amyloid beta protein levels, and diminish plaque deposition in the brain as much as that of donepezil treatment. This study suggests that the 8-herb blend may develop as a therapeutic drug for treatment of Alzheimer's disease patients (Jeon et al., 2011).

22.   Oils of Salvia fruticosa and Salvia officinalis were found to inhibit butyrylcholinesterase, an enzyme that has been studied for its potential role in increasing the chances of developing Alzheimer's disease (Savelev et al., 2004).

23.   Lavender oil was found to be effective at alleviating agitated behaviors in Chinese patients suffering from dementia (Lin et al., 2007).

      Lavandula angustifolia essential oil demonstrated an ability to inhibit GABA-A receptor channels of rat brain cells (Huang et al., 2008).

24.   Subjects who had ylang ylang oil applied to their skin had decreased blood pressure, increased skin temperature, and reported feeling more calm and relaxed, compared to subjects in a control group (Hongratanaworakit et al., 2006).

      In human trials, the aroma of ylang ylang was found to increase calmness (Moss et al., 2008).

25.   In human volunteers wearing breathing masks to prevent aroma inhalation, rose oil applied to the skin was found to significantly decrease breathing rate, blood oxygen saturation, and systolic blood pressure, compared to a placebo. And volunteers receiving rose oil rated themselves more calm and relaxed than did subjects receiving the placebo (Hongratanaworakit et al., 2009).

26.   Melissa (lemon balm) oil applied topically in a lotion was found to reduce agitation and to improve quality of life factors in patients suffering from severe dementia, compared to those receiving a placebo lotion (Ballard et al., 2002).

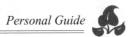

27. Oils with aldehyde or phenol as a major component demonstrated a high level of antibacterial activity (Inouye et al., 2001).

   Tea tree, peppermint, and sage oils were found to inhibit oral bacteria, with thymol and eugenol being the most active components of these oils (Shapiro et al., 1994).

   Subjects using a mouthwash containing thymol, menthol, methyl salicylate, and eucalyptol for 6 months were found to not have developed oral bacteria that were resistant to the oils (Charles et al., 2000).

   Thyme oil demonstrated a strong antibacterial effect against staph and E. coli bacteria (Mohsenzadeh et al., 2007).

   Cinnamon, thyme, and clove essential oils demonstrated an antibacterial effect on several respiratory tract pathogens (Fabio et al., 2007).

   Cinnamon bark, lemongrass, and thyme oils were found to have the highest level of activity against common respiratory pathogens among 14 essential oils tested (Inouye et al., 2001).

28. MRSA (methicillin-resistant staph) and MSSA (methicillin-sensitive staph) in biofilms (plaque/microcolonies) and 5 of 9 CoNS (coagulase-negative staph) were eradicated by a 5% solution of tea tree oil (Brady et al., 2006).

   66 isolates of Staphylococcus aureus (staph), including 64 methicillin-resistant (MRSA) and 33 mupirocin-resistant strains, were inhibited by tea tree essential oil (Carson et al., 1995).

   In a human trial, most patients receiving treatment with Melaleuca alternifolia oil placed topically on boils experienced healing or reduction of symptoms; while of those receiving no treatment (control), half required surgical intervention, and all still demonstrated signs of the infection (Feinblatt, 1960).

   Terpinen-4-ol, found in tea tree oil, was found to effectively inhibit MRSA and CoNS, while not exhibiting toxicity to human fibroblast cells (Loughlin et al., 2008).

   Tea tree oil was found to disrupt the cellular membrane and to inhibit respiration in Candida albicans, gram-negative E. coli, and gram-positive Staphylococcus aureus (staph) (Cox et al., 2000).

   Geranium and tea tree demonstrated strong antibacterial effects on Staphylococcus aureus (Edwards-Jones et al., 2004).

   Among several oils tested, tea tree (tea tree), manuka, and eucalyptus demonstrated strong antibacterial activity against detrimental oral bacteria (Hammer et al., 2008).

   Tea tree oil demonstrated an ability to kill Staphylococcus aureus (staph) bacteria, both within biofilms and in the stationary growth phase at concentrations below 1% (Kwieciński et al., 2009).

   Tea tree oil and its component terpinen-4-ol were found to demonstrate effective antibacterial activity against Staphylococcus aureus (staph) bacteria, superior to the activities of several antibiotic drugs--even against antibiotic resistant strains (Ferrini et al., 2006).

   Tea tree oil and several of its main components were found to be active against Propionibacterium acnes, a bacteria involved in the formation of acne. This oil was also found to be active against 2 types of Staphylococcus bacteria (Raman et al., 1995).

29. Cinnamon oil exhibited a strong antimicrobial activity against 2 detrimental oral bacteria. Manuka, tea tree, and the component thymol also exhibited antimicrobial potency (Filoche et al., 2005).

   Cinnamon, thyme, and clove essential oils demonstrated an antibacterial effect on several respiratory tract pathogens (Fabio et al., 2007).

   Cinnamon bark, lemongrass, and thyme oils were found to have the highest level of activity against common respiratory pathogens among 14 essential oils tested (Inouye et al., 2001).

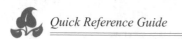 *Quick Reference Guide* **Endnotes** *(cont.)* —

30. A formulation of lemongrass and geranium oil was found to reduce airborne bacteria by 89% in an office environment after diffusion for 15 hours (Doran et al., 2009).

   Lemongrass demonstrated ability to inhibit Helicobacter pylori, a pathogen responsible for gastroduodenal disease. This pathogen also did not develop resistance to lemongrass after 10 passes (it did develop resistance to the antibiotic drug clarithromycin within the same amount of passes) (Ohono et al., 2003).

   Two components of lemongrass demonstrated antibacterial properties; while the addition of a third component, myrcene, enhanced the antibacterial activities even further (Onawunmi et al., 1984).

   Cinnamon bark, lemongrass, and thyme oils were found to have the highest level of activity against common respiratory pathogens among 14 essential oils tested (Inouye et al., 2001).

31. Peppermint and rosemary oils were each found to be more effective at preventing dental biofilm (plaque) formation than chlorhexidine (an antiseptic) (Rasooli et al., 2008).

   Peppermint oil was found to be an effective antibacterial and antioxidant agent (Mimica-Dukić et al., 2003).

   Peppermint oil blended with toothpaste was found to be more effective at lower concentrations in inhibiting the formation of dental plaque than was chlorhexidine (an antiseptic) in human volunteers (Shayegh et al., 2008).

   Peppermint and spearmint oil inhibited resistant strains of Staphylococcus, E. coli, Salmonella, and Helicobacter pylori (Imai et al., 2001).

   Subjects using a mouthwash containing thymol, menthol, methyl salicylate, and eucalyptol for 6 months were found to not have developed oral bacteria that were resistant to the oils (Charles et al., 2000).

32. Oregano oil was found to kill antibiotic resistant strains of staph, E. coli, Klebsiella pneumoniae, Helicobacter pylori, and Mycobacterium terrae (Preuss et al., 2005).

   Oregano oil was found to inhibit MRSA (Nostro et al., 2004).

33. Lemon Myrtle demonstrated antimicrobial inhibition against staph, E. coli, Pseudomonas aeruginosa, Candida, MRSA, black mold, and others (Hayes et al., 2002).

   Four essential oil samples of Backhousia citriodora (lemon myrtle) were found to have antibacterial and antifungal properties (Wilkinson et al., 2003).

34. Basil oil was found to strongly inhibit several multidrug resistant bacteria (Opalchenova et al., 2003).

35. Cinnamon, thyme, and clove essential oils demonstrated an antibacterial effect on several respiratory tract pathogens (Fabio et al., 2007).

36. Peppermint and spearmint oil inhibited resistant strains of Staphylococcus, E. coli, Salmonella, and Helicobacter pylori (Imai et al., 2001).

37. A methanol extract from rosemary with 30% carnosic acid, 16% carnosol, and 5% rosmarinic acid was found to be effective against gram-positive and negative bacteria and yeast (Moreno et al., 2006).

38. Cypress essential oil was found to possess antibacterial activity against Staphlococcus aureus, Klebsiella pneumoniae, and Salmonella indica when tested for antimicrobial properties against 13 microorganisms (Selim et al., 2014).

39. Rose essential oil demonstrated strong antibacterial activity against several pathogenic bacteria (Ulusoy et al., 2009).

40. Schinus molle essential oils demonstrated antibacterial and antifungal activity against a variety of species (Gundidza, 1993).

41. A combination of citricidal and geranium oil demonstrated strong antibacterial effects on MRSA. Geranium and tea tree demonstrated strong antibacterial effects on Staphylococcus aureus (Edwards-Jones et al., 2004).

   A formulation of lemongrass and geranium oil was found to reduce airborne bacteria by 89% in an office environment after diffusion for 15 hours (Doran et al., 2009).

42. Intraperitoneal administration of caraway oil to septic-induced rats effectively reversed kidney damage (including reversal of lipid peroxidation and plasma urea/creatinine ra-tion levels) (Dadkhah et al., 2011).

43. Cinnamaldehyde, the main constituent of cassia oil, showed strong growth inhibiting activity toward five human intestinal bacteria in vitro (Lee et al., 1998).

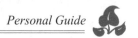

44. Citronella essential oil displayed antibacterial activity against all tested bacteria, including 36 bacterial isolates from various aquatic animals and 7 bacterial strains. These results indicate the potential of citronella oil as an alternative to commercial antibiotics for aquaculture use (Wei et al., 2013).

45. Cumin essential oil exhibited antibacterial activity against Klebsiella pneumoniae, a pathogen frequently associated with hospitals. Cumin's antibacterial activity caused Klebsiella pneumoniae cell elongation, repression of capsule expression, and decreased urease activity (Derakhshan et al., 2008).

46. Goldenrod root essential oil was found to be effective against the tested bacteria (Staphy-lococcus aureus, Bacillus subtilis, Streptococcus faecalis, Escherichia coli, Pseudomonas aeru-ginosa, and Salmonella typhi) at concentrations 500 and 1000 μg/ml. (Mishra et al., 2010).

47. Scanning electron microscopy analysis and zeta potential measurement revealed that lav-ender essential oil's antibacterial action against multi-drug-resistant Escherichia coli oc-curs via two mechanisms: alteration of outer membrane perme-ability and possible inhibi-tion of bacterial quorum sensing (Yap et al., 2014).

48. Eucalyptus oil was found to have an anti-inflammatory and mucin-inhibitory effect in rats with lipopolysaccharide-induced bronchitis (Lu et al., 2004).

49. Tea tree oil inhibited several Candida species in vitro (Vazquez et al., 2000).

    Eleven types of Candida were found to be highly inhibited by tea tree oil (Banes-Marshall et al., 2001).

    Tea tree oil was found to alter the membrane properties and functions of Candida albicans cells, leading to cell inhibition or death (Hammer et al., 2004).

    Tea tree oil was found to disrupt the cellular membrane and to inhibit respiration in Candida albicans, gram-negative E. coli, and gram-positive Staphylococcus aureus (staph) (Cox et al., 2000).

    Terpinen-4-ol, a constituent of tea tree oil, and tea tree oil were found to be effective against several forms of vaginal candida infections in rats, including azole-resistant forms (Mondello et al., 2006).

    Tea tree oil at concentrations of .16% was found to inhibit the transformation of C. albicans from single-cell yeast to the pathogenic mycelial (multi-cellular strands) form (D'Auria et al., 2001).

    Tea tree oil demonstrated fungicidal activity against 4 plant pathogenic fungi (Terzie et al., 2007).

    Tea tree oil was found to inhibit 301 different types of yeasts isolated from the mouths of cancer patients suffering from advanced cancer, including 41 strains that are known to be resistant to antifungal drugs (Bagg et al., 2006).

    When applied as a coating to protect oranges after harvest, a mixture containing chitosan and tea tree essential oil was found to reduce fungal growth by 50% (Cháfer et al., 2012).

50. Vapor of cinnamon bark oil and cinnamic aldehyde was found to be effective against fungi involved in respiratory tract mycoses (fungal infections) (Singh et al., 1995).

    Cinnamon, thyme, oregano, and cumin oils inhibited the production of aflatoxin by Aspergillus fungus (Tantaoui-Elaraki et al., 1994).

    In a test of 9 oils, clove, followed by cinnamon, oregano, and mace oils, was found to be inhibitory to 2 toxin-producing fungi. It was also shown that whole and ground cloves stored with grain reduced the amount of aflatoxin contamination (Juglal et al., 2002).

51. Clove oil was found to display an antifungal effect against tested Candida strains (Chaieb et al., 2007).

    Eugenol from clove and thymol from thyme were found to inhibit the growth of Aspergillus flavus and Aspergillus versicolor at concentrations of .4 mg/ml or less (Hitokoto et al., 1980).

    In a test of 9 oils, clove, followed by cinnamon, oregano, and mace oils, was found to be inhibitory to 2 toxin-producing fungi. It was also shown that whole and ground cloves stored with grain reduced the amount of aflatoxin contamination (Juglal et al., 2002).

52. Mice infected with Candida albicans who were fed origanum oil or carvacrol diluted in olive oil had an 80% survival rate after 30 days, while infected mice fed olive oil alone all died after 10 days (Manohar et al., 2001).

    The vapor of oregano oil was found to be fungicidal against the Trichophyton mentagrophytes fungi (a fungi that causes a skin infection known as Malabar itch) (Inouye et al., 2006).

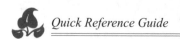

53.   Thyme oil was found to inhibit Candida species by causing lesions in the cell membrane and by inhibiting germ tube (an outgrowth that develops when the fungi is preparing to replicate) formation (Pina-Vaz et al., 2004).

      Cinnamon, thyme, oregano, and cumin oils inhibited the production of aflatoxin by Aspergillus fungus (Tantaoui-elaraki et al., 1994).

      Eugenol from clove and thymol from thyme were found to inhibit the growth of Aspergillus flavus and Aspergillus versicolor at concentrations of .4 mg/ml or less (Hitokoto et al., 1980).

54.   Schinus molle essential oils demonstrated antibacterial and antifungal activity against a variety of species (Gundidza et al., 1993).

      In a screening test of essential oils, Schinus molle oil demonstrated antifungal activity against several pathogenic fungi (Dikshit et al., 1986).

55.   Lemon Myrtle demonstrated antimicrobial inhibition against staph, E. coli, Pseudomonas aeruginosa, Candida, MRSA, black mold, and others (Hayes et al., 2002).

      Lemon myrtle oil was found to effectively inhibit 13 bacteria and 8 fungi (Wilkinson et al., 2003).

56.   Lemon oil was found to be an effective antifungal agent against 2 bread mold species (Caccioni et al., 1998).

57.   Savory oil demonstrated antimicrobial activity against a range of bacteria and yeast, including E. coli, MRSA, and Candida albicans (Skocibusić et al., 2004).

58.   Carrot essential oil was found to demonstrate antifungal activity against yeasts and Aspergillus fungi at concentrations that were not cytotoxic to mouse skin dendritic cells (Tavares et al., 2008).

59.   Cumin essential oil was found to be an effective inhibitor against a broad spectrum of food borne fungi, including Aspergillus flavus (Kedia et al., 2014).

60.   Dorado azul essential oil displayed antifungal activity against various Aspergillus fungal species (Moreira et al., 2010).

61.   Conyza canadensis essential oil from the roots and herbs of the plant displayed antifungal activity in vitro against Candida albicans, Candida glabrata, Candida parapsilosis, Candida tropicalis, Cryptococcus neoformans, Candida kefyr, Rhodotorula glutinis, and Trichophyton interdigitalis (Veres et al., 2012).

62.   Matricaria recutita flower essential oil was shown to be a strong inhibitor of fungal growth for all 10 tested fungal species (Jamalian et al., 2012).

63.   Patients with tinea pedis (athlete's foot) were found to have a higher rate of cure and a higher clinical response when treated topically with 25% or 50% tea tree oil solution, compared to control (Satchell et al., 2002).

64.   Lavender oil demonstrated both fungistatic (stopped growth) and fungicidal (killed) activity against Candida albicans (D'Auria et al., 2005).

65.   Dill essential oil was demonstrated to induce apoptosis (cell death) in Candida albicans in a metacaspase-dependent manner (Chen et al., 2014).

66.   Peppermint oil was found to have a higher fungistatic and fungicidal activity against various fungi (including Candida) than the commercial fungicide bifonazole. Additionally, peppermint oil was found to be an effective antibacterial and antioxidant agent (Mimica-Dukić et al., 2003).

67.   Bergamot essential oil is active in vitro against several common species of ringworm (Sanguinetti et al., 2007).

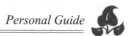

68. Incensole acetate, isolated from frankincense resin, was found to demonstrate an anti-inflammatory and neuro-protective effect in mice with a closed head injury (Moussaieff et al., 2008).

   An acetone extract of frankincense was found to decrease arthritic sores, reduce paw edema (swelling), and suppress proinflammatory cytokines (cellular messengers) (Fan et al., 2005).

   Boswellic acids from frankincense (delivered with sesame seed oil) were found to inhibit TH1 cytokines while potentiating TH2 cytokines, demonstrating their ability to modulate the immune response (Chevrier et al., 2005).

   Boswellic acid reduced induced inflammation and tumors in mice (Huang et al., 2000).

   Compounds from Boswellia serrata were found to carry out anti-inflammatory activity by switching off the proinflammatory cytokines and mediators that initiate the inflammatory process (Gayathri et al., 2007).

   Boswellic acid, from frankincense, was found in vitro to prevent expression and activity of several proteins involved in the inflammatory response. In vivo, boswellic acid was found to protect against experimental arthritis (Roy et al., 2006).

   Triterpene acids isolated from frankincense were found to exhibit a marked anti-inflammatory activity in TPA-induced inflammation in mice (Banno et al., 2006).

   Boswellic extract was found to effect genes related to the inflammatory response in human microvascular cells. Additionally, Boswellic extract was found to reduce inflammation in carrageenan-induced rat paw inflammation (Roy et al., 2005).

69. Inhaled tea tree oil was found to have anti-inflammatory influences on male rats with induced peritoneal inflammation (Golab et al., 2007).

   Tea tree oil applied to histamine-induced edema (swelling) in mice ears was found to significantly reduce swelling (Brand et al., 2002).

   Melaleuca alternifolia oil was found to mediate the reactive oxygen species (ROS) production of leukocytes (white blood cells), indicating a possible anti-inflammatory activity (Caldefie-Chézet et al., 2004).

   Tea tree oil was found to reduce inflammation in the skin of nickel-sensitive human skin exposed to nickel (Pearce et al., 2005).

   Melaleuca alternifolia oil was found to reduce reactive oxygen species (ROS) production in neutrophils (a type of white blood cell), indicating an antioxidant effect. It was also found to decrease interleukin-2 (a chemical messenger that helps trigger an inflammatory response) secretion, while increasing the secretion of interleukin-4 (a chemical messenger involved in turning off the inflammatory response) (Caldefie-Chézet et al., 2006).

   The water soluble terpinen-4-ol component of tea tree was found to suppress the production of proinflammatory mediators in human monocytes (a type of white blood cell that is part of the human immune system (Hart et al., 2000).

70. Eucalyptus oil was shown to ameliorate inflammatory processes by interacting with oxygen radicals and by interfering with leukocyte activation (Grassmann et al., 2000).

   Oils of 3 eucalyptus species (citriodora, tereticornis, and globulus) were found to have analgesic (pain-relieving) and anti-inflammatory properties in rats (Silva et al., 2003).

   Eucalyptus oil was found to have an anti-inflammatory and mucin-inhibitory effect in rats with lipopolysaccharide-induced bronchitis (Lu et al., 2004).

   Extracts from eucalyptus and thyme were found to have high nitrous oxide (NO) scavenging abilities and were found to inhibit NO production in macrophage cells. This could possibly explain their role in aiding respiratory inflammatory diseases (Vigo et al., 2004).

   1,8 cineole (eucalyptol) was found to display an anti-inflammatory effect on rats in several tests and was found to exhibit antinociceptive (pain-reducing) effects in mice, possibly by depressing the central nervous system (Santos et al., 2000).

71. Linalool and linalyl acetate (from lavender and other essential oils) were found to exhibit anti-inflammatory activity in rats subjected to carrageenin-induced edema (inflammation) (Peana et al., 2002).

   Oil from Lavandula angustifolia was found to reduce writhing in induced writhing in rats and to reduce edema (swelling) in carrageenan-induced paw edema, indicating an anti-inflammatory effect (Hajhashemi et al., 2003).

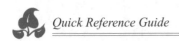

72. Subtoxic levels of myrrh oil were found to inhibit interleukin (chemical messenger involved in inflammation) in part by inhibiting PGE(2) (prostaglandin E, a lipid compound that has several messenger functions in the body, including in the inflammatory response) (Tipton et al., 2006).

    At subtoxic levels, myrrh oil was found to reduce interleukin (chemical signals believed to play a role in the inflammation response) by fibroblast cells in the gums (Tipton et al., 2003).

73. Chamazulene, a chemical in chamomile oil, was found to block formation of leukotriene (a signaling chemical involved in the inflammatory process) in neutrophilic (immune system) granulocytes (white blood cells containing granules). It also demonstrated an antioxidant effect (Safayhi et al., 1994).

74. Methyl salicylate (found in wintergreen or birch oils) was found to inhibit leukotriene C4 (a chemical messenger involved in inflammatory response), while also demonstrating gastroprotective against ethanol-induced gastric injury in rats (Trautmann et al., 1991).

75. In Wistar rats with induced edema, treatment with Eucalyptus citriodora essential oil displayed curative anti-inflammatory action, illustrated by a reduction of edema volume. Eucalyptus citriodora essential oil was also found to have an analgesic effect and the ability to reduce hyperthermia (Gbenou et al., 2013).

76. Ocotea oil was found to demonstrate anti-inflammatory effects in rats, without damaging gastric mucosa (Ballabeni et al., 2009).

77. A combination of peppermint and caraway oil was found to reduce visceral hyperalgesia (pain hypersensitivity in the gastrointestinal tract) after induced inflammation in rats (Adam et al., 2006).

    L-menthol was found to inhibit production of inflammation mediators in human monocytes (a type of white blood cell involved in the immune response) (Juergens et al., 1998).

78. Arzanol, extracted from helichrysum, inhibited HIV-1 replication in T cells and also inhibited the release of proinflammatory cytokines (chemical messengers) in monocytes (Appendino et al., 2007).

79. Chamaecyparis obtusa essential oil displayed anti-inflammatory activity in rats by regulating the production of prostaglandin E_2 and transforming growth factor alpha gene expression (An et al., 2013).

80. Clove oil was found to have very strong radical scavenging activity (antioxidant). It was also found to display an antifungal effect against tested Candida strains (Chaieb et al., 2007).

    Various essential oils demonstrated an antioxidant effect toward skin lipid squalene oxidized by UV irradiation, with a blend of thyme and clove oil demonstrating the highest inhibitory effect (Wei et al., 2007).

81. Aging rats fed thyme oil or the constituent thymol were found to have higher levels of the antioxidant enzymes superoxide dismutase and glutathione peroxidase in the brain than aging rats not fed the oil or constituent (Youdim et al., 2000).

    Older rats whose diets were supplemented with thyme oil were found to have higher levels of the antioxidant enzymes superoxide dismutase and glutathione peroxidase in the heart, liver, and kidneys than did older rats without this supplementation (Youdim et al., 1999).

    Extracts from eucalyptus and thyme were found to have high nitrous oxide (NO) scavenging abilities and were also found to inhibit NO production in macrophage cells. This could possibly explain their role in aiding respiratory inflammatory diseases (Vigo et al., 2004).

    Various essential oils demonstrated an antioxidant effect toward skin lipid squalene oxidized by UV irradiation, with a blend of thyme and clove oil demonstrating the highest inhibitory effect (Wei et al., 2007).

82. Extracts from rosemary were found to have high antioxidant properties. Rosmarinic acid and carnosic acid from rosemary were found to have the highest antioxidant activities of studied components of rosemary (Almela et al., 2006).

    An ethanol extract of rosemary was found to have an antiproliferative and an antioxidant effect on human leukemia and breast carcinoma cells (Cheung et al., 2007).

    Extracts from rosemary were found to have high antioxidant levels. Additionally, a methanol extract with 30% carnosic acid, 16% carnosol, and 5% rosmarinic acid was found to be effective against gram-positive and gram-negative bacteria and yeast (Moreno et al., 2006).

    In patients with chronic bronchitis, rosemary, basil, fir, and eucalyptus oils were found to demonstrate an antioxidant effect. Lavender was found to promote normalization of lipid levels (Siurin, 1997).

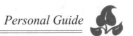

83. Peppermint oil fed to mice prior to exposure to gamma radiation was found to decrease levels of damage from oxidation, compared to mice that were not pretreated with peppermint oil (Samarth et al., 2006).

    Peppermint oil was found to be an effective antibacterial and antioxidant agent (Mimica-Dukić et al., 2003).

    Peppermint extract fed orally to mice demonstrated an ability to protect the testis from gamma radiation damage (Samarth et al., 2009).

84. Melaleuca alternifolia oil was found to reduce reactive oxygen species (ROS) production in neutrophils (a type of white blood cell), indicating an antioxidant effect. It was also found to decrease interleukin-2 (a chemical messenger that helps trigger an inflammatory response) secretion, while increasing the secretion of interleukin-4 (a chemical messenger involved in turning off the inflammatory response) (Caldefie-Chézet et al., 2006).

    Melaleuca alternifolia oil was found to mediate the reactive oxygen species (ROS) production of leukocytes (white blood cells), indicating a possible anti-inflammatory activity (Caldefie-Chézet et al., 2004).

85. Arzanol (extracted from helichrysum), at non-cytotoxic concentrations, showed a strong inhibition of TBH-induced oxidative stress in VERO cells (Rosa et al., 2007).

86. Oil from Abies alba was found to demonstrate antiradical activity against 2 known free radicals (Yang et al., 2009).

87. Lemon oil and one of its components, gamma-terpinene, were found to inhibit oxidation of low-density lipoprotein (LDL). Oxidation of LDL has been found to increase the risk of atherosclerosis and cardiac disease (Grassmann et al., 2001).

88. Extracts from goldenrod were found to have high antioxidant activity, displayed by their high mean peroxyl radical scavenging ability that surpassed that of green tea, ascorbic acid, and Trolox® (an analog of vitamin E) (McCune et al., 2002).

89. The antioxidant activity of oregano essential oil added to extra virgin olive oil at 0.05% was found to retard the lipid oxidation process in olive oil and prolong the olive oil's shelf life (Asensio et al., 2011).

90. Peppermint oil was found to be as effective as Buscopan (an antispasmodic drug) at preventing spasms during a barium enema (a type of enema used to place barium in the colon for X-ray imaging purposes) (Asao et al., 2003).

91. Lavender was found to have a relaxant effect on smooth muscle from guinea-pig ileum (small intestine) (Lis-Balchin et al., 1999).

92. An extract from Artemisia vulgaris (mugwort) was found to have antispasmodic and bronchodilating activities in several different animal and animal tissue tests (Khan et al., 2009).

93. Melissa oil demonstrated inhibition of herpes simplex type 1 and type 2 viruses (Schnitzler et al., 2008).

94. Arzanol, extracted from helichrysum, inhibited HIV-1 replication in T cells and also inhibited the release of proinflammatory cytokines (chemical messengers) in monocytes (Appendino et al., 2007).

    Helichrysum was found to have significant antiviral activity against the herpes virus at non-cytotoxic concentrations (Nostro et al., 2003).

95. Tea tree and eucalyptus oil demonstrated an ability to inhibit herpes simplex virus (Schnitzler et al., 2001).

96. Eugenol was found to be virucidal to herpes simplex and to delay the development of herpes-induced keratitis (inflammation of the cornea) in mice (Benencia et al., 2000).

97. In children with Molluscum contagiosum (a viral infection causing skin lesions), application of a 10% solution of lemon myrtle oil was found to reduce lesions by more than 90% in 56% of patients, while in children receiving application of a control (olive oil), none had a reduction of lesions greater than 90% (Burke et al., 2004).

98. Herpes simplex viruses pretreated with manuka oil before cell infection were significantly inhibited and had plaque formation reduced by over 98% in cultured monkey kidney cells (Reichling et al., 2005).

99. Peppermint oil demonstrated a direct virucidal activity against herpes type 1 and type 2 viruses (Schuhmacher et al., 2003).

    A trial including 80 subjects with Herpes labialis showed that rinsing with an essential oil (menthol, thymol, methyl salicylate, and eucalyptol) containing mouthrinse resulted in effectively zero recoverable virions at 30 seconds post rinse and a significant reduction in saliva viral presence 30 minutes post rinse, suggesting that an essential oil mouthrinse can reduce viral contamination of saliva (Meiller et al., 2005).

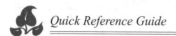

100.   Bergamot extract was found to have potent antiretroviral activity towards HTLV-1 (a human retrovirus that causes T-cell leukemia and lymphoma) and HIV-1 expression in infected cells (Balestrieri et al., 2011).

101.   An office environment featuring a soothing DVD video presentation and diffused lavender oil was found to reduce anxiety in patients awaiting a gastroscopy procedure, compared to a regular office environment (Hoya et al., 2008).

   Oral supplementation of lavender oil was found to decrease anxiety in females in conditions of low anxiety (Bradley et al., 2009).

   In patients admitted to an intensive care unit, those receiving lavender aromatherapy reported a greater improvement in mood and perceived levels of anxiety, compared to those receiving massage or a period of rest (Dunn et al., 1995).

   Patients being treated with chronic hemodialysis demonstrated less anxiety when exposed to lavender aroma (Itai et al., 2000).

   Lavender oil was found to demonstrate anticonflict effects in mice similar to the anxiolytic (antianxiety) drug diazepam (Umezu, 2000).

   Exposure to lavender odor was found to decrease anxiety in gerbils in the elevated plus maze, with a further decrease in anxiety in females after prolonged (2 week) exposure (Bradley et al., 2007).

   A study with 56 percutaneous coronary intervention patients in an intensive care unit found that an aromatherapy blend of lavender, Roman chamomile, and neroli decreased anxiety and improved sleep quality when compared to conventional nursing intervention (Cho et al., 2013).

102.   Female patients waiting for dental treatment were found to be less anxious, more positive, and more calm when exposed to orange oil odor than patients who were not exposed to the orange oil odor (Lehrner et al., 2000).

   Patients waiting for dental treatment were found to be less anxious and to have a better mood when exposed to the odor of lavender or orange oil, compared to control (Lehrner et al., 2005).

   Dental patients (aged 6-9 years) displayed reduce salivary cortisol, pulse rate, and anxiety while undergoing dental treatments when inhaling wild orange essential oil, compared to no aroma (Jafarzadeh et al., 2013).

   Healthy male subjects displayed reduced anxiety after five minutes of inhalation of orange essential oil compared to the inhalation of tea tree essential oil or distilled water when submitted to an anxiety inducing situation (Goes et al., 2012).

   Rats subjected to the elevated plus-maze following exposure to the aroma of orange essential oil for five minutes displayed reduced anxiety as compared to exposure to tea tree essential oil (Faturi et al., 2010).

103.   Lemon oil was found to have an antistress effect on mice involved in several behavioral tasks (Komiya et al., 2006).

   It was found that exposure to lemon oil in rats induced chemical changes in the neuronal circuits involved in anxiety and pain (Ceccarelli et la., 2004).

104.   Massage with a carrier oil including Roman chamomile oil was found to enhance the reduction of anxiety, compared to massage with the carrier oil alone (Wilkinson et al., 1999).

   A study with 56 percutaneous coronary intervention patients in an intensive care unit found that an aromatherapy blend of lavender, Roman chamomile, and neroli decreased anxiety and improved sleep quality when compared to conventional nursing intervention (Cho et al., 2013).

105.   Two chemical components found in valerian were found to have sedative, sleep-enhancing, and anxiolytic (anxiety-lowering) properties (Marder et al., 2003).

106.   Results of a clinical trial indicate that a combination of melissa and valerian oils may have anxiety-reducing properties at some doses (Kennedy et al., 2006).

107.   In the elevated plus-maze, copal oil was found to demonstrate anxiolytic effects in rats comparable to the effects of the antianxiety drug diazepam (Curio et al., 2009).

108.   Oral dosing of successive extracts of Angelica archangelica displayed anti-anxiety activity in rats subjected to two anxiety-inducing tests (elevated T-maze test and the forced swimming test) (Kumar et al., 2012).

   A mixture of non-polar coumarins from Angelica archangelica displayed significant anxiolytic effects on the behavior of rats subjected to three anxiety test models (Kumar et al., 2013).

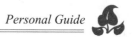

109. Inhalation of bergamot essential oil produced similar anxiolytic results as acute injection of an antianxiety drug, diazepam, administered to mice subjected to two behavioral measurements of anxiety (the elevated plus maze test and the hole-board test) (Saiyudthong et al., 2011). Bergamot essential oil also reduced the corticosterone response to stress exposure of the mice (Saiyudthong et al., 2011).

110. Dietary administration of clary sage oil (from conception) was found to have an anti-anxiety and submissive effect on mice, when compared to administration of sunflower oil (from conception and weaning) and clary sage (from weaning) (Gross et al., 2013).

111. In rats, Chamaecyparis obtusa essential oil (a Japanese plant belonging to the same botanical family as cypress essential oil) decreased anxiety-related behaviors caused by the early life stress of maternal separation. This decrease in anxiety was comparable to the effects of fluoxetine, a drug commonly used to treat depression and anxiety disorders. The same study found that cytokine gene expression in the hippocampus was altered by the inhalation of Chamaecyparis obtusa (Park et al., 2014).

112. Incensole acetate (found in frankincense) was found to open TRPV receptors (a possible channel for emotional regulation) in mice brain (Moussaieff et al., 2008).

113. Inhalation treatment with Chamaecyparis obtusa essential oil reduced anxiety-related behavior shown in maternal separation rats. This behavioral activity was further emphasized by altered expression of cytokine genes in the hippocampus of maternal separation rats treated with essential oil (Park et al., 2014).

114. Carvacrol is a monoterpenic phenol found in thyme and oregano. Oral administration of carvacrol produced antianxiety-like effects in mice (Melo et al., 2010).

115. Results from a randomized, controlled trial suggest that aromatherapy massage can be an effective therapeutic option for the short-term management of mild to moderate anxiety and depression in patients with cancer (Wilkinson et al., 2007).

116. Lemon oil and one of its components, gamma-terpinene, were found to inhibit oxidation of low-density lipoprotein (LDL) in vitro. Oxidation of LDL has been found to increase the risk of atherosclerosis and cardiac disease (Grassmann et al., 2001).

117. Oral administration of ocotea oil in mice was found to prevent collagen-epinephrine induced thrombosis (blood clots) (Ballabeni et al., 2007).

118. Both fennel oil and its constituent, anethole, were found to significantly reduce thrombosis (blood clots) in mice. They were also found to be free from the prohemorrhagic (increased bleeding) side effect that aspirin (acetylsalicylic acid) has (Tognolini et al., 2007).

119. Clove oil demonstrated an ability to prevent the aggregation of platelets that can lead to blood clots and thrombosis both in vivo and in vitro (Saeed et al., 1994).

120. Treatment of rats with 1,8-cineole (or eucalyptol, found in eucalyptus and rosemary) demonstrated an ability to lower mean aortic pressure (blood pressure)through vascular wall relaxation, without decreasing heart rate (Lahlou et al., 2002).

121. Boswellic acid, from frankincense, was found in vitro to prevent expression and activity of several proteins involved in the inflammatory response. In vivo, boswellic acid was found to protect against experimental arthritis (Roy et al., 2006).

     An acetone extract of frankincense was found to decrease arthritic sores, reduce paw edema (swelling), and suppress proinflammatory cytokines (cellular messengers) (Fan et al., 2005).

122. In patients suffering from arthritis, it was found that a blend of lavender, marjoram, eucalyptus, rosemary, peppermint, and carrier oils reduced perceived pain and depression, compared to control (Kim et al., 2005).

123. Eugenol (found in cassia, cinnamon, and clove) was found to ameliorate experimental arthritis in mice by inhibiting mononuclear cell infiltration into the knee joints and lowering cytokine levels (Grespan et al., 2012).

124. Eugenol (found in cassia, cinnamon, and clove) was found to ameliorate experimental arthritis in mice by inhibiting mononuclear cell infiltration into the knee joints and lowering cytokine levels (Grespan et al., 2012).

     The polyphenol fraction from cinnamon bark was found to improve inflammation and pain in animal models of inflammation and rheumatoid arthritis (Rathi et al., 2013).

125. Coriander extract produced a dose dependent inhibition of joint swelling in two mice models of induced arthritis (Nair et al., 2012).

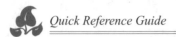

126.   Extracts from eucalyptus and thyme were found to have high nitrous oxide (NO) scavenging abilities and to inhibit NO production in macrophage cells. This could possibly explain their role in aiding respiratory inflammatory diseases (Vigo et al., 2004).

      Therapy with 1,8 cineole (eucalyptol) in both healthy and bronchitis-afflicted humans was shown to reduce production of LTB4 and PGE2 (both metabolites of arachidonic acid, a known chemical messenger involved in inflammation) in white blood cells (Juergens et al., 1998).

127.   L-menthol was found to inhibit production of inflammation mediators in human monocytes (a type of white blood cell involved in the immune response) (Juergens et al., 1998).

128.   The essential oil of rose at concentrations lower than 1% demonstrated relaxant effects on guinea pig trachea comparable to the asthma drug theophylline (Boskabady et al., 2006).

129.   Magnolialide, extracted from laurel leaf, was found to inhibit key factors in the development and amplification of type I hypersensitivity responses (implicated in the cause of allergic asthma)(Lee, T. et al., 2013).

130.   Long-term inhalation of lavender oil was found to suppress allergic airway inflammation and mucous cell hyperplasia in a mouse model of acute asthma (Ueno-Iio et al., 2014

131.   An extract from Artemisia vulgaris (mugwort) was found to have antispasmodic and bronchodilating activities in several different animal and animal tissue tests (Khan et al., 2009).

132.   Clove oil demonstrated an ability to prevent the aggregation of platelets that can lead to blood clots and thrombosis both in vivo and in vitro (Saeed et al., 1994).

133.   Both fennel oil and its constituent, anethole, were found to significantly reduce thrombosis (blood clots) in mice. They were also found to be free from the prohemorrhagic (increased bleeding) side effect that aspirin (acetylsalicylic acid) has (Tognolini et al., 2007).

134.   Inhaled ylang ylang oil was found to decrease blood pressure and pulse rate and to enhance attentiveness and alertness in volunteers, compared to an odorless control (Hongratanaworaki et al., 2004).

      Subjects who had ylang ylang oil applied to their skin had decreased blood pressure, increased skin temperature, and reported feeling more calm and relaxed, compared to subjects in a control group (Hongratanaworakit et al., 2006).

      Eighty-three hypertensive or prehypertensive subjects were divided into the following three groups: a study group (exposed to an essential oil blend containing lavender, ylang ylang, marjoram, and neroli), a placebo group (exposed to artificial fragrance), and a control group (no interventions). The study group was found to have an immediate and long-term decrease in home blood pressure (Kim et al., 2012).

135.   Treatment of rats with 1,8-cineole (or eucalyptol—found in eucalyptus, rosemary, and marjoram) demonstrated an ability to lower mean aortic pressure (blood pressure) through vascular wall relaxation, without decreasing heart rate.

      Eighty-three hypertensive or prehypertensive subjects were divided into the following three groups: a study group (exposed to an essential oil blend containing lavender, ylang ylang, marjoram, and neroli), a placebo group (exposed to artificial fragrance), and a control group (no interventions). The study group was found to have an immediate and long-term decrease in home blood pressure (Kim et al., 2012).

136.   Oral treatment with rosemary essential oil on primary hypotensive subjects was found to increase blood pressure values when compared to the subjects' placebo treatments before and after rosemary treatment (Fernández et al., 2014).

137.   Rats fed dill essential oil were found to have reduced total cholesterol, triglyceride, and low-density lipoprotein (LDL) and to have increased levels of high-density lipoprotein (HDL) (Hajhashemi et al., 2008).

138.   Clove oil demonstrated an ability to prevent the aggregation of platelets that can lead to blood clots and thrombosis both in vivo and in vitro (Saeed et al., 1994).

139.   In mice exposed to whole-body gamma irradiation, only 17% of mice who had been fed peppermint oil died, while 100% of mice who did not receive peppermint oil died. It was also found that mice pre-fed peppermint oil were able to return blood cell levels to normal after 30 days, while control mice were not able to (and, consequently, died), suggesting a protective or stimulating effect of the oil on blood stem cells (Samarth et al., 2004).

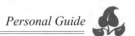

140. In a human trial, most patients receiving treatment with Melaleuca alternifolia oil placed topically on boils experienced healing or reduction of symptoms, while of those receiving no treatment (control), half required surgical intervention, and all still demonstrated signs of the infection (Feinblatt, 1960).

141. Oral intake of rosemary or eucalyptus essential oil (as well as several monoterpenes found in other essential oils) was shown to inhibit bone resorption in rats (Mühlbauer et al., 2003).

142. Subjects exposed to 3 minutes of lavender aroma were more relaxed and able to perform math computations faster and more accurately. Subjects exposed to rosemary aroma were more alert and completed math computations faster (but not more accurately) (Diego et al., 1998).

   Subjects who smelled a cleansing gel with lavender aroma were more relaxed and able to complete math computations faster (DField et al., 2005).

143. Several constituents of lemon oil and their metabolites (chemicals made by these chemicals in the body) were found to increase the release of monoamines (various chemicals responsible for neurotransmission and neuromodulation) in rat brain tissue, indicating a possible effect on brain nerve cell behavior (Fukumoto et al., 2006).

   Pretreatment of human and rat astrocyte cells (cells found in the nerve and brain that support the blood-brain barrier and help repair the brain and spinal cord following injuries) with lemon oil was found to inhibit heat-shock induced apoptosis of these cells (Koo et al., 2002).

144. Three new cadinane sesquiterpenes isolated from myrrh resin were found to have neuroprotective activities against 1-methyl-4-phenylpyridinium induced neuronal cell death in a human derived cell line cells (Xu et al., 2011).

145. The chloroform extract of Rosa damascena was found to cause neurite outgrowth activity in rat cortical neurons subjected to neurotic atrophy conditions. These findings suggest that Rosa damascena possesses neuronal protective properties that may benefit persons with dementia (Awale et al., 2011).

146. Incensole acetate, isolated from frankincense resin, was found to demonstrate an anti-inflammatory and neuro-protective effect in mice with a closed head injury (Moussaieff et al., 2008).

147. Bergamot essential oil was found to reduce excitotoxic neuronal damage caused by exposure of human neuroblastoma cells to NMDA in vitro, displaying the neuroprotection capabilities of bergamot oil (Corasaniti et al., 2007).

148. Peppermint oil was found to inhibit apoptosis of astrocytes (the most abundant glial-type [non-neuronal cells that provide support to neuronal cells and form myelin] cell in the brain) when subjected to heat-shock (Koo et al., 2001).

149. Pretreatment of human and rat astrocyte cells (cells found in the nerve and brain that support the blood-brain barrier and help repair the brain and spinal cord following injuries) with lemon oil was found to inhibit heat-shock induced apoptosis of these cells (Koo et al., 2002).

150. (-)-Linalool (found in basil, bergamot, cinnamon, clary sage, coriander, cypress, eucalyptus, fennel (sweet), geranium, ginger, helichrysum, jasmine, lavender, lemon, lemongrass, lime, marjoram, oregano, peppermint, rosemary, tangerine, thyme, wild orange, and ylang ylang essential oils): In two mice models of chronic pain, inflammatory pain and neuropathic pain, (-)-linalool was able to promote marked and long-lasting reduction in sensitivity to pain when compared to the control (Batista et al., 2010).

   Using a mouse model of neuropathic pain, researchers discovered that injections of bergamot or linalool (a main chemical constituent of bergamot) provided reduction of pain symptoms by inhibiting phosphorylation of the spinal ERK pathway (Kuwahata et al., 2013).

151. Imaging of the brain demonstrated that inhalation of 1,8-cineol (eucalyptol, a constituent of many essential oils—especially eucalyptus, rosemary, and marjoram) increased global cerebral blood flow after an inhalation time of 20 minutes (Nasel et al., 1994).

152. Inhalation of black pepper oil was found to increase cerebral blood flow and to improve the swallowing reflex in elderly patients who had suffered a stroke (Ebihara et al., 2006).

153. Ethanol extract of Boswellia serrata demonstrated antiproliferative effects on 5 leukemia and 2 brain tumor cell lines. It was more potent than one type of boswellic acid (AKBA) on 3 leukemia cell lines (Hostanska et al., 2002).

A=Aromatic   **T**=Topical   **I**=Internal

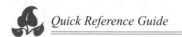

154. Therapy with 1,8 cineole (eucalyptol) in both healthy and bronchitis-afflicted humans was shown to reduce production of LTB4 and PGE2 (both metabolites of arachidonic acid, a known chemical messenger involved in inflammation) in white blood cells (Juergens et al., 1998).

Extracts from eucalyptus and thyme were found to have high nitrous oxide (NO) scavenging abilities and to inhibit NO production in macrophage cells. This could possibly explain their role in aiding respiratory inflammatory diseases (Vigo et al., 2004).

Eucalyptus oil was found to have an anti-inflammatory and mucin-inhibitory effect in rats with lipopolysaccharide-induced bronchitis (Lu et al., 2004).

155. Extracts from eucalyptus and thyme were found to have high nitrous oxide (NO) scavenging abilities and to inhibit NO production in macrophage cells. This could possibly explain their role in aiding respiratory inflammatory diseases (Vigo et al., 2004).

156. Inhaling lavender oil was found to lower agitation in older Chinese adults suffering from dementia (Lin et al., 2007).

Lavandula angustifolia essential oil demonstrated an ability to inhibit GABA-A receptor channels of rat brain cells (Huang et al., 2008).

157. In human trials, ylang ylang aroma was found to increase calmness (Moss et al., 2008).

Subjects who had ylang ylang oil applied to their skin had decreased blood pressure, increased skin temperature, and reported feeling more calm and relaxed (compared to subjects in a control group) (Hongratanaworakit et al., 2006).

In healthy control subjects, inhalation of ylang ylang aroma significantly reduced the P300 (an event-related potential interpreted to reflect attentional allocation and working memory) amplitude when compared to inhalation without aroma. These results suggest that ylang ylang produces a relaxing effect on cognition (Watanabe et al., 2013).

158. In human volunteers wearing breathing masks to prevent aroma inhalation, rose oil applied to the skin was found to significantly decrease breathing rate, blood oxygen saturation, and systolic blood pressure (compared to a placebo). And volunteers receiving rose oil rated themselves as more calm and relaxed than did subjects receiving the placebo (Hongratanaworakit et al., 2009).

Geraniol and eugenol, 2 components of rose oil (among others), were found to demonstrate antianxiety effects on mice in several tests (Umezu et al., 2002).

159. Melissa (lemon balm) oil applied topically in a lotion was found to reduce agitation and to improve quality of life in patients suffering from severe dementia, compared to those receiving a placebo lotion (Ballard et al., 2002).

160. Female patients waiting for dental treatment were found to be less anxious, more positive, and more calm when exposed to orange oil odor than patients who were not exposed to the orange oil odor (Lehrner et al., 2000).

161. A study using 114 subjects found that listening to soft music and/or inhaling Citrus bergamia essential oil were effective methods of relaxation, as indicated by a shift of the autonomic balance toward parasympathetic (Peng et al., 2009).

162. Exposure to lavender oil and to its constituents, linalool and linalyl acetate, was found to decrease normal movement in mice as well as to return mice to normal movement rates after caffeine induced hyperactivity (Buchbauer et al., 1991).

163. Inhaling lavender oil was found to lower agitation in older adults suffering from dementia (Lin et al., 2007).

Exposure to lavender oil, and to its constituents, linalool and linalyl acetate, was found to decrease normal movement in mice and to return mice to normal movement rates after caffeine induced hyperactivity (Buchbauer et al., 1991).

Lavandula angustifolia essential oil demonstrated an ability to inhibit GABA-A receptor channels of rat brain cells (Huang et al., 2008).

Swiss mice fed lavender oil diluted in olive oil were found to be more sedate in several common tests (Guillemain et al., 1989).

164. Lemon oil was found to have an antistress effect on mice involved in several behavioral tasks (Komiya et al., 2006).

165. Two chemical components found in valerian were found to have sedative, sleep-enhancing, and anxiolytic (anxiety-lowering) properties (Marder et al., 2003).

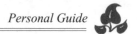

166. Boswellic acids from frankincense were found to induce apoptosis (cell death) in human leukemia cell lines (Xia et al., 2005).

Boswellic acid was found to inhibit DNA and RNA synthesis in human leukemia cells, leading to inhibited cell growth (Shao et al., 1998).

Boswellic acid was found to prevent and to inhibit invasion and metastasis of melanoma (skin pigment) and fibrosarcoma (connective tissue cancer) cells (Zhao et al., 2003).

Boswellic acid was found to cause differentiation in premyelocytic leukemia cells, while inhibiting growth of these cells in mice (Jing et al., 1992).

Boswellic acid was shown to induce apoptosis in 3 leukemia cell lines and to induce differentiation in one leukemia cell line (Jing et al., 1999).

Boswellic acid was found to inhibit the androgen receptors involved in the development and progression of prostate cancer (Yuan et al., 2008).

Boswellic acid induced apoptosis in prostate cancer cells (Lu et al., 2008).

An extract from Boswellia carterii was found to induce apoptosis (cell death) in 2 leukemia cell lines (Hunan et al., 1999).

An extract from frankincense was found to produce apoptosis in human leukemia cells (Bhushan et al., 2007).

Boswellic acids demonstrated an antiproliferative and apoptotic effect on liver cancer cells (Liu et al., Dec 2002).

Boswellic acids demonstrated an antiproliferative and apoptotic effect on liver cancer cells (Liu et al., Oct 2002).

167. Alpha-santalol was found to induce apoptosis in human skin cancer cells (Kaur et al., 2005).

Various concentrations of alpha-santalol (from sandalwood) were tested against skin cancer in mice. All concentrations were found to inhibit skin cancer development (Dwivedi et al., 2005).

Alpha-santalol, derived from sandalwood EO, was found to delay and decrease the incidence and multiplicity of skin tumor (papilloma) development in mice (Swivedi et al., 2003).

Pretreatment with alpha-santalol before UVB (ultraviolet B) radiation significantly reduced skin tumor development and multiplicity and induced proapoptotic and tumor-suppressing proteins (Arasada et al., 2008).

A solution of 5% alpha-santalol (from sandalwood) was found to prevent skin tumor formation caused by ultraviolet B (UVB) radiation in mice (Swivedi et al., 2006).

Sandalwood oil was found to decrease skin papilloma (tumors) in mice (Swivedi et al., 1997).

Oral sandalwood oil use enhanced GST activity (a protein in cell membranes that can help eliminate toxins) and acid-soluble SH levels. This suggests a possible chemopreventive action on carcinogenesis (Banerjee et al., 1993).

168. Rats fed diets containing perillyl alcohol (derived from lavender plants) were found to have less incidence of colon tumors and less multiplicity of tumors in the colon, compared to control. Colon tumors of animals fed perillyl alcohol were found to exhibit increased apoptosis of cells compared to control (Reddy et al., 1997).

In tests for mutagenicity, both tea tree and lavender oils were found to not be mutagenic. Lavender oil was also found to have strong antimutagenic activity, reducing mutations of cells exposed to a known mutagen (Evandri et al., 2005).

Mice treated with perillyl alcohol (found in lavender and mint plants) had a 22% reduction in tumor incidence and a 58% reduction in tumor multiplicity during a mouse lung tumor bioassay (Lantry et al., 1997).

Rats with liver tumors that were treated with perillyl alcohol had smaller tumor sizes than did untreated rats, due to apoptosis of cancer cells in treated rats (Mills et al., 1995).

Perillyl alcohol (found in lavender and caraway) and was found to inhibit hyperproliferation of mammary epithelial cells prior to tumorigenisis. (Katdare et al., 1997).

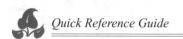

169.   Carnosic acid (derived from rosemary) was found to inhibit the proliferation of human leukemia cells in vitro (Steiner et al., 2001).

Rosemary extracts induced CYP (cytochrome P450) activity in liver cells, suggesting a possibility of increased ability to remove toxins (Debersac et al., 2001).

Rosemary extract injected in rats was found to decrease mammary adenocarcinomas in rats (Singletary et al., 1996).

An ethanol extract of rosemary was found to have an antiproliferative effect on human leukemia and breast carcinoma cells, as well as an antioxidant effect (Cheung et al., 2007).

170.   Supplementation with caraway was found to inhibit development of aberrant crypt foci (precursors to polyps) in the colorectal area of rats induced to develop aberrant crypt foci (Deeptha et al., 2006).

Perillyl alcohol (found in caraway) was found to inhibit hyperproliferation of mammary epithelial cells prior to tumori-genisis (Katdare et al., 1997).

Rats with liver tumors that were treated with perillyl alcohol had smaller tumor sizes than did untreated rats, due to apoptosis of cancer cells in treated rats (Mills et al., 1995).

Carvone, found in dill and caraway oil, was found to induce the glutathione S-transferase enzyme (which helps to remove toxins from the body) in several target mouse tissues (Zheng et al., 1992).

171.   Geraniol (found in lemongrass oil, among others) was found to inhibit colon cancer cell growth, while inhibiting DNA synthesis in these cells (Carnesecchi et al., 2001).

An extract from lemongrass was found to inhibit hepatocarcinogenesis (liver cancer genesis) in rats (Puatanachokchai et al., 2002).

Citral (found in lemongrass, melissa, and verbena oils) was found to induce apoptosis in several cancer cell lines (hemato-poietic cells [stem cells that create blood cells]) (Dudai et al., 2005).

Lemongrass oil and its constituent, isointermedeol, were found to induce apoptosis in human leukemia cells (Kumar et al., 2008).

Lemongrass oil was found to inhibit multiple cancer cell lines, both in vitro and in vivo in mice (Sharma et al., 2009).

172.   Beta-caryophyllene was found to increase the anticancer activities of paclitaxel (a chemotherapy drug derived from the yew tree) (Legault et al., 2007).

173.   Basil and its component, linalool, were found to reduce spontaneous mutagenesis in bacteria cells (Berić et al., 2008).

174.   Geraniol (found in geranium and lemongrass oil, among others) was found to inhibit colon cancer cell growth while inhibiting DNA synthesis in these cells (Carnesecchi et al., 2001).

175.   Sclareol, from clary sage oil, was found to have a cytostatic effect on human leukemia cell lines (Dimas et al., 1999).

176.   In a study of older individuals, it was found that there was a dose-dependent relationship between citrus peel consump-tion (citrus peels are high in d-limonene) and a lower degree of squamous cell carcinoma (SCC) of the skin (Hakim et al., 2000).

177.   Treatment with elemene (found in myrrh oil) was found to increase survival time and to reduce tumor size in patients with malignant brain tumors, as compared with chemotherapy (Tan et al., 2000).

In both in vitro and in vivo studies, elemene (found in myrrh oil) was found to increase apoptosis in laryngeal cancer cells (Tao et al., 2006).

178.   Ethanol extract of Boswellia serrata demonstrated antiproliferative effects on 5 leukemia and on 2 brain tumor cell lines. It was more potent than 1 type of boswellic acid (AKBA) on 3 leukemia cell lines (Hostanska et al., 2002).

179.   Treatment with elemene (found in myrrh oil) was found to increase survival time and to reduce tumor size in patients with malignant brain tumors, as compared with chemotherapy (Tan et al., 2000).

180.   Rosemary extract injected in rats was found to decrease mammary adenocarcinomas in rats (Singletary et al., 1996).

An ethanol extract of rosemary was found to have an antiproliferative and an antioxidant effect on human leukemia and breast carcinoma cells (Cheung et al., 2007).

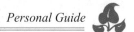

181. Perillyl alcohol (found in lavender and caraway) was found to inhibit hyperproliferation of mammary epithelial cells prior to tumorigenisis. (Katdare et al., 1997).

182. Sclareol, a chemical constituent found in clary sage essential oil, was found to reduce regulatory T cells frequency and also tumor size in a mouse model of breast cancer, suggesting that sclareol can enhance the effect of cancer therapy as an immunostiumlant (Noori et al., 2013).

183. Basil extract was found to inhibit the growth of MCF-7 breast cancer cells, possess antioxidant activity, and protect against DNA damage (Al-Ali et al., 2013).

184. Rats fed diets containing perillyl alcohol (derived from lavender plants) were found to have less incidence of colon tumors and less multiplicity of tumors in the colon, as compared to control. Colon tumors of animals fed perillyl alcohol were found to exhibit increased apoptosis of cells, compared to control (Reddy et al., 1997).

185. Geraniol (found in geranium and lemongrass oil, among others) was found to inhibit colon cancer cell growth, while inhibiting DNA synthesis in these cells (Carnesecchi et al., 2001).

186. Boswellic acids were found to have an antiproliferative and apoptotic effect on human colon cancer cells (Liu et al., 2002).

    Boswellic acids demonstrated an antiproliferative and apoptotic effect on liver cancer cells (Liu et al., 2002).

187. An extract from lemongrass was found to inhibit hepatocarcinogenesis (liver cancer genesis) in rats (Puatanachokchai et al., 2002).

188. Rats with liver tumors that were treated with perillyl alcohol had smaller tumor sizes than untreated rats, due to apoptosis of cancer cells in treated rats (Mills et al., 1995).

189. Mice treated with perillyl alcohol (found in lavender and mint plants) had a 22% reduction in tumor incidence and a 58% reduction in tumor multiplicity during a mouse lung tumor bioassay (Lantry et al., 1997).

190. Alpha-santalol was found to induce apoptosis in human skin cancer cells (Kaur et al., 2005).

    Various concentrations of alpha-santalol (from sandalwood) were tested against skin cancer in mice. All concentrations were found to inhibit skin cancer development (Dwivedi et al., 2005).

    Alpha-santalol, derived from sandalwood EO, was found to delay and decrease the incidence and multiplicity of skin tumor (papilloma) development in mice (Dwivedi et al., 2003).

    Pretreatment with alpha-santalol before UVB (ultraviolet B) radiation significantly reduced skin tumor development and multiplicity and induced proapoptotic and tumor-suppressing proteins (Arasada et al., 2008).

    A solution of 5% alpha-santalol (from sandalwood) was found to prevent skin tumor formation caused by ultraviolet B (UVB) radiation in mice (Dwivedi et al., 2006).

    Sandalwood oil was found to decrease skin papilloma (tumors) in mice (Dwivedi et al., 1997).

191. Boswellic acid was found to prevent and inhibit invasion and metastasis of melanoma (skin pigment) and fibrosarcoma (connective tissue cancer) cells (Zhao et al. 2003).

192. In a human trial in China involving individuals suffering from angina pectoris (heart pain due to restricted blood flow), a preparation of volatile oil fractionated from valerian root was effective in remitting symptoms, decreasing attack frequency, shortening duration, and lowering plasma lipid levels.

193. Older rats whose diets were supplemented with thyme oil were found to have higher levels of the antioxidant enzymes superoxide dismutase and glutathione peroxidase in the heart, liver, and kidneys than did older rats without this supplementation (Youdim et al., 1999).

194. Imaging of the brain demonstrated that inhalation of 1,8-cineol (eucalyptol—a constituent of many essential oils, especially eucalyptus, rosemary, and marjoram) increased global cerebral blood flow after an inhalation time of 20 minutes (Nasel et al., 1994).

195. Melissa essential oil was found to have hypolipidemic effects in transgenic mice. Mice orally administered Melissa essential oil for two weeks had lower plasma triglyceride concentrations and altered metabolic pathways. These results indicate that melissa oil could be beneficial in preventing hypertriglyceridemia, one of the main contributors to the development of cardiovascular disease (Jun et al., 2012).

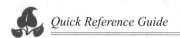

196. Different fractions of Anethum graveolens extract improved hypercholesterolemia in rats fed a high fat diet. Hypercholesterolemia has been found to be a risk factor for the development of atherosclerosis (Bahramikia et al., 2009).

197. A plaque reduction assay showed that eucalyptus essential oil possessed a mild antiviral activity against mumps virus (Cermelli et al., 2008).

198. Colicky infants treated with a fennel oil emulsion were found to exhibit a cessation of colic more frequently than infants treated with the placebo, and the intensity of the colic was significantly lower in the fennel-treated group (Alexandrovich et al., 2003).

     Colicky infants treated with a blend extracted from melissa, German chamomile, and fennel were found to have less crying time than infants treated with a placebo (Savino et al., 2005).

199. Oral administration of German chamomile and melissa extracts was found to delay upper gastrointestinal transit in mice (Capasso et al., 2007).

     Colicky infants treated with a blend extracted from melissa, German chamomile, and fennel were found to have less crying time than infants treated with a placebo (Savino et al., 2005).

200. The use of rosemary, lemon, and peppermint oils in massage demonstrated an ability to reduce constipation and to increase bowel movements in elderly subjects, compared to massage without the oils (Kim et al., 2005).

201. Tea tree oil was found to inhibit 301 different types of yeasts isolated from the mouths of cancer patients suffering from advanced cancer, including 41 strains that are known to be resistant to antifungal drugs (Bagg et al., 2006).

202. Lavender oil demonstrated both fungistatic (stopped growth) and fungicidal (killed) activity against Candida albicans (D'Auria et al., 2005).

203. Thyme oil was found to inhibit Candida species by causing lesions in the cell membrane and was also found to inhibit germ tube (an outgrowth that develops when the fungi is preparing to replicate) formation (Pina-Vaz et al., 2004).

204. Internal lemongrass capsules were found to reduce cholesterol in some subjects (Elson et al., 1989).

205. Inhalation of lavender and monarda oils was found to reduce cholesterol content and atherosclerotic plaques in the aorta (Nikolaevskii et al., 1990).

     Camphene (found in coriander, frankincense, ginger, lavender, lime, peppermint, roman chamomile, rose, rosemary, spearmint, fir): Injection of camphene, a constituent found in many essential oils, was found to reduce plasma cholesterol and triglycerides in naïve and hyperlipidemic rats. Camphene's mechanism of action was different than that of statins (drugs used to lower cholesterol levels) (Vallianou et al., 2011).

206. Rats fed dill essential oil were found to have reduced levels of cholesterol, triglyceride, and low-density lipoprotein (LDL) and increased levels of high-density lipoprotein (HDL) (Hajhashemi et al., 2008).

207. Oral administration of thyme and oregano oil at a dose of 0.2% thyme and 0.1% oregano was found to be effective in decreasing the mortality rate, accelerating body weight gain recovery, and significantly reducing the macroscopic damage of colonic tissue of mice with induced colitis (Bukovska et al., 2007).

208. Rosemary essential oil was found to be effective in reducing colon tissue lesions and colitis indices when administered orally or intraperitoneally to rats induced with colitis, suggesting that rosemary has anti-colitic activity (Minaiyan et al., 2011).

209. Subjects exposed to 3 minutes of lavender aroma were more relaxed and were able to perform math computations faster and more accurately. (Diego et al., 1998).

     Subjects who smelled a cleansing gel with lavender aroma were more relaxed and were able to complete math computations faster (Field et al., 2005).

210. Daily inhalation of lemon essential oil aroma for five minutes was found to have a positive effect on learning in mice (Ogeturk et al., 2010).

211. Incensole acetate, isolated from frankincense resin, was found to demonstrate an anti-inflammatory and neuro-protective effect in mice with closed head injuries (Moussaieff et al., 2008).

212. Eucalyptus oil was found to have an anti-inflammatory and mucin-inhibitory effect on rats with lipopolysaccharide-induced bronchitis (Lu et al., 2004).

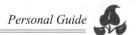

213.　The oral and intraperitoneal administration of caraway essential oil, even at low doses, was effective in reducing colon tissue lesions in the experimental TNBS-induced colitis rat model (Keshavarz et al., 2013).

214.　Basil (Ocimum gratissimum) oil was found to facilitate the healing process of wounds in rabbits to a greater extent than did two antibacterial preparations, Cicatrin and Cetavlex (Orafidiya et al., 2003).

215.　Bergamot extract was found to display inhibitory activity on IL-8 gene expression (IL-8 is involved in the inflammatory processes associated with cystic fibrosis), indicating that bergamot may possess possible anti-inflammatory properties to reduce lung inflammation in cystic fibrosis patients (Borgatti et al., 2011).

216.　Lemon oil vapor was found to have a strong antistress and antidepressant effect on mice subjected to several common stress tests (Komiya et al., 2006).

　　　Lemon oil and its component, citral, were found to decrease depressed behavior in a similar manner to antidepressant drugs in rats involved in several stress tests (Komori et al., Dec. 1995).

　　　In 12 patients suffering from depression, it was found that inhaling citrus aromas reduced the needed doses of antidepressants, normalized neuroendocrine hormone levels, and normalized immune functioning (Komori et al., May 1995).

217.　Incensole acetate (found in frankincense) was found to open TRPV receptors (a possible channel for emotional regulation) in mice brains (Moussaieff et al., 2008).

218.　In patients suffering from arthritis, it was found that a blend of lavender, marjoram, eucalyptus, rosemary, peppermint, and carrier oils reduced perceived pain and depression, compared to control (Kim et al., 2005).

　　　Female students suffering from insomnia were found to sleep better and to have lower levels of depression during weeks they used a lavender fragrance, as compared to weeks they did not use a lavender fragrance (Lee et al., 2006).

219.　In 12 patients suffering from depression, it was found that inhaling citrus aromas reduced the needed doses of antidepressants, normalized neuroendocrine hormone levels, and normalized immune functioning (Komori et al., May 1995).

220.　Transdermal absorption of ylang ylang essential oil altered physiological stress responses, like blood pressure and skin temperature, and subjects reported being more calm and relaxed than the control group (Hongratanaworakit et al., 2006).

221.　Many fractions of Rosmarinus officinalis, including its essential oil, were found to have antidepressant-like effects on mice submitted to two stress tests after oral administration of the rosemary plant fractions (Machado et al., 2013).

222.　Clary sage essential oil displayed antidepressant-like effects via the dopaminergic pathway in rats submitted to the forced swim test (a common stress test) (Seol et al., 2010).

223.　Inhaling lavender oil was found to lower agitation in older adults suffering from dementia (Lin et al., 2007).

　　　Exposure to lavender oil, and to its constituents, linalool and linalyl acetate, was found to decrease normal movement in mice and to return mice to normal movement rates after caffeine-induced hyperactivity (Buchbauer et al., 1991).

　　　Swiss mice fed lavender oil diluted in olive oil were found to be more sedate in several common tests (Guillemain et al., 1989).

224.　Subjects who had ylang ylang oil applied to their skin had decreased blood pressure, increased skin temperature, and reported feeling more calm and relaxed, compared to subjects in a control group (Hongratanaworakit et al., 2006).

225.　Melissa (lemon balm) oil applied topically in a lotion was found to reduce agitation and to improve quality of life in patients suffering from severe dementia, compared to those receiving a placebo lotion (Ballard et al., 2002).

226.　In animal testing, the essential oil of tarragon demonstrated anticonvulsant and sedative properties at low concentrations (Sayyah et al., 2004).

227.　Rosemary extracts induced CYP (cytochrome P450) activity in liver cells, suggesting a possibility of increased ability to remove toxins (Debersac et al., 2001).

228.　Three compounds derived from dill and caraway oil (anethofuran, carvone, and limonene) were found to induce the enzyme glutathione S-transferase (involved in transforming or binding to toxins in tissues) in several mice tissues.

229.　Coriander extract was found to have a protective role against lead toxicity in rat brain (Velaga et al., 2014).

A=Aromatic　　**T**=Topical　　**I**=Internal　　　　　　　　　|

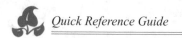

230. Cinnamon bark extract supplementation for three months was found to significantly improve blood glucose control in Chinese patients with type 2 diabetes taking gliclazide (a prescribed antidiabetic medication) (Lu, T. et al., 2012).

Cinnamaldehyde (the major constituent of cinnamon oil) produced protective action against alloxan-induced diabetic nephropathy in rats (Mishra et al., 2010).

231. Oral rosemary extract was found to decrease blood glucose levels, while increasing insulin levels in alloxan-diabetic rabbits (Bakirel et al., 2008).

232. Sage essential oil was found to increase hepatocyte (liver cell) sensitivity to insulin and to inhibit gluconeogenesis (the creation of glucose) in a manner similar to the type 2 diabetes prevention drug, metformin, in mice (Lima et al., 2006).

233. Cuminaldehyde, a component of cumin seed oil, was found to inhibit the activity of aldose reductase (an enzyme that converts glucose into other sugars) and alpha-glucosidase (an enzyme that helps in the digestion of carbohydrates into simple sugars). Inhibiting both of these enzymes has been theorized to aid in controlling diabetes (Lee, 2005).

234. Results from a clinical trial showed that basil leaf extract decreased fasting and postprandial blood glucose in diabetes mellitus patients, suggesting that basil could be used as a dietary therapy in mild to moderate cases of type 2 diabetes mellitus (Agrawal et al., 1996).

235. Dill seed extract suppressed high-fat diet-induced hyperlipidemia through hepatic PPAR-⊠ activation in diabetic obese mice (Takahashi et al., 2013).

D-Limonene (found in lime, lemon, bergamot, dill, grapefruit, lavender, lemongrass, Roman chamomile, tangerine, and orange essential oils): In a recent study oral intake of D-limonene ameliorated insulin resistance in mice fed a high-fat diet (Jing et al., 2013).

236. In vitro data suggest that the constituents of cassia may be appropriate for the treatment of diabetic complications (like cataract and retinopathy) because of the constituents' abil-ity to inhibit aldose reductase and thus prevent the conversion of glucose to corbitol (Lee, 2002).

237. Cinnamon polyphenols were found to restore pancreatic function and exert hypoglycemic and hypolipidemic effects in a diabetic mouse model (Li, R. et al., 2013).

238. Peppermint oil was found to be as effective as Buscopan (an antispasmodic drug) at preventing spasms during a barium enema (a type of enema used to place barium in the colon for X-ray imaging purposes) (Asao et al., 2003).

Peppermint oil in enteric-coated capsules was found to relieve symptoms of irritable bowel syndrome better than a placebo (Rees et al., 1979).

Patients with IBS symptoms who took a peppermint oil formulation in an enteric-coated capsule were found to have a significantly higher reduction of symptoms when compared with IBS patients who took a placebo (Liu et al., 1997).

When taken internally, an enteric-coated capsule with peppermint and caraway oil was found to reduce pain and symptoms of patients with non-ulcer dyspepsia (indigestion), compared to a control (May et al., 1996).

A combination of peppermint and caraway oil was found to reduce visceral hyperalgesia (pain hypersensitivity in the gastrointestinal tract) after induced inflammation in rats (Kim et al., 2005).

The use of rosemary, lemon, and peppermint oils in massage demonstrated an ability to reduce constipation and to increase bowel movements in elderly subjects, compared to massage without the oils (Kim et al., 2005).

239. When taken internally, an enteric-coated capsule with peppermint and caraway oil was found to reduce pain and symptoms in patients with non-ulcer dyspepsia (indigestion), compared to a control (May et al., 1996).

A combination of peppermint and caraway oil was found to reduce visceral hyperalgesia (pain hypersensitivity in the gastrointestinal tract) after induced inflammation in rats (Kim et al., 2005).

240. Colicky infants treated with a fennel oil emulsion were found to exhibit a cessation of colic more frequently than did infants treated with a placebo, and the intensity of the colic was significantly lower in the fennel-treated group (Alexandrovich et al., 2003).

Colicky infants treated with a blend extracted from melissa, German chamomile, and fennel were found to have less crying time than infants treated with a placebo (Savino et al., 2005).

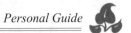
241. Lemongrass demonstrated ability to inhibit Helicobacter pylori, a pathogen responsible for gastroduodenal disease. This pathogen did not develop resistance to lemongrass after 10 passes (it developed resistance to clarithromycin) (Ohno et al., 2003).

242. Ginger root given one hour before major gynecological surgery resulted in less nausea and fewer incidences of vomiting, compared to control (Nanthakomon et al., 2006).

243. Angelica essential oil was found to selectively inhibit the growth of potentially pathogenic microorganisms (mostly Gram positive bacteria and the fungus Candida albicans) while not significantly inhibiting the growth of useful intestinal microflora (specifically bifidobacteria and lactobacilli). These results suggest that the selective antimicrobial activity of angelica essential oil may be useful in the treatment of intestinal dysbiosis (Fraternale et al., 2014).

244. Oregano oil administered orally was found to improve gastrointestinal symptoms in 7 of 11 patients who had tested positive for the parasite Blastocystis hominis, and it was found to cause disappearance of this parasite in 8 cases (Force et al., 2000).

245. The use of rosemary, lemon, and peppermint oils in massage demonstrated an ability to reduce constipation and to increase bowel movements in elderly subjects, compared to massage without the oils (Kim et al., 2005).

246. In irritable bowel syndrome patients (IBS) without bacterial overgrowth, lactose intolerance, or celiac disease, peppermint oil was found over a period of 8 weeks to reduce IBS symptoms significantly more than a placebo (Cappello et al., 2007).

247. Peppermint oil was found to be as effective as Buscopan (an antispasmodic drug) at preventing spasms during a barium enema (a type of enema used to place barium in the colon for X-ray imaging purposes) (Asao et al., 2003).

248. In isolated rat ileum tissue, galbanum oil demonstrated an antispasmodic effect against contractions induced by KCl (potassium chloride) (Sadraei et al., 2001).

249. Lavender was found to have a relaxant effect on smooth muscle from guinea pig ileum (small intestine) (Lis-Balchin et al., 1999).

250. Rose essential oil and its main constituents were found to inhibit rat isolated ileum (a section of the small intestine), suggesting that rose oil can be used as an antispasmodic remedy for treatment of abdominal spasm (Sadraei et al., 2013).

251. Oregano oil administered orally was found to improve gastrointestinal symptoms in 7 of 11 patients who had tested positive for the parasite Blastocystis hominis, and it was found to cause disappearance of this parasite in 8 cases (Force et al., 2000).

252. Palmarosa oil and its constituent, geraniol, demonstrated antiparasitic activity against the parasitic roundworm, Caenorhabditis elegans, in vitro (Kumaran et al., 2003).

253. Essential oil from Lavandula angustifolia demonstrated ability to eliminate protozoal pathogens Giardia duodenalis, Trichomonas vaginalis, and Hexamita inflata at concentrations of 1% or less (Moon et al., 2006).

254. In patients with dyspepsia (indigestion), treatments with capsules containing peppermint and caraway oil were found to decrease pain and pain frequency (Freise et al., 1999).

     Children suffering from irritable bowel syndrome (IBS) who received peppermint oil in enteric-coated capsules (encapsulated so the capsules wouldn't open until they reached the intestines) reported a reduced severity of pain associated with IBS (Kline et al., 2001).

     Patients with IBS symptoms who took a peppermint oil formulation in an enteric-coated capsule were found to have a significantly higher reduction of symptoms when compared to IBS patients taking a placebo (Liu et al., 1997).

     In irritable bowel syndrome (IBS) patients without bacterial overgrowth, lactose intolerance, or celiac disease, peppermint oil was found over a period of 8 weeks to reduce IBS symptoms significantly more than a placebo (Cappello et al., 2007).

255. In patients with dyspepsia (indigestion), treatments with capsules containing peppermint and caraway oil were found to decrease pain and pain frequency (Freise et al., 1999).

256. The scent of grapefruit oil and its component, limonene, was found to affect the autonomic nerves and to reduce appetite and body weight in rats exposed to the oil for 15 minutes 3 times per week (Shen et al., 2005).

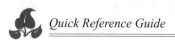

257. A quasi experiment comparing exercise performance before and after consumption of mineral water containing peppermint essential oil for 10 days found that exercise performance improved after consumption of peppermint oil (including increases in respiratory efficiency, energy expenditure, time to exhaustion, and distance during exercise and decreases in resting and exercise heart rates) (Meamarbashi et al., 2013).

258. Inhalation of black pepper oil was found to increase cerebral blood flow and to improve the swallowing reflex in elderly patients who had suffered a stroke (Nasel et al., 1994).

259. Inhalation of linalool or Lavandula burnatii super-derived essential oil (composed from the five main lavender oils and containing a high level of linalool) was found to aid in the recovery of ether-inhalation induced decrease in adrenaline, noradrenaline, and dopamine levels in female menopausal model rats. The researchers stated that these results suggest that lavender or linalool may contribute to relieving tension and may be applicable to the treatment of menopausal disorders (Yamada et al., 2005).

260. Using a mouse model of postmenopausal bone loss researchers found that oral administration of fennel oil for six weeks had an intermediate effect on the prevention of femoral bone mineral density and bone mineral content when compared to controls. These findings suggest that fennel oil has potential in preventing bone loss in postmenopausal osteoporosis (Kim et al., 2012).

261. In an experiment with 67 female college students, an aromatherapy massage with lavender, clary sage, and rose essential oils proved to be more effective at treating dysmenorrhea than a placebo treatment of almond oil or the control (Han et al., 2006).

    Compared to a synthetic fragrance, dysmenorrhea pain decreased and shortened in duration when subjects massaged a blend of lavender, marjoram, and clary sage essential oils (in a ratio of 2:1:1) daily on the abdomen between menstruations (Ou et al., 2012).

262. Compared to a synthetic fragrance, dysmenorrhea pain decreased and shortened in duration when subjects massaged a blend of lavender, marjoram, and clary sage essential oils (in a ratio of 2:1:1) daily on the abdomen between menstruations (Ou et al., 2012).

263. A study with 92 university age female students with primary dysmenorrhea found that ingestion of a capsule containing 200 mg of Rosa damascena extract every 6 hours at the first 3 days of menstruation was as effective as administration of Mefenamic acid (a drug with possible adverse reactions and side effects) (Bani et al., 2014).

    In an experiment with 67 female college students, an aromatherapy massage with lavender, clary sage, and rose essential oils proved to be more effective at treating dysmenorrhea than a placebo treatment of almond oil or the control (Han et al., 2006).

264. Fennel oil was found to reduce contraction frequency and intensity in rat uterus induced to contract (Ostad et al., 2001).

265. Subjects exposed to 3 minutes of lavender aroma were more relaxed and were able to perform math computations faster and more accurately (Diego et al., 1998).

    Subjects who smelled a cleansing gel with lavender aroma were more relaxed and were able to complete math computations faster (Field et al., 1995).

266. Patients with alopecia areata (hair loss) that massaged carrier oils containing a blend of thyme, rosemary, lavender, and cedarwood oils into their scalps were more likely to show improvement when compared to a control group that massaged carrier oils alone into their scalps (Hay et al., 1998).

267. A combination of peppermint oil and ethanol was found to have a significant analgesic effect, reducing sensitivity to headache; while a combination of peppermint, eucalyptus, and ethanol was found to relax muscles and to increase cognitive performance in humans (Göbel et al., 1994).

268. Inhalation of lavender essential oil was found to be more effective than inhalation of a placebo for reducing the severity of headaches in subjects diagnosed with migraine headaches (Sasannejad et al., 2012).

269. Peppermint oil demonstrated a direct virucidal activity against herpes type 1 and type 2 viruses (Schuhmacher et al., 2003).

270. Tea tree and eucalyptus oil demonstrated an ability to inhibit the herpes simplex virus (Schnitzler et al., 2001).

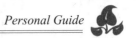
271. Helichrysum was found to have significant antiviral activity against the herpes virus at non-cytotoxic concentrations (Nostro et al., 2003).

272. Eugenol was found to be virucidal to herpes simplex and was found to delay the development of herpes-induced keratitis (inflammation of the cornea) in mice (Benencia et al., 2000).

273. Melissa oil demonstrated inhibition of herpes simplex type 1 and type 2 viruses (Schnitzler et al., 2008).

274. Herpes simplex viruses pretreated with manuka oil before cell infection were significantly inhibited and had plaque formation reduced by over 98% in cultured monkey kidney cells (Reichling et al., 2005).

275. Tea tree oil applied to histamine-induced weal and flare in human volunteers was found to decrease the mean weal volume when compared to a control (Koh et al., 2002).

    Tea tree oil applied to histamine-induced edema (swelling) in mice ears was found to significantly reduce swelling (Brand et al., 2002).

    Tea tree oil was found to reduce inflammation in the skin of nickel-sensitive human skin exposed to nickel (Pearce et al., 2005).

276. L-menthol was found to inhibit production of inflammation mediators in human monocytes (a type of white blood cell involved in the immune response) (Juergens et al., 1998).

277. Lavender oil was found to inhibit immediate-type allergic reactions in mice and rats by inhibiting mast cell degranulation (Kim et al., 1999).

278. Inhaling lavender oil was found to lower agitation in older adults suffering from dementia (Lin et al., 2007).

279. Growth-retarded pigs receiving a supplementation of oregano leaves and flowers enriched with cold-pressed oregano oil were found to have increased growth, decreased mortality, and higher numbers of immune-system cells and compounds when compared to control pigs who did not receive supplementation (Walter et al., 2004).

280. Boswellic acids from frankincense (delivered with sesame seed oil) were found to inhibit TH1 cytokines while potentiating TH2 cytokines, demonstrating their ability to modulate the immune response (Chevrier et al., 2005).

281. In 12 patients suffering from depression, it was found that inhaling citrus aromas reduced the needed doses of antidepressants, normalized neuroendocrine hormone levels, and normalized immune function (Komori et al, 1995).

282. Basil (Ocimum gratissimum) oil was found to facilitate the healing process of wounds in rabbits to a greater extent than did two antibacterial preparations, Cicatrin and Cetavlex (Orafidiya et al., 2003).

283. In vitro research has found that Melaleuca alternifolia concentrate can disturb the normal viral membrane fusion of the influenza virus and inhibit entry of influenza virus into the host cell (Li et al., 2013).

284. Cumin essential oil was found to possess insecticidal activity against the German cockroach, showing 100% fumigant toxicity and 100% contact toxicity at 10-20 mg/mL and 1 mg/cockroach concentrations, respectively (Yeom et al., 2012).

285. In a test of 34 different essential oils, patchouli (Pogostemon cablin) oil proved to be the insecticide that was most effective against the common house fly (Pavela, 2008).

    Both patchouli oil and its constituent, patchouli alcohol (patchoulol), were found to be repellent and insecticidal when applied topically to Formosan termites (Zhu et al., 2003).

286. Clove oil was found to be highly termiticidal (Zhu et al., 2001).

    A blend of eugenol, alpha-terpineol, and cinnamic alcohol was found to be insecticidal against American cockroaches, carpenter ants, and German cockroaches (Enan et al., 2001).

287. Lavandula angustifolia oil was found to be a potent topical insecticide for the African cotton leafworm larvae (Pavela, 2005).

288. Two basil oils (Ocimum basilicum and O. gratissimum) were found to be insecticidal against the cowpea weevil (an agricultural pest) beetle and eggs in both a diffused and aromatized powder form (Kéita et al., 2001).

289. Essential oil of Melaleuca alternifolia was found to be lethal to more than 80% of Ixodes ricinus tick nymphs (carriers or Lyme disease) when they inhaled a 10 microl dose of the oil for 90 minutes or more (Iori et al., 2005).

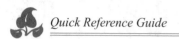

290. The leaf and fruit oils of Schinus molle (pink pepper) demonstrated a repellent and insecticidal activity against two beetles that commonly damage and consume stored grains (Abdel-Sattar et al., 2009).

291. Prepared microcapsules containing rosemary oil were found to be toxic to the larvae of gypsy moths, pests that causes massive defoliation of forests (Moretti et al., 2002).

292. Researchers found that an 8% eucalyptus oil spray was the most effective treatment (when compared against other concentrations of eucalyptus and clove oil sprays) against lice and insecticide-resistant head lice (Choi et al., 2010).

293. Caraway essential oil displayed insecticidal activity against two species of grain storage insects (maize weevil and red flour beetle), indicating the oils potential as a natural fumigant for stored products (Fang et al., 2010).

294. Eucalyptus Citriodora essential oil was found to possess insecticidal activity against Aedes aegypti mosquito larvae (Vera et al., 2014).

295. Topical application of dorado azul essential oil decreased the percentage of mosquitoes that landed and blood fed on the forearm of volunteers in a laboratory test. In a field test, within the first 15 minutes of essential oil application no mosquitoes landed on the treated subject, while 493 mosquitoes landed on the control subject (Abagli et al., 2012).

     Dorado azul essential oil displayed larvicidal and repellent activity against Aedes albopictus mosquito larvae (Conti et al., 2012).

296. A slow-release citronella formula was found to significantly reduce infection with head lice in elementary school children, compared to a control (Mumcuoglu et al., 2004).

     Citronella oil applied in high concentration was found to effectively repel nymphs of Amblyomma cajennense (a type of tick known to carry Rocky Mountain spotted fever) for up to 35 hours (Soares et al., 2009).

     Clove, citronella, and patchouli oils were found to effectively repel 3 species of mosquitoes (with clove being the most effective—demonstrating 100% repellency for 2–4 hours) (Trongtokit et al., 2005).

297. Clove, citronella, and patchouli oils were found to effectively repel 3 species of mosquitoes (with clove being the most effective—demonstrating 100% repellency for 2–4 hours) (Trongtokit et al., 2005).

298. Both patchouli oil and its constituent, patchouli alcohol (patchoulol), were found to be repellent and insecticidal when applied topically to Formosan termites (Zhu et al., 2003).

     Clove, citronella, and patchouli oils were found to effectively repel 3 species of mosquitoes (with clove being the most effective—demonstrating 100% repellency for 2–4 hours) (Trongtokit et al., 2005).

299. Lavender oil was found to be comparable to DEET in its ability to repel ticks (Hyalomma marginatum) (Mkolo et al., 2007).

     The infestation of the red bud borer pest was reduced by more than 95% in the grafted buds of apple trees by application of the essential oil of Lavandula angustifolia (van Tol et al., 2007).

300. Citrus hystrix essential oil was found to be an effective repellent against three types of cockroaches—exhibiting 100% repellency against two types and 87% repellency against the third (Thavara et al., 2007).

301. The leaf and fruit oils of Schinus molle (pink pepper) demonstrated repellent and insecticidal activity against two beetles that commonly damage and consume stored grains (Abdel-Sattar et al., 2009).

302. Cassia oil and its components were found to repel adult female mosquitoes for about 50 minutes post-application when applied to human subjects (Chang et al., 2006).

303. A sesquiterpene alcohol from geranium essential oil proved to be an effective repellant of the lone star tick (Amblyomma americanum) and at concentrations greater than 0.052 mg the oil was comparable to the repellant capability of DEET (Tabanca et al., 2013).

304. In a small clinical trial, diffusion of lavender oil was found to improve sleep in patients with insomnia more than diffusion of sweet almond oil, which was used as a control (Lewith et al., 2005).

     Female students suffering from insomnia were found to sleep better and to have lower levels of depression during weeks they used a lavender fragrance, compared to weeks they did not use a lavender fragrance (Lee et al., 2006).

     Twenty-four sessions of lavender essential oil aromatherapy was found to improve sleep quality in midlife women with insomnia up to one week after the end of the intervention when compared to the control group (Chien et al., 2012).

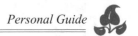

305. Subjects suffering from insomnia who took an extract from valerian demonstrated results similar to those of subjects who took oxazepam (an anti-anxiety and anti-insomnia drug) (Ziegler et al., 2002).

306. Older rats whose diets were supplemented with thyme oil were found to have higher levels of the antioxidant enzymes superoxide dismutase and glutathione peroxidase in the heart, liver, and kidneys than did older rats without this supplementation (Youdim et al., 1999).

307. The antioxidant activity of bergamot juice was found to have protective action against renal (kidney) injury of diet-induced hypercholesterolemia in rats (Trovato et al., 2010).

308. The use of rosemary, lemon, and peppermint oils in massage demonstrated an ability to reduce constipation and to increase bowel movements in elderly subjects, compared to massage without the oils (Kim et al., 2005).

309. Tea tree oil was found to be effective against both lice and dust mites in a mite chamber assay (Williamson et al., 2007).

Tea tree oil was found to prevent some blood feeding by lice on treated skin; and while not highly effective at the studied dosages, tea tree oil was found to be more effective than DEET at repelling head lice (Canyon et al., 2007).

310. A slow-release citronella formula was found to significantly reduce infection with head lice in elementary school children, compared to a control (Mumcuoglu et al., 2004).

311. Three compounds derived from dill and caraway oil—anethofuran, carvone, and limonene—were found to induce the enzyme glutathione S-transferase (involved in transforming or binding to toxins in tissues) in several mice tissues (Zheng et al., 1992).

312. Rosemary extracts induced CYP (cytochrome P450) activity in liver cells, suggesting a possible increased ability to remove toxins (Debersac et al., 2001).

313. Older rats whose diets were supplemented with thyme oil were found to have higher levels of the antioxidant enzymes superoxide dismutase and glutathione peroxidase in the heart, liver, and kidneys than did older rats without this supplementation (Youdim et al., 1999).

314. Daily oral administration of ginger (Z. officinale R.) essential oil and isolated citral (the main constituent of ginger essential oil) displayed preventative effects on the formation alcohol fatty liver disease in mice administered an alcoholic liquid diet for four weeks (Liu et al., 2013).

315. Daily administration of rosemary essential oil displayed a protective effect against chemical-induced liver injury in rats (Ra Kovi et al., 2014).

316. Oral administration of cypress methanolic extract displayed preventive action against CCl4-induced hepatotoxicity in rats. These results suggest that the antioxidant activity of the flavonoid content of cypress could have potential use as a treatment for liver diseases (Ali et al., 2010).

317. A methanol extract of Boswellia carterii was found to have a high inhibition rate of hepatitis C virus protease (Hussein et al., 2000).

318. Cinnamon bark essential oil was found to have a protective effect against damages in male rat reproductive organs and cells induced by carbon tetrachloride (a common toxic substance) (Yüce et al., 2014).

319. Male mice exposed to a harmful insecticide, known to cause sperm damage, were successfully treated with geranium essential oil through its antioxidant effects. Compared to the control group, the oral administration of geranium oil prevented testicular oxidative damage, reduced lipid peroxidation, and improved total sperm motility, viability, and morphology in mice spermatozoa (Slima et al., 2013).

320. Volunteers completing a battery of tests were found to be more content when exposed to lavender and rosemary aromas. Rosemary aroma also was found to enhance quality of memory, compared to control (Moss et al., 2003).

321. In a small human trial, oral administration of sage lavender oil was found to improve speed of memory as well as alertness and calmness in healthy volunteers, compared to a placebo (Tildesley et al., 2005).

322. In human trials, the aroma of peppermint was found to enhance memory and to increase alertness, while ylang ylang aroma was found to increase calmness (Moss et al., 2008).

323. A study evaluating memory retention and retrieval of mice revealed that the hydroalcoholic extract of Ocimum basilicum significantly increased memory retention and retrieval. The memory enhancing effects were attributed to the antioxidant activity of flavonoids, tannins and terpenoids in the basil extract (Sarahroodi et al., 2012).

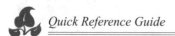

324. Administration of clove essential oil for three weeks before treatment with scopolamine (a known agent causing memory impairment) was shown to significantly reverse the scopolamine-induced memory deficit, when compared to pretreatment with saline only (Halder et al., 2011).

325. Oral administration of Rosa damascena extract for one month was found to enhance adult neurogenesis, hippocampal volume, and synaptic plasticity, as well as reverse the amyloid-beta-associated memory abnormalities in a rat model of amyloid-beta-induced Alzheimer's disease. These results indicate that rose extract may have memory-enhancing ability (Esfandiary et al., 2014).

326. A combined extract of Cissampelos pareira and Anethum graveolens was found to produce cognitive-enhancing and neuroprotective effects on spatial memory in memory deficit induced rats (Thukham-Mee et al., 2012).

327. Subjects who had learned a list of 24 words while exposed to an odor had an easier time relearning the list when exposed to the same odor, compared to those who were exposed to an alternate odor (Smith et al., 1992).

328. The overproduction of oxygen radicals, specifically NO and H_2O_2, and cytokines (both involved in the etiology of M.S.) by mouse splenocytes was significantly inhibited by copaiba oil (Dias et al., 2014).

329. A combination of peppermint oil and ethanol was found to have a significant analgesic effect, reducing sensitivity to headache; while a combination of peppermint, eucalyptus, and ethanol was found to relax muscles and to increase cognitive performance in humans (Göbel et al., 1994).

330. Rosemary oil demonstrated a relaxant effect on smooth muscle from the trachea of rabbit and guinea pig (Aqel, 1991).

331. Topical application of 100% tea tree oil was found to produce results similar to topical application of 1% clotrimazole (an antifungal drug) solution on onychomycosis (also known as tinea or fungal nail infection) (Buck et al., 1994).

332. Ginger root given orally to pregnant women was found to decrease the severity of nausea and the frequency of vomiting, compared to control (Vutyavanich et al., 2001).

     In a trial of women receiving gynaecological surgery, women receiving ginger root had less incidences of nausea than those who received a placebo. Ginger root has similar results to the antiemetic drug (a drug effective against vomiting and nausea) metoclopramide (Bone et al., 1990).

     Ginger root given one hour before major gynecological surgery resulted in lower nausea and fewer incidences of vomiting as compared to the control (Nanthakomon et al., 2006).

333. Oral administration of capsules containing two drops of either spearmint or peppermint oil to cancer patients during chemotherapy cycles was found to reduce the intensity of nausea when compared to the control (Tayarani-Najaran et al., 2013).

334. Pretreatment of human and rat astrocyte cells (cells found in the nerve and brain that support the blood-brain barrier and that help repair the brain and spinal cord following injuries) with peppermint oil was found to inhibit heat-shock induced apoptosis of these cells (Koo et al., 2001).

335. Lavender oil was found to inhibit sympathetic nerve activity, while exciting parasympathetic nerve activity in rats. Linalool, a component of lavender, was shown to have similar effects (Shen et al., 2005).

     Lavender oil scent was found to lower sympathetic nerve activity and blood pressure in rats, while elevating parasympathetic nerve activity. It was further found that applying an anosmia-inducing agent (something that causes a loss of smell) eliminated the effects of the lavender oil scent (Tanida et al., 2006).

336. Inhalation of the aroma of lemon essential oil was found to decrease pain response in rats and was also found to modulate the neuronal response to formalin-induced pain (Aloisi et al., 2002).

     Several constituents of lemon oil and their metabolites (chemicals made by these chemicals in the body) were found to increase the release of monoamines (various chemicals responsible for neurotransmission and neuromodulation) in rat brain tissue, indicating a possible effect on brain nerve cell behavior (Fukumoto et al., 2006).

     Pretreatment of human and rat astrocyte cells (cells found in the nerves and brain that support the blood-brain barrier and help repair the brain and spinal cord following injuries) with lemon oil was found to inhibit heat-shock induced apoptosis of these cells (Koo et al., 2002).

337. In healthy adults, inhalation of essential oils such as pepper, estragon, fennel, and grapefruit had a stimulating effect on sympathetic activity; while inhalation of essential oils of rose or patchouli caused a decrease in sympathetic activity (Haze et al., 2002).

    The scent of grapefruit oil and its component, limonene, was found to affect the autonomic nerves, exciting the sympathetic nervous system, and to reduce appetite and body weight of rats exposed to the oil for 15 minutes 3 times per week (Shen et al., 2005).

338. Incensole acetate, isolated from frankincense resin, demonstrated an anti-inflammatory and neuro-protective effect on mice with closed head injuries (Moussaieff et al., 2008).

339. Oral administration of copaiba oil demonstrated antinociceptive (blocks transmission of pain-causing stimuli) activity in rodents (Gomes et al., 2007).

340. Pretreatment of human and rat astrocyte cells (cells found in the nerves and the brain that support the blood-brain barrier and help repair the brain and spinal cord following injuries) with juniper oil was found to inhibit heat-shock induced apoptosis of these cells (Na et al., 2001).

341. 1,8 cineole (eucalyptol) displayed an anti-inflammatory effect on rats in several tests and exhibited antinociceptive (pain-reducing) effects in mice, possibly by depressing the central nervous system (Santos et al., 2000).

342. Female patients waiting for dental treatment were found to be less anxious, more positive, and more calm when exposed to orange oil odor than were patients who were not exposed to the orange oil odor (Lehrner et al., 2000).

343. A study including 100 patients (ages 3 to 79) suffering from vasomotor allergic rhinopathy, showed that topical application of a citrus lemon based spray resulted in a total reduction of eosinophils granulocytes and mast cells. These results suggest that the lemon-based nasal spray is a good alternative to conventional medicine for the treatment of perennial and seasonal allergic and vasomotor rhinopathy (Ferrara et al., 2012).

344. The scent of grapefruit oil and its component, limonene, was found to affect the autonomic nerves, exciting the sympathetic nervous system, and to reduce appetite and body weight of rats exposed to the oil for 15 minutes 3 times per week (Shen et al., 2005).

    Grapefruit essential oil was found to directly inhibit adipogenesis of adipocytes, indicating that grapefruit has an antiobesity effect (Haze et al., 2010).

    Oral intake of D-limonene (found in lime, lemon, bergamot, dill, grapefruit, lavender, lemongrass, Roman chamomile, tangerine, and orange essential oils) effectively protects against the development of hyperglycemia and dyslipidemia in mice fed a high-fat diet (Jing et al., 2013). This study also found evidence suggesting that D-limonene may prevent lipid accumulation in the livers of mice fed a high-fat diet and improve metabolic dysfunctions by ameliorating glucose tolerance in obese mice (Jing et al., 2013).

345. After 10 weeks of feeding, the body weight gain, visceral fat-pad weights, and final body weights of mice fed a high-fat diet and carvacrol (found in oregano and thyme essential oils) were significantly lower than that of mice fed a high-fat diet without carvacrol (specifically a 24% decrease in final body weight, a 43% decrease in body weight gain, and a 36% decrease in total visceral fat-pad weight was observed when carvacrol was ingested)(Cho et al., 2012). Interestingly, the food intake during the 10-week feeding period did not differ among the groups and mRNA expressions were different among the two groups (Cho et al., 2012).

346. Tea tree, peppermint, and sage oils were found to inhibit oral bacteria—with thymol and eugenol being the most active components of these oils (Shapiro et al., 1994).

347. Among several oils tested, tea tree (tea tree), manuka, and eucalyptus demonstrated strong antibacterial activity against detrimental oral bacteria (Takarada et al., 2004).

    Tea tree, peppermint, and sage oils were found to inhibit oral bacteria—with thymol and eugenol being the most active components of these oils (Shapiro et al., 1994).

    Cinnamon oil exhibited strong antimicrobial activity against two detrimental oral bacteria. Manuka, tea tree, and the component thymol also exhibited antimicrobial potency (Filoche et al., 2005).

    In 34 patients with fixed orthodontic appliances, a dental gel containing 5% tea tree essential oil performed better than Colgate Total gel when comparing microbial biofilm and quantification of Streptococcus mutans in the patients' saliva (Santamaria et al., 2014).

A=Aromatic   **T**=Topical   **I**=Internal

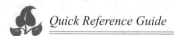

348. Peppermint oil blended with toothpaste was more effective at lower concentrations in inhibiting the formation of dental plaque than was chlorhexidine (an antiseptic) in human volunteers (Shayegh et al., 2008).

Subjects using a mouthwash containing thymol, menthol, methyl salicylate, and eucalyptol for 6 months were found to not have developed oral bacteria that were resistant to the oils (Charles et al., 2000).

349. Lavender oil was found to work as an anaesthetic (reducing pain) in rabbit reflex tests (Ghelardini et al., 1999).

Oil from Lavandula angustifolia was found to reduce writhing in induced writhing in rats and to reduce edema (swelling) in carrageenan-induced paw edema, indicating an anti-inflammatory effect (Hajhashemi et al., 2003).

In patients suffering from arthritis, it was found that a blend of lavender, marjoram, eucalyptus, rosemary, peppermint, and carrier oils reduced perceived pain and depression, compared to control (Kim et al., 2005).

The odor of lavender combined with relaxing music was found to lessen the intensity of pain following a vascular wound dressing change (Kane et al., 2004).

350. Oils of three eucalyptus species (citriodora, tereticornis, and globulus) were found to have analgesic (pain-relieving) and anti-inflammatory properties in rats (Silva et al., 2003).

1,8 cineole (eucalyptol) was found to have antinociceptive (pain-reducing) properties similar to morphine. Beta-pinene was found to reverse the effects of morphine in a degree similar to naloxone (a drug used to counter the effects of morphine overdose) (Liape et al., 2007).

1,8 cineole (eucalyptol) was found to display an anti-inflammatory effect on rats in several tests and was found to exhibit antinociceptive (pain-reducing) effects in mice, possibly by depressing the central nervous system (Santos et al., 2000).

In Wistar rats with induced edema, treatment with Eucalyptus citriodora essential oil displayed curative anti-inflammatory action, illustrated by a reduction of edema volume. Eucalyptus citriodora essential oil was also found to have an analgesic effect and the ability to reduce hyperthermia (Gbenou et al., 2013).

351. Inhalation of the aroma of lemon essential oil was found to decrease pain response in rats and was also found to modulate the neuronal response to formalin-induced pain (Aloisi et al., 2002).

Rats exposed long-term to lemon essential oil were found to demonstrate different anxiety and pain threshold levels than did untreated rats. It was also found that exposure to lemon oil induced chemical changes in the neuronal circuits involved in anxiety and pain (Ceccarelli et al., 2004).

352. An ethanol extract of rosemary was found to demonstrate antinociceptive (pain-blocking) and anti-inflammatory activity in mice and rats (González-Trujano et al., 2007).

Rosemary oil was found to have anti-inflammatory and peripheral antinociceptive (pain sensitivity–blocking) properties in mice (Takaki et al., 2008).

1,8 cineole (eucalyptol) displayed an anti-inflammatory effect on rats in several tests, and exhibited antinociceptive (pain-reducing) effects on mice, possibly by depressing the central nervous system (Santos et al., 2000).

In patients suffering from arthritis, it was found that a blend of lavender, marjoram, eucalyptus, rosemary, peppermint, and carrier oils reduced perceived pain and depression compared to control (Kim et al., 2005).

353. Beta-caryophyllene (found in clove and copaiba oils) demonstrated anaesthetic (pain-reducing) activity in rats and rabbits (Ghelardini et al., 2001).

354. Oral administration of copaiba oil demonstrated antinociceptive (blocks transmission of pain-causing stimuli) activity in rodents (Gomes et al., 2007).

Beta-caryophyllene (found in clove and copaiba oils) demonstrated anaesthetic (pain-reducing) activity in rats and rabbits (Ghelardini et al., 2001).

355. The essential oil of laurel (Laurus nobilis) reduced pain and inflammation in rats in a manner similar to morphine and piroxicam (an anti-inflammatory drug) in mice and rats (Sayyah et al., 2003).

356. A double-blind, placebo-controlled study demonstrated that aroma massage with ginger and orange essential oils relieved knee joint pain in elderly subjects more than the placebo (massage with olive oil) or the control (conventional treatment without massage) (Yip et al., 2008).

357. Oregano oil administered orally improved gastrointestinal symptoms in 7 of 11 patients who had tested positive for the parasite Blastocystis hominis and caused the disappearance of this parasite in 8 of the patients (Force et al., 2000).

358. Essential oil from Lavandula angustifolia demonstrated ability to eliminate protozoal pathogens Giardia duodenalis, Trichomonas vaginalis, and Hexamita inflata at concentrations of 1% or less (Moon et al., 2006).

359. Copaiba oil was found to inhibit the parasite Leishmania amazonensis (a protozoa that causes skin lesions) (Santos et al., 2008).

360. Eucalyptus citriodora essential oil inhibited egg hatching and larval development of goat gastrointestinal nematodes in vivo and in vitro (Macedo et al., 2011).

361. Tea tree oil was effective at killing anisakis simplex larva in vitro. Data suggests that the mechanism of action against anisakis involves inhibition of acetylcholinesterase (Gómez-Rincón et al., 2014).

362. The process of alpha-syn protein aggregation is a major component of Parkinson's disease. Preventing alpha-syn aggregation may help in the treatment of Parkinson's disease. Research-ers have discovered that an aqueous cinnamon extract precipitation has a curative effect on alpha-syn aggregation in a Drosophila model of Parkinson's disease. Furthermore, in vitro tests have revealed that the cinnamon extract has an inhibitory effect on the process of alpha-syn fibrillation (Shaltiel-Karyo et al., 2012).

    Eugenol (found in cassia, cinnamon, and clove) administration was found to pre-vent induced dopamine depression and lipid peroxidation inductivity in the mouse stria-tum model, suggesting that eugenol may be useful in the treatment of Parkinson's disease (Kabuto et al., 2007).

363. Cinnamon, thyme, and clove essential oils demonstrated an antibacterial effect on several respiratory tract pathogens (Fabio et al., 2007).

    Oils with aldehyde or phenol as a major component demonstrated a high level of antibacterial activity (Inouye et al., 2001).

364. Oregano oil was found to kill antibiotic resistant strains of Staph, E. coli, Klebsiella pneumoniae, Helicobacter pylori, and Mycobacterium terrae (Preuss et al., 2005).

365. In rats with induced pulmonary fibrosis oral treatment of hydrodistilled tangerine essential oil suppressed body weight loss and significantly improved scores of alveolitis and fibrosis of lung tissue. The effects of tangerine essential oil on lung fibrosis were associated with free radical scavenging and antioxidant activity (Zhou et al., 2012).

366. A triple blind randomized placebo-controlled trial, consisting of 60 subjects and evaluating the use of lavender oil for Cesarean postoperative pain management, found that inhalation of lavender (when compared to inhalation of a placebo) decreased postoperative pain and increased patient satisfaction. Furthermore, patients inhaling lavender oil required significantly lower dosages of Diclofenac suppository as a supplemental analgesic drug than the placebo group. The researchers state that lavender essential oil is not recommended as the sole analgesic treatment (Olapour et al., 2013).

367. Inhaled ylang ylang oil was found to decrease blood pressure and pulse rate and to enhance attentiveness and alertness in volunteers, compared to an odorless control (Hongratanaworakit et al., 2004).

    Subjects who had ylang ylang oil applied to their skin had decreased blood pressure, increased skin temperature, and reported feeling more calm and relaxed, compared to subjects in a control group (Hongratanaworakit et al., 2006).

368. Patchouli alcohol (a tricyclic sesquiterpene and an essential oil of Pogostemon cablin) was found to inhibit chemically in-duced mastitis in a mouse model by inhibiting inflammation, suggesting patchouli may prevent mastitis (Li et al., 2014).

369. Ginger root given orally to pregnant women was found to decrease the severity of nausea and frequency of vomiting, compared to control (Vutyavanich et al., 2001).

    Ginger root given one hour before major gynecological surgery resulted in lower nausea and fewer incidences of vomiting, compared to control (Nanthakomon et al., 2006).

    In a trial of women receiving gynaecological surgery, women receiving ginger root had fewer incidences of nausea than did those who received a placebo. Ginger root showed results similar to those of the antiemetic drug (a drug effective against vomiting and nausea) metoclopramide (Bone et al., 1990).

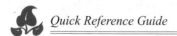

370. A randomized clinical trial carried out on 100 pregnant women suffering from mild to moderate nausea found inhalation of lemon essential oil to be more effective at preventing nausea than inhalation of a carrier oil on days two and four of a four day trial (Yavari kia et al., 2014).

371. Jasmine flowers applied to the breast were found to be as effective as the antilactation drug bromocriptine in reducing breast engorgement, milk production, and analgesic (pain relieving drug) intake in women after giving birth (Shrivastave et al., 1988).

372. Female students suffering from insomnia were found to sleep better and to have lower levels of depression during weeks they used a lavender fragrance, compared to weeks they did not use a lavender fragrance (Lee et al., 2006).

 In patients suffering from arthritis, a blend of lavender, marjoram, eucalyptus, rosemary, peppermint, and carrier oils was found to reduce perceived pain and depression, compared to control (Kim et al., 2005).

373. In 12 patients suffering from depression, it was found that inhaling citrus aromas reduced the needed doses of antidepressants, normalized neuroendocrine hormone levels, and normalized immune functioning (Komori et al., May 1995).

 Lemon oil and its component, citral, were found to decrease depressed behavior in rats involved in several stress tests in a manner similar to antidepressant drugs (Komori et al., Dec. 1995).

 Lemon oil vapor was found to have strong antistress and antidepressant effects on mice subjected to several common stress tests (Komiya et al., 2006).

374. Peppermint extract fed orally to mice demonstrated an ability to protect the testis from gamma radiation damage (Samarth et al., 2009).

 In mice exposed to whole-body gamma irradiation, only 17% of mice who had been fed peppermint oil died, while 100% of mice who did not receive peppermint oil died. It was also found that mice pre-fed peppermint oil were able to return blood cell levels to normal after 30 days, while control mice were not able to (and consequently died), suggesting a protective or stimulating effect of the oil on blood stem cells (Samarth et al., 2004).

 Mice treated with an oral administration of peppermint extract demonstrated a higher ability to tolerate gamma radiation than did untreated mice (Samarth et al., 2003).

375. Pretreatment with alpha-santalol before UVB (ultraviolet-B) radiation significantly reduced skin tumor development and multiplicity and induced proapoptotic and tumor-suppressing protein (Arasada et al., 2008).

 A solution of 5% alpha-santalol (from sandalwood) was found to prevent skin-tumor formation caused by ultraviolet-B (UVB) radiation in mice (Dwivedi et al., 2006).

376. Calophyllum inophyllum (tamanu) oil was found to demonstrate UV filtering properties in the SPF 18-22 range at low concentrations and was also found to not be cytotoxic to human eye cells at concentrations up to 1% (Said et al., 2007).

377. Subjects who smelled a cleansing gel with lavender aroma were more relaxed and were able to complete math computations faster (Field et al., 2005).

 Nurses working in an ICU setting demonstrated decreased perception of stress when receiving a topical application of Lavandula angustifolia and Salvia sclarea essential oils (Pemberton et al., 2008).

 Subjects exposed to 3 minutes of lavender aroma were more relaxed and able to perform math computations faster and more accurately (Diego et al., 1998).

378. Subjects who had ylang ylang oil applied to their skin had decreased blood pressure, increased skin temperature, and reported feeling more calm and relaxed, compared to subjects in a control group (Hongratanaworakit et al., 2006).

379. Lemon oil was found to have an antistress effect on mice involved in several behavioral tasks (Komiya et al., 2006).

380. In human volunteers wearing breathing masks to prevent aroma inhalation, rose oil applied to the skin was found to significantly decrease breathing rate, blood oxygen saturation, and systolic blood pressure, compared to a placebo. And volunteers receiving rose oil rated themselves as more calm and relaxed than did subjects receiving the placebo (Hongratanaworakit et al., 2009).

381. Extracts from eucalyptus and thyme were found to have high nitrous oxide (NO) scavenging abilities and to inhibit NO production in macrophage cells. This could possibly explain their role in aiding respiratory inflammatory diseases (Vigo et al., 2004).

    Eucalyptus oil was found to have an anti-inflammatory and mucin-inhibitory effect on rats with lipopolysaccharide-induced bronchitis (Lu et al., 2004).

382. L-menthol was found to inhibit production of inflammation mediators in human monocytes (a type of white blood cell involved in the immune response) (Juergens et al., 1998).

383. Vapor of cinnamon bark oil and cinnamic aldehyde was found to be effective against fungi involved in respiratory tract mycoses (fungal infections) (Singh et al., 1995).

    Cinnamon bark, lemongrass, and thyme oils were found to have the highest level of activity against common respiratory pathogens among 14 essential oils tested (Inouye et al., 2001).

384. Linalool, found in several essential oils, was found to inhibit induced convulsions in rats by directly interacting with the NMDA receptor complex (Brum et al., 2001).

385. Myrrh essential oil was shown to be an efficient quencher of singlet oxygen (a type of antioxidant action) by its ability to decrease formation of squalene peroxide in UV irradiated sebum on the facial skin of human subjects. These findings suggest that topical application of myrrh essential oil can help decrease sebum damage and in turn protect skin from aging (Auffray 2007).

386. An in vitro study using human fibroblast cells from adult skin showed that dill extract was able to stimulate LOXL gene expression to induce elastogenesis in adult skin cells. These findings suggest that dill extract may be able to increase skin elasticity and firming (Cenizo et al., 2006).

387. In a small clinical trial, diffusion of lavender oil was found to improve sleep in patients with insomnia than diffusion of sweet almond oil as a control (Lewith et al., 2005).

    Female students suffering from insomnia were found to sleep better and have a lower level of depression during weeks they used a lavender fragrance when compared to weeks they did not use a lavender fragrance (Lee et al., 2006).

    A study with 56 percutaneous coronary intervention patients in an intensive care unit found that an aromatherapy blend of lavender, Roman chamomile, and neroli decreased anxiety and improved sleep quality when compared to conventional nursing intervention (Cho et al., 2013).

388. Two chemical components found in valerian were found to have sedative, sleep-enhancing, and anxiolytic (anxiety lowering) properties (Marder et al., 2003).

389. A study with 56 percutaneous coronary intervention patients in an intensive care unit found that an aromatherapy blend of lavender, Roman chamomile, and neroli decreased anxiety and improved sleep quality when compared to conventional nursing intervention (Cho et al., 2013).

390. The scent of grapefruit oil and its component, limonene, was found to affect the autonomic nerves, exciting the sympathetic nervous system, and to reduce appetite and body weight of rats exposed to the oil for 15 minutes three times per week (Shen et al., 2005).

391. Carnosic acid, a diterpene extracted from sage, taken orally was found to significantly inhibit lipid absorption, reduce triglyceride elevation, and reduced the gain of body weight in mice fed a high-fat (olive oil) diet. (Ninomiya et al., 2004).

392. Inhaled vapor of black pepper oil was found to reduce craving for cigarettes and symptoms of anxiety in smokers deprived from smoking compared to a control (Rose et al., 1994).

393. Basil (Ocimum gratissimum) oil was found to facilitate the healing process of wounds in rabbits to a greater extent than two antibacterial preparations, Cicatrin and Cetavlex (Kane et al., 2004).

394. Imaging of the brain demonstrated that inhalation of 1,8-cineol (eucalyptol, a constituent of many essential oils, especially eucalyptus, rosemary, and marjoram) increased global cerebral blood flow after an inhalation-time of 20 minutes (Nasel et al., 1994).

395. In a trial of women receiving gynaecological surgery, women receiving ginger root had less incidences of nausea compared to a placebo. Ginger root has similar results to the antiemetic drug (a drug effective against vomiting and nausea), metoclopramide (Bone et al., 1990).

A=Aromatic   **T**=Topical   **I**=Internal

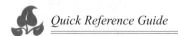
Ginger root given one hour before major gynecological surgery resulted in lower nausea and fewer incidences of vomiting compared to control (Nanthakomon et al., 2006).

396. Lavender odor was found to reduce mental stress while increasing arousal (Motomura et al., 2001).

    Nurses working in an ICU setting demonstrated decreased perception of stress when receiving a topical application of Lavandula angustifolia and Salvia sclaria essential oils (Pemberton et al, 2008).

    An office environment featuring a soothing DVD video presentation and diffused lavender oil was found to reduce anxiety in patients awaiting a gastroscopy procedure compared to a regular office environment (Hoya et al., 2008).

397. Subjects who had ylang ylang oil applied to their skin had decreased blood pressure, increased skin temperature, and reported feeling more calm and relaxed compared to subjects in a control group (Hongratanaworakit et al., 2006).

398. Lemon oil vapor was found to have a strong anti-stress and antidepressant effects on mice subjected to several common stress tests (Komiya et al., 2006).

399. Both fennel oil, and its constituent, anethole, were found to significantly reduce thrombosis (blood clots) in mice. They were also found to be free from the prohemorrhagic (increased bleeding) side effect that aspirin (acetylsalicylic acid) has (Tognolini et al., 2007).

400. Oral pretreatment of basil extract was found to protect against brain damage induced by bilateral carotid artery occlusion in mice by reducing tissue death size and the oxidative degradation of lipids and restoring antioxidant content and motor functions. The researchers state that these results suggest that basil could be useful clinically in the prevention of stroke (Bora et al., 2011).

401. Inhalation of black pepper oil was found to increase cerebral blood flow and improve the swallowing reflex in elderly patients who had suffered a stroke (Ebihara et al., 2006).

402. Calophyllum inophyllum (tamanu) oil was found to demonstrate UV filtering properties in the SPF 18-22 range at low concentrations, and was also found to not be cytotoxic to human eye cells at concentrations up to 1% (Said et al., 2007).

403. The ethanolic extract of vetiver root was found to inhibit both virulent and avirulent strains of M. tuberculosis, suggesting that vetiver could be useful in treating tubercular infections (Saikia et al., 2012).

404. Eucalyptus citriodora essential oil showed airborne tuberculosis inhibition at levels greater than 90%, suggesting that this essential oil could manage tuberculosis through inhalation therapy (Ramos et al., 2014).

405. A formulation of lemongrass and geranium oil was found to reduce airborne bacteria by 89% in an office environment after diffusion for 15 hours (Doran et al., 2009).

406. Oral administration of marjoram extract was shown to significantly decrease the incidence of ulcers, basal gastric secretion, and acid output in rats (Al-Howiriny et al., 2009).

407. Lemon essential oil and its majority compound (limonene) exhibited a gastroprotective effect against induced gastric ulcers in rats (Rozza et al., 2011).

408. Oral administration of dill seed extract was found to have effective antisecretory and anti-ulcer activity against HCl- and ethanol-induced stomach lesions in mice (Hosseinzadeh et al., 2002).

409. Lemon odor was found to enhance the positive mood of volunteers exposed to a stressor (Kiecolt-Glaser et al., 2008).

410. Ginger root given orally to pregnant women was found to decrease the severity of nausea and frequency of vomiting compared to control (Vutyavanich et al., 2001).

    Ginger root given one hour before major gynecological surgery resulted in lower nausea and fewer incidences of vomiting compared to control (Nanthakomon et al., 2006).

411. The scent of grapefruit oil and its component, limonene, was found to affect the autonomic nerves, exciting the sympathetic nervous system, and to reduce appetite and body weight of rats exposed to the oil for 15 minutes three times per week (Shen et al., 2005).

412. Basil (Ocimum gratissimum) oil was found to facilitate the healing process of wounds in rabbits to a greater extent than two antibacterial preparations, Cicatrin and Cetavlex (Orafindiya et al., 2003).

APPENDIX

BODY SYSTEMS CHART

The following chart lists all of the products discussed within this book and indicates which body systems they primarily affect. While this chart does not include every system that could possibly be affected by each product, it attempts to list the primary systems that are most often affected. It is provided to give the beginning aromatherapy student a starting point for personal use and analysis.

Essential Oil/ Blend/Product	Cardiovascular System	Digestive System	Emotional Balance	Hormonal System	Immune System	Muscles and Bones	Nervous System	Respiratory System	Skin and Hair
3 Wise Men			X						
Abundance			X		X			X	
Acceptance			X				X		
AlkaLime	X	X				X			
Allerzyme		X						X	
Angelica			X				X		
Animal Scents Blends	X	X			X	X	X		X
Animal Scents Products									X
Anise	X	X		X				X	
AromaEase		X	X	X					
Aroma Life	X								
Aroma Siez						X		X	
AromaSleep			X	X			X		
AromaGuard Deodorants									X
A•R•T System									X
Australian Blue			X						
Awaken			X						
Balance Complete		X							
Basil	X						X		
Believe			X						

Essential Oil/ Blend/Product	Cardiovascular System	Digestive System	Emotional Balance	Hormonal System	Immune System	Muscles and Bones	Nervous System	Respiratory System	Skin and Hair
Bergamot		X	X						X
Bite Buster									X
BLM						X			
Blue Agave				X		X			
Boswellia Wrinkle Cream									X
Brain Power			X				X		
Breathe Again					X			X	
Build Your Dream			X	X			X		X
Cajeput	X							X	
Cardamom		X							
Carrot	X						X		X
Cedar, Western Red									X
Cedarwood							X	X	
Cel-Lite Magic									X
Celery Seed		X				X	X		
Chamomile, German			X				X		X
Chamomile, Roman			X				X		X
Christmas Spirit	X		X				X		
Cinnamint Lip Balm									X
Cinnamon Bark					X				
Cistus					X				X
Citronella						X			X
Citrus Fresh			X		X				
ClaraDerm									X
Clarity			X				X		
Clary Sage				X					
Clove	X	X			X			X	
ComforTone		X			X				
Cool Azul Blend/Gel						X			X
Copaiba	X		X			X	X	X	X
Common Sense			X				X		
Coriander		X		X					
CortiStop				X					
Cumin		X			X				
Cypress	X					X			
Cypress, Blue		X			X				

Essential Oil/ Blend/Product	Cardiovascular System	Digestive System	Emotional Balance	Hormonal System	Immune System	Muscles and Bones	Nervous System	Respiratory System	Skin and Hair
Davana				X					
Deep Relief						X	X		
Detoxzyme		X			X				
Di-Gize		X							
Digest + Cleanse		X							
Dill		X							
Divine Release			X	X			X		
Dorado Azul				X			X	X	
Dragon Time			X	X					
Dream Catcher			X						
Elemi									X
Egyptian Gold			X		X				
En-R-Gee			X				X		
EndoFlex				X					
EndoGize		X		X					
Envision			X						
Essentialzyme		X							
Essentialzymes-4		X							
Estro				X					
Eucalyptus						X		X	
Eucalyptus Blue					X			X	
Eucalyptus citriodora								X	
Eucalyptus radiata								X	X
Eucalyptus staigeriana						X		X	X
Evening Peace									X
Evergreen Essence			X						
Exodus II					X				
FemiGen				X					
Fennel		X		X					
Fir								X	
Fir, Balsam						X	X		
Fir, Douglas						X		X	
Fir, White			X			X		X	
Fleabane (Conyza)	X			X					
Forgiveness			X						
Frankincense			X		X		X		X

Essential Oil/ Blend/Product	Cardiovascular System	Digestive System	Emotional Balance	Hormonal System	Immune System	Muscles and Bones	Nervous System	Respiratory System	Skin and Hair
Frankincense, Sacred			X		X		X		X
Freedom			X	X			X		
Galbanum					X				
Gathering			X						
Genesis Lotion			X						X
GeneYus			X				X		
Gentle Baby			X						X
Geranium			X						X
Ginger		X					X		
GLF		X							
Goldenrod	X			X					
Grapefruit	X								
Grapefruit Lip Balm									X
Gratitude			X						
Grounding			X						
Harmony			X						
Helichrysum	X					X			
Highest Potential			X						
Hinoki			X		X			X	X
Hong Kuai			X		X			X	
Hope			X						
Humility			X						
Hyssop	X						X	X	
ICP	X	X							
Idaho Blue Spruce			X				X	X	
ImmuPower					X				
ImmuPro					X				
Inner Child			X						
Inner Harmony			X				X		
Inspiration			X						
Into the Future			X						
InTouch			X				X		
Jade Lemon		X			X			X	
Jasmine			X	X					
Joy			X						
Juniper		X	X				X		X
Juva Cleanse		X							
JuvaFlex		X							

Essential Oil/ Blend/Product	Cardiovascular System	Digestive System	Emotional Balance	Hormonal System	Immune System	Muscles and Bones	Nervous System	Respiratory System	Skin and Hair
JuvaPower		X							
JuvaSpice		X							
JuvaTone		X			X				
K&B		X							
KidScents MightyVites	X		X		X		X		
Lady Sclareol			X						X
Laurel		X			X			X	
LavaDerm Cooling Mist			X						X
Lavandin	X					X		X	
Lavender	X		X				X		X
Lavender Lotion			X						X
LBrianté			X	X					X
Ledum		X			X				X
Legacy		X							
Lemon		X			X			X	
Lemongrass					X	X			
Light the Fire			X				X		
Lime		X			X			X	
Live with Passion			X				X		
Longevity	X		X						
Longevity Capsules	X				X		X		X
M-Grain						X	X		
Magnify Your Purpose			X				X		
Majestic Essence	X	X			X		X		
Mandarin		X							X
Manuka						X		X	X
Marjoram	X					X			
Master Formula	X		X		X		X		
Mastrante						X	X		X
MegaCal	X					X	X		
Melaleuca					X	X		X	X
Melaleuca Ericifolia								X	X
Melaleuca Quinquenrvia						X		X	
Melissa			X						X
Melrose								X	X
Micromeria					X				

Essential Oil/ Blend/Product	Cardiovascular System	Digestive System	Emotional Balance	Hormonal System	Immune System	Muscles and Bones	Nervous System	Respiratory System	Skin and Hair
MindWise	X				X		X	X	
Mineral Essence	X		X	X	X	X	X		
Mister				X					
Morning Start			X						X
Motivation			X				X		
Mountain Savory					X				
MultiGreens	X	X			X	X	X		
Myrrh				X	X		X		X
Myrtle		X		X		X		X	
Neroli		X							X
NingXia Nitro	X	X							
NingXia Red					X				
NingXia Wolfberries		X			X	X			
Nutmeg				X	X		X		
Ocotea	X		X						X
Omega Blue	X						X		
OmegaGize³	X						X		
Onycha	X		X						X
Oola Balance/Grow			X	X			X		
Orange		X	X		X				X
Orange Blossom Facial Wash									X
Oregano					X	X		X	
Ortho Ease						X			
Ortho Sport						X			
Owie					X				X
Palmarosa	X		X						X
Palo Santo			X		X		X		
PanAway						X	X		
ParaFree		X			X				
Patchouli									X
PD 80/20	X		X	X	X	X			
Peace & Calming			X				X		
Pepper, Black		X					X		
Pepper, Pink					X			X	X
Peppermint		X				X	X	X	X
Petitgrain			X						
Pine			X					X	

Essential Oil/ Blend/Product	Cardiovascular System	Digestive System	Emotional Balance	Hormonal System	Immune System	Muscles and Bones	Nervous System	Respiratory System	Skin and Hair
Plectranthus Oregano					X	X			
Power Meal	X	X			X	X			
Prenolone			X	X		X	X		X
Present Time			X						
ProGen				X					
Progessence			X	X		X	X		X
Progessence Plus			X	X		X	X		X
Protec				X					
Pure Protein Complete						X			
Purification		X	X						X
Raven								X	X
Ravintsara					X			X	
RC								X	
Reconnect			X	X			X		
Regenolone			X			X	X		X
Rehemogen	X	X							
Relaxation			X			X			X
Release			X						
Relieve It						X			
Rose			X						X
Rose Ointment									X
Rosemary camphor	X	X				X			
Rosemary cineol					X		X	X	
Rosemary verbenon		X		X					X
Rosewood									X
RutaVaLa			X				X		
Sacred Mountain			X						
Sage				X	X				
Sage Lavender			X	X		X	X	X	X
Sandalwood			X			X	X		X
Sandalwood Moisture Cream									X
SARA			X						
Satin Facial Scrubs									X
SclarEssence		X		X					
Sensation Lotion									X
Sensation Oil Blend			X	X					

Essential Oil/ Blend/Product	Cardiovascular System	Digestive System	Emotional Balance	Hormonal System	Immune System	Muscles and Bones	Nervous System	Respiratory System	Skin and Hair
Shutran			X	X					
SleepEssence	X	X	X			X			
SleepyIze			X	X			X		
Slique Bar		X							
Slique Essence		X	X						
Slique Gum		X							
Slique Tea		X		X					
Slique Slim Caps		X		X					
SniffleEase					X			X	
Spearmint		X	X						
Spikenard			X						X
Spruce			X				X	X	
Stevia	X	X			X				
Stress Away			X		X				
Sulfurzyme					X	X	X		X
Super B	X					X	X		
Super C					X			X	
Super C Chewable					X	X			
Super Cal	X		X			X	X		
Surrender			X				X		
Tangerine			X		X				X
Tansy, Blue							X		
Tansy, Idaho					X				
Tarragon		X					X		
The Gift					X	X			X
Thieves					X				
Thieves Cleaning Prod					X				
Thieves Lozenges					X				
Thyme					X	X			
Thyme linalol								X	X
Thyromin				X					
T.R. Care			X				X		
Tranquil			X				X		
Transformation			X						
Trauma Life			X						
True Source	X				X	X			X
Tsuga	X							X	
TummyGize		X			X				

Essential Oil/ Blend/Product	Cardiovascular System	Digestive System	Emotional Balance	Hormonal System	Immune System	Muscles and Bones	Nervous System	Respiratory System	Skin and Hair
Ultra Young+				X	X				
Valerian							X		
Valor			X			X	X		X
Vetiver			X	X			X		X
White Angelica			X						
White Lotus					X				
Wintergreen						X			
Wolfberry Crisp Bars		X			X	X			
Wolfberry Eye Cream									X
Xiang Mao		X			X	X			
Yarrow				X	X				X
Ylang Ylang	X		X	X					
Yuzu		X			X				X

SINGLE OIL SUMMARY INFORMATION

The following chart displays summary information for each of the single oils: botanical name, safety data, and the products (blends, personal care products, bath and shower gels, tinctures, massage oils, and supplements) that contain the single oil. The safety data includes possible skin reactions and conditions where use of that particular oil should be limited or completely avoided (refer to the legend following the Blend Summary Information). **Note:** This safety data is provided for **external use only!**

Single Oil Name	Botanical Name	Safety Data	Products Containing Single Oil
Angelica	*Angelica archangelica* (Umbelliferae)	(GRAS), D, P, PH Dilute 1:1	Awaken, Forgiveness, Grounding, Harmony, Live with Passion, Surrender
Anise	*Pimpinella anisum* (Umbelliferae)	(GRAS), CS Dilute 1:1	Awaken, Di-Gize, Dream Catcher, Allerzyme, ComforTone, Detoxzyme, Digest + Cleanse, Essentialzyme, ICP, JuvaPower, JuvaSpice, ParaFree, Power Meal
Basil	*Ocimum basilicum* (Labiatae)	(GRAS), E*, P*, SI, Dilute 1:1	Aroma Siez, Clarity, M-Grain
Bergamot	*Citrus bergamia* (Rutaceae)	(GRAS), CS*, PH* Dilute 1:1	A·R·T Renewal Serum, Awaken, Believe, Clarity, Dream Catcher, Forgiveness, Gentle Baby, Harmony, Joy, White Angelica, Genesis Hand & Body Lotion, Prenolone, Prenolone+, Progessence, Progessence Plus, Rosewood Moisturizing Shampoo, Rosewood Moisturizing Conditioner, Sandalwood Moisture Cream, Dragon Time Bath Gel, Evening Peace Bath Gel
Cajeput	*Melaleuca leucadendra* (Myrtaceae)	(FA/FL), SI Dilute 1:1	
Calamus	*Acorus calamus* (Araceae)	Dilute 1:4	Exodus II
Caraway	*Carum carvi* (Umbelliferae)	(GRAS), CS, SI, P* Dilute 1:1	Digest + Cleanse

Single Oil Name	Botanical Name	Safety Data	Products Containing Single Oil
Cardamom	*Elettaria cardamomum* (Zingiberaceae)	(GRAS) Dilute 1:1	Clarity, Transformation
Carrot	*Daucus carota* (Umbelliferae)	(GRAS) Dilute 1:1	Animal Scents Pet Ointment, Rose Ointment
Cassia	*Cinnamomum cassia* (Lauraceae)	(GRAS), CS*, SI*, Dilute 1:4	Exodus II, EndoGize
Cedar, Western Red	*Thuja plicata* (Cupressaceae)	Dilute 1:1	Evergreen Essence, KidScents Lotion
Cedar Leaf	*Thuja occidentalis* (Cupressaceae)	Dilute 1:1	
Cedarwood	*Cedrus atlantica* (Pinaceae)	P	A·R·T Beauty Masque, Australian Blue, Brain Power, Egyptian Gold, Grounding, Inspiration, Into the Future, Live with Passion, Sacred Mountain, SARA, Tranquil, Essential Beauty Serums - Dry Skin Blend & Acne-Prone Skin Blend, KidScents Bath Gel, KidScents Lotion, Sacred Mountain Bar Soap, Peppermint Cedarwood Bar Soap, Progessence Plus, Cel-Lite Magic Massage Oil
Celery Seed	*Apium graveolens* (Umbelliferae)	(GRAS), CS, SI, P, Dilute 1:1	GLF, Juva Cleanse
Chamomile (German/Blue)	*Matricaria chamomilla/ recutita* (Compositae)	(GRAS), P, SI	EndoFlex, Surrender, K&B Tincture, A·R·T Day Activator, A·R·T Night Reconstructor, ComforTone, JuvaTone, Omega Blue, OmegaGize³
Chamomile (Roman)	*Chamaemelum nobile* (Compositae)	(GRAS), SI	Clarity, Forgiveness, Gentle Baby, Harmony, Joy, JuvaFlex, M-Grain, Motivation, Surrender, Tranquil, ClaraDerm, Genesis Hand & Body Lotion, KidScents Tender Tush, Lemon Sage Clarifying Shampoo, Lemon Sage Clarifying Conditioner, Wolfberry Eye Cream, Dragon Time Bath Gel, Evening Peace Bath Gel, K&B Tincture, Rehemogen Tincture

Single Oil Name	Botanical Name	Safety Data	Products Containing Single Oil
Cinnamon Bark	*Cinnamomum verum* (Lauraceae)	CS*, P*, SI* Dilute 1:4	Christmas Spirit, Egyptian Gold, Exodus II, Gathering, Magnify Your Purpose, Thieves, Cinnamint Lip Balm, Slique Bar, Thieves Dentarome/Dentarome Plus Toothpaste, Thieves Dentarome Ultra Toothpaste, Thieves Fresh Essence Plus Mouthwash, Thieves Bar Soap, Mineral Essence, Thieves Lozenges
Cistus	*Cistus ladanifer* (Cistaceae)	(FA/FL), P	ImmuPower, The Gift, KidScents Tender Tush
Citronella	*Cymbopogon nardus* (Gramineae)	(GRAS), CS*, P, SI, Dilute 1:1	Purification, Animal Scents Pet Shampoo
Clary Sage	*Salvia sclarea* (Labiatae)	(GRAS), A, P Dilute 1:1	Dragon Time, Into the Future, Lady Sclareol, Live with Passion, SclarEssence, Transformation, Lavender Volume Shampoo, Lavender Volume Conditioner, Prenolone, Prenolone+, Rosewood Moisturizing Shampoo, Rosewood Moisturizing Conditioner, Dragon Time Bath Gel, Evening Peace Bath Gel, Estro Tincture, Cel-Lite Magic Massage Oil, Dragon Time Massage Oil, Ortho Ease Massage Oil, CortiStop (Women's), EndoGize, FemiGen, Transformation
Clove	*Syzygium aromaticum* (Myrtaceae)	(GRAS), CS*, P, SI, Dilute 1:4	Abundance, Deep Relief, En-R-Gee, ImmuPower, Longevity, Melrose, PanAway, Thieves, AromaGuard Deodorants, Essential Beauty Serum - Dry Skin Blend, KidScents Toothpaste, Thieves Dentarome/Dentarome Plus Toothpaste, Thieves Dentarome Ultra Toothpaste, Thieves Fresh Essence Plus Mouthwash, Thieves Bar Soap, K&B Tincture, BLM, Essentialzyme, Longevity Capsules, Omega Blue, OmegaGize[3], ParaFree, Thieves Lozenges
Copaiba	*Copaifera reticulata or Copaifera L. genus* (Leguminosae)	CS	A·R·T Beauty Masque, Deep Relief, Progessence Plus
Coriander	*Coriandrum sativum* L. (Umbelliferae)	(GRAS), ST Dilute 1:1	A·R·T Renewal Serum, Believe
Cumin	*Cuminus cyminum* (Umbelliferae)	(GRAS), P, PH* Dilute 1:1	ImmuPower, Detoxzyme, ParaFree, Protec

Single Oil Name	Botanical Name	Safety Data	Products Containing Single Oil
Cypress	*Cupressus sempervirens* (Cupressaceae)	P Dilute 1:1	Aroma Life, Aroma Siez, RC, Cel-Lite Magic Massage Oil, Super Cal
Cypress, Blue	*Callitris intratropica* (Cupressaceae)		Australian Blue, Brain Power, Essential Beauty Serum - Dry Skin Blend
Davana	*Artemisia pallens* (Compositae)	(FA/FL), P Dilute 1:1	A·R·T Creme Masque, Trauma Life, Lavender Hand & Body Lotion, Lavender Bath Gel
Dill	*Anethum graveolens* (Umbelliferae)	(GRAS), E Dilute 1:1	
Dorado Azul	*Guayafolis officinalis* (Labiatae)		Common Sense
Elemi	*Canarium luzonicum* (Burseraceae)	(FA/FL)	Ortho Sport Massage Oil
Eucalyptus	*Eucalyptus globulus* (Myrtaceae)	(FA/FL) Dilute 1:1	RC, Ortho Ease Massage Oil, Ortho Sport Massage Oil
Eucalyptus Blue	*Eucalyptol natriol azul* (Myrtaceae)		Breathe Again Roll-On
Eucalyptus Citriodora	*Eucalyptus citriodora* (Myrtaceae)	CS Dilute 1:1	RC
Eucalyptus Dives	*Eucalyptus dives* (Myrtaceae)	Dilute 1:1	
Eucalyptus Polybractea	*Eucalyptus polybractea* (Myrtaceae)	Dilute 1:1	

Single Oil Name	Botanical Name	Safety Data	Products Containing Single Oil
Eucalyptus Radiata	*Eucalyptus radiata* (Myrtaceae)	Dilute 1:1	Raven, RC, Thieves, AromaGuard Deodorants, Ortho Ease Massage Oil, Thieves Dentarome/Dentarome Plus Toothpaste, Thieves Dentarome Ultra Toothpaste, Thieves Fresh Essence Plus Mouthwash, Thieves Bar Soap, Thieves Lozenges
Eucalyptus Staigeriana	*Eucalyptus staigeriana* (Myrtaceae)	Dilute 1:1	Essential Beauty Serum - Acne-Prone Skin Blend
Fennel	*Foeniculum vulgare* (Umbelliferae)	(GRAS), CS, E, P Dilute 1:1	Di-Gize, Dragon Time, JuvaFlex, Mister, SclarEssence, Allerzyme, Detoxzyme, Essentialzyme, JuvaPower, JuvaSpice, Prenolone, Prenolone+, Progessence Cream, Dragon Time Bath Gel, Estro Tincture, K&B Tincture, Dragon Time Massage Oil, CortiStop (Women's), Digest + Cleanse, FemiGen, ParaFree, Power Meal, ProGen
Fir	*Abies alba* (Pinaceae)	(FA/FL), SI Dilute 1:1	Sacred Mountain
Fir, Balsam (Idaho Balsam Fir)	*Abies balsamea* (Pinaceae)	(FA/FL), SI Dilute 1:1	Deep Relief, Egyptian Gold, En-R-Gee, The Gift, Transformation, Animal Scents Pet Ointment, Sacred Mountain Bar Soap, BLM, Slique Slim Caps
Fir, Douglas	*Pseudotsuga menziesii* (Pinaceae)	SI Dilute 1:1	Regenolone
Fir, Red	*Abies magnifica* (Pinaceae)	SI Dilute 1:1	Evergreen Essence
Fir, White	*Abies grandis or Abies concolor* (Pinaceae)	SI Dilute 1:1	Australian Blue, Believe, Evergreen Essence, Gratitude, Grounding, Into the Future, AromaGuard Deodorants
Fleabane	*Conyza canadensis* (Compositae)	Dilute 1:1	CortiStop (Women's), EndoGize, Ultra Young+

Single Oil Name	Botanical Name	Safety Data	Products Containing Single Oil
Frankincense	*Boswellia carterii* (Burseraceae)	(FA/FL)	Abundance, Acceptance, Believe, Brain Power, Common Sense, Egyptian Gold, Exodus II, Forgiveness, Gathering, Gratitude, Harmony, Humility, ImmuPower, Inspiration, Into the Future, Longevity, The Gift, 3 Wise Men, Transformation, Trauma Life, Valor, A·R·T Day Activator, A·R·T Gentle Foaming Cleanser, A·R·T Night Reconstructor, A·R·T Purifying Toner, Boswellia Wrinkle Cream, ClaraDerm, KidScents Tender Tush, Progessence Plus, Protec, Wolfberry Eye Cream, Valor Bar Soap, CortiStop (Women's), Longevity Capsules
Frankincense, Sacred	*Boswellia sacra* (Burseraceae)	(FA/FL)	Transformation
Galbanum	*Ferula gummosa* (Umbelliferae)	(FA/FL)	Exodus II, Gathering, Gratitude, The Gift
Geranium	*Pelargonium graveolens* (Geraniaceae)	(GRAS), CS	A·R·T Creme Masque, A·R·T Renewal Serum, Acceptance, Believe, Clarity, EndoFlex, Envision, Forgiveness, Gathering, Gentle Baby, Harmony, Humility, Joy, JuvaFlex, Lady Sclareol, Release, SARA, Trauma Life, White Angelica, Animal Scents Pet Ointment, AromaGuard Deodorants, Boswellia Wrinkle Cream, Genesis Hand & Body Lotion, Lemon Sage Clarifying Shampoo, Lemon Sage Clarifying Conditioner, Prenolone, Prenolone+, Progessence Cream, Rosewood Moisturizing Shampoo, Rosewood Moisturizing Conditioner, Wolfberry Eye Cream, Animal Scents Pet Shampoo, Dragon Time Bath Gel, Evening Peace Bath Gel, KidScents Bath Gel, KidScents Lotion, Melaleuca Geranium Bar Soap, K&B Tincture, JuvaTone
Ginger	*Zingiber officinale* (Zingiberaceae)	(GRAS), CS, PH Dilute 1:1	Abundance, Di-Gize, Live with Passion, Magnify Your Purpose, Allerzyme, ComforTone, Digest + Cleanse, EndoGize, ICP
Goldenrod	*Solidago canadensis* (Asteraceae)	Dilute 1:1	Common Sense
Grapefruit	*Citrus x paradisi* (Rutaceae)	(GRAS) Dilute 1:1	Citrus Fresh, GLF, Cel-Lite Magic Massage Oil, Power Meal, Slique Essence, Super C

Quick Reference Guide for Using Essential Oils

Single Oil Name	Botanical Name	Safety Data	Products Containing Single Oil
Helichrysum	*Helichrysum italicum* (Compositae)	(GRAS)	Aroma Life, Brain Power, Deep Relief, Forgiveness, GLF, Juva Cleanse, JuvaFlex, Live with Passion, M-Grain, PanAway, Trauma Life, ClaraDerm
Hinoki	*Chamaecyparis obtusa* (Cupressaceae)	Dilute 1:1	
Hong Kuai	*Chamaecyparis formosensis* (Cupressaceae)	P*, Dilute 1:1	
Hyssop	*Hyssopus officinalis* (Labiatae)	(GRAS), E*, HBP*, P*, D-1:1	Egyptian Gold, Exodus II, GLF, Harmony, ImmuPower, Relieve It, White Angelica
Jasmine	*Jasminum officinale* (Oleaceae)	(GRAS)	A·R·T Creme Masque, A·R·T Renewal Serum, Clarity, Dragon Time, Forgiveness, Gentle Baby, Harmony, Highest Potential, Inner Child, Into the Future, Joy, Lady Sclareol, Live with Passion, Sensation, The Gift, Genesis Hand & Body Lotion, Lavender Volume Shampoo, Lavender Volume Conditioner, Sensation Hand & Body Lotion, Dragon Time Bath Gel, Evening Peace Bath Gel, Sensation Bath Gel, Dragon Time Massage Oil, Sensation Massage Oil
Juniper	*Juniperus osteosperma* and/ or *J. scopulorum* (Cupressaceae)	Dilute 1:1	Di-Gize, Dream Catcher, En-R-Gee, Grounding, Hope, Into the Future, 3 Wise Men, Allerzyme, Morning Start Bath Gel, Morning Start Bar Soap, K&B Tincture, Cel-Lite Magic Massage Oil, Ortho Ease Massage Oil
Laurel	*Laurus nobilis* (Lauraceae)	(GRAS), CS, P* Dilute 1:1	ParaFree
Lavandin	*Lavandula x hybrida* (Labiatae)	(GRAS), E, P*	Purification, Release, Animal Scents Pet Shampoo

Single Oil Name	Botanical Name	Safety Data	Products Containing Single Oil
Lavender	*Lavandula angustifolia* CT linalool (Labiatae)		A·R·T Beauty Masque, Aroma Siez, Brain Power, Dragon Time, Egyptian Gold, Envision, Forgiveness, Gathering, Gentle Baby, Harmony, M-Grain, Mister, Motivation, RC, RutaVaLa, SARA, Surrender, Tranquil, Trauma Life, A·R·T Gentle Foaming Cleanser, A·R·T Purifying Toner, AromaGuard Deodorants, ClaraDerm, Essential Beauty Serum - Dry Skin Blend, LavaDerm Cooling Mist, Lavender Hand & Body Lotion, Lavender Volume Shampoo, Lavender Volume Conditioner, KidScents Tender Tush, Orange Blossom Facial Wash, Sandalwood Moisture Cream, Wolfberry Eye Cream, Dragon Time Bath Gel, Lavender Bath Gel, Lavender Rosewood Bar Soap, Estro Tincture, Dragon Time Massage Oil, Relaxation Massage Oil, ProGen
Ledum	*Ledum groenlandicum* (Ericaceae)		GLF, Juva Cleanse
Lemon	*Citrus limon* (Rutaceae)	(GRAS), PH*, SI* Dilute 1:1	Citrus Fresh, Clarity, Deep Relief, Forgiveness, Gentle Baby, Harmony, Joy, Raven, Surrender, Thieves, Transformation, A·R·T Gentle Foaming Cleanser, A·R·T Purifying Toner, AromaGuard Deodorants, Genesis Hand & Body Lotion, Animal Scents Pet Shampoo, KidScents Shampoo, Lavender Hand & Body Lotion, Lavender Volume Shampoo, Lavender Volume Conditioner, Lemon Sage Clarifying Shampoo, Lemon Sage Clarifying Conditioner, NingXia Red, Orange Blossom Facial Wash, Thieves Dentarome/Dentarome Plus Toothpaste, Thieves Dentarome Ultra Toothpaste, Thieves Fresh Essence Plus Mouthwash, Dragon Time Bath Gel, Evening Peace Bath Gel, Lavender Bath Gel, Thieves Bar Soap, Lemon Sandalwood Bar Soap, AlkaLime, Digest + Cleanse, JuvaTone, MegaCal, Mineral Essence, MultiGreens, NingXia Red, Power Meal, Slique Essence, Super C, Super C Chewable, Thieves Lozenges, Transformation
Lemongrass	*Cymbopogon flexuosus* (Gramineae)	(GRAS), SI* Dilute 1:4	Di-Gize, En-R-Gee, Inner Child, Purification, Allerzyme, Evening Peace Bath Gel, Morning Start Bath Gel, Morning Start Bar Soap, Ortho Ease Massage Oil, Ortho Sport Massage Oil, ICP, MultiGreens, Omega Blue, Slique Slim Caps, Super C, Super Cal
Lime	*Citrus aurantifolia* (Rutaceae)	(GRAS), PH* Dilute 1:1	A·R·T Beauty Masque, Common Sense, Lemon Sage Clarifying Shampoo, Lemon Sage Clarifying Conditioner, AlkaLime, KidScents Mighty Vites

Single Oil Name	Botanical Name	Safety Data	Products Containing Single Oil
Limette (Combava)	Citrus hystrix (Rutaceae)	PH* Dilute 1:1	Trauma Life
Mandarin	*Citrus reticulata* (Rutaceae)	(GRAS), PH Dilute 1:1	Citrus Fresh, Joy, Dragon Time Bath Gel, KidScents Mighty Vites
Manuka	*Leptospermum scoparium* (Myrtaceae)	Dilute 1:1	Essential Beauty Serum - Acne-Prone Skin Blend
Marjoram	*Origanum majorana* (Labiatae)	(GRAS), P Dilute 1:1	Aroma Life, Aroma Siez, Dragon Time, M-Grain, RC, Dragon Time Bath Gel, Ortho Ease Massage Oil, Ortho Sport Massage Oil, Super Cal
Mastrante	*Lippia Alba* (Verbenaceae)		Light the Fire
Melaleuca (Tea Tree)	*Melaleuca alternifolia* (Myrtaceae)	(FA/FL), CS Dilute 1:1	Melrose, Purification, Animal Scents Pet Ointment, AromaGuard Deodorants, ClaraDerm, Essential Beauty Serum - Acne-Prone Skin Blend, Rose Ointment, Melaleuca Geranium Bar Soap, Rehemogen Tincture, ParaFree
Melaleuca ericifolia (Rosalina)	*Melaleuca ericifolia* (Myrtaceae)	(FA/FL) Dilute 1:1	Melaleuca Geranium Bar Soap
Melaleuca quinquenervia (Niaouli)	*Melaleuca quinquenervia* (Myrtaceae)	(FA/FL), CS Dilute 1:1	Melrose, AromaGuard Deodorants
Melissa	*Melissa officinalis* (Labiatae)	(GRAS)	Brain Power, Forgiveness, Hope, Humility, Live with Passion, White Angelica, A·R·T Gentle Foaming Cleanser, A·R·T Purifying Toner, MultiGreens
Micromeria	*Micromeria fruticosa* (Labiatae)	P*, SI* Dilute 1:2	
Mountain Savory	*Satureja montana* (Labiatae)	(GRAS), P*, SI* Dilute 1:4	ImmuPower, Surrender
Mugwort	*Artemisia vulgaris* (Asteraceae)	P* Dilute 1:1	Inspiration, ComforTone

Single Oil Name	Botanical Name	Safety Data	Products Containing Single Oil
Myrrh	*Commiphora myrrha* (Burseraceae)	(FA/FL), P	Abundance, Egyptian Gold, Exodus II, Gratitude, Hope, Humility, The Gift, 3 Wise Men, White Angelica, Animal Scents Pet Ointment, Boswellia Wrinkle Cream, ClaraDerm, Essential Beauty Serum - Dry Skin Blend, Lavender Hand & Body Lotion, Protec, Rose Ointment, Sandalwood Moisture Cream, Lavender Bath Gel, EndoGize, Omega Blue, Thyromin
Myrrh , Biblical Sweet	*Commiphora erythraea* (Burseraceae)	(FA/FL), P	
Myrtle	*Myrtus communis* (Myrtaceae)	Dilute 1:1	EndoFlex, Inspiration, Mister, Purification, RC, JuvaTone, ProGen, Super Cal, Thyromin
Myrtle, Lemon	*Backhousia citriodora* (Myrtaceae)	CS, SI Dilute 1:4	Slique Slim Caps
Neroli	*Citrus aurantium bigaradia* (Rutaceae)	(GRAS) Dilute 1:1	Acceptance, Humility, Inner Child, Live with Passion, Present Time
Nutmeg	*Myristica fragrans* (Myristicaceae)	(GRAS), E*, P Dilute 1:2	EndoFlex, En-R-Gee, Magnify Your Purpose, NingXia Nitro, ParaFree, Power Meal
Ocotea	*Ocotea quixos* (Lauraceae)	Dilute 1:1	A·R·T Beauty Masque, A·R·T Creme Masque, Common Sense, Slique Essence, Stress Away Roll-On, Transformation
Onycha	*Styrax benzoin* (Styracaceae)	(FA/FL)	
Orange	*Citrus sinensis* (Rutaceae)	(GRAS), PH* Dilute 1:1	Abundance, Christmas Spirit, Citrus Fresh, Envision, Harmony, Inner Child, Into the Future, Lady Sclareol, Longevity, NingXia Red, Peace & Calming, SARA, Cinnamint Lip Balm, Balance Complete, ImmuPro, Longevity Capsules, Pure Protein Complete, KidScents Mighty Vites, NingXia Red, Power Meal, Slique Bar, Super C, Thieves Lozenges
Oregano	*Origanum compactum* (Labiatae)	(GRAS), SI* Dilute 1:4	ImmuPower, Regenolone, Ortho Sport Massage Oil

Single Oil Name	Botanical Name	Safety Data	Products Containing Single Oil
Palmarosa	*Cymbopogon martinii* (Gramineae)	(GRAS) Dilute 1:1	Clarity, Forgiveness, Gentle Baby, Harmony, Joy, Animal Scents Pet Ointment, Genesis Hand & Body Lotion, Rose Ointment, Dragon Time Bath Gel, Evening Peace Bath Gel
Palo Santo	*Bursera graveolens* (Burseraceae)		Deep Relief, Transformation
Patchouli	*Pogostemon cablin* (Labiatae)	(FA/FL)	Abundance, Di-Gize, Live with Passion, Magnify Your Purpose, Peace & Calming, Allerzyme, Animal Scents Pet Ointment, Orange Blossom Facial Wash, Rose Ointment
Pepper, Black	*Piper nigrum* (Piperaceae)	(GRAS), SI* Dilute 1:1	Dream Catcher, En-R-Gee, Relieve It, Cel-Lite Magic Massage Oil, NingXia Nitro
Pepper, Pink	*Schinus molle* (Anacardiaceae)	(GRAS), P* Dilute 1:1	
Peppermint	*Mentha piperita* (Labiatae)	(GRAS), CS, HBP, P Dilute 1:2	Aroma Siez, Clarity, Deep Relief, Di-Gize, M-Grain, Mister, PanAway, Raven, RC, Relieve It, SclarEssence, Transformation, A·R·T Purifying Toner, AromaGuard Deodorants, Cinnamint Lip Balm, Lemon Sage Clarifying Conditioner, Mint Satin Facial Scrub, Progessence Plus, Regenolone, Thieves Dentarome/Dentarome Plus Toothpaste, Thieves Dentarome Ultra Toothpaste, Thieves Fresh Essence Plus Mouthwash, Morning Start Bath Gel, Peppermint Cedarwood Bar Soap, Ortho Ease Massage Oil, Ortho Sport Massage Oil, Relaxation Massage Oil, Allerzyme, ComforTone, CortiStop (Women's), Digest + Cleanse, Essentialzyme, Mineral Essence, NingXia Nitro, ProGen, Slique Gum, Thieves Lozenges, Thyromin, Transformation
Petitgrain	*Citrus aurantium* (Rutaceae)	(GRAS) Dilute 1:1	
Pine	*Pinus sylvestris* (Pinaceae)	(FA/FL), SI Dilute 1:1	Evergreen Essence, Grounding, RC, Lemon Sage Clarifying Shampoo, Lemon Sage Clarifying Conditioner
Pine, Black	*Pinus nigra* (Pinaceae)	SI	Evergreen Essence

Single Oil Name	Botanical Name	Safety Data	Products Containing Single Oil
Pine, Lodge Pole	*Pinus contorta* (Pinaceae)	SI	Evergreen Essence
Pine, Piñon	*Pinus edulis* (Pinaceae)	SI	Evergreen Essence
Pine, Ponderosa (Yellow Pine)	*Pinus ponderosa* (Pinaceae)	SI	Evergreen Essence
Plectranthus Oregano	*Plectranthus amboinicus* (Lauraceae)	SI*	
Ravensara	*Ravensara aromatica* (Lauraceae)		ImmuPower, Raven
Rose (Bulgarian)	*Rosa damascena* (Rosaceae)	(GRAS), P	Egyptian Gold, Envision, Forgiveness, Gathering, Gentle Baby, Harmony, Humility, Joy, SARA, Trauma Life, White Angelica, Rose Ointment
Rosehip	*Rosa canina or Rosa rubiginosa* (Rosaceae)	(GRAS)	Animal Scents Pet Ointment, Rose Ointment, Sandalwood Moisture Cream, Wolfberry Eye Cream
Rosemary Cineol	*Rosmarinus officinalis* CT 1,8 cineol (Labiatae)	(GRAS), E*, HBP*, P* Dilute 1:1	En-R-Gee, JuvaFlex, Melrose, Purification, Thieves, Transformation, AromaGuard Deodorants, Thieves Dentarome/Dentarome Plus Toothpaste, Thieves Dentarome Ultra Toothpaste, Thieves Fresh Essence Plus Mouthwash, Evening Peace Bath Gel, Morning Start Bath Gel, Morning Start Bar Soap, Rehemogen Tincture, ComforTone, ICP, JuvaTone, MultiGreens, Thieves Lozenges
Rosemary Verbenon	*Rosmarinus officinalis* CT verbenon (Labiatae)	(GRAS), E*, HBP, P Dilute 1:1	Clarity, Orange Blossom Facial Wash, Sandalwood Moisture Cream

Single Oil Name	Botanical Name	Safety Data	Products Containing Single Oil
Rosewood	*Aniba rosaeodora* (Lauraceae)	(GRAS)	Acceptance, Clarity, Forgiveness, Gentle Baby, Gratitude, Harmony, Humility, Inspiration, Joy, Lady Sclareol, Magnify Your Purpose, Sensation, Valor, White Angelica, Animal Scents Pet Ointment, AromaGuard Deodorants, Genesis Hand & Body Lotion, KidScents Lotion, KidScents Tender Tush, Progessence Plus, Rose Ointment, Rosewood Moisturizing Shampoo, Rosewood Moisturizing Conditioner, Sandalwood Moisture Cream, Sensation Hand & Body Lotion, Wolfberry Eye Cream, Dragon Time Bath Gel, Evening Peace Bath Gel, Sensation Bath Gel, Lavender Rosewood Bar Soap, Valor Bar Soap, Relaxation Massage Oil, Sensation Massage Oil
Ruta (Rue)	*Ruta graveolens* (Rutaceae)	P*, PH*, SI*	Common Sense, RutaVaLa
Sage	*Salvia officinalis* (Labiatae)	(GRAS), E*, HBP*, P* Dilute 1:1	EndoFlex, Envision, Magnify Your Purpose, Mister, Progessence Cream, Protec, Lemon Sage Clarifying Shampoo, Lemon Sage Clarifying Conditioner, Dragon Time Bath Gel, K&B Tincture, Dragon Time Massage Oil, FemiGen, ProGen
Sage, Spanish (Sage Lavender)	*Salvia lavandulifolia* (Labiatae)	(GRAS) Dilute 1:1	Harmony, Lady Sclareol, SclarEssence
Sandalwood	*Santalum album* (Santalaceae)	(FA/FL)	Acceptance, Brain Power, Dream Catcher, Forgiveness, Gathering, Harmony, Inner Child, Inspiration, Lady Sclareol, Live with Passion, Magnify Your Purpose, Release, 3 Wise Men, Transformation, Trauma Life, White Angelica, A·R·T Day Activator, A·R·T Gentle Foaming Cleanser, A·R·T Night Reconstructor, A·R·T Purifying Toner, Boswellia Wrinkle Cream, Essential Beauty Serum - Dry Skin Blend, KidScents Tender Tush, Rosewood Moisturizing Shampoo, Rosewood Moisturizing Conditioner, Sandalwood Moisture Cream, Evening Peace Bath Gel, Lemon Sandalwood Bar Soap, Transformation, Ultra Young+
Sandalwood, Royal Hawaiian	*Santalum paniculatum* (Santalaceae)	(FA/FL)	Animal Scents T-Away, Build Your Dream, Divine Release, Inner Harmony, InTouch, KidScents GeneYus, Reconnect, T.R. Care

Single Oil Name	Botanical Name	Safety Data	Products Containing Single Oil
Spearmint	*Mentha spicata* (Labiatae)	(GRAS), P Dilute 1:2	Citrus Fresh, EndoFlex, GLF, Cinnamint Lip Balm, Thieves Fresh Essence Plus Mouthwash, NingXia Nitro, OmegaGize³, Relaxation Massage Oil, Slique Essence, Slique Gum, Thyromin
Spikenard	*Nardostachys jatamansi* (Valerianaceae)		Egyptian Gold, Exodus II, Humility, The Gift, Animal Scents Pet Shampoo
Spruce	*Picea mariana* (Pinaceae)	(FA/FL) Dilute 1:1	Abundance, Christmas Spirit, Envision, Gathering, Grounding, Harmony, Hope, Inner Child, Inspiration, Motivation, Present Time, Relieve It, Sacred Mountain, Surrender, 3 Wise Men, Trauma Life, Valor, White Angelica, Sacred Mountain Bar Soap, Valor Bar Soap
Spruce, Colorado Blue	*Picea pungens* (Pinaceae)		Evergreen Essence
Spruce, Idaho Blue	*Picea Pungens* (Pinaceae)	(FA/FL), Dilute 1:1	Believe, Transformation
Tangerine	*Citrus nobilis* (Rutaceae)	(GRAS) Dilute 1:1	Citrus Fresh, Dream Catcher, Inner Child, Peace & Calming, KidScents Shampoo, Relaxation Massage Oil, ComforTone, Slique Essence, Super C
Tansy, Blue	*Tanacetum annuum* (Compositae)	Dilute 1:1	Acceptance, Australian Blue, Dream Catcher, JuvaFlex, NingXia Red, Peace & Calming, Release, SARA, Valor, KidScents Shampoo, KidScents Tender Tush, Dragon Time Bath Gel, Evening Peace Bath Gel, Valor Bar Soap, JuvaTone
Tansy, Idaho	*Tanacetum vulgare* (Compositae)	Dilute 1:1	ImmuPower, Into the Future, Lady Sclareol, ParaFree
Tarragon	*Artemisia dracunculus* (Compositae)	(GRAS), E*, P* Dilute 1:1	Di-Gize, Allerzyme, ComforTone, ICP, Essentialzyme
Thyme	*Thymus vulgaris* (Labiatae)	(GRAS), HBP Dilute 1:4	Longevity, Essential Beauty Serum - Acne-Prone Skin Blend, KidScents Toothpaste, Rehemogen, Longevity Capsules, ParaFree
Thyme linalool	*Thymus vulgaris* CT Linalool (Labiatae)	(GRAS) Dilute 1:2	

Single Oil Name	Botanical Name	Safety Data	Products Containing Single Oil
Thyme, Red	*Thymus serpyllum* (Labiatae)	(GRAS)	Ortho Ease
Tsuga	*Tsuga canadensis* (Pinaceae)	(FA/FL), SI* Dilute 1:1	RC
Valerian	*Valeriana officinalis* (Valerianaceae)	(FA/FL), CS	RutaVaLa, Trauma Life
Vetiver	*Vetiveria zizanioides* (Gramineae)	P	A·R·T Creme Masque, Deep Relief, Lady Sclareol, Thieves Fresh Essence Plus Mouthwash, Melaleuca Geranium Bar Soap, Ortho Ease Massage Oil, Ortho Sport Massage Oil, ParaFree
White Lotus	*Nymphaea lotus* (Nymphaeaceae)		SARA
Wintergreen	*Gaultheria procumbens* (Ericaceae)	E*, P* Dilute 1:2	Deep Relief, PanAway, Raven, Regenolone, Rosewood Moisturizing Shampoo, Rosewood Moisturizing Conditioner, Thieves Dentarome/Dentarome Plus Toothpaste, Thieves Dentarome Ultra Toothpaste, Ortho Ease Massage Oil, Ortho Sport Massage Oil, BLM, Super Cal
Xiang Mao (Red Lemongrass)	*Cymbopogon citratus* (Gramineae)	(GRAS), SI* Dilute 1:4	
Yarrow	*Achillea millefolium* (Compositae)	CS, P Dilute 1:1	Dragon Time, Mister, Prenolone/ Prenolone+, Progessence Cream, Dragon Time Massage Oil, ProGen

Single Oil Name	Botanical Name	Safety Data	Products Containing Single Oil
Ylang Ylang	*Cananga odorata* (Annonaceae)	(GRAS), CS Dilute 1:1	Aroma Life, A·R·T Creme Masque, A·R·T Renewal Serum, Australian Blue, Clarity, Common Sense, Dream Catcher, Forgiveness, Gathering, Gentle Baby, Gratitude, Grounding, Harmony, Highest Potential, Humility, Inner Child, Into the Future, Joy, Lady Sclareol, Motivation, Peace & Calming, Present Time, Release, Sacred Mountain, SARA, Sensation, White Angelica, Boswellia Wrinkle Cream, Genesis Hand & Body Lotion, Lemon Sage Clarifying Shampoo, Lemon Sage Clarifying Conditioner, Prenolone/Prenolone+, Sensation Hand & Body Lotion, Dragon Time Bath Gel, Evening Peace Bath Gel, Sensation Bath Gel, Sacred Mountain Bar Soap, Dragon Time Massage Oil, Relaxation Massage Oil, Sensation Massage Oil, FemiGen
Ylang Ylang, Amazonian	*Cananga odorata equitoriana* (Annonaceae)	(GRAS), CS Dilute 1:1	Believe
Yuzu	*Citrus junos* (Rutaceae)	PH, Dilute 1:1	NingXia Red

Safety Data Legend:

A	**Avoid** during and after consumption of **alcohol**
CS	Could possibly result in **contact sensitization** (redness or irritation of the skin due to repeated application of a substance) (rotate or use different oils)
CS*	Repeated use can result in **extreme contact sensitization** (rotate between different oils)
D	**Avoid** if **diabetic**
E	Use with **caution** if susceptible to **epilepsy** (small amounts or in dilution)
E*	**Avoid** if susceptible to **epilepsy** (can trigger a seizure)
HBP	Use with **caution** if dealing with **high blood pressure** (small amounts)
HBP*	**Avoid** if dealing with **high blood pressure**
P	Use with **caution** during **pregnancy** (small amounts or in dilution)
P*	**Avoid** during **pregnancy**
PH	**Photosensitivity**–direct exposure to sunlight after use could cause dermatitis (test first)
PH*	**Extreme Photosensitivity**–direct exposure to sunlight after use can cause severe dermatitis (avoid exposing affected area of skin to direct sunlight for 12 hours)
SI	Could possibly result in **skin irritation** (dilution may be necessary)
SI*	Can cause **extreme skin irritation** (dilution highly recommended)
ST	Can cause **stupefaction** in high doses (use only small amounts or in dilution)

Dilute - Dilution ratios shown equal Essential Oil:Vegetable Oil

BLEND SUMMARY INFORMATION

The following chart displays summary information for each of the oil blends: single oils contained in the blend, possible uses or areas of application, and safety data. The safety data includes possible skin reactions and conditions where use of that particular blend should be limited or completely avoided (refer to the legend following the chart). **Note:** This safety data is provided for **external use only!**

Blend Name	Single Oil Contents	Uses/Application Areas	Safety Data
Abundance	Myrrh, frankincense, patchouli, orange, clove, ginger, spruce	Diffuse; Wrists, ears, neck, face; Wallet/urse; Painting; Perfume	CS*, SI Dilute 1:1
Acceptance	Geranium, blue tansy, frankincense, sandalwood, neroli, rosewood (Carrier: Almond oil)	Diffuse; *Liver*, heart, *chest*, face, ears, neck, thymus, wrists; Sacral chakra; Perfume	
Animal Scents Infect Away	Myrrh, patchouli, dorado azul, palo santo, plectranthus oregano, ocotea (Carrier: Coconut oil)	Topically on location (dilute for small animals); Spray over affected area	
Animal Scents Mendwell	Geranium, lavender, hyssop, myrrh, frankincense, hinoki (Carrier: Coconut oil)	Topically on location (dilute for small animals)	
Animal Scents ParaGize	Ginger, anise, peppermint, cumin, spearmint, rosemary, juniper, fennel, lemongrass, patchouli (Carrier: Coconut oil)	Abdominal area (dilute for small animals)	
Animal Scents PuriClean	Patchouli, lavender, mountain savory, cistus, palo santo, lemongrass, rosemary, melaleuca, lavandin, myrtle (Carrier: Coconut oil)	Topically on location (dilute for small animals); Spray over affected area	
Animal Scents RepelAroma	Citronella, Idaho Tansy, Palo Santo, Melaleuca (Carrier: Coconut oil)	Diffuse; Spray over animal; Topically on animal's coat (dilute for small animals)	
Animal Scents T-Away	Tangerine, lavender, royal Hawaiian sandalwood, German chamomile, frankincense, valerian, ylang ylang, black spruce, geranium, davana, orange, angelica, *Ruta graveolens* (rue), helichrysum, hyssop, Spanish sage, limette (combova), patchouli, coriander, blue tansy, bergamot, rose, lemon, jasmine, Roman chamomile, palmarosa (Carrier: Coconut oil)	Diffuse; Ears, bottom of paws, flank (dilute for small animals)	PH*
AromaEase	Peppermint, spearmint, ginger, cardamom, fennel	Diffuse; Stomach, solar plexus, Vita Flex points on feet	P

Blend Name	Single Oil Contents	Uses/Application Areas	Safety Data
Aroma Life	Cypress, marjoram, helichrysum, ylang ylang (Carrier: Sesame seed oil)	Heart; Vita Flex heart points—under left ring finger, under left ring toe, above left elbow, arteries; Spine	
Aroma Siez	Basil, marjoram, lavender, peppermint, cypress	Muscles; Neck; Heart; Vita Flex points; Full-body massage; Bath	Dilute 1:1
AromaSleep	Lavender, geranium, Roman chamomile, bergamot, tangerine, sacred frankincense, valerian, *Ruta graveolens* (rue)	Diffuse; Internally in a capsule; Topically as desired (dilute)	P Dilute 1:1
Australian Blue	Blue cypress, ylang ylang, cedarwood, blue tansy, white fir	Diffuse; Perfume; Forehead	CS, SI
Awaken	Oil Blends of Joy, Forgiveness, Dream Catcher, Present Time, Harmony	Diffuse; Chest, heart, *forehead*, neck, temples, wrists; Perfume; Full-body massage; Bath	
Believe	Idaho Balsam fir, coriander, bergamot, frankincense, Idaho Blue Spruce, Ylang Ylang, Geranium	Diffuse; *Heart, forehead, temples*; Perfume	Dilute 1:1
Brain Power	Cedarwood, sandalwood, frankincense, melissa, blue cypress, lavender, helichrysum	Diffuse; Neck, throat, nose; Inside of cheeks; Perfume	
Breathe Again *(Roll-on)*	*Eucalyptus staigeriana, Eucalyptus globulus,* laurel, rose hip, peppermint, copaiba, *Eucalyptus radiata,* myrtle, manuku, eucalyptus blue	Chest; Under nose	SI, P
Build Your Dream	Lavender, ylang ylang, blue cypress, sacred frankincense, hong kuai, melissa, Idaho blue spruce, balsam fir, royal Hawaiian sandalwood, coriander, mandarin, black pepper, bergamot, frankincense, juniper, anise, blue tansy, geranium, blue lotus	Diffuse; Topically on location (dilute)	P, PH*
Christmas Spirit	Orange, cinnamon bark, spruce	Diffuse; Crown; Perfume; Place on pine boughs or fireplace logs; Add to potpourri	CS*, SI* Dilute 1:1
Citrus Fresh	Orange, tangerine, mandarin, grapefruit, lemon, spearmint	Diffuse; Ears, heart, wrists; Perfume; Full-body massage; Bath; Purify drinking water	SI*, PH* Dilute 1:1
Clarity	Basil, cardamom, rosemary verbenon, peppermint, rosewood, geranium, lemon, palmarosa, ylang ylang, bergamot, Roman chamomile, jasmine	Diffuse; Forehead, neck, temples, wrists; Perfume; Bath	SI, P, PH*

Blend Name	Single Oil Contents	Uses/Application Areas	Safety Data
Common Sense	Frankincense, ylang ylang, ocotea, goldenrod, rue, dorado azul, lime	Diffuse	SI, P, PH*
Cool Azul	Wintergreen, peppermint, sage, plectranthus oregano, balsam copaiba, melaleuca quinquenervia, lavender, blue cypress, elemi, vetiver, caraway, dorado azul, German chamomile	Roll on stiff or sore muscles	CS, SI, P*
Deep Relief *(Roll-on)*	Peppermint, lemon, balsam fir, copaiba, clove, wintergreen, helichrysum, vetiver, palo santo (Carriers: Fractionated coconut oil and virgin coconut oil)	Directly on pain location; Forehead, neck, temples	
Di-Gize	Tarragon, ginger, peppermint, juniper, anise, fennel, lemongrass, patchouli	Vita Flex points—feet and ankles; Stomach; Abdomen, bottom of throat; Compress	P, E
Divine Release	Royal Hawaiian sandalwood, Roman chamomile, frankincense, melissa, geranium, grapefruit, blue cypress, hinoki, helichrysum, bergamot, rose, ledum, angelica	Diffuse; Topically where desired	SI, P
Dragon Time	Clary sage, fennel, lavender, marjoram, yarrow, jasmine	Vita Flex points; Diffuse; Abdomen, lower back, location	P
Dream Catcher	Sandalwood, bergamot, ylang ylang, juniper, blue tansy, tangerine, black pepper, anise	Diffuse; Forehead, eyebrows, *temples*, ears, throat chakra; Perfume; Pillow; Bath or sauna	PH
Egyptian Gold	Frankincense, lavender, balsam fir, myrrh, spikenard, hyssop, cedarwood, rose, cinnamon bark	Diffuse; Wrists, ears, neck, temples; Perfume	SI, E Dilute 1:4
En-R-Gee	Rosemary cineol, juniper, nutmeg, balsam fir, black pepper, lemongrass, clove	Diffuse; Wrists, ears, neck, temples, feet; Full-body massage; Perfume	SI*, E Dilute 1:1
EndoFlex	Spearmint, sage, geranium, myrtle, nutmeg, German chamomile (Carrier: Sesame seed oil)	Thyroid, kidneys, liver, pancreas, glands; Vita Flex points	SI, E
Envision	Spruce, geranium, orange, lavender, sage, rose	Vita Flex points; Diffuse; Wrists, *temples*; Bath; Massage	HBP, E, P
Evergreen Essence	Colorado blue spruce (*Picea pungens*), ponderosa pine (*Pinus ponderosa*), pine, red fir (*Abies magnifica*), western red cedar, white fir, black pine (*Pinus nigra*), pinyon pine (*Pinus edulis*), lodgepole pine (*Pinus contorta*), and other conifers	*Diffuse*; Hands, bottoms of feet	CS, SI Dilute 1:1

Blend Name	Single Oil Contents	Uses/Application Areas	Safety Data
Exodus II	Cassia, myrrh, cinnamon bark, calamus, hyssop, galbanum, frankincense, spikenard (Carrier: Olive oil)	Vita Flex points; Spine (dilute well)	CS*, SI*, P* Dilute 1:1
Forgiveness	Melissa, geranium, frankincense, rosewood, sandalwood, angelica, lavender, lemon, jasmine, Roman chamomile, bergamot, ylang ylang, palmarosa, helichrysum, rose (Carrier: Sesame seed oil)	Diffuse; *Navel*, heart, ears, wrists; Perfume	
Freedom	Copaiba, sacred frankincense, Idaho blue spruce, vetiver, lavender, peppermint, palo santo, valerian, *Ruta graveolens* (rue)	Diffuse; Topically on disired area	SI Dilute 1:1
Gathering	Lavender, galbanum, frankincense, geranium, ylang ylang, spruce, cinnamon bark, rose, sandalwood	Diffuse; *Forehead, heart, temples*, neck, thymus, face, chest; Perfume	
Gentle Baby	Rosewood, geranium, palmarosa, lavender, Roman chamomile, ylang ylang, lemon, jasmine, bergamot, rose	Diffuse; Ankles, lower back, abdomen, feet, face, neck; Massage; Perfume; Bath	
GLF	Grapefruit, helichrysum, celery seed, ledum, hyssop, spearmint.	Liver; Vita Flex points on feet	
Gratitude	Balsam fir, frankincense, rosewood, myrrh, galbanum, ylang ylang	Diffuse; *Heart, forehead, temples*; Perfume	Dilute 1:1
Grounding	Fir, spruce, ylang ylang, pine, cedarwood, angelica, juniper	Diffuse; *Brain stem, back of neck, sternum*, temples	SI
Harmony	Lavender, sandalwood, ylang ylang, frankincense, orange, angelica, geranium, hyssop, spruce, sage lavender, rosewood, lemon, jasmine, Roman chamomile, bergamot, palmarosa, rose	Diffuse; Each chakra; Ears, feet, heart; *Energy meridians*, crown; Perfume	P, E*, HBP, PH
Highest Potential	Oil blends of Australian Blue and Gathering, and single oils of jasmine and ylang ylang	Diffuse; *Heart, forehead, temples*; Perfume	Dilute 1:1
Hope	Melissa, myrrh, juniper, spruce (Carrier: Almond oil)	Diffuse; *Ears*; Chest, heart, temples, solar plexus, neck, feet, wrists; Perfume	
Humility	Rosewood, ylang ylang, geranium, melissa, frankincense, spikenard, myrrh, rose, neroli (Carrier: Sesame seed oil)	Diffuse; *Heart, neck, temples*	
ImmuPower	Hyssop, mountain savory, cistus, ravensara, frankincense, oregano, clove, cumin, Idaho tansy	Diffuse; Throat, chest, spine, feet; Thymus; Veins in neck, under arm pits	SI, P, E Dilute 1:1

Blend Name	Single Oil Contents	Uses/Application Areas	Safety Data
Inner Child	Orange, tangerine, jasmine, ylang ylang, spruce, sandalwood, lemongrass, neroli	Diffuse; *Navel, chest, temples, nose*	SI
Inner Harmony	Geranium, lavender, royal Hawaiian sandalwood, sacred frankincense, ylang ylang, Idaho blue spruce, Roman chamomile, galbanum, orange, tangerine, melissa, angelica, rose, myrrh	Diffuse; Internally in a capsule; Topically where desired	SI, P Dilute 1:1
Inspiration	Cedarwood, spruce, rosewood, myrtle, sandalwood, frankincense, mugwort	Diffuse; *Horns*, crown, shoulders, back of neck	
Into the Future	Clary sage, ylang ylang, white fir, Idaho tansy, juniper, jasmine, frankincense, orange, cedarwood (Carrier: Almond oil)	Diffuse; Bath; Heart, wrists, neck; Compress; Full-body massage	
InTouch	Vetiver, melissa, royal Hawaiian sandalwood, cedarwood, Idaho blue spruce (Carrier: Coconut oil)	Diffuse; Topically where desired	SI Dilute 1:1
Joy	Bergamot, ylang ylang, geranium, rosewood, lemon, mandarin, jasmine, Roman chamomile, palmarosa, rose	Diffuse; *Heart*, ears, neck, thymus, temples, forehead, wrists; Bath; Compress; Massage; Perfume	PH*
Juva Cleanse	Helichrysum, ledum, celery seed	Liver; Vita Flex points on feet	SI
JuvaFlex	Fennel, geranium, rosemary cineol, Roman chamomile, blue tansy, helichrysum (Carrier: Sesame seed oil)	Vita Flex points; Feet, spine, LIVER; Full-body massage	SI Dilute 1:1
KidScents Bite Buster	Idaho tansy, citronella, palo santo (Carrier: Coconut oil)	Diffuse; Skin	
KidScents GeneYus	Sacred frankincense, blue cypress, cedarwood, melissa, Idaho blue spruce, palo santo, galbanum, bergamot, myrrh, royal Hawaiian sandalwood, geranium, rosewood, ylang ylang, hyssop, spruce, rose (Carrier: Coconut oil)	Diffuse; Back of ears, feet	PH*
KidScents Owie	Idaho balsam fir, melaleuca, helichrysum, elemi, cistus, hinoki, clove (Carrier: Coconut oil)	Topically on location	
KidScents SleepyIze	Lavender, geranium, Roman chamomile, tangerine, bergamot, sacred frankincense, valerian, *Ruta graveolens* (rue) (Carrier: Coconut oil)	Diffuse; Spray on bed linens; Massage on back, feet, arms	PH*
KidScents SniffleEase	Eucalyptus blue, palo santo, lavender, dorado azul, ravintsara, myrtle, eucalyptus, marjoram, pine, *Eucalyptus citriodora*, cypress, *Eucalyptus radiata*, spruce, peppermint (Carrier: Coconut oil)	Diffuse; Neck, chest, forehead, back of the ears	

Blend Name	Single Oil Contents	Uses/Application Areas	Safety Data
KidScents TummyGize	Spearmint, peppermint, tangerine, fennel, anise, ginger, cardamom (Carrier: Coconut oil)	Diffuse; Abdominal area, Vita Flex points on feet	
Lady Sclareol	Rosewood, vetiver, geranium, orange, clary sage, ylang ylang, sandalwood, sage lavender, jasmine, Idaho tansy	On location (by male partner); Massage; Bath; Compress over abdomen; Diffuse, *Perfume*	
Legacy	Ninety-one different essential oils	Vita Flex points; Diffuse; Topically on location	E, P, CS, SI
Light the Fire	Nutmeg, cassia, mastrante, ocotea, fleabane, lemon, black pepper, hinoki, Northern Lights black spruce	Feet, wrists, heart; Diffuse; Massage	P, CS, SI Dilute 1:1
Live with Passion	Clary sage, ginger, sandalwood, jasmine, angelica, cedarwood, helichrysum, patchouli, neroli, melissa	Wrists, *temples, chest, forehead*; Bath; Perfume or cologne	
Longevity	Thyme, orange, clove, frankincense	Internally as Dietary Supplement	CS, SI, PH Dilute 1:4
M-Grain	Basil, marjoram, lavender, peppermint, Roman chamomile, helichrysum	DIFFUSE; Forehead, crown, shoulders, neck, temples; Vita Flex points; Massage	Dilute 1:1
Magnify Your Purpose	Sandalwood, rosewood, sage, nutmeg, patchouli, cinnamon bark, ginger	Vita Flex points; Feet, wrists, *temples*; Diffuse; Bath; Massage	E, P, CS, SI
Melrose	Melaleuca (*alternifolia* & *quinquenervia*), rosemary cineol, clove	Diffuse; Forehead, liver; Topically on location	CS, SI Dilute 1:1
Mister	Sage, fennel, lavender, myrtle, peppermint, yarrow (Carrier: Sesame seed oil)	Vita Flex points; Ankles, lower pelvis, prostate (dilute); Compress	P*, E
Motivation	Roman chamomile, spruce, ylang ylang, lavender	Diffuse; Chest, neck; *Solar plexus*, sternum, feet, navel, ears; wrists, palms; Perfume	
Oola Balance	Lavender, frankincense, ocotea, sandalwood, ylang ylang, orange, angelica, geranium, hyssop, sage, spruce, coriander, bergamot, lemon, jasmine, Roman chamomile, palmarosa, rose, balsam fir, myrrh, cistus, spikenard, blue spruce	Diffuse; Topically on location	P, PH* Dilute 1:1
Oola Grow	Ylang ylang, white fir, blue tansy, cedarwood, blue cypress, jasmine, galbanum, frankincense, sandalwood, lavender, cinnamon bark, rose, geranium, coriander, bergamot, neroli, Roman chamomile, spruce, rosewood, clary sage, juniper, Idaho tansy, orange (Carrier: Almond oil, fractionated coconut oil)	Diffuse; Topically where desired	P, PH* Dilute 1:1

Quick Reference Guide for Using Essential Oils

Blend Name	Single Oil Contents	Uses/Application Areas	Safety Data
PanAway	Wintergreen, helichrysum, clove, peppermint	Compress on spine; Vita Flex on feet; Topically on location	Dilute 1:1
Peace & Calming	Tangerine, orange, ylang ylang, patchouli, blue tansy	Diffuse; Navel, nose, neck, feet; Bath; Perfume	PH
Present Time	Neroli, spruce, ylang ylang (Carrier: Almond oil)	*Thymus*; Neck, forehead	
Purification	Citronella, lemongrass, rosemary cineol, melaleuca, lavandin, myrtle	Diffuse; Vita Flex points; Ears, feet, temples; Topically on location	CS, SI
Raven	Ravensara, lemon, wintergreen, peppermint, *Eucalyptus radiata*	Diffuse; Vita Flex points; Lungs, throat; Pillow; Suppository (diluted)	SI Dilute 1:1
RC	Eucalyptus (*E. globulus*), myrtle, pine, marjoram, *Eucalyptus radiata*, *Eucalyptus citriodora*, lavender, cypress, tsuga, peppermint	DIFFUSE; Chest, back, feet; Sinuses, nasal passages; Ears, neck, throat; Compress; Massage	
Reconnect	Sacred frankincense, bergamot, myrrh, lavender, geranium, blue cypress, royal Hawaiian sandalwood, ylang ylang, cedarwood, rosewood, melissa, Idaho blue spruce, spruce, hyssop, rose (Carrier: Coconut oil, sweet almond oil)	Diffuse; Topically where desired	PH*, SI Dilute 1:1
Release	Ylang ylang, lavandin, geranium, sandalwood, blue tansy (Carrier: Olive oil)	*Compress on liver*; Ears, feet, Vita Flex points; Perfume	Dilute 1:1
Relieve It	Spruce, Black pepper, hyssop, peppermint	Apply on location of pain	SI, P, E, HBP Dilute 1:1
RutaVaLa	Ruta, valerian, lavender	***Aromatic Use Only!*** Diffuse; Direct inhalation	P*, PH*
Sacred Mountain	Spruce, ylang ylang, fir, cedarwood	Diffuse; *Solar plexus, brain stem*, crown, neck, ears, thymus, wrists; Perfume	SI
SARA	Ylang ylang, geranium, lavender, orange, blue tansy, cedarwood, rose, white lotus (Carrier: Almond oil)	*Energy centers*; Vita Flex points; *Temples, nose*; Places of abuse	
SclarEssence	Clary sage, peppermint, sage lavender, fennel	Internally as dietary supplement	
Sensation	Rosewood, ylang ylang, jasmine	Diffuse; Apply on location; Massage; Bath	

Blend Name	Single Oil Contents	Uses/Application Areas	Safety Data
Shutran	Idaho blue spruce, ocotea, hinoki, ylang ylang, coriander, davana, cedarwood, lemon, lavender	Cologne	PH*
Stress Away *(Roll-on)*	Copaiba, lime, cedarwood, ocotea, lavender	Wrists, temples, neck; Other desired areas	P, SI
Surrender	Lavender, Roman chamomile, German chamomile, angelica, mountain savory, lemon, spruce	*Forehead, rim of ears, nape of neck, chest, solar plexus*; Bath	P, SI
The Gift	Frankincense, balsam fir, jasmine, galbanum, myrrh, cistus, spikenard	Diffuse; Skin, wound location, feet, temples, neck; Bath	SI, P
Thieves	Clove, lemon, cinnamon bark, *Eucalyptus radiata*, rosemary cineol	Diffuse; Feet, throat, stomach, intestines; Thymus, arm pits (Dilute well for topical uses!)	CS*, SI, P Dilute 1:4
3 Wise Men	Sandalwood, juniper, frankincense, spruce, myrrh (Carrier: Almond oil)	Diffuse; *Crown of head*; Neck, forehead, solar plexus, thymus; Perfume	
Tranquil *(Roll-on)*	Lavender, cedarwood, Roman chamomile (Carriers: Fractionated coconut oil and virgin coconut oil)	Forehead, temples, neck, wrists	
Transformation	Lemon, pepperming, clary sage, sandalwood, Idaho blue spruce, sacred frankincense, cardamom, palo santo, ocotea	Diffuse; *Forehead, heart*	
Trauma Life	Frankincense, sandalwood, valerian, lavender, davana, spruce, geranium, helichrysum, *Citrus hystrix* (leech lime), rose	Diffuse; Spine; Feet, chest, ears, neck, forehead	
T.R. Care	Blue cypress, ylang ylang, lavender, Roman chamomile, tangerine, jasmine, royal Hawaiian sandalwood, bergamot, frankincense, cedarwood, geranium, valerian, galbanum, spruce, orange, blue tansy, white fir, davana, *Ruta graveolens* (rue), angelica, helichrysum, hyssop, Spanish sage, limette (combova), cinnamon bark, coriander, lemon, rose	Diffuse; Topically where desired	P, PH*
Valor	Spruce, rosewood, blue tansy, frankincense (Carrier: Almond oil)	*FEET*; Diffuse; Heart, wrists, solar plexus, neck to thymus, spine; Perfume	
Valor *(Roll-on)*	Spruce, rosewood, frankincense, blue tansy (Carriers: Fractionated coconut oil and virgin coconut oil)	Wrists, solar plexus, neck, spine	

Blend Name	Single Oil Contents	Uses/Application Areas	Safety Data
White Angelica	Bergamot, geranium, myrrh, sandalwood, rosewood, ylang ylang, spruce, hyssop, melissa, rose (Carrier: Almond oil)	Diffuse; *Shoulders*, crown, chest, ears, neck, forehead, wrists; Bath; Perfume	PH*

Note: Italicized application areas represent the most effective areas for **emotional applications**.

Safety Data Legend:

A   **Avoid** during and after consumption of **alcohol**

CS   Could possibly result in **contact sensitization** (redness or irritation of the skin due to repeated application of a substance) (rotate or use different oils)

CS*   Repeated use may result in **extreme contact sensitization** (rotate between different oils)

D   **Avoid** if **diabetic**

E   Use with **caution** if susceptible to **epilepsy** (small amounts or in dilution)

E*   **Avoid** if susceptible to **epilepsy** (can trigger a seizure)

HBP   Use with **caution** if dealing with **high blood pressure** (small amounts)

HBP*   **Avoid** if dealing with **high blood pressure**

P   Use with **caution** during **pregnancy** (small amounts or in dilution)

P*   **Avoid** during **pregnancy**

PH   **Photosensitivity**–direct exposure to sunlight after use could cause dermatitis (test first)

PH*   **Extreme Photosensitivity**–direct exposure to sunlight after use can cause severe dermatitis (avoid exposing affected area of skin to direct sunlight for 12 hours)

SI   Could possibly result in **skin irritation** (dilution may be necessary)

SI*   Can cause **extreme skin irritation** (dilution highly recommended)

ST   Can cause **stupefication** in high doses (use only small amounts or in dilution)

Dilute - Dilution ratios shown equal Essential Oil:Vegetable Oil

RESEARCH REFERENCES

Abagli, A. Z., Alavo, T. B., Avlessi, F., & Moudachirou, M. (2012). Potential of the bush mint, Hyptis suaveolens essential oil for personal protection against mosquito biting. J Am Mosq Control Assoc, 28(1), 15-19.

Abdel-Sattar E, Zaitoun AA, Farag MA, El Gayed SH, Harraz FM (2009 Feb 25). "Chemical composition, insecticidal and insect repellent activity of Schinus molle L. leaf and fruit essential oils against Trogoderma granarium and Tribolium castaneum," Nat Prod Res. Epub ahead of print:1-10.

Abrams SA, Griffin IJ, Hawthorne KM, Liang L, Gunn SK, Darlington G, Ellis KJ (2005 Aug). "A combination of prebiotic short- and long-chain inulin-type fructans enhances calcium absorption and bone mineralization in young adolescents," Am J Clin Nutr. 82(2):471-6.

Agrawal, P., Rai, V., & Singh, R. B. (1996 Sep). Randomized placebo-controlled, single blind trial of holy basil leaves in patients with noninsulin-dependent diabetes mellitus. Int J Clin Pharmacol Ther, 34(9), 406-409.

Al-Ali, K. H., El-Beshbishy, H. A., El-Badry, A. A., & Alkhalaf, M. (2013 Dec). Cytotoxic activity of methanolic extract of Mentha longifolia and Ocimum basilicum against human breast cancer. Pak J Biol Sci, 16(23), 1744-1750.

Alexandrovich I, Rakovitskaya O, Kolmo E, Sidorova T, Shushunov S (2003 Jul-Aug). "The effect of fennel (Foeniculum Vulgare) seed oil emulsion in infantile colic: a randomized, placebo-controlled study," Altern Ther Health Med. 9(4):58-61.

Al-Howiriny, T., Alsheikh, A., Alqasoumi, S., Al-Yahya, M., ElTahir, K., & Rafatullah, S. (2009 Aug). Protective Effect of Origanum majorana L. 'Marjoram' on various models of gas-tric mucosal injury in rats. Am J Chin Med, 37(3), 531-545.

Ali, S. A., Rizk, M. Z., Ibrahim, N. A., Abdallah, M. S., Sharara, H. M., & Moustafa, M. M. (2010 Dec). Protective role of Juniperus phoenicea and Cupressus sempervirens against CCl(4). World J Gastrointest Pharmacol Ther, 1(6), 123-131.

Almela L, Sánchez-Muñoz B, Fernández-López JA, Roca MJ, Rabe V (2006 Jul). "Liquid chromatograpic-mass spectrometric analysis of phenolics and free radical scavenging activity of rosemary extract from different raw material," J Chromatogr A. 1120(1-2):221-9.

al-Zuhair H, el-Sayeh B, Ameen HA, al-Shoora H (1996 Jul-Aug). "Pharmacological studies of cardamom oil in animals," Pharmacol Res. 34(1-2):79-82.

An, B. S., Kang, J. H., Yang, H., Jung, E. M., Kang, H. S., Choi, I. G., ... Jeung, E. B. (2013). Anti-inflammatory effects of essential oils from Chamaecyparis obtusa via the cyclooxygenase-2 pathway in rats. Mol Med Rep, 8(1), 255-259.

Anderson R.C., Krueger N.A., Byrd J.A., Harvey R.B., Callaway T.R., Edrington T.S., Nisbet D.J. (2009) Effects of thymol and diphenyliodonium chloride against Campylobacter spp. during pure and mixed culture in vitro. Journal of Applied Microbiology. 107: 1258-1268.

Andrews R.E., Parks L.W., Spence K.D. (1980) Some Effects of Douglas Fir Terpenes on Certain Microorganisms. Applied and Environmental Microbiology. 40: 301-304.

Andrian E., Grenier D., Rouabhia M. (2006) Porphyromonas gingivalis-Epithelial Cell Interactions in Periodontitis. Journal of Dental Research. 85: 392-403.

Appendino G, Ottino M, Marquez N, Bianchi F, Giana A, Ballero M, Sterner O, Fiebich BL, Munoz E (2007 Apr). "Arzanol, an anti-inflammatory and anti-HIV-1 phloroglucinol alpha-Pyrone from Helichrysum italicum ssp. microphyllum," J Nat Prod. 70(4):608-12.

Arasada BL, Bommareddy A, Zhang X, Bremmon K, Dwivedi C. (2008 Jan-Feb). "Effects of alpha-santalol on proapoptotic caspases and p53 expression in UVB irradiated mouse skin," Anticancer Res. 28(1A):129-32.

Arias P., Cudeiro J. (2008) Effects of rhythmic sensory stimulation (auditory, visual) on gait in Parkinson's disease patients. Experimental Brain Research. 186: 589-601.

Ariyoshi T., Arakaki M., Ideguchi K., Ishizuka Y. (1975) Studies on the Metabolism of d-Limonene (?-Mentha-1,8-diene). III. Effects of d-Limonene on the Lipids and Drug-Metabolizing Enzmes in Rat Livers. Xenobiotica. 5: 33-38.

Asensio, C. M., Nepote, V., & Grosso, N. R. (2011 Sep). Chemical stability of extra-virgin olive oil added with oregano essential oil. J Food Sci, 76(7), S445-450.

Atkinson D.C., Hicks R. (1971) Relationship between the anti-inflammatory and irritant properties of inflammatory exudate. British Journal of Pharmacology. 41: 480-487.

Auffray, B. (2007 Feb). Protection against singlet oxygen, the main actor of sebum squalene peroxidation during sun exposure, using Commiphora myrrha essential oil. Int J Cosmet Sci, 29(1), 23-29.

Awale, S., Tohda, C., Tezuka, Y., Miyazaki, M., & Kadota, S. (2011). Protective Effects of Rosa damascena and Its Active Constituent on Abeta(25-35)-Induced Neuritic Atrophy. Evid Based Complement Alternat Med, 2011, 1-8.

Badia P, Wesensten N, Lammers W, Culpepper J, Harsh J (1990 Jul). "Responsiveness to olfactory stimuli presented in sleep," Physiol Behav. 48(1):87-90.

Bahramikia, S., & Yazdanparast, R. (2009 Aug). Efficacy of different fractions of Anethum graveolens leaves on serum lipoproteins and serum and liver oxidative status in ex-perimentally induced hypercholesterolaemic rat models. Am J Chin Med, 37(4), 685-699.

Bakirel T, Bakirel U, Keleş OU, Ulgen SG, Yardibi H (2008 Feb 28). "In vivo assessment of antidiabetic and antioxidant activities of rosemary (Rosmarinus officinalis) in alloxan-diabetic rabbits," J Ethnopharmacol. 116(1):64-73.

Bakkai F., Averbeck S., Averbeck D., Idaomar M. (2008) Biological effects of essential oils - A review. Food and Chemical Toxicology. 46: 446-475.

Balanehru S., Nagarajan B. (1991) Protective Effect of Oleanolic Acid and Ursolic Acid Against Lipid Peroxidation. Biochemistry International. 24: 981-990.

Balestrieri, E., Pizzimenti, F., Ferlazzo, A., Giofre, S. V., Iannazzo, D., Piperno, A., . . . Macchi, B. (2011 Mar). Antiviral activity of seed extract from Citrus bergamia towards human retroviruses. Bioorg Med Chem, 19(6), 2084-2089.

Ballabeni V, Tognolini M, Giorgio C, Bertoni S, Bruni R, Barocelli E (2009 Oct 13). "Ocotea quixos Lam. essential oil: In vitro and in vivo investigation on its anti-inflammatory properties," Fitoterapia. Epub ahead of print.

Balzer J, Rassaf T, Heiss C, Kleinbongard P, Lauer T, Merx M, Heussen N, Gross HB, Keen CL, Schroeter H, Kelm M (2008 Jun 3). "Sustained benefits in vascular function through flavanol-containing cocoa in medicated diabetic patients a double-masked, randomized, controlled trial," J Am Coll Cardiol. 51(22):2141-9.

Banerjee S, Ecavade A, Rao AR (1993 Feb). "Modulatory influence of sandalwood oil on mouse hepatic glutathione S-transferase activity and acid soluble sulphydryl level," Cancer Lett. 68(2-3):105-9.

Bani, S., Hasanpour, S., Mousavi, Z., Mostafa Garehbaghi, P., & Gojazadeh, M. (2014 Jan). The Effect of Rosa Damascena Extract on Primary Dysmenorrhea: A Double-blind Cross-over Clinical Trial. Iran Red Crescent Med J, 16(1), 1-6.

Banno N, Akihisa T, Yasukawa K, Tokuda H, Tabata K, Nakamura Y, Nishimura R, Kimura Y, Suzuki T (2006 Sep 19). "Anti-inflammatory activities of the triterpene acids from the resin of Boswellia carterii," J Ethnopharmacol. 107(2):249-53.

Barthelman M., Chen W., Gensler H.L., Huang C., Dong Z., Bowden G.T. (1998) Inhibitory Effects of Perillyl Alcohol on UVB-induced Murine Skin Cancer and AP-1 Transactivation. Cancer Research. 58: 711-716.

Basketter D.A., Wright Z.M., Colson N.R., Patewicz G.Y., Pease C.K.S. (2002) Investigation of the skin sensitizing activity of linalool. Contact Dermatitis. 47: 161-164.

Bastos J.F.A., Moreira I.J., Ribeiro T.P., Medeiros I.A., Antoniolli A.R., de Sousa D.P., Santos M.R.V. (2009) Hypotensive and Vasorelaxant Effects of Cirtonellol, a Monoterpene Alcohol, in Rats. Basic & Clinical Pharmacology & Toxicology. 106: 331-337.

Batista, P. A., Werner, M. F., Oliveira, E. C., Burgos, L., Pereira, P., Brum, L. F., . . . Santos, A. R. (2010 Nov). The antinociceptive effect of (-)-linalool in models of chronic inflammatory and neuropathic hypersensitivity in mice. J Pain, 11(11), 1222-1229.

Behnam S, Farzaneh M, Ahmadzadeh M, Tehrani AS (2006). "Composition and antifungal activity of essential oils of Mentha piperita and Lavandula angustifolia on post-harvest phytopathogens," Commun Agric Appl Biol Sci. 71(3 Pt B):1321-6.

Berchtold N.C., Cotman C.W. (1997) Evolution in the Conceptulization of Dementia and Alzheimer's Disease: Greco-Roman Period to the 1960s. Neurobiology of Aging. 19: 173-189.

Berić T, Nikolić B, Stanojević J, Vuković-Gacić B, Knezević-Vukcević J (2008 Feb). "Protective effect of basil (Ocimum basilicum L.) against oxidative DNA damage and mutagenesis," Food Chem Toxicol. 46(2):724-32.

Bezanilla F. (2006) The action potential: From voltage-gated conductances to molecular structures. Biological Research. 39: 425-435.

Birari R.B., Bhutani K.K. (2007) Pancreatic lipase inhibitors from natural sources: unexplored potential. Drug Discovery Today. 12: 879-889.

Bone ME, Wilkinson DJ, Young JR, McNeil J, Charlton S (1990 Aug). "Ginger root--a new antiemetic. The effect of ginger root on postoperative nausea and vomiting after major gynaecological surgery," Anaesthesia. 45(8):669-71.

Bora, K. S., Arora, S., & Shri, R. (2011 Oct). Role of Ocimum basilicum L. in prevention of ischemia and reperfusion-induced cerebral damage, and motor dysfunctions in mice brain. J Ethnopharmacol, 137(3), 1360-1365.

Borgatti, M., Mancini, I., Bianchi, N., Guerrini, A., Lampronti, I., Rossi, D., . . . Gambari, R. (2011 Apr). Bergamot (Citrus bergamia Risso) fruit extracts and identified components alter expression of interleukin 8 gene in cystic fibrosis bronchial epithelial cell lines. BMC Biochem, 12, 15.

Bouwstra J.A., Gooris G.S., Dubbelaar F.E.R., Weeheim A.M., Ijzerman A.P., Ponec M. (1998) Role of ceramide 1 in the molecular organization of the stratum corneum lipids. Journal of Lipid Research. 39: 186-196.

Bradford H.F. (1995) Glutamate, GABA, and Epilepsy. Progress in Neurobiology. 47: 477-511.

Bradley BF, Brown SL, Chu S, Lea RW (2009 Jun). "Effects of orally administered lavender essential oil on responses to anxiety-provoking film clips," Hum Psychopharmacol. 24(4):319-30.

Brady A, Loughlin R, Gilpin D, Kearney P, Tunney M (2006 Oct). "In vitro activity of tea-tree oil against clinical skin isolates of methicillin-resistant and -sensitive Staphylococcus aureus and coagulase-negative staphylococci growing planktonically and as biofilms," J Med Microbiol. 55(Pt 10):1375-80.

Brand C, Grimbaldeston MA, Gamble JR, Drew J, Finlay-Jones JJ, Hart PH (2002 May). "Tea tree oil reduces the swelling associated with the efferent phase of a contact hypersensitivity response," Inflamm Res. 51(5):236-44.

Brum LF, Elisabetsky E, Souza D (2001 Aug). "Effects of linalool on [(3)H]MK801 and [(3)H] muscimol binding in mouse cortical membranes," Phytother Res. 15(5):422-5.

Buchbauer G, Jirovetz L, Jäger W, Dietrich H, Plank C (1991 Nov-Dec). "Aromatherapy: evidence for sedative effects of the essential oil of lavender after inhalation," Z Naturforsch [C]. 46(11-12):1067-72.

Bukovska, A., Cikos, S., Juhas, S., Il'kova, G., Rehak, P., & Koppel, J. (2007 Feb). Effects of a combination of thyme and oregano essential oils on TNBS-induced colitis in mice. Mediators Inflamm, 2007, 23296.

Bulbring E. (1946) Observations on the Isolated Phrenic Nerve Diaphragm Preparation of the Rat. British Journal of Pharmacology. 1: 38-61.

Burke BE, Baillie JE, Olson RD (2004 May). "Essential oil of Australian lemon myrtle (Backhousia citriodora) in the treatment of molluscum contagiosum in children," Biomed Pharmacother. 58(4):245-7.

Burke Y.D., Stark J., Roach S.L., Sen S.E., Crowell P.L. (1997) Inhibition of Pancreatic Cancer Growth by the Dietary Isoprenoids Farnesol and Geraniol. Lipids. 32: 151-156.

Burt S. (2004) Essential oils: their antibacterial properties and potential applications in foods - a reivew. International Journal of Food Microbiology. 94: 223-253.

Caldefie-Chézef F, Fusillier C, Jarde T, Laroye H, Damez M, Vasson MP, Guillot J (2006 May). "Potential anti-inflammatory effects of Melaleuca alternifolia essential oil on human peripheral blood leukocytes," Phytother Res. 20(5):364-70.

Campelo, L. M., Goncalves, F. C., Feitosa, C. M., & de Freitas, R. M. (2011 Jul). Antioxidant activity of Citrus limon essential oil in mouse hippocampus. Pharm Biol, 49(7), 709-715.

Candan F, Unlu M, Tepe B, Daferera D, Polissiou M, Sökmen A, Akpulat HA (2003 Aug). "Antioxidant and antimicrobial activity of the essential oil and methanol extracts of Achillea millefolium subsp. millefolium Afan. (Asteraceae)," J Ethnopharmacol. 87(2-3):215-20.

Capasso R, Savino F, Capasso F (2007 Oct). "Effects of the herbal formulation ColiMil on upper gastrointestinal transit in mice in vivo," Phytother Res. 21(10):999-1101.

Carlsson L., Larsson A., Lindman H. (2009) Elevated levels of thymidine kinase 1 peptide in serum from patients with breast cancer. Upsala Journal of Medical Sciences. 114: 116-120.

Carnesecchi S., Bradaia A., Fischer B., Coelho D., Scholler-Guinard M., Gosse F., Raul F. (2002) Perturbation by Geraniol of Cell Membrane Permeability and Signal Transduction Pathways in Human Colon Cancer Cells. The Journal of Pharmacology and Experimental Therapeutics. 303: 711-715.

Carnesecchi S., Bras-Goncalves R., Bradaia A., Zeisel M., Gosse F., Poupon M-F., Raul F. (2004) Geraniol, a component of plant essential oils, modulates DNA synthesis and potentiates 5-fluorouracil efficacy on human colon tumor xenografts. Cancer Letters. 215: 53-59.

Carnesecchi S., Langley K., Exinger F., Gosse F., Raul F. (2002) Geraniol, a Component of Plant Essential Oils, Sensitizes Human Colonic Cancer Cells to 5-Flurouracil Treatment. The Journal of Pharmacology and Experimental Therapeutics. 301: 625-630.

Carnesecchi S, Schneider Y, Ceraline J, Duranton B, Gosse F, Seiler N, Raul F (2001 Jul). "Geraniol, a component of plant essential oils, inhibits growth and polyamine biosynthesis in human colon cancer cells," J Pharmacol Exp Ther. 298(1):197-200.

Carreras C.W., Santi D.V. (1995) The Catalytic Mechanism and Structure of Thymidylate Synthase. Anuual Review of Biochemistry. 64: 721-762.

Carroll M.C. (2004) The complement system in regulation of adaptive immunity. Nature Immunology. 5: 981-986.

Carvalho-Freitas MI, Costa M (2002 Dec). "Anxiolytic and sedative effects of extracts and essential oil from Citrus aurantium L," Biol Pharm Bull. 25(12):1629-33.

Cavalieri E., Bergamini C., Mariotto S., Leoni S., Perbellini G., Darra E., Suzuki H., Fato R., Lenaz G. (2009) Involvement of mitochondrial permeability transition pore opening in ?-bisabolol induced apoptosis. FEBS Journal. 276: 3990-4000.

Cavalieri E., Mariotto S., Fabrizi C., de Prati A.C., Gottardo R., Leone S., Berra L.V., Lauro G.M., Ciampa A.R., Suzuki H. (2004) ?-Bisabolol, a nontoxic natural compound, strongly induced apoptosis in glioma cells. Biochemical and Biophysical Research Communications. 315: 589-594.

Ceccarelli I, Lariviere WR, Fiorenzani P, Sacerdote P, Aloisi AM (2004 Mar 19). "Effects of long-term exposure of lemon essential oil odor on behavioral, hormonal and neuronal parameters in male and female rats," Brain Res. 1001(1-2):78-86.

Cenizo, V., Andre, V., Reymermier, C., Sommer, P., Damour, O., & Perrier, E. (2006 Aug). LOXL as a target to increase the elastin content in adult skin: a dill extract induces the LOXL gene expression. Exp Dermatol, 15(8), 574-581.

Cermelli, C., Fabio, A., Fabio, G., & Quaglio, P. (2008 Jan). Effect of eucalyptus essential oil on respiratory bacteria and viruses. Curr Microbiol, 56(1), 89-92.

Cháfer, M., Sanchez-Gonzalez, L., Gonzalez-Martinez, C., & Chiralt, A. (2012 Aug). Fungal decay and shelf life of oranges coated with chitosan and bergamot, thyme, and tea tree essential oils. J Food Sci, 77(8), E182-187.

Chaieb K, Zmantar T, Ksouri R, Hajlaoui H, Mahdouani K, Abdelly C, Bakhrouf A (2007 Sep). "Antioxidant properties of the essential oil of Eugenia caryophyllata and its antifungal activity against a large number of clinical Candida species," Mycoses. 50(5):403-6.

Chambers H.F. (2001) The Changing Epidemiology of Staphylococcus aureus?. Emerging Infectious Diseases. 7: 178-182.

Chang, K. S., Tak, J. H., Kim, S. I., Lee, W. J., & Ahn, Y. J. (2006 Nov). Repellency of Cinnamomum cassia bark compounds and cream containing cassia oil to Aedes aegypti (Diptera: Culicidae) under laboratory and indoor conditions. Pest Manag Sci, 62(11), 1032-1038.

Chapman A.G. (1998) Glutamate receptors in epilepsy. Progress in Brain Research. 116: 371-383.

Chapman A.G. (2000) Glutamate and Epilepsy. The Journal of Nutrition. 130: 1043S-1045S.

Charles CH, Vincent JW, Borycheski L, Amatnieks Y, Sarina M, Qaqish J, Proskin HM (2000 Sep). "Effect of an essential oil-containing dentifrice on dental plaque microbial composition," Am J Dent. 13:26C-30C.

Chen, Y., Zeng, H., Tian, J., Ban, X., Ma, B., & Wang, Y. (2014 Apr). Dill (Anethum graveolens L.) seed essential oil induces Candida albicans apoptosis in a metacaspase-dependent manner. Fungal Biol, 118(4), 394-401.

Cheung S, Tai J (2007 Jun). "Anti-proliferative and antioxidant properties of rosemary Rosmarinus officinalis," Oncol Rep. 17(6):1525-31.

Chien, L. W., Cheng, S. L., & Liu, C. F. (2012 Aug). The effect of lavender aromatherapy on autonomic nervous system in midlife women with insomnia. Evid Based Complement Alternat Med, 2012.

Chinou IB, Roussis V, Perdetzoglou D, Loukis A (1996 Aug). "Chemical and biological studies on two Helichrysum species of Greek origin," Planta Med. 62(4):377-9.

Cho, M. Y., Min, E. S., Hur, M. H., & Lee, M. S. (2013 Feb). Effects of aromatherapy on the anxiety, vital signs, and sleep quality of percutaneous coronary intervention patients in intensive care units. Evid Based Complement Alternat Med, 2013, 1-6.

Cho, S., Choi, Y., Park, S., & Park, T. (2012 Feb). Carvacrol prevents diet-induced obesity by modulating gene expressions involved in adipogenesis and inflammation in mice fed with high-fat diet. J Nutr Biochem, 23(2), 192-201.

Choi, H. Y., Yang, Y. C., Lee, S. H., Clark, J. M., & Ahn, Y. J. (2010 May). Efficacy of spray formulations containing binary mixtures of clove and eucalyptus oils against susceptible and pyrethroid/ malathion-resistant head lice (Anoplura: Pediculidae). J Med Entomol, 47(3), 387-391.

Chow H.H.S., Salazar D., Hakim I.A. (2002) Pharmacokinetics of Perillic Acid in Humans after a Single Dose Administration of a Citrus Preparation Rich in d-Limonene Content. Cancer Epidemiology, Biomarkers & Prevention. 11: 1472-1476.

Ciftci O., Ozdemir I., Tanyildizl S., Yildiz S., Oguzturk H. (2011) Antioxidative effects of curcumin, ?-myrcene and 1,8-cineole against 2,3,7,8-tetracholorodibenzo-p-dioxin - induced oxidative stress in rats liver. Toxicology and Industrial Health. 27: 447-453.

Cioanca, O., Hritcu, L., Mihasan, M., & Hancianu, M. (2013 Aug). Cognitive-enhancing and antioxidant activities of inhaled coriander volatile oil in amyloid beta(1-42) rat model of Alzheimer's disease. Physiol Behav, 120, 193-202.

Cioanca, O., Hritcu, L., Mihasan, M., Trifan, A., & Hancianu, M. (2014 May). Inhalation of co-riander volatile oil increased anxiolytic-antidepressant-like behaviors and decreased oxidative status in beta-amyloid (1-42) rat model of Alzheimer's disease. Physiol Be-hav, 131, 68-74.

Clericuzio M., Alagona G., Ghio C., Toma L. (2000) Ab Initio and Density Functional Evaluations of the Molecular Conformations of ?-Caryophyllene and 6-Hydroxycaryophyllene. Journal of Organic Chemistry. 65: 6910-6916.

Coderch L., Lopez O., de la Maza A., Parra J.L. (2003) Ceramides and Skin Function. American Journal of Clinical Dermatology. 4: 107-129.

Conti, B., Benelli, G., Flamini, G., Cioni, P. L., Profeti, R., Ceccarini, L., . . . Canale, A. (2012). Larvicidal and repellent activity of Hyptis suaveolens (Lamiaceae) essential oil against the mosquito Aedes albopictus Skuse (Diptera: Culicidae). Parasitol Res, 110(5), 2013-2021.

Contractor A., Swanson G.T., Sailer A., O'Gorman S., Heinemann S.F. (2000) Identification of the Kainate Receptor Subunits Underlying Modulation of Excitatory Synaptic Transmission in the CA3 Region of the Hippocampus. The Journal of Neuroscience. 20: 8260-8278.

Cooke B., Ernst E. (2000) Aromatherapy: a systematic review. British Journal of General Practice. 50: 493-496.

Corasaniti, M. T., Maiuolo, J., Maida, S., Fratto, V., Navarra, M., Russo, R., . . . Bagetta, G. (2007 Jun). Cell signaling pathways in the mechanisms of neuroprotection afforded by bergamot essential oil against NMDA-induced cell death in vitro. Br J Pharmacol, 151(4), 518-529.

Crestell T., Monsarrat B., Alvinerie P., Treluyer J.M., Vieira I., Wright M. (1994) Taxol Metabolism by Human Liver Microsomes: Identification of Cytochrome P450 Isozymes Involved in Its Biotransformation. Cancer Research. 54: 386-392.

Cross SE, Russell M, Southwell I, Roberts MS (2008 May). "Human skin penetration of the major components of Australian tea tree oil applied in its pure form and as a 20% solution in vitro," Eur J Pharm Biopharm. 69(1):214-22.

Crowell P.L. (1997) Monoterpenes in breast cancer chemoprevention. Breast Cancer Research and Treatment. 46: 191-197.

Crowell P.L. (1999) Prevention and Therapy of Cancer by Dietary Monoterpenes. J. Nutr. 129:775S-778S.

Crowell P.L., Chang R.R., Ren Z., Elson C.E., Gould M.N. (1991) Selective Inhibition of Isoprenylation of 21-26kDa Proteins by the Anticarcinogen d-Limonene and Its Metabolites. J. Biol. Chem. 266: 17679-17685.

Dadkhah, A., & Fatemi, F. (2011 Jul). Heart and kidney oxidative stress status in septic rats treated with caraway extracts. Pharm Biol, 49(7), 679-686.

D'Auria FD, Laino L, Strippoli V, Tecca M, Salvatore G, Battinelli L, Mazzanti G (2001 Aug). "In vitro activity of tea tree oil against Candida albicans mycelial conversion and other pathogenic fungi," J Chemother. 13(4):377-83.

Damiani C.E.N., Rossoni L.V., Vassallo D.V. (2003) Vasorelaxant effects of eugenol on rat thoracic aorta. Vascular Pharmacology. 40: 59-66. "

Darra E., Abdel-Azeim S., Manara A., Shoji K., Marechal J-D., Mariotto S., Cavalieri E., Perbellini L., Pizza C., Perahia D., Crimi M., Suzuki H. (2008) Insight into the apoptosis-inducing action of ?-bisabolol towards malignant tumor cells: Involvement of lipid rafts and Bid. Archives of Biochemistry and Biophysics. 476: 113-123.

de Almeida R.N., Araujo D.A.M., Goncalvevs J.C.R., Montenegro F.C., de Sousa D.P., Leite J.R., Mattei R., Benedito M.A.C., de Carvalho J.G.B., Cruz J.S., Maia J.G.S. (2009) Rosewood oil induces sedation and inhibits compound action petential in rodents. Journal of Ethanopharmacology. 124: 440-443.

de Almeida R.N., de Sousa D.P., Nobrega F.F.F., Claudino F.S., Araujo D.A.M., Leite J.R., Mattei R. (2008) Anticonvulsant effect of a natural compound ?,?-epoxy-carvone and its actioin on the nerve excitability. Neuroscience Letters. 443: 51-55.

de Araujo D.A.M., Freitas C., Cruz J.S. (2011) Essential oils components as a new path to understand ion channel molecular pharmacology. Life Sciences. doi: 10.1016/j.lfs.2011.04.020

Debersac P, Heydel JM, Amiot MJ, Goudonnet H, Artur Y, Suschetet M, Siess MH (2001 Sep). "Induction of cytochrome P450 and/or detoxication enzymes by various extracts of rosemary: description of specific patterns," Food Chem Toxicol. 39(9):907-18.

De Carvalho C.C.C.R., da Fonseca M.M.R. (2006) Carvone: Why and how should one bother to produce this terpene. Food Chemistry. 95: 413-422.

de Gruijl F.R. (1999) Skin Cancer and Solar UV Radiation. European Journal of Cancer. 35: 2003-2009.

de Sousa D.P. (2011) Analgesic-like Activity of Essential Oils Constituents. Molecules. 16: 2233-2252.

de Sousa D.P., Goncalves J.C.R., Quintanas-Junior L., Cruz J.S., Araujo D.A.M., de Almeida R.N. (2006) Study of anticonvulsant effect of citronellol, a monoterpene alcohol, in rodents. Neuroscience Letters. 401: 231-235.

Decker K. (1990) Biologically active products of stimulated liver macrophages (Kupffer cells). European Journal of Biochemistry. 192: 245-261.

DeLeo F.R., Otto M., Kreiswirth B.N., Chambers H.F. (2010) Community-associated meticillin-resistant Staphylococcus aureus. The Lancet. 375: 1557-1568.

De-Oliveira A.C.A.X., Ribeiro-Pinto L.F., Paumgartten F.J.R. (1997) In vitro inhibition of CYP2B1 monooxygenase by ?-myrcene and other monoterpenoid compounds. Toxicology Letters. 92: 39-46.

Derakhshan, S., Sattari, M., & Bigdeli, M. (2008). Effect of subinhibitory concentrations of cumin (Cuminum cyminum L.) seed essential oil and alcoholic extract on the morphol-ogy, capsule expression and urease activity of Klebsiella pneumoniae. International Journal of Antimicrobial Agents, 32(5), 432-436.

Dias, D. S., Fontes, L. B., Crotti, A. E., Aarestrup, B. J., Aarestrup, F. M., da Silva Filho, A. A., & Correa, J. O. (2014). Copaiba Oil Suppresses Inflammatory Cytokines in Splenocytes of C57Bl/6 Mice Induced with Experimental Autoimmune Encephalomyelitis (EAE). Molecules, 19(8), 12814-12826.

Díaz C, Quesada S, Brenes O, Aguilar G, Cicció JF (2008). "Chemical composition of Schinus molle essential oil and its cytotoxic activity on tumour cell lines," Nat Prod Res. 22(17):1521-34.

Dichter M.A. (1997) Basic Mechanisms of Epilepsy: Targets for Therapeutic Intervention. Epilepsia. 38: S2-S6.

Diggins K.C. (2008) Treatment of mild to moderate dehydration in children with oral rehydration therapy. Journal of the American Academy of Nurse Practitioners. 20: 402-406.

Dikshit A, Naqvi AA, Husain A. (1986 May). "Schinus molle: a new source of natural fungitoxicant," Appl Environ Microbiol. 51(5):1085-8.

Dimpfel W, Pischel I, Lehnfeld R (2004 Sep 29). "Effects of lozenge containing lavender oil, extracts from hops, lemon balm and oat on electrical brain activity of volunteers," Eur J Med Res. 9(9):423-31.

Dolder S., Hofstetter W., Wetterwald A., Muhlbauer R., Felix R. (2006) Effect of Monoterpenes on the Formation and Activation of Osteoclasts In Vitro. Journal of Bone and Mineral Research. 21: 647-655.

Dorman H.J.D., Deans S.G. (2000) Antimicrobial agents from plants: antibacterial activity of plant volatile oils. Journal of Applied Microbiology. 88: 308-316.

Duarte MC, Leme EE, Delarmelina C, Soares AA, Figueira GM, Sartoratto A (2007 May 4). "Activity of essential oils from Brazilian medicinal plants on Escherichia coli," J Ethnopharmacol. 111(2):197-201.

Dunn C, Sleep J, Collett D (1995 Jan). "Sensing an improvement: an experimental study to evaluate the use of aromatherapy, massage and periods of rest in an intensive care unit," J Adv Nurs. 21(1):34-40.

Dwivedi C, Guan X, Harmsen WL, Voss AL, Goetz-Parten DE, Koopman EM, Johnson KM, Valluri HB, Matthees DP (2003 Feb). "Chemopreventive effects of alpha-santalon on skin tumor development in CD-1 and SENCAR mice," Cancer Epidemiol Biomarkers Prev. 12(2):151-6.

Dwivedi C, Valluri HB, Guan X, Agarwal R (2006 Sep). "Chemopreventive effects of alpha-santalol on ultraviolet B radiation-induced skin tumor development in SKH-1 hairless mice," Carcinogenesis. 27(9):1917-22.

Edwards-Jones V, Buck R, Shawcross SG, Dawson MM, Dunn K (2004 Dec). "The effect of essential oils on methicillin-resistant Staphylococcus aureus using a dressing model," Burns. 30(8):772-7.

Enan E (2001 Nov). "Insecticidal activity of essential oils: octopaminergic sites of action," Comp Biochem Physiol C Toxicol Pharmacol. 130(3):325-37.

Engel J. (2001) A Proposed Diagnostic Scheme for People with Epileptic Seizures and with Epilepsy: Report of the ILAE Task Force on Classification and Terminology. Epilepsia. 42: 796-803.

Eriksson K., Levin J.O. (1996) Gas chromatographic-mass spectrometric identification of metabolites from ?-pinene in human urine after occupational exposure to sawing fumes. J. Chromatography B. 677: 85-98.

Esfandiary, E., Karimipour, M., Mardani, M., Alaei, H., Ghannadian, M., Kazemi, M., . . . Esmaeili, A. (2014 Apr). Novel effects of Rosa damascena extract on memory and neurogenesis in a rat model of Alzheimer's disease. J Neurosci Res, 92(4), 517-530.

Evandri MG, Battinelli L, Daniele C, Mastrangelo S, Bolle P, Mazzanti G (2005 Sep). "The antimutagenic activity of Lavandula angustifolia (lavender) essential oil in the bacterial reverse mutation assay," Food Chem Toxicol. 43(9):1381-7.

Evans J.D., Martin S.A. (2000) Effects of Thymol on Ruminal Microorganisms. Current Microbiology. 41: 336-340.

Fan AY, Lao L, Zhang RX, Zhou AN, Wang LB, Moudgil KD, Lee DY, Ma ZZ, Zhang WY, Berman BM (2005 Oct 3). "Effects of an acetone extract of Boswellia carterii Birdw. (Burseraceae) gum resin on adjuvant-induced arthritis in lewis rats," J Ethnopharmacol. 101(1-3):104-9.

Fang, R., Jiang, C. H., Wang, X. Y., Zhang, H. M., Liu, Z. L., Zhou, L., . . . Deng, Z. W. (2010 Dec). Insecticidal activity of essential oil of Carum Carvi fruits from China and its main components against two grain storage insects. Molecules, 15(12), 9391-9402.

Faturi, C. B., Leite, J. R., Alves, P. B., Canton, A. C., & Teixeira-Silva, F. (2010 May). Anxiolytic-like effect of sweet orange aroma in Wistar rats. Prog Neuropsychopharmacol Biol Psychiatry, 34(4), 605-609.

Fearon D.T., Locksley R.M. (1996) The Instructive Role of Innate Immunity in the Acquired Immune Response. Science. 272: 50-54.

Fernandez, L. F., Palomino, O. M., & Frutos, G. (2014 Jan). Effectiveness of Rosmarinus of-ficinalis essential oil as antihypotensive agent in primary hypotensive patients and its influence on health-related quality of life. J Ethnopharmacol, 151(1), 509-516.

Ferrante M, Andreeta A, Landoni MF (2009 Oct 6). "Effect of different penetration enhancers on diclofenac permation across horse skin," Vet J. (Epub ahead of print).

Ferrara, L., Naviglio, D., & Armone Caruso, A. (2012). Cytological aspects on the effects of a nasal spray consisting of standardized extract of citrus lemon and essential oils in allergic rhinopathy. ISRN Pharm, 2012, 1-6.

Ferreira-da-Silva F.V., Barbosa R., Moreira-Junior L., dos Santos-Nascimento T., de Oliveira-Martins M.D., Coelho-de-Souza A.N., Cavalcante F.S.A., Ceccatto V.M., de Lemos T.L.G., Magalhaes P.J.C., Lahlou S., Leal-Cardoso J.H. (2009) Effects of 1,8-Cineole on Electrophysiological Parameters of Neurons of the Rat Superior Cervical Ganglion. Clinical and Experimental Pharamacology and Physiology. 36: 1068-1073.

Ferrini AM, Mannoni V, Aureli P, Salvatore G, Piccirilli E, Ceddia T, Pontieri E, Sessa R, Oliva B (2006 Jul-Sep). "Melaleuca alternifolia essential oil possesses potent anti-staphylococcal activity extended to strains resistant to antibiotics," Int J Immunopathol Pharmacol. 19(3):539-44.

Filoche SK, Soma K, Sissons CH (2005 Aug). "Antimicrobial effects of essential oils in combination with chlorhexidine digluconate," Oral Microbiol Immunol. 20(4):221-5.

Force M, Sparks WS, Ronzio RA (2000 May). "Inhibition of enteric parasites by emulsified oil of oregano in vivo," Phytother Res. 14(3):213-4.

Fraternale, D., Flamini, G., & Ricci, D. (2014 May). Essential Oil Composition and Antimicrobial Activity of Angelica archangelica L. (Apiaceae) Roots. J Med Food.

Freitas F.P., Freitas S.P., Lemos G.C.S., Vieira I.J.C., Gravina G.A., Lemos F.J.A. (2010) Comparative Larvicial Activity of Essential Oils from Three Medicinal Plants against Aedes aeypti L. Chemistry & Biodiversity. 7: 2801-2807.

Freitas J.C.B.R., Presgrave O.A.F., Fingola F.F., Menezes M.A.C., Paumgartten F.J.R. (1993) Effect of ?-myrcene on pentobarbital sleeping time. Brazilian Journal of Medicine and Biological Research. 26: 519-523.

Fujisawa S., Atsumi T., Kadoma Y., Sakagami H. (2002) Antioxidant and prooxidant action of eugenol-related compounds and their cytotoxicity. Toxicology. 177: 39-54.

Fukumoto S, Sawasaki E, Okuyama S, Miyake Y, Yokogoshi H (2006 Feb-Apr). "Flavor components of monoterpenes in citrus essential oils enhance the release of monoamines from rat brain slices," Nutr Neurosci. 9(1-2):73-80.

Frydman-Marom, A., Levin, A., Farfara, D., Benromano, T., Scherzer-Attali, R., Peled, S., . . . Ovadia, M. (2011 Feb). Orally administered cinnamon extract reduces beta-amyloid oligomerization and corrects cognitive impairment in Alzheimer's disease animal models. PLoS ONE, 6(1), 1-11.

Gaetani G.F., Ferraris A.M., Rolfo M., Mangerini R., Arena S., Kirkman H.N. (1996) Predominant role of catalase in the disposal of hydrogen peroxide within human erythrocytes. Blood. 87: 1595-1599.

Gaunt L.F., Higgins S.C., Hughes J.F. (2005) Interaction of air ions and bactericidal vapours to control micro-organisms. Journal of Applied Microbiology. 99: 1324-1329.

Gbenou, J. D., Ahounou, J. F., Akakpo, H. B., Laleye, A., Yayi, E., Gbaguidi, F., . . . Kotchoni, S. O. (2013). Phytochemical composition of Cymbopogon citratus and Eucalyptus citriodora essential oils and their anti-inflammatory and analgesic properties on Wistar rats. Mol Biol Rep, 40(2), 1127-1134.

Gehrmann J., Matsumoto Y., Kreutzberg G.W. (1995) Microglia: intrinsic immuneffector cell of the brain. Brain Research Reviews. 20: 269-287.

Gertsch J. (2008) Anti-inflammatory cannabinoids in diet. Communicative & Integrative Biology. 1: 26-28.

Gertsch J., Leonti M., Raduner S., Racz I., Chen J-Z., Xie X-Q., Altmann K-H., Karsak M., Zimmer A. (2008) Beta-caryophyllene is a dietary cannabinoid. Proceedings of the National Academy of Sciences. 105: 9099-9104.

Ghelardini C, Galeotti N, Di Cesare Mannelli L, Mazzanti G, Bartolini A (2001 May-Jul). "Local anaesthetic activity of beta-caryophyllene," Farmaco. 56(5-7):387-9.

Ghelardini C, Galeotti N, Salvatore G, Mazzanti G (1999 Dec). "Local anaesthetic activity of the essential oil of Lavandula angustifolia," Planta Med. 65(8):700-3.

Goes, T. C., Antunes, F. D., Alves, P. B., & Teixeira-Silva, F. (2012 Aug). Effect of sweet orange aroma on experimental anxiety in humans. J Altern Complement Med, 18(8), 798-804.

Golab M, Skwarlo-Sonta K (2007 Mar). "Mechanisms involved in the anti-inflammatory action of inhaled tea tree oil in mice," Exp Biol Med (Maywood). 232(3):420-6.

Gomes-Carneiro M.R., Dias D.M.M., De-Oliveira A.C.A.X., Paumgartten F.J.R. (2005) Evaluation of mutagenic and antimutagenic activities of ?-bisabolol in the Salmonella/microsome assay. Genetic Toxicology and Environmental Mutagenesis. 585: 105-112.

Gómez-Rincón, C., Langa, E., Murillo, P., Valero, M. S., Berzosa, C., & López, V. (2014 May). Activity of Tea Tree (Melaleuca alternifolia) Essential Oil against L3 Larvae of Anisakis simplex. 2014, 1-6.

Goncalves J.C.R., Alves A.M.H., de Araujo A.E.V., Cruz J.S., Araujo D.A.M. (2010) Distinct effects of carvone analogues on the isolated nerve of rats. European Journal of Pharmacology. 645: 108-112.

Goncalves J.C.R., Oliveira F.S., Benedito R.B., de Sousa D.P., de Almeida R.N., Araujo D.A.M. (2008) Antinociceptive Activity of (-)-Carvone: Evidence of Association with Decreased Peripheral Nerve Excitability. Biological and Parmaceutical Bulletin. 31: 1017-1020.

González-Trujano ME, Peña EI, Martínez AL, Moreno J, Guevara-Fefer P, Déciga-Campos M, López-Muñoz FJ (2007 May 22). "Evaluation of the antinociceptive effect of Rosmarinus officinalis L. using three different experimental models in rodents," J Ethnopharmacol. 111(3):476-82.

Goodwin J.S., Atluru D., Sierakowski S., Lianos E.A. (1986) Mechanism of Action of Glucocorticosteroids: Inhibition of T Cell Proliferation and Interleukin 2 Production by Hydrocortisones Is Reversed by Leukotriene B4. Journal of Clinical Investigation. 77: 1244-1250.

Gorwitz R.J., Kruszon-Moran D., McAllister S.K., McQuillan G., McDougal L.K., Fosheim G.E., Jensen B.J., Killgore G., Tenover F.C., Kuehnert M.J. (2008) Changes in the Prevalence of Nasal Colonization with Staphylococcus aureusin the United States, 2001-2004. Journal of Infectious Diseases. 197: 1226-1234.

Grassmann J, Hippeli S, Dornisch K, Rohnert U, Beuscher N, Elstner EF (2000 Feb). "Antioxidant properties of essential oils. Possible explanations for their anti-inflammatory effects," Arzneimittelforschung. 50(2):135-9.

Grespan, R., Paludo, M., Lemos Hde, P., Barbosa, C. P., Bersani-Amado, C. A., Dalalio, M. M., & Cuman, R. K. (2012 Oct). Anti-arthritic effect of eugenol on collagen-induced arthritis experimental model. Biol Pharm Bull, 35(10), 1818-1820.

Griesmacher A., Kindhauser M., Andert S.E., Schreiner W., Toma C., Knoebl P., Pietschmann P., Prager R., Schnack C., Schernthaner G., Mueller M.M. (1995) Enhanced Serum Levels of Thiobarbituric-Acid-Reactve Substances in Diabetes Mellitus. The American Journal of Medicine. 98: 469-475.

Grigoleit HG, Grigoleit P (2005 Aug). "Peppermint oil in irritable bowel syndrome," Phytomedicine. 12(8):601-6.

Gross, M., Nesher, E., Tikhonov, T., Raz, O., & Pinhasov, A. (2013 Mar). Chronic food administration of Salvia sclarea oil reduces animals' anxious and dominant behavior. J Med Food, 16(3), 216-222.

Gundidza M (1993 Nov). "Antimicrobial activity of essential oil from Schinus molle Linn," Cent Afr J Med. 39(11):231-4.

Guo X., Longnecker M.P., Michalek J.E. (2001) Relation of serum tetrachlorodibenzo-p-dioxin concentration to diet among veterans in the Air Force health study with background-level exposure. Journal of Toxicology and Environmental Health, Part A. 63: 159-172.

Gupta A., Myrdal P.B. (2004) Development of perillyl alcohol topical cream formulation. Internation Journal of Pharmaceutics. 269: 373-383.

Gurney A.M. (1994) Mechanisms of Drug-induced Vasodilation. Journal of Pharmacy and Pharmacology. 46: 242-251.

Haag J.D., Lindstrom M.J., Gould M.N. (1992) Limonene-induced Regression of Mammary Carcinomas. Cancer Research. 52: 4021-4026.

Haghparast, A., Shams, J., Khatibi, A., Alizadeh, A.-M., & Kamalinejad, M. (2008). Effects of the fruit essential oil of Cuminum cyminum Linn. (Apiaceae) on acquisition and expression of morphine tolerance and dependence in mice. Neurosci Lett, 440(2), 134-139.

Hajhashemi V, Abbasi N (2008 Mar). "Hypolipidemic activity of Anethum graveolens in rats," Phytother Res. 22(3):372-5.

Hakim IA, Harris RB, Ritenbaugh C (2000). "Citrus peel use is associated with reduced risk of squamous cell carcinoma of the skin," Nutr Cancer. 37(2):161-8.

Halder, S., Mehta, A. K., Kar, R., Mustafa, M., Mediratta, P. K., & Sharma, K. K. (2011 May). Clove oil reverses learning and memory deficits in scopolamine-treated mice. Planta Med, 77(8), 830-834.

Halder, S., Mehta, A. K., Mediratta, P. K., & Sharma, K. K. (2011 Aug). Essential oil of clove (Eugenia caryophyllata) augments the humoral immune response but decreases cell mediated immunity. Phytother Res, 25(8), 1254-1256.

Han, S. H., Hur, M. H., Buckle, J., Choi, J., & Lee, M. S. (2006 Aug). Effect of aromatherapy on symptoms of dysmenorrhea in college students: A randomized placebo-controlled clinical trial. J Altern Complement Med, 12(6), 535-541.

Hammer KA, Carson CF, Riley TV (1996 Jun). "Susceptibility of transient and commensal skin flora to the essential oil of Melaleuca alternifolia (tea tree oil)," J Antimicrob Chemother. 24(3):186-9.

Hart PH, Brand C, Carson CF, Riley TV, Prager RH, Finlay-Jones JJ (2000 Nov). "Terpinen-4-ol, the main component of the essential oil of Melaleuca alternifolia (tea tree oil), suppresses inflammatory mediator production by activated human monocytes," Inflamm Res. 49(11):619-26.

Hay IC, Jamieson M, Ormerod AD (1998 Nov). "Randomized trial of aromatherapy. Successful treatment for alopecia areata," Arch Dermatol. 135(5):1349-52.

Haze, S., Sakai, K., Gozu, Y., & Moriyama, M. (2010 Jul). Grapefruit oil attenuates adipogenesis in cultured subcutaneous adipocytes. Planta Med, 76(10), 950-955.

Hiramatsu N, Xiufen W, Takechi R, Itoh Y, Mamo J, Pal S (2004). "Antimutagenicity of Japanese traditional herbs, gennoshoko, yomogi, senburi and iwa-tobacco," Biofactors. 22(1-4):123-5.

Holt E. (2005) Doctor sues clinic over Yushchenko poisoning claims. The Lancet. 365: 1375.

Hongratanaworakit T (2009 Feb). "Relaxing effect of rose oil on humans," Nat Prod Commun. 4(2):291-6.

Hongratanaworakit T, Buchbauer G (2006 Sep). "Relaxing effect of ylang ylang oil on humans after transdermal absorption," Phytother Res. 20(9):758-63.

Hosseinzadeh, H., Karimi, G. R., & Ameri, M. (2002 Dec). Effects of Anethum graveolens L. seed extracts on experimental gastric irritation models in mice. BMC Pharmacol, 2, 1-5.

Howard J., Hyman A.A. (2003) Dynamics and mechanics of the microtubule plus end. Nature. 422: 753-758.

Hoya Y, Matsumura I, Fujita T, Yanaga K. (2008 Nov-Dec). "The use of nonpharmacological interventions to reduce anxiety in patients undergoing gastroscopy in a setting with an optimal soothing environment," Gastroenterol Nurs. 31(6):395-9.

Hsu H-Y., Yang J-J., Lin C-C. (1997) Effects of oleanolic acid and ursolic acid in inhibiting tumor growth and enhancing the recovery of hematopoietic system postirradiation in mice. Cancer Letters. 111: 7-13.

Huang MT, Badmaev V, Ding Y, Liu Y, Xie JG, Ho CT (2000). "Anti-tumor and anti-carcinogenic activities of triterpenoid, beta-boswellic acid," Biofactors. 13(1-4):225-30.

Hummel T., Fuschik T., Frasnelli J., Huttenbrink K-B. (2003) Effects of olfactory function, age, and gender on trigeminally mediated sensations: a study based on the lateralization of chemosensory stimuli. Toxicology Letters. 140-141: 273-280.

Hussein G, Miyashiro H, Nakamura N, Hattori M, Kakiuchi N, Shimotohno K (2000 Nov). "Inhibitory effects of sudanese medicinal plant extracts on hepatitis C virus (HCV) protease," Phytother Res. 14(7):510-6.

Ichihashi M., Ueda M., Budiyanto A., Bito T., Oka M., Fukuaga M., Tsuru K., Horikawa T. (2003) UV-induced skin damage. Toxicology. 189: 21-39.

Imai H, Osawa K, Yasuda H, Hamashima H, Arai T, Sasatsu M (2001). "Inhibition by the essential oils of peppermint and spearmint of the growth of pathogenic bacteria," Microbios. 106(Suppl 1):31-9.

Inouye S, Takizawa T, Yamaguchi H (2001 May). "Antibacterial activity of essential oils and their major constituents against respiratory tract pathogens by gaseous contact," J Antimicrob Chemother. 47(5):565-73.

Iori A, Grazioli D, Gentile E, Marano G, Salvatore G (2005 Apr 20). "Acaricidal properties of the essential oil of Melaleuca alternifolia Cheel (tea tree oil) against nymphs of Ixodes ricinus," Vet Parasitol. 129(1-2):173-6.

Itai T, Amayasu H, Kuribayashi M, Kawamura N, Okada M, Momose A, Tateyama T, Narumi K, Uematsu W, Kaneko S (2000 Aug). "Psychological effects of aromatherapy on chronic hemodialysis patients," Psychiatry Clin Neurosci. 54(4):393-7.

Jafarzadeh, M., Arman, S., & Pour, F. F. (2013 Aug). Effect of aromatherapy with orange essential oil on salivary cortisol and pulse rate in children during dental treatment: A randomized controlled clinical trial. Adv Biomed Res, 2, 1-10.

Jamal, A., Javed, K., Aslam, M., & Jafri, M. A. (2006 Jan). Gastroprotective effect of cardamom, Elettaria cardamomum Maton. fruits in rats. J Ethnopharmacol, 103(2), 149-153.

Jamalian, A., Shams-Ghahfarokhi, M., Jaimand, K., Pashootan, N., Amani, A., & Razzaghi-Abyaneh, M. (2012). Chemical composition and antifungal activity of Matricaria recutita flower essential oil against medically important dermatophytes and soil-borne pathogens. J Mycol Med, 22(4), 308-315.

Janahmadi M, Niazi F, Danyali S, Kamalinejad M (2006 Mar 8). "Effects of the fruit essential oil of Cuminum cyminum Linn. (Apiaceae) on pentylenetetrazol-induced epileptiform activity in F1 neurones of Helix aspersa," J Ethnopharmacol. 104(1-2):278-82.

Jankovic J. (2008) Parkinson's disease: clinical features and diagnosis. Journal of Neurology, Neurosurgery & Psychiatry. 79: 368-376.

Jefferies H., Coster J., Khalil A., Bot J., McCauley R.D., Hall J.C. (2003) Glutathione. ANZ Journal of Surgery. 73: 517-522.

Jeon, S., Bose, S., Hur, J., Jun, K., Kim, Y. K., Cho, K. S., & Koo, B. S. (2011 Sep). A modified formulation of Chinese traditional medicine improves memory impairment and reduces Abeta level in the Tg-APPswe/PS1dE9 mouse model of Alzheimer's disease. J Ethnopharmacol, 137(1), 783-789.

Jeong H.G. (1999) Inhibition of cytochrome P450 2E1 expression by oleanolic acid: hepatoprotective effects against carbon tetrachloride-induced hepatic injury. Toxicology Letters. 105: 215-222.

Jing, L., Zhang, Y., Fan, S., Gu, M., Guan, Y., Lu, X., . . . Zhou, Z. (2013 Sep). Preventive and ameliorating effects of citrus D-limonene on dyslipidemia and hyperglycemia in mice with high-fat diet-induced obesity. Eur J Pharmacol, 715(1-3), 46-55.

Jing Y, Xia L, Han R (1992 Mar). "Growth inhibition and differentiation of promyelocytic cells (HL-60) induced by BC-4, an active principle from Boswellia carterii Birdw," Chin Med Sci J. 7(1):12-5.

Juergens U.R., Dethlefsen U., Steinkamp G., Gillissen A., Repges R., Vetter H. (2003) Anti-inflammatory activity of 1.8-cineol (eucalyptol) in bronchial asthma: a double-blind placebo-controlled trial. Respiratory Medicine. 97: 250-256.

Juergens UR, Stöber M, Vetter H (1998 Dec 16). "The anti-inflammatory activity of L-menthol compared to mint oil in human monocytes in vitro: a novel perspective for its therapeutic use in inflammatory diseases," Eur J Med Res. 3(12):539-45.

Jun, H. J., Lee, J. H., Jia, Y., Hoang, M. H., Byun, H., Kim, K. H., & Lee, S. J. (2012 Mar). Melissa officinalis essential oil reduces plasma triglycerides in human apolipoprotein E2 transgenic mice by inhibiting sterol regulatory element-binding protein-1c-dependent fatty acid synthesis. J Nutr, 142(3), 432-440.

Jungersted J.M., Hellgren L.I., Hogh J.K., Drachmann T., Jemec G.B.E., Agner T. (2010) Ceramides and Barrier Function in Healthy Skin. Acta Dermato-Venereologica. 90: 350-353.

Kabuto, H., Tada, M., & Kohno, M. (2007 Mar). Eugenol [2-methoxy-4-(2-propenyl)phenol] prevents 6-hydroxydopamine-induced dopamine depression and lipid peroxidation inductivity in mouse striatum. Biol Pharm Bull, 30(3), 423-427.

Kalemba D., Kunicka A. (2003) Antibacterial and Antifungal properties of Essential Oils. Current Medicinal Chemistry. 10: 813-829.

Kamatou G.P.P., Viljoen A.M. (2010) A Review of the Application and Pharmacological Properties of ?-Bisabolol and ?-Bisabolol-Rich Oils. Journal of the American Oil Chemists' Society. 87: 1-7.

Kane FM, Brodie EE, Coull A, Coyne L, Howd A, Milne A, Niven CC, Robbins R (2004 Oct 28-Nov 10). "The analgesic effect of odour and music upon dressing change," Br J Nurs. 13(19):S4-12.

Kapil A., Sharma S. (1994) Anti-complement activity of oleanolic acid: an inhibitor of C3-convertase of the classical complement pathway. Journal of Pharmacy and Pharmacology. 46: 922-923.

Kato K., Cox A.D., Hisaka M.M., Graham S.M., Buss J.E., Der C.J. (1992) Isoprenoid addition to Ras protein is the critical modification for its membrane association and transforming activity. Proc. Natl. Sci. USA. 89: 6403-6407.

Kaur M, Agarwal C, Singh RP, Guan X, Dwivedi C, Agarwal R (2005 Feb). "Skin cancer chemopreventive agent, [alpha]-santalol, induces apoptotic death of human epidermoid carcinoma A431 cells via caspase activation together with dissipation of mitochondrial membrane potential and cytochrome c release," Carcinogenesis. 26(2):369-80.

Kedia, A., Prakash, B., Mishra, P. K., & Dubey, N. K. (2014). Antifungal and antiaflatoxigenic properties of Cuminum cyminum (L.) seed essential oil and its efficacy as a preservative in stored commodities. Int J Food Microbiol, 168-169, 1-7.

Kennedy DO, Little W, Haskell CF, Scholey AB (2006 Feb). "Anxiolytic effects of a combination of Melissa officinalis and Valeriana officinalis during laboratory induced stress," Phytother Res. 20(2):96-102.

Keshavarz, A., Minaiyan, M., Ghannadi, A., & Mahzouni, P. (2013 Jan). Effects of Carum carvi L. (Caraway) extract and essential oil on TNBS-induced colitis in rats. Res Pharm Sci, 8(1), 1-8.

Khatibi A, Haghparast A, Shams J, Dianati E, Komaki A, Kamalinejad M (2008 Dec 19). "Effects of the fruit essential oil of Cuminum cyminum L. on the acquisition and expression of morphine-induced conditioned place preference in mice," Neurosci Lett. 448(1):94-8.

Kiecolt-Glaser JK, Graham JE, Malarkey WB, Porter K, Lemeshow S, Glaser R (2008 Apr). "Olfactory influences on mood and autonomic, endocrine, and immune function," Psychoneuroendocrinology. 33(3):328-39.

Kim, I. H., Kim, C., Seong, K., Hur, M. H., Lim, H. M., & Lee, M. S. (2012 Dec). Essential oil inhalation on blood pressure and salivary cortisol levels in prehypertensive and hypertensive subjects. Evid Based Complement Alternat Med, 2012, 1-9.

Kim K-A., Lee J-S., Park H-J., Kim J-W., Kim C-J., Shim I-S., Kim N-J., Han S-M., Lim S. (2004) Inhibition of cytochrome P450 activities by oleanolic acid and ursolic acid in human liver microsomes. Life Sciences. 74: 2769-2779.

Kim MA, Sakong JK, Kim EJ, Kim EH, Kim EH (2005 Feb). "Effect of aromatherapy massage for the relief of constipation in the elderly,"Taehan Kanho Hakhoe Chi. 35(1):56-64.

Kim S., Lee J., Jung E., Huh S., Park J-O., Lee J-W., Byun S.Y., Park D. (2008) Mechanisms of depigmentation by ?-bisabolol. Journal of Dermatological Science. doi: 10.1016/j.jdermsci.2008.06.005.

Kim, T. H., Kim, H. J., Lee, S. H., & Kim, S. Y. (2012 Jun). Potent inhibitory effect of Foeniculum vulgare Miller extract on osteoclast differentiation and ovariectomy-induced bone loss. Int J Mol Med, 29(6), 1053-1059.

Kite SM, Maher EJ, Anderson K, Young T, Young J, Wood J, Howells N, Bradburn J (1998 May). "Development of an aromatherapy service at a Cancer Centre," Palliat Med. 12(3):171-80.

Klein T.W. (2005) Cannabinoid-Based Drugs As Anti-Inflammatory Therapeutics. Nature Reviews. 5: 400-411.

Kobayashi Y, Takahashi R, Ogino F (2005 Oct 3). "Antipruritic effect of the single oral administration of German chamomile flower extract and its combined effect with antiallergic agents in ddY mice,"J Ethnopharmacol. 101(1-3):308-12.

Kocevski, D., Du, M., Kan, J., Jing, C., Lacanin, I., & Pavlovic, H. (2013 May). Antifungal effect of Allium tuberosum, Cinnamomum cassia, and Pogostemon cablin essential oils and their components against population of Aspergillus species. J Food Sci, 78(5), M731-737.

Komiya M, Takeuchi T, Harada E (2006 Sep 25). "Lemon oil vapor causes an anti-stress effect via modulating the 5-HT and DA activities in mice," Behav Brain Res. 172(2):240-9.

Komori T, Fujiwara R, Tanida M, Nomura J (1995 Dec). "Potential antidepressant effects of lemon odor in rats," Eur Neuropsychopharmacol. 5(4):477-80.

Koo HN, Hong SH, Kim CY, Ahn JW, Lee YG, Kim JJ, Lyu YS, Kim HM (2002 Jun). "Inhibitory effect of apoptosis in human astrocytes CCF-STTG1 cells by lemon oil," Pharmacol Res. 45(6):469-73.

Koo HN, Jeong HJ, Kim CH, Park ST, Lee SJ, Seong KK, Lee SK, Lyu YS, Kim HM (2001 Dec). "Inhibition of heat shock-induced apoptosis by peppermint oil in astrocytes," J Mol Neurosci. 17(3):391-6.

Kosaka K., Mimura J., Itoh K., Satoh T., Shimojo Y., Kitajima C., Maruyama A., Yamamoto M., Shirasawa T. (2010) Role of Nrf2 and p62/ZIP in the neurite outgrowth by carnosic acid in PC12h cells. Journal of Biochemistry. 147: 73-81.

Kosaka K., Yokoi T. (2003) Carnosic Acid, a Component of Rosemary (Rosmarinus officinalis L.), Promotes Synthesis of Nerve Growth Factor in T98G Human Glioblastoma Cells. Biological & Phareuatical Bulletin. 26: 1620-1622.

Kozam G., Mantell G.M. (1978) The Effect of Eugenol on Oral Mucous Membranes. Journal of Dental Research. 57: 954-957.

Kumar A, Malik F, Bhushan S, Sethi VK, Shahi AK, Kaur J, Taneja SC, Qazi GN, Singh J (2008 Feb 15). "An essential oil and its major constituent isointermedeol induce apoptosis by increased expression of mitochondrial cytochrome c and apical death receptors in human leukaemia HL-60 cells," Chem Biol Interact. 171(3):332-47.

Kumar, D., Bhat, Z. A., & Shah, M. Y. (2012 Sep). Anti-anxiety activity of successive extracts of Angelica archangelica Linn. on the elevated T-maze and forced swimming tests in rats. J Tradit Chin Med, 32(3), 423-429.

Kumari, S., & Dutta, A. (2013 Jul). Protective effect of Eleteria cardamomum (L.) Maton against Pan masala induced damage in lung of male Swiss mice. Asian Pac J Trop Med, 6(7), 525-531.

Kuwahata, H., Komatsu, T., Katsuyama, S., Corasaniti, M. T., Bagetta, G., Sakurada, S., . . . Takahama, K. (2013 Feb). Peripherally injected linalool and bergamot essential oil attenuate mechanical allodynia via inhibiting spinal ERK phosphorylation. Pharmacol Biochem Behav, 103(4), 735-741.

Kwieciński J, Eick S, Wójcik K (2009 Apr). "Effects of tea tree (Melaleuca alternifolia) oil on Staphylococcus aureus in biofilms and stationary growth phase," Int J Antimicrob Agents. 33(4):343-7.

Lahlou S., Figueiredo A.F., Magalaes P.J.C., Leal-Cardoso J.H. (2002) Cardiovascular effects of 1,8-cineole, a terpenoid oxide present in many plant essential oils, in normotensive rats. Canadian Journal of Physiology and Pharmacology. 80: 1125-1131.

Lahlou S., Interaminense L.F.L., Magalhaes P.J.C., Leal-Cardoso J.H., Duarte G.P. (2004) Cardiovascular Effects of Eugenol, a Phenolic Compound Present in Many Plant Essential Oils, in Normotensive Rats. Journal of Cardiovascular Pharmacology. 43: 250-257.

Lambert R.J.W., Skandamis P.N., Coote P.J., Nychas G-J.E. (2001) A study of the minimun inhibitory concentration and mode of action of oregano essential oil, thymol and carvacrol. Journal of Applied Microbiology. 91: 453-462.

Lampronti I, Saab AM, Gambari R (2006 Oct). "Antiproliferative activity of essential oils derived from plants belonging to the Magnoliophyta division," Int J Oncol. 29(4):989-95.

Lapczynski A., Bhatia S.P., Letizia C.S., Api A.M. (2008) Fragrance material review on dl-citronellol. Food and Chemical Toxicology. 46: S103-S109.

Larder B.A., Kemp S.D., Harrigan P.R. (1995) Potential Mechanism for Sustained Antiretroviral Efficacy of AZT-3TC Combination Therapy. Science. 269: 696-699.

Lawrence, H. A., & Palombo, E. A. (2009 Dec). Activity of essential oils against Bacillus subtilis spores. J Microbiol Biotechnol, 19(12), 1590-1595.

Leal-Cardoso J.H., Lahlou S., de Souza A.N.C., Criddle D.N., Duarte G.I.B.P., Santos M.A.V., Magalhaes P.J.C. (2002) Inhibitory actions of eugenol on rat isolated ileum. Canadian Journal of Physiology and Pharmacology. 80: 901-906.

Lee, H. S., & Ahn, Y. J. (1998 Jan). Growth-Inhibiting Effects of Cinnamomum cassia Bark-Derived Materials on Human Intestinal Bacteria. J Agric Food Chem, 46(1), 8-12.

Lee, H. S. (2002 Dec). Inhibitory activity of Cinnamomum cassia bark-derived component against rat lens aldose reductase. J Pharm Pharm Sci, 5(3), 226-230.

Lee HS (2005 Apr 6). "Cuminaldehyde: Aldose Reductase and alpha-Glucosidase Inhibitor Derived from Cuminum cyminum L. Seeds," J Agric Food Chem. 53(7):2446-50.

Lee J., Jun H., Jung E., Ha J., Park D. (2010) Whitening effect of ?-bisabolol in Asian women subjects. International Journal of Cosmetic Science.

Lee SU, Shim KS, Ryu SY, Min YK, Kim SH (2009 Feb). "Machilin A isolated from Myristica fragrans stimulates osteoblast differentiation," Planta Med. 75(2):152-7.

Lee, T., Lee, S., Ho Kim, K., B., Shin, J., & Mar, W. (2013 Sep). Effects of magnolialide isolated from the leaves of Laurus nobilis L. (Lauraceae) on immunoglobulin E-mediated type I hypersensitivity in vitro. J Ethnopharmacol, 149(2), 550-556.

Legault J, Dahl W, Debiton E, Pichette A, Madelmont JC (2003 May). "Antitumor activity of balsam fir oil: production of reactive oxygen species induced by alpha-humulene as possible mechanism of action," Planta Med. 69(5):402-7.

Legault J., Pichette A. (2007) Potentiating effect of ?-caryophyllene on anticancer activity of ?-humulene, isocaryophyllene, and paclitaxel. Journal of Pharmacy and Pharmacology. 59: 1643-1647.

Lehrner J, Eckersberger C, Walla P, Pötsch G, Deecke L (2000 Oct 1-15). "Ambient odor of orange in a dental office reduces anxiety and improves mood in female patients," Physiol Behav. 71(1-2):83-6.

Lewith GT, Godfrey AD, Prescott P (2005 Aug). "A single-blinded, randomized pilot study evaluating the aroma of Lavandula angustifolia as a treatment for mild insomnia," J Altern Complement Med. 11(4):631-7.

Li, R., Liang, T., Xu, L., Li, Y., Zhang, S., & Duan, X. (2013 Jan). Protective effect of cinnamon polyphenols against STZ-diabetic mice fed high-sugar, high-fat diet and its underlying mechanism. Food Chem Toxicol, 51, 419-425.

Li, Y. P., Yuan, S. F., Cai, G. H., Wang, H., Wang, L., Yu, L., . . . Yun, J. (2014 May). Patchouli Alcohol Dampens Lipopolysaccharide Induced Mastitis in Mice. Inflammation.

Li, X., Duan, S., Chu, C., Xu, J., Zeng, G., Lam, A. K., . . . Jiang, L. (2013 Aug). Melaleuca alternifolia concentrate inhibits in vitro entry of influenza virus into host cells. Molecules, 18(8), 9550-9566.

Lie J. (2005) Oleanolic acid and ursolic acid: Research perspectives. Journal of Ethnopharmacology. 100: 92-94.

Lim PF, Liu XY, Kang L, Ho PC, Chan YW, Chan SY (2006 Mar 27). "Limonene GP1/PG organogel as a vehicle in transdermal delivery of haloperidol," Int J Pharm 311(12):157-64.

Lima-Accioly P.M., Lavor-Porto P.R., Cavalcante F.S., Magalhaes P.J.C., Lahlou S., Morais S.M., Leal-Cardoso J.H. (2006) Essential Oil of Croton Nepetaefolius and Its Main Constituent, 1,8-Cineole, Block Excitability of Rat Sciatic Nerve In Vitro. Clinical and Experimental Pharmacology and Physiology. 33: 1158-1163.

Lima CF, Azevedo MF, Araujo R, Fernandes-Ferreira M, Pereira-Wilson C (2006 Aug). "Metformin-like effect of Salvia officinalis (common sage): is it useful in diabetes prevention?," Br J Nutr. 96(2):326-33.

Linck V.M., da Silva A.L., Figueiro M., Caramao E.B., Moreno P.R.H., Elisabetsky E. (2010) Effects of inhaled Linalool in anxiety, social interaction and aggressive behavior in mice. Phytomedicine. 17: 679-683.

Linck V.M., da Silva A.L., Figueiro M., Piato A.L., Herrmann A.P., Birck F.D., Moreno P.R.H., Elisabetsky E. (2009) Inhaled linalool-induced sedation in mice. Phytomedicine. 16: 303-307.

Lin PW, Chan WC, Ng BF, Lam LC (2007 May). "Efficacy of aromatherapy (Lavandula angustifolia) as an intervention for agitated behaviours in Chinese older persons with dementia: a cross-over randomized trial," Int J Geriatr Psychiatry. 22(5):405-10.

Lis-Balschin M., Hart S. (1999) Studies on the Mode of Action of the Essential Oil of Lavender (Lavandula angustifolia P. Miller). Phytotherapy Research. 13: 540-542.

Lis-Balchin M, Hart S, Wan Hang Lo B (2002 Aug). "Jasmine absolute (Jasminum grandiflora L.) and its mode of action on guinea-pig ileum in vitro," Phyther Res. 16(5):437-9.

Liu, C. T., Raghu, R., Lin, S. H., Wang, S. Y., Kuo, C. H., Tseng, Y. J., & Sheen, L. Y. (2013 Nov). Metabolomics of ginger essential oil against alcoholic fatty liver in mice. J Agric Food Chem, 61(46), 11231-11240.

Liu J. (1995) Pharmacology of oleanolic acid and ursolic acid. Journal of Ethnopharmacology. 49: 57-68.

Liu JJ, Nilsson A, Oredsson S, Badmaev V, Duan RD (2002 Oct). "Keto- and acetyl-keto-boswellic acids inhibit proliferation and induce apoptosis in Hep G2 cells via a caspase-8 dependent pathway," Int J Mol Med. 10(4):501-5.

Liu Y., Hartley D.P., Liu J. (1998) Protection against carbone tetrachloride hepatotoxicity by oleanolic acid is not mediated through metallothionein. Toxicology Letters. 95: 77-85.

Livermore D.M. (2002) Multiple Mechanisms of Antimicrobial Resistance in Pseudomonas aeruginosa: Our Worst Nightmare?. Clinical Infectious Diseases. 34: 634-640.

Loew O. (1900) A New Enzyme of General Occurrence in Organisms. Science. 11: 701-702.

Loizzo MR, Tundis R, Menichini F, Saab AM, Statti GA, Menichini F (2007 Sep-Oct). "Cytotoxic activity of essential oils from labiatae and lauraceae families against in vitro human tumor models," Anticancer Res. 27(5A):3293-9.

Longley D.B., Harkin D.P., Johnston P.G. (2003) 5-Fluorouracil: Mechanisms of Action and Clinical Strategies. Nature Reviews. 3: 330-338.

Lu M, Battinelli L, Daniele C, Melchioni C, Salvatore G, Mazzanti G (2002 Mar). "Muscle relaxing activity of Hyssopus officinalis essential oil on isolated intestinal preparations," Planta Med. 68(3):213-6.

Lu, T., Sheng, H., Wu, J., Cheng, Y., Zhu, J., & Chen, Y. (2012 Jun). Cinnamon extract improves fasting blood glucose and glycosylated hemoglobin level in Chinese patients with type 2 diabetes. Nutr Res, 32(6), 408-412.

Lu XQ, Tang FD, Wang Y, Zhao T, Bian RL (2004 Feb). "Effect of Eucalyptus globulus oil on lipopolysaccharide-induced chronic bronchitis and mucin hypersecretion in rats," Zhongguo Zhong Yao Za Zhi. 29(2):168-71.

Macedo, I. T., Bevilaqua, C. M., de Oliveira, L. M., Camurca-Vasconcelos, A. L., Vieira Lda, S., & Amora Sdos, S. (2011). Evaluation of Eucalyptus citriodora essential oil on goat gastrointestinal nematodes. Rev Bras Parasitol Vet, 20(3), 223-227.

Machado, D. G., Cunha, M. P., Neis, V. B., Balen, G. O., Colla, A., Bettio, L. E., . . . Rodrigues, A. L. (2013 Jan). Antidepressant-like effects of fractions, essential oil, carnosol and betulinic acid isolated from Rosmarinus officinalis L. Food Chem, 136(2), 999-1005.

Macilwain C. (1993) US Congress urged to back further Agent Orange studies. Nature. 364: 373.

Manohar V, Ingram C, Gray J, Talpur NA, Echard BW, Bagchi D, Preuss HG (2001 Dec). "Antifungal activities of origanum oil against Candida albicans," Mol Cell Biochem. 228(1-2):111-7.

Mans D.R.A., Grivicich I., Peters G.J., Schwartsmann G. (1999) Sequence-dependent Growth Inhibition and DNA Damage Formation by t he Irinotecan-5-Fluorouracil Combination in Human Colon Carcinoma Cell Lines. European Journal of Cancer. 35: 1851-1861.

Marks R. (1995) An Overview of Skin Cancers: Incidence and Causation. Cancer. 75: 607-612.

Maruyama N, Sekimoto Y, Ishibashi H, Inouye S, Oshima H, Yamaguchi H, Abe S (2005 Feb 10). "Suppression of neutrophil accumulation in mice by cutaneous application of geranium essential oil," J Inflamm (Lond). 2(1):1.

Masuda T., Inaba Y., Takeda Y. (2001) Antioxidant Mechanism of Carnosic Acid: Structural Identification of Two Oxidation Products. Journal of Agricultural and Food Chemistry. 49: 5560-5565.

Masukawa Y., Narita H., Sato H., Naoe A., Kondo N., Sugai Y., Oba T., Homma R., Ishikawa J., Takagi Y., Kitahara T. (2009) Comprehensive quantification of ceramide species in human stratum corneum. Journal of Lipid Research. 50: 1708-1719.

Mathews G.C. (2007) The Dual Roles of GABA in Seizures and Epilepsy Generate More Excitement. Epilepsy Currents 7: 28-30.

Mayer M.L. (2005) Glutamate receptor ion channels. Current Opinion in Neurobiology. 15: 282-288.

McCord J.M., Fridovich I. (1969) Superoxide Dismutase: an enzymic function for erytrocuprein (hemocuprein). The Journal of Biological Chemistry. 244: 6049-6055.

McCune, L. M., & Johns, T. (2002). Antioxidant activity in medicinal plants associated with the symptoms of diabetes mellitus used by the indigenous peoples of the North American boreal forest. J Ethnopharmacol, 82(2-3), 197-205.

McGarvey D.J., Croteau R. (1995) Terpenoid Metabolism. The Plant Cell. 7: 1015-1026.

McGeady P., Wansley D.L., Logan D.A. (2002) Carvone and Perillaldehyde Interfere with the Serum-Induced Formation of Filamentous Structures in Candida albicansat Substantially Lower Concentrations than Those Causing Significant Inhibition of Growth. Journal of Natural Products. 65: 953-955.

McKee M. (2009) The poisoning of Victor Yushchenko. The Lancet. 374: 1131-1132.

Meamarbashi, A., & Rajabi, A. (2013 Mar). The effects of peppermint on exercise performance. J Int Soc Sports Nutr, 10(1), 15.

Medzhitov R., Janeway C.A. (1997) Innate Immunity: Impact on the adaptive Immune response. Current Opinion in Immunology. 9: 4-9.

Meiller, T. F., Silva, A., Ferreira, S. M., Jabra-Rizk, M. A., Kelley, J. I., & DePaola, L. G. (2005 Apr). Efficacy of Listerine Antiseptic in reducing viral contamination of saliva. J Clin Periodontol, 32(4), 341-346.

Meisler M.H., Kearney J.A. (2005) Sodium channel mutations in epilepsy and other neurological disorders. The Journal of Clinical Investigation. 115: 2010-2017.

Meldrum B.S. (1994) The role of glutamate in epilepsy and other CNS disorders. Neurology. 44: S14-S23.

Meldrum B.S., Akbar M.T., Chapman A.G. (1999) Glutamate receptors and transporters in genetic and acquired models of epilepsy. Epilepsy Research. 36: 189-204.

Melo, F. H., Venancio, E. T., de Sousa, D. P., de Franca Fonteles, M. M., de Vasconcelos, S. M., Viana, G. S., & de Sousa, F. C. (2010 Aug). Anxiolytic-like effect of Carvacrol (5-isopropyl-2-methylphenol) in mice: involvement with GABAergic transmission. Fundam Clin Pharmacol, 24(4), 437-443.

Melov S., Ravenscroft J., Malik S., Gill M.S., Walker D.W., Clayton P.E., Wallace D.C., Malfroy B., Doctrow S.R., Lithgow G.J. (2000) Extension of Life-Span with Superoxide Dismutase/Catalase Mimetics. Science. 289: 1567-1569.

Mercier B., Prost J., Prost M. (2009) The Essential Oil of Turpentine and Its Major Volatile Fraction (?- and ?-Pinenes): A Review. International Journal of Occupational Medicine and Environmental Health. 22: 331-342.

Mills JJ, Chari RS, Boyer IJ, Gould MN, Jirtle RL (1995 Mar 1). "Induction of apoptosis in liver tumors by the monoterpene perillyl alcohol," Cancer Res. 55(5):979-83.

Milross C.G., Mason K.A., Hunter N.R., Chung W-K., Peters L.J., Milas L. (1996) Relationship of Mitotic Arrest and Apoptosis to Antitumor Effect of Paclitaxel. Journal of the National Cancer Institute. 88: 1308-1314.

Mimura J., Kosaka K., Maruyama A., Satoh T., Harada N., Yoshida H., Satoh K., Yamamoto M., Itoh K. (2011) Nrf2 regulates NGF mRNA induction by carnosic acid in T98G gliobastoma cells and normal human astrocytes. The Journal of Biochemistry. 150: 209-217.

Minaiyan, M., Ghannadi, A. R., Afsharipour, M., & Mahzouni, P. (2011 Jan). Effects of extract and essential oil of Rosmarinus officinalis L. on TNBS-induced colitis in rats. Res Pharm Sci, 6(1), 13-21.

Mishra, A., Bhatti, R., Singh, A., & Singh Ishar, M. P. (2010 Mar). Ameliorative effect of the cinnamon oil from Cinnamomum zeylanicum upon early stage diabetic nephropathy. Planta Med, 76(5), 412-417.

Mishra, D., Joshi, S., Bisht, G., & Pilkhwal, S. (2010). Chemical composition and antimicrobial activity of solidago canadensis linn. Root essential oil. J Basic Clin Pharm, 1(3), 187-190.

Mitic-Culafic D., Zegura B., Nikolic B., Vukovic-Gacic B., Knezevic-Vukcevic J., Filipic M. (2008) Protective effect of linalool, myrcene and eucalyptol against t-butyl hydroperoxide induced genotoxicity in bacteria and cultured human cells. Food and Chemical Toxicology. 47: 260-266.

Mkolo MN, Magano SR (2007 Sep). "Repellent effects of the essential oil of Lavandula angustifolia against adults of Hyalomma marginatum rufipes," J S Afr Vet Assoc. 78(3):149-52.

Mondello F, De Bernardis F, Girolamo A, Cassone A, Salvatore G (2006 Nov 3). "In vivo activity of terpinen-4-ol, the main bio-active component of Melaleuca alternifolia Cheel (tea tree) oil against azole-susceptible and -resistant human pathogenic Candida species," BMC Infect Dis. 6:158.

Monti D, Chetoni P, Burgalassi S, Najarro M, Saettone MF, Boldrini E (2002 Apr 26). "Effect of different terpene-containing essential oils on permeation of estradiol through hairless mouse skin," Int j Pharm. 237(1-2):209-14.

Monzo M., Rosell R., Sanchez J.J., Lee J.S., O'Brate A., Gonzalex-Larriba J.L., Alberola V., Lorenzo J.C., Nunez L., Ro J.Y., Martin C. (1999) Paclitaxel Resistance in Non-Small Cell Lung Cancer Associated With Beta-Tubulin Gene Mutations. Journal of Clincial Oncology. 17: 1786-1793.

Moreira, A. C., de Oliveira Lima, E., Wanderley, P. A., Carmo, E. S., & de Souza, E. L. (2010). Chemical composition and antifungal activity of Hyptis Suaveolens (L.) Poit leaves essential oil against Aspergillus species. Braz J Microbiol, 41(1), 28-33.

Moreira-Lobo D.C.A., Linhares-Siqueira E.D., Cruz G.M.P., Cruz J.S., de Souza J.L.C., Lahlou S., de Souza A.N.C., Barbosa R., Magalhaes P.J.C., Leal-Cardoso J.H. (2010) Eugenol modifies the excitability of rat sciatic nerve and superior cervical ganglion neurons. Neuroscience Letters. 472: 220-224.

Moreno S, Scheyer T, Romano CS, Vojnov AA (2006 Feb). "Antioxidant and antimicrobial activities of rosemary extracts linked to their polyphenol composition," Free Radic Res. 40(2):223-31.

Morse M.A., Stoner G.D. (1993) Cancer chemoprevention: principles and prospects. Carcinogenesis. 14: 1737-1746.

Moss M, Cook J, Wesnes K, Duckett P (2003 Jan). "Aromas of rosemary and lavender essential oils differentially affect cognition and mood in healthy adults," Int J Neurosci. 113(1):15-38.

Motomura N, Sakurai A, Yotsuya Y (2001 Dec). "Reduction of mental stress with lavender odorant," Percept Mot Skills. 93(3):713-8.

Moussaieff A, Rimmerman N, Bregman T, Straiker A, Felder CC, Shoham S, Kashman Y, Huang SM, Lee H, Shohami E, Mackie K, Caterina MJ, Walker JM, Fride E, Mechoulam R (2008 Aug). "Incensole acetate, an incense component, elicits psychoactivity by activating TRPV3 channels in the brain," FASEB J. 22(8):3024-34.

Muhlbauer R.C., Lozano A., Palacio S., Reinli A., Felix R. (2003) Common herbes, essential oils, and monoterpenes potently modulate bone metabolism. Bone. 32: 372-380.

Mukherjee P.K., Chandra J., Kuhn D.M., Ghannoum M.A. (2003) Mechanism of Fluconazole Resistance in Candida albicansB-iofilms: Phase-Specific Role of Efflux Pumps and Membrane Sterols. Infection and Immunity. 71: 4333-4340.

Muller M., Pape H-C., Speckmann E-J., Gorji A. (2006) Effect of Eugenol on Spreading Depression and Epileptiform Discharges in Rat Neocortical and Hippocampal Tissues. Neuroscience. 140: 743-751.

Mumcuoglu KY, Magdassi S, Miller J, Ben-Ishai F, Zentner G, Helbin V, Friger M, Kahana F, Ingber A (2004 Dec). "Repellency of citronella for head lice: double-blind randomized trial of efficacy and safety," Isr Med Assoc J. 6(12):756-9.

Munzel T., Feil R., Mulsch A., Lohmann S.M., Hofmann F., Walter U. (2003) Physiology and Pathophysiology of Vascular Signaling Controlled by Cyclic Guanosine 3′,5′-Cyclic Monophosphate-Dependent Protein Kinase. Circulation. 108: 2172-2183.

Nair B. (2001). "Final report on the safety assessment of Mentha Piperita (Peppermint) Oil, Mentha Piperita (Peppermint) Leaf Extract, Mentha Piperita (Peppermint) Leaf, and Mentha Piperita (Peppermint) Leaf Water," Int J Toxicol. 20(Suppl 3):61-73..

Nair, V., Singh, S., & Gupta, Y. K. (2012 Mar). Evaluation of disease modifying activity of Coriandrum sativum in experimental models. Indian J Med Res, 135, 240-245.

Narishetty S.T.K., Panchagnula R. (2004) Transdermal delivey of zidovudine: effect of terpenes and their mechanism of action. Journal of Controlled Release. 95: 367-379.

Narishetty S.T.K., Panchagnula R. (2005) Effects of L-menthol and 1,8-cineole on phase behavior and molecular organization of SC lipids and skin permeation of zidovudine. Journal of Controlled Release. 102: 59-70.

Nasel C, Nasel B, Samec P, Schindler E, Buchbauer G (1994 Aug). "Functional imaging of effects of fragrances on the human brain after prolonged inhalation," Chem Senses. 19(4):359-64.

Nikitin E.S., Balaban P.M. (2000) Optical Recording of Odor-Evoked Responses in the Olfactory Brain of the Naïve and Aversively Trained Terrestrial Snails. Learning & Memory 7: 422-432.

Ninomiya K, Matsuda H, Shimoda H, Nishida N, Kasajima N, Yoshino T, Morikawa T, Yoshikawa M (2004 Apr 19). "Carnosic acid, a new class of lipid absorption inhibitor from sage," Bioorg Med Chem Lett. 14(8):1943-6. Nebert D.W., Russell D.W. (2002) Clinical importance of the cytochromes P450. The Lancet. 360: 1155-1162.

Noori, S., Hassan, Z. M., & Salehian, O. (2013 Mar). Sclareol reduces CD4+ CD25+ FoxP3+ Treg cells in a breast cancer model in vivo. Iran J Immunol, 10(1), 10-21.

Nostro A, Blanco AR, Cannatelli MA, Enea V, Flamini G, Morelli I, Sudano Roccaro A, Alonzo V (2004 Jan 30). "Susceptibility of methicillin-resistant staphylococci to oregano essential oil, carvacrol and thymol," FEMS Microbiol Lett. 230(2):191-5.

Nyadjeu, P., Nguelefack-Mbuyo, E. P., Atsamo, A. D., Nguelefack, T. B., Dongmo, A. B., & Kamanyi, A. (2013 Feb). Acute and chronic antihypertensive effects of Cinnamomum zeylanicum stem bark methanol extract in L-NAME-induced hypertensive rats. BMC Complement Altern Med, 13, 1-10.

Oboh, G., Olasehinde, T. A., & Ademosun, A. O. (2014 Mar). Essential oil from lemon peels inhibit key enzymes linked to neurodegenerative conditions and pro-oxidant induced lipid peroxidation. J Oleo Sci, 63(4), 373-381.

Ogeturk, M., Kose, E., Sarsilmaz, M., Akpinar, B., Kus, I., & Meydan, S. (2010 Oct). Effects of lemon essential oil aroma on the learning behaviors of rats. Neurosciences (Riyadh), 15(4), 292-293.

Ohkubo T., Shibata M. (1997) The Selective Capsaicin Antagonist Capsazepine Abolishes the Antinociceptive Action of Eugenol and Guaiacol. Journal of Dental Research. 76: 848-851.

Ohno T, Kita M, Yamaoka Y, Imamura S, Yamamoto T, Mitsufuji S, Kodama T, Kashima K, Imanishi J (2003 Jun). "Antimicrobial activity of essential oils against Helicobacter pylori," Helicobacter. 8(3):207-15.

Olajide OA, Ajayi FF, Ekhelar AI, Awe SO, Makinde JM, Alada AR (1999 Jun). "Biological effects of Myristica fragrans (nutmeg) extract," Phytother Res. 13(4):344-5.

Olapour, A., Behaeen, K., Akhondzadeh, R., Soltani, F., Al Sadat Razavi, F., & Bekhradi, R. (2013 Nov). The Effect of Inhalation of Aromatherapy Blend containing Lavender Essential Oil on Cesarean Postoperative Pain. Anesth Pain Med, 3(1), 203-207.

Opalchenova G, Obreshkova D (2003 Jul). "Comparative studies on the activity of basil--an essential oil from Ocimum basilicum L.--against multidrug resistant clinical isolates of the genera Staphylococcus, Enterococcus and Pseudomonas by using different test methods," J Microbiol Methods. 54(1):105-10.

Ostad SN, Soodi M, Shariffzadeh M, Khorshidi N, Marzban H (2001 Aug). "The effect of fennel essential oil on uterine contraction as a model for dysmenorrhea, pharmacology and toxicology study," J Ethnopharmacol. 76(3):299-304.

Ou, M. C., Hsu, T. F., Lai, A. C., Lin, Y. T., & Lin, C. C. (2012 May). Pain relief assessment by aromatic essential oil massage on outpatients with primary dysmenorrhea: a randomized, double-blind clinical trial. J Obstet Gynaecol Res, 38(5), 817-822.

Paduch R., Kanderfer-Szerszen M., Trytek M., Feidurek J. (2007) Terpenes: substances useful in human healthcare. Archivum Immunologiae et Therapia Experimentalis. 55: 315-327.

Paoletti P., Neyton J. (2007) NMDA receptor subunits: functions and pharmacology. Current Opinion in Pharmacology. 7: 39-47.

Park, H. J., Kim, S. K., Kang, W. S., Woo, J. M., & Kim, J. W. (2014 Feb). Effects of essential oil from Chamaecyparis obtusa on cytokine genes in the hippocampus of maternal separation rats. Can J Physiol Pharmacol, 92(2), 95-101.

Pavela R (2005 Dec). "Insecticidal activity of some essential oils against larvae of Spodoptera littoralis," Fitoterapia. 76(7-8):691-6.

Peana A.T., D'Aquila P.S., Chessa M. L., Moretti M.D.L., Serra G., Pippia P. (2003) (-)-Linalool produces antinociception in two experimental models of pain. European Journal of Pharmacology. 460: 37-41.

Peana A.T., D'Aquila P.S., Panin F., Serra G., Pippia P., Moretti M.D.L. (2002) Anti-inflammatory activity of linalool and linalyl acetate constituents of essential oils. Phytomedicine. 9: 721-726.

Pearce AL, Finlay-Jones JJ, Hart PH (2005 Jan). "Reduction of nickel-induced contact hypersensitivity reactions by topical tea tree oil in humans," Inflamm Res. 54(1):22-30.

Peng SM, Koo M, Yu ZR (2009 Jan). "Effects of music and essential oil inhalation on cardiac autonomic balance in healthy individuals," J Altern Complement Med. 15(1):53-7.

Peters G.J., Backus H.H.J., Freemantle S., van Triest B., Codacci-Pisanelli G., van der Wilt C.L., Smid K., Lunec J., Calvert A.H., Marsh S., McLeod H.L., Bloemena E., Meijer S., Jansen G., van Groeningen C.J., Pinedo H.M. (2002) Induction of thymidylate synthase as a 5-fluorouracil resistance mechanism. Biochimica et Biophysica Acta. 1587: 194-205.

Pichette A, Larouche PL, Lebrun M, Legault J (2006 May). "Composition and antibacterial activity of Abies balsamea essential oil," Phytother Res. 20(5):371-3.

Politano V.T., Lewis E.M., Hoberman A.M., Christian M.S., Diener R.M., Api A.M. (2008) Evaluation of the Developmental Toxicity of Linalool in Rats. International Journal of Toxicology. 27: 183-188.

Preuss HG, Echard B, Enig M, Brook I, Elliott TB (2005 Apr). "Minimum inhibitory concentrations of herbal essential oils and monolaurin for gram-positive and gram-negative bacteria," Mol Cell Biochem. 272(1-2):29-34.

Puatanachokchai R, Kishida H, Denda A, Murata N, Konishi Y, Vinitketkumnuen U, Nakae D (2002 Sep 8). "Inhibitory effects of lemongrass (Cymbopogon citratus, Stapf) extract on the early phase of hepatocarcinogenesis after initiation with diethylnitrosamine in male Fischer 344 rats," Cancer Lett. 183(1):9-15.

Querfurth H.W., LaFeria F.M. (2010) Alzheimer's Disease. The New England Journal of Medicine. 362: 329-344.

Qureshi A.A., Mangels W.R., Din A.A., Elson C.E. (1988) Inhibition of Hepatic Mevalonate Biosynthesis by the Monoterpene, d-Limonene. J. Agric. Food Chem. 36: 1220-1224.

Ra Kovi, A., Milanovi, I., Pavlovi, N. A., Ebovi, T., Vukmirovi, S. A., & Mikov, M. (2014 Jul). Antioxidant activity of rosemary (Rosmarinus officinalis L.) essential oil and its hepatoprotective potential. BMC Complement Altern Med, 14(1), 1-20.

Ramos Alvarenga, R. F., Wan, B., Inui, T., Franzblau, S. G., Pauli, G. F., & Jaki, B. U. (2014). Airborne antituberculosis activity of Eucalyptus citriodora essential oil. J Nat Prod, 77(3), 603-610.

Rao S., Krauss N.E., Heerding J.M., Swindell C.S., Ringel I., Orr G.A., Horwitz S.B. (1994) 3'-(p-Azidobenzamido)taxol Photolabels the N-terminal 31 AminoAcids of ?-Tubulin. The Journal of Biological Chemistry. 269: 3132-3134.

Rao S., Orr G.A., Chaudhary A.G., Kingston D.G.I., Horwitz S.B. (1995) Characterization of the Taxol Binding Site on the Microtubule. The Journal of Biological Chemistry. 270: 20235-20238.

Raphael T.J., Kuttan G. (2003) Effect of naturally occurring triterpenoids glycyrrhizic acid, ursolic acid, oleanolic acid and nomilin on the immune system. Phytomedicine. 10: 483-489.

Rasooli I, Fakoor MH, Yadegarinia D, Gachkar L, Allameh A, Rezaei MB (2008 Feb 29). "Antimycotoxigenic characteristics of Rosmarinus officinalis and Trachyspermum copticum L. essential oils," Int J Food Microbiol. 122(1-2):135-9.

Rathi, B., Bodhankar, S., Mohan, V., & Thakurdesai, P. (2013 Jun). Ameliorative Effects of a Polyphenolic Fraction of Cinnamomum zeylanicum L. Bark in Animal Models of Inflammation and Arthritis. Sci Pharm, 81(2), 567-589.

Reddy AC, Lokesh BR (1994). "Studies on anti-inflammatory activity of spice principles and dietary n-3 polyunsaturated fatty acids on carrageenan-induced inflammation in rats," Ann Nutr Metab. 38(6):349-58.

Rees WD, Evans BK, Rhodes J (1979 Oct 6). "Treating irritable bowel syndrome with peppermint oil," Br Med J. 2(6194):835-6.

Reichling J, Koch C, Stahl-Biskup E, Sojka C, Schnitzler P (2005 Dec). "Virucidal activity of a beta-triketone-rich essential oil of Leptospermum scoparium (manuka oil) against HSV-1 and HSV-2 in cell culture," Planta Med. 71(12):1123-7.

Re L., Barocci S., Sonnino S., Mencarelli A., Vivani C., Paolucci G., Scarpantonio A., Rinaldi L., Mosca E. (2000) Linalool modifies the nicotinic receptor-ion channel kinetics at the mouse neuromuscular junction. Pharmacological Research. 42: 177-181.

Reddy B.S., Wang C-X., Samaha H., Lubet R., Steele V.E., Kelloff G.J., Rao C.V. (1997) Chemoprevention of Colon Carcinogenesis by Dietary Perillyl Alcohol. Cancer Research. 57: 420-425.

Ripple G.H., Gould M.N., Stewart J.A., Tutsch K.D., Arzoomanian R.Z., Alberti D., Feierabend C., Pomplun M., Wilding G., Bailey H.H. (1998) Phase I Clinical Trial of Perillyl Alcohol Administered Daily. Clinical Cancer Research. 4: 1159-1164.

Romero-Jiménez M, Campos-Sánchez J, Analla M, Muñoz-Serrano A, Alonso-Moraga A (2005 Aug 1). "Genotoxicity and anti-genotoxicity of some traditional medicinal herbs," Mutat Res. 585(1-2):147-55.

Rose JE, Behm FM (1994 Feb). "Inhalation of vapor from black pepper extract reduces smoking withdrawal symptoms," Drug Alcohol Depend. 34(3):225-9.

Rowinsky E.K., Donehower R.C. (1995) Paclitaxel (Taxol). The New England Journal of Medicine. 332: 1004-1014.

Roy S, Khanna S, Shah H, Rink C, Phillips C, Preuss H, Subbaraju GV, Trimurtulu G, Krishnaraju AV, Bagchi M, Bagchi D, Sen CK (2005 Apr). "Human genome screen to identify the genetic basis of the anti-inflammatory effects of Boswellia in microvascular endothelial cells," DNA Cell Biol. 24(4):244-55.

Rozza, A. L., Moraes Tde, M., Kushima, H., Tanimoto, A., Marques, M. O., Bauab, T. M., ... Pellizzon, C. H. (2011 Jan). Gastroprotective mechanisms of Citrus lemon (Rutaceae) essential oil and its majority compounds limonene and beta-pinene: involvement of heat-shock protein-70, vasoactive intestinal peptide, glutathione, sulfhydryl compounds, nitric oxide and prostaglandin E(2). Chem Biol Interact, 189(1-2), 82-89.

Saeed SA, Gilani AH (1994 May). "Antithrombotic activity of clove oil," J Pak Med Assoc. 44(5):112-5.

Sadraei, H., Asghari, G., & Emami, S. (2013 Jan). Inhibitory effect of Rosa damascena Mill flower essential oil, geraniol and citronellol on rat ileum contraction. Res Pharm Sci, 8(1), 17-23.

Said T, Dutot M, Martin C, Beaudeux JL, Boucher C, Enee E, Baudouin C, Warnet JM, Rat P (2007 Mar). "Cytoprotective effect against UV-induced DNA damage and oxidative stress: role of new biological UV filter," Eur J Pharm Sci. 30(3-4):203-10.

Saikia, D., Parveen, S., Gupta, V. K., & Luqman, S. (2012 Dec). Anti-tuberculosis activity of Indian grass KHUS (Vetiveria zizanioides L. Nash). Complement Ther Med, 20(6), 434-436.

Saiyudthong, S., & Marsden, C. A. (2011 Jun). Acute effects of bergamot oil on anxiety-related behaviour and corticosterone level in rats. Phytother Res, 25(6), 858-862.

Samaila D., Toy B.J., Wang R.C., Elegbede J.A. (2004) Monoterpenes Enhanced the Sensitivity of Head and Neck Cancer Cells to Radiation Treatment In Vitro. Anticancer Research. 24: 3089-3096.

Samarth RM, Goyal PK, Kumar A (2004 Jul). "Protection of swiss albino mice against whole-body gamma irradiation by Mentha piperita (Linn.)," Phytother Res. 18(7):546-50.

Samarth RM, Panwar M, Kumar M, Kumar A (2006 May). "Radioprotective influence of Mentha piperita (Linn) against gamma irradiation in mice: Antioxidant and radical scavenging activity," Int J Radiat Biol. 82(5):331-7.

Sampaio, L.F.S., Maia J.G.S., de Parijos A.M., de Souza R.Z., Barata L.E.S. (2011) Linalool from Rosewood (Aniba rosaeodora Ducke) Oil Inhibits Adenylate Cyclase in the Retina, Contributing to Understanding its Biological Activity. Phytotherapy Research. doi: 10.1002/ptr.3518.

Sanguinetti, M., Posteraro, B., Romano, L., Battaglia, F., Lopizzo, T., De Carolis, E., & Fadda, G. (2007 Feb). In vitro activity of Citrus bergamia (bergamot) oil against clinical isolates of dermatophytes. J Antimicrob Chemother, 59(2), 305-308.

Santamaria, M., Jr., Petermann, K. D., Vedovello, S. A., Degan, V., Lucato, A., & Franzini, C. M. (2014 Feb). Antimicrobial effect of Melaleuca alternifolia dental gel in orthodontic patients. Am J Orthod Dentofacial Orthop, 145(2), 198-202.

Santos AO, Ueda-Nakamura T, Dias Filho BP, Veiga Junior VF, Pinto AC, Nakamura CV (2008 Nov 20). "Effect of Brazilian copaiba oils on Leishmania amazonensis," J Ethnopharmacol. 120(2):204-8.

Santos FA, Rao VS (2000 Jun). "Anti-inflammatory and antinociceptive effects of 1,8-cineole a terpenoid oxide present in many plant essential oils," Phytother Res. 14(4):240-4.

Santos F.A., Rao V.S.N. (1997) Mast cell involvement in the rat paw oedema response to 1,8-cineole, the main constituent of eucalyptus and rosemary oils. European Journal of Pharmacology. 331: 253-258.

Santos F.A., Rao V.S.N. (2001) 1,8-Cineol, a Food Flavoring Agent, Prevents Ethanol-Induced Gastric Injury in Rats. Digestive Diseases and Sciences. 46: 331-337.

Sarahroodi, S., Esmaeili, S., Mikaili, P., Hemmati, Z., & Saberi, Y. (2012 Apr). The effects of green Ocimum basilicum hydroalcoholic extract on retention and retrieval of memory in mice. Anc Sci Life, 31(4), 185-189.

Sasannejad, P., Saeedi, M., Shoeibi, A., Gorji, A., Abbasi, M., & Foroughipour, M. (2012 Apr). Lavender essential oil in the treatment of migraine headache: a placebo-controlled clinical trial. Eur Neurol, 67(5), 288-291.

Satoh T., Kosaka K., Itoh K., Kobayashi A., Yamamoto M., Shimoho Y., Kitajima C., Cui J., Kamins J., Okamoto S-I., Izumi M., Shirasawa T., Lipton S.A. (2008) Carnosic acid, a catechol-type electrophilic compound, protects neurons both in vitro and in vivothrough activation of the Keap1/Nrf2 pathway via S-alkylation of targeted cysteines on Keap1. Journal of Neurochemistry. 104: 1116-1131.

Savelev SU, Okello EJ, Perry EK (2004 Apr). "Butyryl- and acetyl-cholinesterase inhibitory activities in essential oils of Salvia species and their constituents," Phytother Res. 18(4):315-24.

Sayyah M, Nadjafnia L, Kamalinejad M (2004 Oct). "Anticonvulsant activity and chemical composition of Artemisia dracunculus L. essential oil," J Ethnopharmacol. 94(2-3):283-7.

Sayyah M, Saroukhani G, Peirovi A, Kamalinejad M (2003 Aug). "Analgesic and anti-inflammatory activity of the leaf essential oil of Laurus nobilis Linn," Phytother Res. 17(7):733-6.

Schecter A., Birnbaum L., Ryan J., Constable J.D. (2006) Dioxins: An overview. Environmental Research. 101: 419-428.

Schmitt S, Schaefer UF, Doebler L, Reichling J (2009 Oct). "Cooperative interaction of monoterpenes and phenylpropanoids on the in vitro human skin permeation of complex composed essential oils," Planda Med. 75(13):1381-5.

Schnitzler P, Schön K, Reichling J (2001 Apr). "Antiviral activity of Australian tea tree oil and eucalyptus oil against herpes simplex virus in cell culture," Pharmazie. 56(4):343-7.

Schroeter H, Heiss C, Balzer J, Kleinbongard P, Keen CL, Hollenberg NK, Sies H, Kwik-Uribe C, Schmitz HH, Kelm M (2006 Jan 24). "(-)-Epicatechin mediates beneficial effects of flavanol-rich cocoa on vascular function in humans," Proc Natl Acad Sci USA. 103(4):1024-9.

Schroter A., Kessner D., Kiselev M.A., Haub T., Dante S., Neubert R.H.H. (2009) Basic Nanostructure of Stratum Corneum Lipid Matrices Based on Ceramides [EOS] and [AP]: A Neutron Diffraction Study. Biophysical Journal. 97: 1104-1114.

Schuhmacher A, Reichling J, Schnitzler P (2003). "Virucidal effect of peppermint oil on the enveloped viruses herpes simplex virus type 1 and type 2 in vitro," Phytomedicine. 10(6-7):504-10.

Sedmak D.D., Davis D.H., Singh U., van de Winkel J.G.J., Anderson C.L. (1991) Expression of IgG Fc Receptor Antigens in Placenta and on Endothelial Cells in Humans: An Immunohistochemical Study. American Journal of Pathology. 138: 175-181.

Selim, S. A., Adam, M. E., Hassan, S. M., & Albalawi, A. R. (2014). Chemical composition, antimicrobial and antibiofilm activity of the essential oil and methanol extract of the Mediterranean cypress (Cupressus sempervirens L.). BMC Complement Altern Med, 14(1), 1-8.

Semah F., Picot M-C., Adam C., Broglin D., Arzimanoglou A., Bazin B., Cavalcanti D., Baulac M. (1998) Is the underlying cause of epilepsy a major prognostic factor for recurrence? Neurology. 51: 1256-1262.

Seol, G. H., Shim, H. S., Kim, P. J., Moon, H. K., Lee, K. H., Shim, I., . . . Min, S. S. (2010 Jul). Antidepressant-like effect of Salvia sclarea is explained by modulation of dopamine activities in rats. J Ethnopharmacol, 130(1), 187-190.

Shapiro S., Guggenheim B. (1995) The action of thymol on oral bacteria. Oral Microbiology and Immunology. 10: 241-246.

Shapiro S, Meier A, Guggenheim B (1994 Aug). "The antimicrobial activity of essential oils and essential oil components towards oral bacteria," Oral Microbiol Immunol. 9(4):202-8.

Sharma PR, Mondhe DM, Muthiah S, Pal HC, Shahi AK, Saxena AK, Qazi GN (2009 May 15). "Anticancer activity of an essential oil from Cymbopogon flexuosus," Chem Biol Interact. 179(2-3):160-8.

Shaltiel-Karyo, R., Davidi, D., Frenkel-Pinter, M., Ovadia, M., Segal, D., & Gazit, E. (2012 Oct). Differential inhibition of alpha-synuclein oligomeric and fibrillar assembly in parkinson's disease model by cinnamon extract. Biochim Biophys Acta, 1820(10), 1628-1635.

Shen J, Niijima A, Tanida M, Horii Y, Maeda K, Nagai K (2005 Jun 3). "Olfactory stimulation with scent of grapefruit oil affects autonomic nerves, lipolysis and appetite in rats," Neurosci Lett. 380(3):289-94.

Sherry E, Boeck H, Warnke PH (2001). "Percutaneous treatment of chronic MRSA osteomyelitis with a novel plant-derived antiseptic," BMC Surg. 1:1.

Shibata M., Ohkubo T., Takahashi H., Inoki R. (1989) Modified formalin test: characteristic biphasic pain response. Pain. 38: 347-352.

Sikkema J., de Bont J.A.M., Poolman B. (1995) Mechanisms of Membrane Toxicity of Hydrocarbons. Microbiological Reviews. 59: 201-222.

Silva Brum L.F., Elisabetsky E., Souza D. (2001) Effects of Linalool on [3H] MK801 and [3H] Muscimol Binding in Mouse Cortical Membranes. Phytotherapy Research. 15: 422-425.

Silva Brum L.F., Emanuelli T., Souza D.O., Elisabetsky E. (2001) Effects of Linalool on Glutamate Release and Uptake in Mouse Cortical Synaptosomes. Neurochemical Research. 26: 191-194.

Silva J, Abebe W, Sousa SM, Duarte VG, Machado MI, Matos FJ (2003 Dec). "Analgesic and anti-inflammatory effects of essential oils of Eucalyptus," J Ethnopharmacol. 89(2-3):277-83.

Simons K., Toomre D. (2000) Lipid Rafts and Signal Transduction. Nature Reviews. 1: 31-41.

Singletary K, MacDonald C, Wallig M (1996 Jun 24). "Inhibition by rosemary and carnosol of 7,12-dimethylbenz[a]anthracene (DMBA)-induced rat mammary tumorigenesis and in vivo DMBA-DNA adduct formation," Cancer Lett. 104(1):43-8.

Skocibusić M, Bezić N (2004 Dec). "Phytochemical analysis and in vitro antimicrobial activity of two Satureja species essential oils," Phytother Res. 18(12):967-70.

Skold M., Borje A., Harambasic E., Karlberg A-T. (2004) Contact Allergens Formed on Air Exposure of Linalool. Identification and Quantification of Primary and Secondary Oxidation Products and the Effect on Skin Sensitization. Chemical Research in Toxicology. 17: 1697-1705.

Skold M., Borje A., Matura M., Karlberg A-T. (2002) Studies on the autoxidation and sensitizing capacity of the fragrance chemical linalool, identifying a linalool hydroperoxide. Contact Dermatitis. 46: 267-272.

Skold M., Karlberg A-T., Matura M., Borje A. (2006) The fragrace chemical ?-caryophyllene - air oxidation and skin sensitation. Food and Chemical Toxicology. 44: 538-545.

Slima, A. B., Ali, M. B., Barkallah, M., Traore, A. I., Boudawara, T., Allouche, N., & Gdoura, R. (2013 Mar). Antioxidant properties of Pelargonium graveolens L'Her essential oil on the reproductive damage induced by deltamethrin in mice as compared to alpha-tocopherol. Lipids Health Dis, 12(1), 30.

Smith DG, Standing L, de Man A (1992 Apr). "Verbal memory elicited by ambient odor," Percept Mot Skills. 74(2):339-43.

Soares SF, Borges LM, de Sousa Braga R, Ferreira LL, Louly CC, Tresvenzol LM, de Paula JR, Ferri PH (2009 Oct 7). "Repellent activity of plant-derived compounds against Amblyomma cajennense (Acari: Ixodidae) nymphs," Vet Parasitol. Epub ahead of print.

Sorentino S., Landmesser U. (2005) Nonlipid-lowering Effects of Statins. Current Treatment Options to Cardiovascular Medicine. 7: 459-466.

Sorg O., Zennegg M., Schmid P., Dedosyuk R., Valikhnovskyi R., Gaide O., Kniazevych V., Saurat J-H. (2009) 2,3,7,8-tetrachlorodibenzo-p-dioxin (TCDD) poisoning in Victor Yushchenko: identification and measurement of TCDD metabolites. The Lancet. 374: 1179-1185.

Staubach S., Hanisch F-G. (2011) Lipid rafts: signaling and sorting platforms of cells and their roles in cancer. Expert Review of Proteomics. 8: 263-277.

Steiner M, Priel I, Giat J, Levy J, Sharoni Y, Danilenko M (2001). "Carnosic acid inhibits proliferation and augments differentiation of human leukemic cells induced by 1,25-dihydroxyvitamin D3 and retinoic acid," Nutr Cancer. 41(1-2):135-44.

Stellman J.M., Stellman S.D., Christian R., Weber T., Tomasallo C. (2003) The extent and patterns of usage of Agent Orange and other herbicides in Vietnam. Nature. 422: 681-687.

Stratton S.P., Alberts D.S., Einspahr J.G. (2010) A Phase 2a Study of Topical Perillyl Alcohol Cream for Chemoprevention of Skin Cancer. Cancer Prevention Research. 3: 160-169.

Stratton S.P., Saboda K.L., Myrdal P.B., Gupta A., McKenzie N.E., Brooks C., Salasche S.J., Warneke J.A., Ranger-Moore J., Bozzo P.D., Blanchard J., Einspahr J.G. (2008) Phase 1 Study of Topical Perillyl Alcohol Cream for Chemoprevention of Skin Cancer. Nutrition and Cancer. 60: 325-330.

Sun Y., Olson R., Horning M., Armstrong N., Mayer M., Gouaux E. (2002) Mechanism of glutamate receptor desensitization. Nature. 417: 245-253.

Tabanca, N., Wang, M., Avonto, C., Chittiboyina, A. G., Parcher, J. F., Carroll, J. F., . . . Khan, I. A. (2013 May). Bioactivity-guided investigation of geranium essential oils as natural tick repellents. J Agric Food Chem, 61(17), 4101-4107.

Taherian, A. A., Vafaei, A. A., & Ameri, J. (2012 Apr). Opiate System Mediate the Antinociceptive Effects of Coriandrum sativum in Mice. Iran J Pharm Res, 11(2), 679-688.

Takada K., Nakane T., Masuda K., Ishii H. (2010) Ursolic acid and oleanolic acid, members of pentacyclic triterpenoid acids, suppress TNF-?-induced E-selectin expression by cultured umbilical vein endothelial cells. Phytomedicine. 17: 1114-1119.

Takahashi, N., Yao, L., Kim, M., Sasako, H., Aoyagi, M., Shono, J., . . . Kawada, T. (2013 Jul). Dill seed extract improves abnormalities in lipid metabolism through peroxisome proliferator-activated receptor-alpha (PPAR-alpha) activation in diabetic obese mice. Mol Nutr Food Res, 57(7), 1295-1299.

Takarada K, Kimizuka R, Takahashi N, Honma K, Okuda K, Kato T (2004 Feb). "A comparison of the antibacterial efficacies of essential oils against oral pathogens," Oral Microbiol Immunol. 19(1):61-4.

Tanida M, Niijima A, Shen J, Nakamura T, Nagai K (2006 May 1). "Olfactory stimulation with scent of lavender oil affects autonomic neurotransmission and blood pressure in rats," Neurosci Lett. 398(1-2):155-60.

Tantaoui-Elaraki A, Beraoud L (1994). "Inhibition of growth and aflatoxin production in Aspergillus parasiticus by essential oils of selected plant materials," J Environ Pathol Toxicol Oncol. 13(1):67-72.

Tare V, Deshpande S, Sharma RN (2004 Oct). "Susceptibility of two different strains of Aedes aegypti (Diptera: Culicidae) to plant oils," J Econ Entomol. 97(5):1734-6.

Tayarani-Najaran, Z., Talasaz-Firoozi, E., Nasiri, R., Jalali, N., & Hassanzadeh, M. (2013 Jan). Antiemetic activity of volatile oil from Mentha spicata and Mentha x piperita in chemotherapy-induced nausea and vomiting. Ecancermedicalscience, 7, 1-6.

Terzi V, Morcia C, Faccioli P, Valè G, Tacconi G, Malnati M (2007 Jun). "In vitro antifungal activity of the tea tree (Melaleuca alternifolia) essential oil and its major components against plant pathogens," Lett Appl Microbiol. 44(6):613-8.

Thomas E.D., Ramberg R.E., Sale G.E., Sparkes R.S., Golde D.W. (1976) Direct Evidence for a Bone Marrow Origin of the Alveolar Macrophages in Man. Science. 192: 1016-1018.

Thorsen M.A., Hildebrandt K.S. (2003) Quantitative determination of phenolic diterpenes in rosemary extracts: Aspects of accurate quantification. Journal of Chromatography A. 995: 119-125.

Thukham-Mee, W., & Wattanathorn, J. (2012). Evaluation of Safety and Protective Effect of Combined Extract of Cissampelos pareira and Anethum graveolens (PM52) against Age-Related Cognitive Impairment. Evid Based Complement Alternat Med, 2012, 1-10.

Tildesley NT, Kennedy DO, Perry EK, Ballard CG, Wesnes KA, Scholey AB (2005 Jan 17). "Positive modulation of mood and cognitive performance following administration of acute doses of Salvia lavandulaefolia essential oil to healthy young volunteers," Physiol Behav. 83(5):699-709.

Tipton DA, Lyle B, Babich H, Dabbous MKh (2003 Jun). "In vitro cytotoxic and anti-inflammatory effects of myrrh oil on human gingival fibroblasts and epithelial cells," Toxicol In Vitro. 17(3):301-10.

Trautmann M, Peskar BM, Peskar BA (1991 Aug 16). "Aspirin-like drugs, ethanol-induced rat gastric injury and mucosal eicosanoid release," Eur J Pharmacol. 201(1):53-8.

Trongtokit Y, Rongsriyam Y, Komalamisra N, Apiwathnasorn C (2005 Apr). "Comparative repellency of 38 essential oils against mosquito bites," Phytother Res. 19(4):303-9.

Trouw L.A., Daha M.R. (2011) Role of complement in innate immunity and host defense. Immunology Letters. 138: 35-37.

Trovato, A., Taviano, M. F., Pergolizzi, S., Campolo, L., De Pasquale, R., & Miceli, N. (2010 Apr). Citrus bergamia Risso & Poiteau juice protects against renal injury of diet-induced hypercholesterolemia in rats. Phytother Res, 24(4), 514-519.

Turrens J.F. (2003) Mitochondrial formation of reactive oxygen species. Journal of Physiology.552: 335-344.

Tuszynski M.H. (2007) Nerve Growth Factor Gene Therapy in Alzheimer Disease. Alzheimer Disease & Associated Disorders. 21: 179-189.

Tuszynski M.H., Thal L., Pay M., Salmon D.P., Hoi S.U., Bakay R., Patel P., Blesch A., Vahlsing H.L., Ho G., Tong G., Potkin S.G., Fallon J., Hansen L., Mufson E.J., Kordower J.H., Gall C., Conner J. (2005) A phase 1 clinical trial of nerve growth factor gene therapy in Alzheimer disease. Nature Medicine. 11: 551-555.

Udagawa N., Takahashi N., Akatsu T., Tanaki H., Sasaki T., Nishihara T., Koga T., Martin T.J., Suda T. (1990) Origin of osteoclasts: Mature monocytes and macrophages are capable of differentiating into osteoclasts under a suitable microenvironment prepared by bone marrow-derived stromal cells. Proceedings of the National Academy of Science, USA. 87: 7260-7264.

Ueno-Iio, T., Shibakura, M., Yokota, K., Aoe, M., Hyoda, T., Shinohata, R., . . . Kataoka, M. (2014 Jun). Lavender essential oil inhalation suppresses allergic airway inflammation and mucous cell hyperplasia in a murine model of asthma. Life Sci.

Umezu T (2000 Jun). "Behavioral effects of plant-derived essential oils in the geller type conflict test in mice," Jpn J Pharmacol. 83(2):150-3.

Umezu T (1999 Sep). "Anticonflict effects of plant-derived essential oils," Pharmacol Biochem Behav. 64(1):35-40.

Uribe S., Ramirez J., Pena A. (1985) Effects of ?-Pinene on Yeast Membrane Functions. Journal of Bacteriology. 161: 1195-1200.

Vaka S.R.K., Murthy S.N., Repka M.A., Nagy T. (2011) Upregulation of Endogenous Neurotophin Levels in the Brain by Intranasal Administration of Carnosic Acid. Journal of Pharmaceutical Sciences. 100: 3139-3145.

Vallianou, I., Peroulis, N., Pantazis, P., & Hadzopoulou-Cladaras, M. (2011 Nov). Camphene, a plant-derived monoterpene, reduces plasma cholesterol and triglycerides in hyperlipidemic rats independently of HMG-CoA reductase activity. PLoS ONE, 6(11), e20516.

van Tol RW, Swarts HJ, van der Linden A, Visser JH (2007 May). "Repellence of the red bud borer Resseliella oculiperda from grafted apple trees by impregnation of rubber budding strips with essential oils," Pest Manag Sci. 63(5):483-90.

Velaga, M. K., Yallapragada, P. R., Williams, D., Rajanna, S., & Bettaiya, R. (2014 Jun). Hydroalcoholic Seed Extract of Coriandrum sativum (Coriander) Alleviates Lead-Induced Oxidative Stress in Different Regions of Rat Brain. Biol Trace Elem Res, 159(1-3), 351-363.

Vera, S. S., Zambrano, D. F., Mendez-Sanchez, S. C., Rodriguez-Sanabria, F., Stashenko, E. E., & Duque Luna, J. E. (2014). Essential oils with insecticidal activity against larvae of Aedes aegypti (Diptera: Culicidae). Parasitol Res, 113(7), 2647-2654.

Veres, K., Csupor-Loffler, B., Lazar, A., & Hohmann, J. (2012). Antifungal activity and composition of essential oils of Conyza canadensis herbs and roots. ScientificWorldJournal, 2012, 489646.

Vigo E, Cepeda A, Gualillo O, Perez-Fernandez R (2004 Feb). "In-vitro anti-inflammatory effect of Eucalyptus globulus and Thymus vulgaris: nitric oxide inhibition in J774A.1 murine macrophages," J Pharm Pharmacol. 56(2):257-63.

Vigushin DM, Poon GK, Boddy A, English J, Halbert GW, Pagonis C, Jarman M, Coombes RC (1998). "Phase I and pharmacokinetic study of D-limonene in patients with advanced cancer. Cancer Research Campaign Phase I/II Clinical Trials Committee," Cancer Chemother Pharmacol. 42(2):111-7.

Vuković-Gaćić B, Nikcević S, Berić-Bjedov T, Knezević-Vukcević J, Simić D (2006 Oct). "Antimutagenic effect of essential oil of sage (Salvia officinalis L.) and its monoterpenes against UV-induced mutations in Escherichia coli and Saccharomyces cerevisiae," Food Chem Toxicol. 44(10):1730-8.

Vutyavanich T, Kraisarin T, Ruangsri R (2001 Apr). "Ginger for nausea and vomiting in pregnancy: randomized, double-masked, placebo-controlled trial," Obstet Gynecol. 97(4):577-82.

Wallace R.J. (2004) Antimicrobial properties of plant secondary metabolites. Proceedings of the Nutrition Soiciety. 63: 621-629.

Wang T., Takikawa Y., Satoh T., Yoshioka Y., Kosaka K., Tatemichi Y., Suzuki K. (2011) Carnosic acid prevents obesity and hepatic steatosis in ob/ob mice. Hepatology Research. 41: 87-92.

Watanabe, S., Hara, K., Ohta, K., Iino, H., Miyajima, M., Matsuda, A., . . . Matsushima, E. (2013 Jan). Aroma helps to preserve information processing resources of the brain in healthy subjects but not in temporal lobe epilepsy. Seizure, 22(1), 59-63.

Wei A, Shibamoto T (2007). "Antioxidant activities of essential oil mixtures toward skin lipid squalene oxidized by UV irradiation," Cutan Ocul Toxicol. 26(3):227-33.

Wei, L. S., & Wee, W. (2013 Jun). Chemical composition and antimicrobial activity of Cymbopogon nardus citronella essential oil against systemic bacteria of aquatic animals. Iran J Microbiol, 5(2), 147-152.

Wilkinson JM, Hipwell M, Ryan T, Cavanagh HM (2003 Jan 1). "Bioactivity of Backhousia citriodora: antibacterial and antifungal activity," J Agric Food Chem. 51(1):76-81.

Wilkinson, S. M., Love, S. B., Westcombe, A. M., Gambles, M. A., Burgess, C. C., Cargill, A., . . . Ramirez, A. J. (2007 Feb). Effectiveness of aromatherapy massage in the management of anxiety and depression in patients with cancer: a multicenter randomized controlled trial. Journal of Clinical Oncology, 25(5), 532-539.

Williamson EM, Priestley CM, Burgess IF (2007 Dec). "An investigation and comparison of the bioactivity of selected essential oils on human lice and house dust mites," Fitoterapia. 78(7-8):521-5.

Wintersberger E. (1996) DNA Damage and Mutagenesis. Biochemical Society Transactions. 25: 303-308.

Wong K-K. (2009) Recent Developments in Anti-Cancer Agents Targeting the Ras/Raf/MEK/ERK Pathway. Recent Patents on Anti-Cancer Drug Discovery. 4: 28-35.

Woolf A. (1999) Essential Oil Poisoning. Clinical Toxicology. 37: 721-727.

Xia L, Chen D, Han R, Fang Q, Waxman S, Jing Y (2005 Mar). "Boswellic acid acetate induces apoptosis through caspase-mediated pathways in myeloid leukemia cells," Mol Cancer Ther. 4(3):381-8.

Xu J., Zhou F., Ji B-P., Pei R-S., Xu N. (2008) The antibacterial mechanism of carvacrol and thymol against Escherichia coli. Letters in Applied Microbiology. 47: 174-179.

Xu, J., Guo, Y., Zhao, P., Xie, C., Jin, D. Q., Hou, W., & Zhang, T. (2011 Dec). Neuroprotective cadinane sesquiterpenes from the resinous exudates of Commiphora myrrha. Fitoterapia, 82(8), 1198-1201.

Yamada, K., Mimaki, Y., & Sashida, Y. (2005 Feb). Effects of inhaling the vapor of Lavandula burnatii super-derived essential oil and linalool on plasma adrenocorticotropic hormone (ACTH), catecholamine and gonadotropin levels in experimental menopausal female rats. Biol Pharm Bull, 28(2), 378-379.

Yamato K, Takahashi Y, Akiyama H, Tsuji K, Onishi H, Machida Y (2009 Apr). "Effect of penetration enhancers on transdermal delivery of propofol," Biol Pharm Bull. 32(4):677-83.

Yang GY, Wang W (1994 Sep). "[Clinical studies on the treatment of coronary heart disease with Valeriana officinalis var latifolia]," Zhongguo Zhong Xi Yi Jie He Za Zhi. 14(9):540-2.

Yang SA, Jeon SK, Lee EJ, Im NK, Jhee KH, Lee SP, Lee IS (2009 May). "Radical Scavenging Activity of the Essential Oil of Silver Fir (Abies alba)," J Clin Biochem Nutr. 44(3):253-9.

Yap, P. S., Krishnan, T., Yiap, B. C., Hu, C. P., Chan, K. G., & Lim, S. H. (2014 May). Membrane disruption and anti-quorum sensing effects of synergistic interaction between Lavandula angustifolia (lavender oil) in combination with antibiotic against plasmid-conferred multi-drug-resistant Escherichia coli. J Appl Microbiol, 116(5), 1119-1128.

Yavari Kia, P., Safajou, F., Shahnazi, M., & Nazemiyeh, H. (2014 Mar). The effect of lemon inhalation aromatherapy on nausea and vomiting of pregnancy: a double-blinded, randomized, controlled clinical trial. Iran Red Crescent Med J, 16(3).

Yeom, H. J., Kang, J. S., Kim, G. H., & Park, I. K. (2012). Insecticidal and acetylcholine esterase inhibition activity of Apiaceae plant essential oils and their constituents against adults of German cockroach (Blattella germanica). J Agric Food Chem, 60(29), 7194-7203.

Yeruva L., Pierre K.J., Elegbede A., Wang R.C., Carper S.W. (2007) Perillyl alcohol and perillic acid induced cell cycle arrest and apoptosis in non small cell lung cancer cells. Cancer Letters. 257: 216-226.

Yip, Y. B., & Tam, A. C. (2008 Jun). An experimental study on the effectiveness of massage with aromatic ginger and orange essential oil for moderate-to-severe knee pain among the elderly in Hong Kong. Complement Ther Med, 16(3), 131-138.

Yoshikawa M., Matsuda H. (2000) Antidiabetogenic activity of oleanolic acid glycosides from medicinal foodstuffs. Biofactors. 13: 231-237.

Youdim KA, Deans SG (1999 Sep 8). "Dietary supplementation of thyme (Thymus vulgaris L.) essential oil during the lifetime of the rat: its effects on the antioxidant status in liver, kidney and heart tissues," Mech Ageing Dev. 109(3):163-75.

Youn L.J., Yoon J.W., Hovde C.J. (2010) A Brief Overview of Escherichia coli O157:H7 and Its Plasmid O157. Journal of Microbiology and Biotechnology. 20: 1-10.

Yu B.P. (1994) Cellular Defenses Against Damage From Reactive Oxygen Species. Physiological Reviews. 74: 139-162.

Yu S.G., Hildebrandt L.A., Elson C.E. (1995) Geraniol, and Inhibitor of Mevalonate Biosynthesis, Suppresses the Growth of Hepatomas and Melanomas Transplanted to Rats and Mice. Journal of Nutrition. 125: 2763-2767.

Yu Y-M., Lin H-C., Chang W-C. (2008) Carnosic acid prevents the migration of human aortic smooth muscle cells by inhibiting the activation and expression of matrix metalloproteinase-9. British Journal of Nutrition. 100: 731-738.

Yuan HQ, Kong F, Wang XL, Young CY, Hu XY, Lou HX (2008 Jun 1). "Inhibitory effect of acetyl-11-keto-beta-boswellic acid on androgen receptor by interference of Sp1 binding activity in prostate cancer cells," Biochem Pharmacol. 75(11):2112-21.

Yüce, A., Turk, G., Ceribasi, S., Guvenc, M., Ciftci, M., Sonmez, M., . . . Aksakal, M. (2014 Apr). Effectiveness of cinnamon (Cinnamomum zeylanicum) bark oil in the prevention of carbon tetrachloride-induced damages on the male reproductive system. Andrologia, 46(3), 263-272.

Yun, J. (2014 Jan). Limonene inhibits methamphetamine-induced locomotor activity via regulation of 5-HT neuronal function and dopamine release. Phytomedicine. Retrieved from http://dx.doi.org/10.1016/j.phymed.2013.12.004

Zamith H.P.S., Vidal M.N.P., Speit G., Paumgartten F.J.R (1993) Absence of genotoxic activity of ?-myrcene in the in vivo cytogenetic bone marrow assay. Brazilian Journal of Medical and Biological Research. 26: 93-98.

Zha C., Brown G.B., Brouillette W.J. (2004) Synthesis and Structure-Activity Relationship Studies for Hydantoins and Analogues as Voltage-Gasted Sodium Channel Ligands. Journal of Medicinal Chemistry. 47: 6519-6528.

Zheng GQ, Kenney PM, Lam LK (1992 Aug). "Anethofuran, carvone, and limonene: potential cancer chemopreventive agents from dill weed oil and caraway oil," Planta Med. 58(4):338-41.

Zheng GQ, Kenney PM, Zhang J, Lam LK (1993). "Chemoprevention of benzo[a]pyrene-induced forestomach cancer in mice by natural phthalides from celery seed oil," Nutr Cancer. 19(1):77-86.

Zhou, J., Tang F., Bian R. (2004) Effect of ?-pinene on nuclear translocation of NF-?B in THP-1 cells. Acta Pharmacol Sin. 25: 480-484.

Zhou, X. M., Zhao, Y., He, C. C., & Li, J. X. (2012 Feb). Preventive effects of Citrus reticulata essential oil on bleomycin-induced pulmonary fibrosis in rats and the mechanism. Zhong Xi Yi Jie He Xue Bao, 10(2), 200-209.

Zhu BC, Henderson G, Yu Y, Laine RA (2003 Jul 30). "Toxicity and repellency of patchouli oil and patchouli alcohol against Formosan subterranean termites Coptotermes formosanus Shiraki (Isoptera: Rhinotermitidae)," J Agric Food Chem. 51(16):4585-8.

Zore G.B., Thakre A.D., Jadhav S., Karuppayil S.M. (2011) Terpenoids inhibit Candida albicans growth by affecting membrane integrity and arrest of cell cycle. Phytomedicine. doi: 10.1016/j.phymed.2011.03.008.

BIBLIOGRAPHY

Balch, M.D., James, and Phyllis Balch, C.N.C. *Prescription for Nutritional Healing.* Garden City Park, NY: Avery Publishing Group, 1990.

Becker, M.D., Robert O. *The Body Electric.* New York, NY: Wm. Morrow, 1985.

Brown T.L., LeMay H.E., Bursten B.E. Chemistry: The Central Science. 10th ed. Upper Saddle River: Pearson Prentice Hall, 2006.

Burroughs, Stanley. *Healing for the Age of Enlightenment.* Auburn, CA: Burroughs Books, 1993.

Burton Goldberg Group, The. *Alternative Medicine: The Definitive Guide.* Fife, WA: Future Medicine Publishing, Inc., 1994.

Cowan M.K., Talaro K.P. *Microbiology: A Systems Approach. 2nd ed.* New York: McGraw Hill, 2009.

DeVita, Sabina M. *Electromagnetic Pollution. A Hidden Stress to Your System.* Marble Hill, MO: Stewart Publishing Company, 2000.

---------------. *Essential Oils Desk Reference.* Essential Science Publishing. Third Edition, First Printing March 2004.

Fischer-Rizzi, Suzanne. *Complete Aromatherapy Handbook.* New York, NY: Sterling Publishing, 1990.

Foley, Marcy. *Embraced by the Essence! Your Journey into Wellness Using Pure Quality Essential Oils.* Boulder, Colorado: Holistic Wellness Foundation I, April 2000.

Freeman S. *Biological Science. 2nd ed.* Upper Saddle River: Pearson Prentice Hall, 2005.

Gattefosse, Ph.D., Rene-Maurice. *Gattefosse's Aromatherapy.* Essex, England: The C.W. Daniel Company Ltd., 1937 English translation.

Green, Mindy. *Natural Perfumes: Simple Aromatherapy Recipes.* Loveland CO: Interweave Press Inc., 1999.

Guyton A.C., Hall J.E. *Textbook of Medical Physiology. 10th ed.* Philadelphia: W.B. Saunders Company, 2000.

---------------. *Integrated Aromatic Medicine.* Proceedings from the First International Symposium, Grasse, France. Essential Science Publishing, March 2000.

Klug W.S., Cummings M.R., Spencer C., Palladino M.A. *Concepts of Genetics.* San Francisco: Pearson Custom Publishing, 2009.

Lawless, Julia. *The Encyclopaedia of Essential Oils.* Rockport, MA: Element, Inc., 1992.

Lee, M.D., John R. *Natural Progesterone: The Multiple Roles of a Remarkable Hormone.* Sebastopol, CA: BLL Publishing, 1995.

Lewin B. *Essential Genes.* Upper Saddle River: Pearson Prentice Hall, 2006.

Maury, Marguerite. *Marguerite Maury's Guide to Aromatherapy.* C.W. Daniel, 1989.

Pènoël, M.D., Daniel and Pierre Franchomme. *L'aromatherapie exactement.* Limoges, France: Jollois, 1990.

Price, Shirley, and Len Price. *Aromatherapy for Health Professionals.* New York, NY: Churchill Livingstone Inc., 1995.

Price, Shirley, and Penny Price Parr. *Aromatherapy for Babies and Children.* San Francisco, CA: Thorsons, 1996.

Rose, Jeanne. *The Aromatherapy Book: Applications and Inhalations.* Berkeley, CA: North Atlantic Books, 1992.

Ryman, Danièle. *Aromatherapy: The Complete Guide to Plant & Flower Essences for Health and Beauty.* New York: Bantam Books, 1993.

Sheppard-Hanger, Sylla. *The Aromatherapy Practitioner Reference Manual.* Tampa, FL: Atlantic Institute of Aromatherapy, Twelfth Printing February 2000.

Stewart, Ph.D., R.A., David. *A Statistical Validation of Raindrop Technique.* Marble Hill, MO: Care Publications, 2003

Tisserand, Maggie. *Aromatherapy for Women: a Practical Guide to Essential Oils for Health and Beauty.* Rochester, VT: Healing Arts Press, 1996.

Tisserand, Robert. *Aromatherapy: to Heal and Tend the Body.* Wilmot, WI: Lotus Press, 1988.

Tisserand, Robert. *The Art of Aromatherapy.* Rochester, VT: Healing Arts Press, 1977.

Tisserand, Robert, and Tony Balacs. *Essential Oil Safety: A Guide for Health Care Professionals.* New York, NY: Churchill

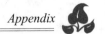
Tortora G.J., Funke B.R., Case C.L. *Microbiology: An Introduction. 9th ed.* San Francisco: Pearson Benjamin Cummings, 2007.

Livingstone, 1995. Valnet, M.D., Jean. *The Practice of Aromatherapy: a Classic Compendium of Plant Medicines and their Healing Properties.*

Rochester, VT: Healing Arts Press, 1980.

Watson, Franzesca. *Aromatherapy Blends & Remedies.* San Francisco, CA: Thorsons, 1995.

Weaver R.F. *Molecular Biology. 4th ed.* New York: McGraw Hill, 2008.

Wilson, Roberta. *Aromatherapy for Vibrant Health and Beauty: a practical A-to-Z reference to aromatherapy treatments for health, skin, and hair problems.* Honesdale, PA: Paragon Press, 1995.

Worwood, Valerie Ann. *The Complete Book of Essential Oils & Aromatherapy.* San Rafael, CA: New World Library, 1991.

Young, N.D., D. Gary. *An Introduction to Young Living Essential Oils.* Payson, UT: Young Living Essential Oils, 2000.

Young, N.D., D. Gary. *Aromatherapy: The Essential Beginning.* Salt Lake City, UT: Essential Press Publishing, 1995.

Young, Ph.D., Robert O. *One Sickness, One Disease, One Treatment.* Alpine, UT: Self-published, 1995.

Video Listing

--------------. Essential Tips for Happy, Healthy Pets. The Vision Firm, LLC, 2000.

Eaton, Cathy. Raindrop Therapy. Health is Your Wealth Enterprises, 1997.

Woloshyn, Tom. Vita Flex Instruction. Vita-Gem Enterprises, 1998.

Young, ND, D. Gary. Raindrop Technique. Young Living Essential Oils, 2000.

INDEX

Quick Reference Guide for Using Essential Oils

B

Quick Reference Guide for Using Essential Oils

F

G

H

I

J

K

L

M

N

Quick Reference Guide for Using Essential Oils

R

Quick Reference Guide for Using Essential Oils

T

U

V

W

Quick Reference Guide for Using Essential Oils

Z

NOTES & NEW PRODUCTS

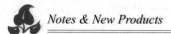

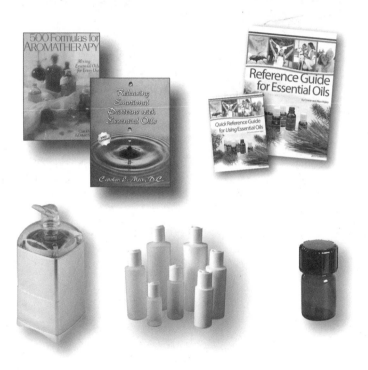